I0066001

Urology Handbook

Urology Handbook

Edited by **Karl Meloni**

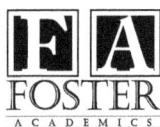

FA

FOSTER
ACADEMICS

New Jersey

Published by Foster Academics,
61 Van Reypen Street,
Jersey City, NJ 07306, USA
www.fosteracademics.com

Urology Handbook
Edited by Karl Meloni

© 2016 Foster Academics

International Standard Book Number: 978-1-63242-438-9 (Hardback)

This book contains information obtained from authentic and highly regarded sources. Copyright for all individual chapters remain with the respective authors as indicated. All chapters are published with permission under the Creative Commons Attribution License or equivalent. A wide variety of references are listed. Permission and sources are indicated; for detailed attributions, please refer to the permissions page and list of contributors. Reasonable efforts have been made to publish reliable data and information, but the authors, editors and publisher cannot assume any responsibility for the validity of all materials or the consequences of their use.

The publisher's policy is to use permanent paper from mills that operate a sustainable forestry policy. Furthermore, the publisher ensures that the text paper and cover boards used have met acceptable environmental accreditation standards.

Trademark Notice: Registered trademark of products or corporate names are used only for explanation and identification without intent to infringe.

Printed in the United States of America.

Contents

Preface

Urology is the field of medicine that studies the diseases of the male and female urinary tract systems and the male reproductive organs. Urology has advanced over the years by including cutting edge technologies like laser-assisted surgeries, laparoscopic surgeries, robotic surgeries etc. The objective of this book is to give a general view of the different areas of this discipline, and its applications. It is a compilation of chapters that discuss the most vital concepts and emerging trends in the area of urology. It aims to shed light on some of the unexplored aspects of urology and the recent researches in this field. Coherent flow of topics, student-friendly language and extensive use of examples make this book an invaluable source of knowledge.

Significant researches are present in this book. Intensive efforts have been employed by authors to make this book an outstanding discourse. This book contains the enlightening chapters which have been written on the basis of significant researches done by the experts.

Finally, I would also like to thank all the members involved in this book for being a team and meeting all the deadlines for the submission of their respective works. I would also like to thank my friends and family for being supportive in my efforts.

Editor

Nested Variant of Urothelial Carcinoma

Anthony Kodzo-Grey Venyo

Department of Urology, North Manchester General Hospital, Delaunays Road, Crumpsall, Manchester, UK

Correspondence should be addressed to Anthony Kodzo-Grey Venyo; akodzogrey@yahoo.co.uk

Academic Editor: Nazareno Suardi

Background. Nested variant of urothelial carcinoma was added to the WHO's classification in 2004. *Aims.* To review the literature on nested variant of urothelial carcinoma. *Results.* About 200 cases of the tumour have been reported so far and it has the ensuing morphological features: large numbers of small confluent irregular nests of bland-appearing, closely packed, haphazardly arranged, and poorly defined urothelial cells infiltrating the lamina propria and the muscularis propria. The tumour has a bland histomorphologic appearance, has an aggressive biological behaviour, and has at times been misdiagnosed as a benign lesion which had led to a significant delay in the establishment of the correct diagnosis and contributing to the advanced stage of the disease. Immunohistochemically, the tumour shares some characteristic features with high-risk conventional urothelial carcinomas such as high proliferation index and loss of p27 expression. However, p53, bcl-2, or EGF-r immunoreactivity is not frequently seen. The tumour must be differentiated from a number of proliferative lesions of the urothelium. *Conclusions.* Correct and early diagnosis of this tumour is essential to provide early curative treatment to avoid diagnosis at an advanced stage. A multicentre trial is required to identify treatment options that would improve the outcome of this tumour.

1. Introduction

Carcinoma of the urinary bladder is the most common malignancy involving the urinary tract system. Urothelial carcinomas can also occur in the renal pelvis, ureter, or urethra but their occurrence is far less common than in the urinary bladder. The histology of urothelial carcinoma is variable. On the whole about 70% of urothelial carcinomas of the urinary bladder are noninvasive or superficially invasive and these tumours are usually papillary and exhibit different degrees of differentiation; on the other hand, most muscle-invasive urothelial carcinomas are nonpapillary and usually exhibit high-grade cytomorphology. These types of classic urothelial carcinomas can be easily diagnosed histologically and they do not pose a problem to the pathologist.

A number of systems have been utilized to grade and classify urinary bladder tumours. In 1972, the World Health Organization (WHO) adopted a system which distinguished papillomas from grades I, II, and III papillary transitional cell carcinomas. Subsequently in 1998, The World Health Organization in a collaborative effort conjointly with the International Society of Urological Pathologists (ISUP) published a consensus opinion classification system for urothelial

(transitional cell) tumours. Studies that were carried out after 1998 were supportive of/validated the clinical significance of the classification scheme, and in view of this in 2004, the classification system was accepted as the standard classification system. According to this classification system, urothelial carcinoma has been classified into (a) low grade and (b) high grade depending upon the degree of nuclear anaplasia and architectural abnormalities with exception of some tumours, for example, tubular or nested/tubular variant. Invasive urothelial carcinoma is of high grade.

A number of variants of urothelial carcinoma were added to the World Health Organization classification in 2004 and some of these include lymphoepithelioma-like cell variant, sarcomatoid variant, plasmacytoid variant, microcystic variant, micropapillary variant, nested variant, and small cell type. These variants of urothelial carcinoma have varied biological behaviours but small cell carcinoma of the urinary bladder is a very aggressive tumour with very poor prognosis. Nested variant of urothelial carcinoma is characterized by an unusual, bland morphology which mimics some benign urinary bladder lesions and it has a clinical behaviour which simulates the clinical behaviour of high-grade conventional urothelial carcinomas. Nested variant of urothelial carcinoma was first reported by Stern [1, 2]. The first reported case of nested variant of urothelial carcinoma was interpreted as a benign lesion, but this lesion subsequently recurred. Pursuant to this Talbert and Young [3] reported 3 cases of nested variant of urothelial carcinoma in 1989 which they described as the carcinomas of the urinary bladder with deceptively benign-appearing foci. Murphy and Deana in 1992 [4] coined for this tumour the terminology of nested variant of transitional cell carcinoma, as it resembles von Brunn's nests. There are reports which indicate that such tumours are diagnosed at an advanced stage and they are associated with inferior prognosis. There is no consensus opinion regarding the optimum management of nested variant of urothelial carcinoma. The ensuing paper contains a review of the literature on nested variant of urothelial carcinoma.

2. Methods

Extensive literature search was done using various internet search engines to identify case reports, case series, and review manuscripts as well as conference abstracts on nested variant of urothelial carcinoma using the following terms: nested variant of urothelial carcinoma and nested variant of transitional cell carcinoma. The identified documentations were thoroughly read in order to ascertain the presentation, investigation, diagnostic features, tumour stage, management, and outcome of nested variant of urothelial carcinoma. Details of diagnostic features, tumour details and outcome were not detailed in few of the identified documentations on nested variant of urothelial carcinoma; however, enough information was gathered to summarize the presentation, diagnosis, management, and outcome of patients in most cases (see Tables 1 and 2).

3. Results/Literature Review

3.1. Definition. Nested variant of urothelial carcinoma is one of the variants of urothelial carcinoma that was added to the WHO classification in 2004. This variant of urothelial carcinoma exhibits a deceptively bland-appearing invasion by nests of cells [5]. They are rare tumours which are composed of irregular and confluent small nests and abortive tubules which are made up of urothelial cells infiltrating the lamina propria or muscularis propria, usually without any evidence of surface epithelium [3]. Nested variant of urothelial carcinoma was first described in 1989 by Talbert and Young [3] who reported the cases of 3 men aged from 53 to 77, and who had carcinoma of the urinary bladder which was characterized by foci with a deceptively benign histologic appearance. In two cases this feature led to a significant delay in the establishment of the correct diagnosis. The diagnostic difficulty in these cases resulted from the resemblance of foci of infiltrating carcinoma von Brunn's nests, cystitis glandularis, cystitis cystica, and nephrogenic adenoma, alone or in combination. The features that helped in distinguishing these foci from benign processes were an irregular distribution, the presence of large numbers of closely packed epithelial aggregates, focal-to-moderate cytologic atypia, and

transitions to unequivocal carcinoma. In the third case, the superficial component of a carcinoma closely resembled an inverted papilloma [3].

3.2. Epidemiology. Nested variant of urothelial carcinoma usually occurs in men who are older than 60 years which is similar to the occurrence of classic urothelial carcinoma [6].

3.3. Age. Nested variant of urothelial carcinomas has been reported in patients aged between 42 years and 90 years.

3.4. Clinical Features. Nested variant of urothelial carcinoma is either rare or underreported with a reported incidence of 0.3% of invasive bladder tumours [6]. Lin and associates [7] stated that the nested variants of urothelial carcinoma exhibit aggressive behaviour despite their bland cytologic features. Wasco and associates [8] stated that the clinical outcome of pure or mixed nested variant with usual urothelial carcinoma is similar. Often nested variant of urothelial carcinoma at first presentation is diagnosed in an advanced stage and the tumour often involves the ureteric orifices [6].

It has been stated that the neoplasm resembles von Brunn's nest [4] and it may be misinterpreted as benign [9].

3.5. Treatment. Radical surgical resection is the treatment of choice [6].

3.6. Macroscopic Features. Quite often there is no evidence of a clearly defined tumour.

3.7. Microscopic Features. The described microscopic features of nested variant of urothelial carcinoma include the following.

(i) Irregular and confluent small nests and abortive tubules are composed of urothelial cells infiltrating the lamina propria or muscularis propria, usually without surface involvement [2].

(ii) The tumour cells usually exhibit mild atypia (mild pleomorphism, slightly increased nuclear/cytoplasmic ratios, occasional prominent nucleoli, and rare mitotic figures) and resemble cystitis glandularis and cystitis cystica [5].

(iii) Deep tumour-stroma interface is jagged and infiltrative [6].

(iv) Often more atypia and focal anaplasia with increasing depth of invasion are one of the features [6].

(v) Typical urothelial is often present [10].

(vi) Retraction artefact may be seen [6].

(vii) By definition these tumours cannot be high grade or have overlying surface carcinoma *in situ* [6].

3.8. Cytology. It has been stated that subtle features are not diagnostic themselves—these subtle features include medium sized round/polygonal cells with abundant, dense, slightly granular basophilic cytoplasm and well-defined cell borders,

TABLE 1: A list of some of the reported cases of nested variant of urothelial carcinoma and their outcome.

Patient	Reference	Age/sex	Pathologic stage	AJCC stage	Treatment	Status	Follow-up	Associated CUC (WHO/ISUP 1998)
1	Lin et al. [7]	90/F	pT1	1	Cystectomy	NED	30	No
2	Lin et al. [7]	73/F	pT3b	III	Cystectomy + chemotherapy	NED	5	No
3	Lin et al. [7]	65/M	pT2b	IV	Cystectomy + chemotherapy	AWM	16	Flat CIS
4	Lin et al. [7]	70/M	pT3b	III	Cystectomy + chemotherapy	AWM	15	Flat CIS
5	Lin et al. [7]	61/M	pT3b	IV	Cystectomy + chemotherapy	NED	19	Flat CIS
6	Lin et al. [7]	80/M	pT3b	III	Cystectomy	NED	27	Flat CIS
7	Lin et al. [7]	66/M	pT1	I	Cystectomy	NED	22	No
8	Lin et al. [7]	53/M	pT1	I	Cystectomy	NED	19	No
9	Lin et al. [7]	51/M	pT2	IV	Radiotherapy	DOD	3	No
10	Lin et al. [7]	59/M	pT2a	II	Cystectomy	NED	24	No
11	Lin et al. [7]	42/F	pT2a	II	Cystectomy	NED	20	No
12	Lin et al. [7]	75/M	pT2a	I	TUR	NED	12	Low-grade papillary UC
13	Wang et al. [11]	49/F	G3pT4M1		Partial cystectomy; en bloc resection of distal ileum, caecum; resection of transplanted pancreas; right salpingo-oophorectomy; repair of ileocolostomy anastomosis; chemotherapy	DOD	12 months	Plus conventional high-grade TCC
14	Tatsura et al. [12]	70/M	G3pT3b Nx M0	>III	Bladder adherent and cystectomy abandoned; open bladder total layer biopsy + bilateral ureterocutaneostomy; chemotherapy	Alive with disease	12 months	Small tumour atypical cells positive for cytokeratin
15	Terada [13]	80/F	pT1		TUR	Alive with no tumour	6 months	Atypical cells forming nests and tubules in lamina propria without surface urothelial involvement
16	Terada [13]	78/M	pT1		TUR	Alive with no tumour	15 months	Atypical cells forming nests and tubules in lamina propria without surface urothelial involvement

TABLE 1: Continued.

Patient	Reference	Age/sex	Pathologic stage	AJCC stage	Treatment	Status	Follow-up	Associated CUC (WHO/ISUP 1998)
17	De Berardinis et al. [14]	70/M	pT2aN+		TUR twice + BCG for initial conventional G3pT1b tumour and cystectomy + lymphadenectomy + chemotherapy for nested variant was started	Alive 12 months after initial diagnosis of conventional urothelial carcinoma	12 months after initial diagnosis and exact duration of follow-up after cystectomy not stated but patient just started on chemotherapy after cystectomy	
18, 19, 20, 21, 22, 23, 24	Cardillo et al. [15]	5 M 2 F 7 cases Age range 53–90 years		3 stage 1; 2 stage II; 1 stage III; 1 stage IV with metastasis	6 patients with stages 1 to III tumours underwent cystectomy; 1 patient with stage IV tumour had radiotherapy	Follow-up outcome data not provided	Follow-up outcome data not provided in paper	
25	Dundar et al. [16]	78/M	pT4N1		Cystoprostatectomy and chemotherapy planned but not given at time of publication	Alive	Follow-up data not available at time of publication	
26	Dundar et al. [16]	56/M	pT2 at least		TURBT he refused radical cystoprostatectomy	Alive but had 3 recurrences of nested variant urothelial carcinoma resected over 23 months	23 months	
27	Badoual et al. [17]	Details not available	Details not available in English	Details not available	Details not available to author	Details not available	Details not available	Details not available
28	Badoual et al. [17]	Details not available	Details not available	Details not available	Details not available	Details not available	Details not available	Details not available
29	Krishnamoorthy et al. [18]	45 F	pT1		TUR	Alive	No follow-up paper soon after TUR	
30	Ozdemir et al. [19]	65 M	pT2 at least		TUR biopsy Further details of treatment not mentioned in paper	Alive no data provided on follow-up case reported after biopsy	Data not available	
31	Holmäng and Johansson 2001 [20]	10 patients	Details not available to author		Details not available to author	7 died of disease or treatment complications (4 months–40 months); 1 died of unrelated cause after 90 months; follow-up ≤1 year for the remaining 2		
32	Ooi et al. [21]	74/M	Bladder tumour with ureteric involvement		TUR + bilateral local resection of ureter and chemotherapy	Alive with tumour (partial response)	12 months	

TABLE 1: Continued.

Patient	Reference	Age/sex	Pathologic stage	AJCC stage	Treatment	Status	Follow-up	Associated CUC (WHO/ISUP 1998)
33–86	Linder et al. [22]	52 patients Mean age 69.5 years Range 62–74	36 (69%) with pT3–T4 10 (19%) with nodal invasion		All had radical cystectomy 8 had additional perioperative (15%) chemotherapy	Analysis in the comparison of patients with nested variant matched with a cohort of conventional urothelial carcinoma showed no significant differences in the 10-year local recurrence free survival (83% versus 80%, $P = 0.46$) or 10-year cancer specific survival (41% versus 46%, $P = 0.75$)	Median follow-up 10.8 months Range 9.3–11.3	
87	Tripodi et al. [23]	49/F	Renal pelvis pT1		Nephrectomy and upper ureterectomy	Alive	No long-term follow-up at time of publication	
88	Cerda et al. [24]	53/M	pT3b pN1		TUR and radical cystoprostatectomy, radiotherapy, and chemotherapy	Died due to advanced metastatic disease	12 months	
89	Cerda et al. [24]	83/F	pT2		TUR (surgical procedure not done due to advanced age)	Died of disease	3 years (36 months)	
90	Yildiz et al. [25]	60/M	T2 at least (muscle invasion)		TUR further details in Turkish language	Not found in data		
91	Pusztaszeri et al. [26]		Renal pelvis and ureter		Details not available to author	Details not available to author	Details not available to author	
92	Lau [27]		Renal pelvis	Locally advanced	Details not available to author	Details not available to author	Details not available to author	
93	Stern [1]	45/M	Details not available to author	Details not available to author	TUR	Alive tumour recurred 18 months later	18 months	
94, 95, 96	Talbert and Young [3]	3 men Aged 53–73 years	Details not available to author		Details not available to author	Details not available to author		
97, 98, 99, 100	Murphy and Deana [4]	4 cases	Details not available to author	Details not available to author	Details not available to author	Tumours persisted/recurred	Details not available to author	

TABLE 1: Continued.

Patient	Reference	Age/sex	Pathologic stage	AJCC stage	Treatment	Status	Follow-up	Associated CUC (WHO/ISUP 1998)
101–130	Wasco et al. [8]	30 cases Aged 41–83 years Average 63 Male-female 2.3:1	All but 1 invasive tumours (9% pT1; pT2-3a; 65% pT3b; 17% pT4)		All had cystectomy and 15 had cystectomy and chemotherapy	3 (10%) died of disease; 16 (55%) alive with persistent or recurrent disease; 10 (34%) alive without disease Response to chemotherapy observed in 2 (13%) of 15 patients	Follow-up in 29 patients (97%) with median 12 months (range 1–31 months)	Focal atypia in 90% and focal high-grade cytological atypia at tumour base in 40%
131–134	Young and Oliva [9]	4 patients Age range 70–85 years	Details not available to author		Details not available to author	Details not available to author		1 or more specimens were misinterpreted as benign
135–150	Drew et al. [10]	16 cases with marked male predominance	Details not available to author		Details not available to author	3 with no disease	Average follow-up 16.6 months	A few cells in every case with cytological atypia
151 and 152	Xiao et al. [28]	69/M 70/M	pT4 N1 pT2/3 + perineural and vascular invasion + Gleason 3 + 3 adenoca of prostate		Radical cystoprostatectomy and chemotherapy Radical cystoprostatectomy	Developed bone and soft tissue metastases in 4 months	4 months Lost to follow-up at 2 months	Focal urothelial CIS and multiple foci of urothelial atypia Focus of urothelial CIS
153	Huang et al. [29]	83/M	G3pT2-3		Cystoprostatectomy	Alive no long-term follow-up data available to author		
154–164	Volmar et al. [30]	11 patients	5 pT2-3 N0 1 pT2-3 M1; 1 pT4 stage of remaining not available to author			Details not available to author	Details not available	
165–174	Holmäng and Johansson [20]	10 patients	Details not available		Locoregional therapy	7 died of disease or treatment complications 4–40 months after diagnosis; 1 died of unrelated cause after 90 months; Follow-up ≤1 year for the remaining 2		

TABLE 1: Continued.

Patient	Reference	Age/sex	Pathologic stage	AJCC stage	Treatment	Status	Follow-up	Associated CUC (WHO/ISUP 1998)
175–177	Liedberg et al. [31]	3 patients		Advanced muscle-invasive 2 with lymph node involvement	Final outcome not available			
178–200	Cox and Epstein [32]	23 cases Mean age 63.7 years; Range 39–89; 86% male	20 T2-T3 2 pT1 1a pT1b		18 had TURBT 2 nephroureterectomy 3 radical cystectomy	3 of 17 patients developed metastasis 2 lung 1 unknown with 2 of the 3 dead of disease; 1 patient died of disease with no known details	Follow-up for 17 patients Mean 43 months Range 5 months to 9 years	

Abbreviations: M: male; F: female; NED: alive with no evidence of disease; AWM: alive with metastasis; DOD: dead of disease; CIS: carcinoma *in situ*; CUC: conventional urothelial carcinoma; TUR: transurethral resection of tumour; and Lin et al.: Lin O, Cardillo M, Dalbagni G, Linkov I, Hutchinson B, and Reuter V E. Nested variant of urothelial carcinoma: a clinicopathologic and immunohistochemical study of 12 cases. Modern Pathology 2003; 16(12): 1289-1298.

TABLE 2: Nested variant of urothelial carcinoma: example of results and geographic distribution of several markers in nested variant of urothelial carcinoma taken from Lin O, Cardillo M, Dalbagni G, Linkov I, Hutchinson B, and Reuter V E. Nested variant of urothelial carcinoma: a clinicopathologic and immunohistochemical study of 12 cases. Modern Pathology 2003;16(12): 1289–1298.

Case	Ref.	P21 result	P21 location	P27 result	P27 location	P53 result	P53 location	EGF-R result	Bcl2 result	Bcl2 location	MIB-1%	MIB1 location	Other comments
1	Lin et al. [7]	+	Diffuse	+	Surface	−		−	−		20	Diffuse	
2	Lin et al. [7]	+	Diffuse	+	Diffuse	−		−	−		15	Diffuse	
3	Lin et al. [7]	+	Diffuse	−		−		−	−		35	Diffuse	
4	Lin et al.[7]	+	Diffuse	+	Surface	−		−	−		35	Diffuse	
5	Lin et al. [7]	+	Base	+	Surface	+	Base	−	+	Surface	2	Base	
6	Lin et al. [7]	−		+	Surface	−		−	−		20	Diffuse	
7	Lin et al. [7]	+	Base	+	Surface	−		−	+	Surface	35	Diffuse	
8	Lin et al. [7]	+	Base	+	Surface	+		−	−		15	Base	
9	Lin et al. [7]	−	Diffuse	+	Surface	+	Diffuse	−	−		30	Diffuse	
10	Lin et al. [7]	+	Diffuse	+	Surface	−		−	−		30	Base	
11	Lin et al. [7]	+	Base	+	Surface	−		−	−		20	Diffuse	
12	Lin et al. [7]	+	Base	+	Surface	+	Base	−	−		15	Base	
13	Wang et al. [11]	Not done		Not done		−		Not done	Not done		Not done		
14	Tatsura et al. [12]	Not done		Not done		Not done		Not done	Not done		Not done		Cytokeratin+
15	Terada [13]	Not done		Not done		+		Not done					Ki-67 labeling = 15%; +cytokeratins; +EMA; α-methylacyl CoA racemase; +Ca19-9; MUC1
16	Terada [13]	Not done		Not done		+		Not done					Ki-67 labeling = 30%; +cytokeratins; +EMA, +p63, +p53, +Cl0, +CEA, +MUC1
17	De Berardinis et al. [14]	Not done		Not done		Strongly+		Not done					Ki-67 +high expression
18, 19, 20, 21, 22, 23, 24	Cardillo et al. [15] (7 cases)	Not done		Not done		Not done		Not done					
25	Dundar et al. [16]	Not done		+40%		+40%		Not done					Ki-67 20%; 34βE12; −PSA; −AE1
26	Dundar et al. [16]	Not done		+50%		+40%		Not done					Ki-67 15%; +34βE12; −PSA; −AE1

TABLE 2: Continued.

Case	Ref.	P21 result	P21 location	P27 result	P27 location	P53 result	P53 location	EGF-R result	Bcl2 result	Bcl2 location	MIB-1%	MIB1 location	Other comments
27	Badoual et al. [17]	Details not available	Details not available	Details not available	Details not available	Details not available	Details not available	Details not available	Details not available	Details not available	Details not available	Details not available	Details not available
28	Badoual et al. [17]	Details not available	Details not available	Details not available	Details not available	Details not available	Details not available	Details not available	Details not available	Details not available	Details not available	Details not available	Details not available
29	Krishnamoorthy et al. [18]	Details not available	Details not available	Details not available	Details not available	Details not available	Details not available	Details not available	Details not available	Details not available	Details not available	Details not available	Irregular nests of tubules in lamina propria
30.	Ozdemir et al. [19]	Not done		Not done	Not done	Not done		Not done				Not done	Details not available to author
31	Holmäng and Johansson [20]	Details not available to author	Details not available to author	Details not available to author	Details not available to author	Details not available to author	Details not available to author	Details not available to author	Details not available to author	Details not available to author	Details not available to author	Details not available to author	
32	Ooi et al. [21]	Details not available to author	Details not available to author	Details not available to author	Details not available to author	Details not available to author	Details not available to author	Details not available to author	Details not available to author	Details not available to author	Details not available to author	Details not available to author	
33 to 86	Linder et al. [22]	52 patients	Details not availabe	Details not availabe	Details not availabe	Details not availabe	Details not availabe	Details not availabe	Details not availabe	Details not availabe	Details not availabe	Details not availabe	
87	Tripodi et al. [23]	Not done		Not done		Not done							+P63
88	Cerda et al. [24]	Not done		Not done		Not done		Not done	Not done	Not done	Not done		+CK7, +CK20, +34βE12, +P63
89	Cerda et al. [24]	Not done		Not done		Not done		Not done	Not done	Not done	Not done		+CK7, +CK20, +34βE12, +P63
90	Yildiz et al. [25]	Details unavailable		Details unavailable		Details unavailable		Details unavailable	Details unavailable	Details unavailable	Details unavailable	Details unavailable	
91	Pusztaszeri et al. [26]	Details not available to author		Details not available to author		Details not available to author		Details not available to author	Details not available to author	Details not available to author	Details not available to author	Details not available to author	
92	Lau [27]	Details not available to author	Details not available to author	Details not available to author	Details not available to author	Details not available to author	Details not available to author	Details not available to author	Details not available to author	Details not available to author	Details not available to author	Details not available to author	
93	Stern [1]	Details not available to author	Details not available to author	Details not available to author	Details not available to author	Details not available to author	Details not available to author	Details not available to author	Details not available to author	Details not available to author	Details not available to author	Details not available to author	

TABLE 2: Continued.

Case	Ref.	P21 result	P21 location	P27 result	P27 location	P53 result	P53 location	EGF-R result	Bcl2 result	Bcl2 location	MIB-1%	MIB1 location	Other comments
94–96	Talbert and Young [3]	Details not available to author	Details not available to author	Details not available to author	Details not available to author	Details not available to author	Details not available to author	Details not available to author	Details not available to author	Details not available to author	Details not available to author	Details not available to author	
97–100	Murphy and Deana [4]	Details not available to author	Details not available to author	Details not available to author	Details not available to author	Details not available to author	Details not available to author	Details not available to author	Details not available to author	Details not available to author	Details not available to author	Details not available to author	
101–130	Wasco et al. [8]												CK7+ (93%); CK20+ (68%); P63+ (92%); CK903+ (92%)
131–134	Young and Oliva [9]	Details not available to author	Details not available to author	Details not available to author	Details not available to author	Details not available to author	Details not available to author	Details not available to author	Details not available to author	Details not available to author	Details not available to author	Details not available to author	
135–150	Drew et al. [10]	Details not available to author	Details not available to author	Details not available to author	Details not available to author	Details not available to author	Details not available to author	Details not available to author	Details not available to author	Details not available to author	Details not available to author	Details not available to author	
151 and 152	Xiao et al. [28]					High +p53								Both Strongly+ for 63; and High Ki-67 indices Case 1 +CK 903; +CK7 +CK20; −PSA; −prostatic acid phosphatase; Strongly +p63; +p53 40% to 50%; +Ki-6730 to Case 2 +CK903; +CK7; −PSA; −prostatic acid phosphatase; −S100; −chromogranin; +p63 30 to 40%; Focally +p53; Focally +Ki-67

TABLE 2: Continued.

Case	Ref.	P21 result	P21 location	P27 result	P27 location	P53 result	P53 location	EGF-R result	Bcl2 result	Bcl2 location	MIB-1%	MIB1 location	Other comments
153	Huang et al. [29]												+CK7; +CK20; +thrombomodulin; +34βE12
154–164	Volmar et al. [30]										8.8%		+p53 4.2%; +P27 4.7%;
165–174	Holmäng and Johansson [20] 10 cases	Details not available	Details not available to author	Details not available to author	Details not available to author	Details not available to author	Details not available to author	Details not available to author	Details not available to author	Details not available to author	Details not available to author	Details not available to author	
175–177	Liedberg et al. [31]	Details not available	Details not available to author	Details not available to author	Details not available to author	Details not available to author	Details not available to author	Details not available to author	Details not available to author	Details not available to author	Details not available to author	Details not available to author	
178–200	Cox and Epstein [32]	Details not available	Details not available to author	Details not available to author	Details not available to author	Details not available to author	Details not available to author	Details not available to author	Details not available to author	Details not available to author	Details not available to author	Details not available to author	

irregular cell counters, increased nuclear/cytoplasmic ratio, coarse chromatin, and occasional prominent nucleoli [15].

3.9. Positive Immunohistochemical Stains. Nested variants of urothelial carcinoma stain positively for the following:

(i) CK7, CK20, p63, Ki-67, and CK903 [28],

(ii) variable P53 [6].

3.10. Negative Immunohistochemical Stains. Nested variants of urothelial carcinoma stain negatively with

(i) Bcl2, EGFR, and PSA [6].

3.11. Differential Diagnosis. Some of the listed differential diagnoses of nested variant of urothelial carcinoma include the following.

(i) Adenocarcinoma: colonic differentiation and more prominent atypia [6].

(ii) Cystitis cystica/cystitis glandularis: this has no atypia and no invasion [6].

(iii) Inverted papilloma: this has no deep invasion [6].

(iv) Nephrogenic metaplasia/adenoma: this usually has papillary component, prominent tubular, or cystic structures lined by single layer of cuboidal cells, no atypia, and no invasion [6].

(v) Adenocarcinoma of prostate: this is centred in the prostate gland and immunohistochemically stains positively with PSA and PSAP [6].

(vi) Urothelial carcinoma with small tubules: this is an invasive carcinoma with small gland-like spaces lined by urothelial cells without intracellular mucin or columnar lining; some authors have considered this as part of nested variant of urothelial carcinoma [29].

(vii) von Brunn's nests: these have no invasion, no prominent atypia, and no focal anaplasia as stated by some authors [30].

3.12. Characteristic Diagnostic Criteria Used to Confirm Nested Variant of Urothelial Carcinoma. Rouse [5] summarized the diagnostic features that could be used to confirm the diagnosis of nested variant of urothelial carcinoma as follows.

(1) Infiltrative pattern: it is worth noting that (a) the infiltrative pattern may sometimes be difficult to assess on biopsies that are small; (b) deep foci of classical jagged invasion quite often exist; (c) if present evidence of muscularis propria involvement is definitional (d) the stroma may be desmoplastic or normal.

(2) Predominant pattern—variably sized nests are seen and these are most often small sized and fused.

(3) Frequent forms of lumens or spaces—(a) the lumens are quite often empty; however, necrotic debris may be found in them or PASd stainable material; (b) the carcinoma cells forming and lining the spaces do not

have secretory/glandular cytoplasmic differentiation; (c) the lining cells of the spaces tend to be transitional or squamous PASd negative; (d) There is no absence of goblet cells; and (e) if extensive then the terminology of microcytic urothelial carcinoma can be used.

Cytologically predominantly bland—the cytological features of this tumour include the following (a) focal cytologic atypia is almost invariably present but sometimes this is only present in deeper tissues; (b) the overlying mucosa is often normal or there may be a papillary component; (c) nested variant of urothelial carcinoma often involves the ureteric orifices; and (d) despite the bland cytology these tumours are usually aggressive and invasive tumours [5].

3.13. Salient Points from Reported Cases and Case Series. Lin and associates [7] stated the following.

(i) Nested variant of urothelial carcinoma is characterized by confluent small nests and abortive tubules of mildly atypical neoplastic cells infiltrating the lamina propria and/or muscularis propria of the bladder.

(ii) Despite its deceptively bland histomorphologic appearance, the lesion is reported to have an aggressive behaviour. The collective immunohistochemical expression of suppressor genes, growth factor, and proliferation activity marker had not been previously studied in this disease.

(iii) They had stained formalin-fixed, paraffin-embedded archival tissues from 12 cases of nested variant of urothelial carcinoma with monoclonal antibodies to p21, p27, p53, EGF-R, and bcl-2, as well as the proliferation marker MIB-1. They also evaluated the area of predominant immunoreactivity. They also compared the pattern of immunostaining with the clinical parameters.

(iv) p21 was positive in 10 of 12 cases and located at the deepest portion of the tumour in 5 of 10 positive cases. Immunoreactivity for p27 was seen in 11 of 12 cases and limited to the superficial portion of the tumor in 9 of 11 positive cases. Only 3 and 2 of 12 cases were positive for p53 and bcl-2, respectively. MIB-1 immunoreactivity ranged from 2 to 35% of the neoplastic cells, with most tumors showing a proliferation index of >15%. Follow-up ranged from 3 to 30 months (mean, 17.6 months). All patients except one were alive, although three patients developed metastases. Nested variant of urothelial carcinoma is a deceptively benign-appearing neoplasm with potential of deep invasion and metastases. Immunohistochemically, nested variant of urothelial carcinoma shares some features with high-risk conventional urothelial carcinomas, such as loss of p27 expression and high proliferation index. Nevertheless, p53, bcl-2, or EGF-r immunoreactivity is not frequently seen.

Wang and associates [11] reported a case of urothelial carcinoma which had directly involved a pancreatic allograft with metastasis that occurred in a 49-year-old pancreas and kidney transplant recipient. Her initial clinical presentation and findings of computed tomography scan of the abdomen suggested pancreatitis with features worrisome for rejection. A biopsy of her pancreatic allograft was obtained and histological examination of the specimen revealed that the specimen contained poorly differentiated carcinoma and cystoscopic biopsy disclosed an invasive high-grade urothelial carcinoma arising in the background of extensive urothelial carcinoma *in situ*. She underwent exploratory laparotomy which revealed extensive tumor invading the right ovary and tube, the caecum, and the transplant pancreas with extensive retroperitoneal involvement. Subsequently, she underwent en bloc resection of distal ileum and caecum, resection of transplanted pancreas, partial cystectomy, right salpingo-oophorectomy, and repair of ileocolostomy anastomosis. Pathological examination of the resected specimen disclosed a 4.9 cm mass within the bladder cuff near the allograft that directly invaded the right ovary, fallopian tube, caecum, and pancreas allograft, as well as extensive retroperitoneal involvement. The tumour demonstrated a prominent nested growth pattern reminiscent of the nested variant of urothelial carcinoma (NVUC) with other areas showing features more typical of conventional invasive high-grade urothelial carcinoma. The neoplastic cells were positive for pancytokeratin and OC125 (cytoplasmic) while being negative for chromogranin, synaptophysin, CD56, CK7, CK20, CDX2, TTF1, ER, PR, p53, and BRST2. While not entirely specific, the staining pattern combined with the presence of adjacent urothelial carcinoma *in situ* was supportive of a urothelial origin. In addition, the lesions resected from her abdominal wall were positive for metastatic urothelial carcinoma. Postoperatively, she received four cycles of gemcitabine and carboplatin, which she completed, with no measurable disease noted radiographically following therapy. One year later, she was admitted to hospital for the worsening abdominal pain. She had a computed tomography (CT) scan which revealed multiple intra-abdominal and peritoneal nodules consistent with metastatic disease. She went into a hospice and died shortly after her admission to the hospice.

Wang and associates [11] stated that carcinoma of the urinary bladder developing in organ transplant recipients remains a challenging disease to manage as it has been demonstrated by some authors [33–36] that the clinical course seems worse than that in the general population as reported in [33–36]. Other authors stated that the immunosuppressed status of the transplant recipients renders the therapy and posttreatment surveillance very difficult [37]. With the increase of organ transplantation, urological cancer (including bladder cancer) may pose a critical problem affecting the survival of these patients.

Nested variant of urothelial carcinoma was classified by the World Health Organization in 2004 as an "uncommon aggressive tumor," with few reported cases and a 70% mortality rate 4 to 40 months after diagnosis despite therapy [38]. Holmäng and Johansson [20] stated that the incidence of nested variant of urothelial carcinoma has been estimated to be 0.8% of all invasive bladder carcinoma [20] and less than 100 cases had been reported [4, 9, 29, 31]. Liedberg

and associates [31] stated that nested variant of urothelial carcinoma exhibits aggressive clinical behaviour with rapid spread along the lymphatics in the lamina propria of the urinary bladder and along lymphatic channels into the peritoneum [4, 9, 29, 31].

While the degree of cytologic atypia noted in this case is not typically described in NVUC, this feature can be seen in these lesions and NVUC is associated with areas of conventional high-grade urothelial carcinoma in the majority of instances [8]. In the present case, her pancreas is bladder drained and it is possible that the atypia noted may be related to the effect of exocrine pancreatic secretions. Indeed, clinical behaviour and pattern of spread are compatible with NVUC and cases with nested features have a poor outcome [8].

Wang and associates [11] stated that to their knowledge, their case was the first case of urothelial carcinoma demonstrating NVUC features reported in the transplant receipt; the tumour invaded the transplanted pancreas with extensive retroperitoneal involvement. This is a unique presentation that clinically mimicked pancreatitis and/or rejection. The rapid progression from a clinically nonapparent lesion widely invasive disease may be related to the patient's immunosuppressive status, although as noted above lesions with nested growth patterns often demonstrate an aggressive phenotype.

Some authors [7, 20] stated that the optimal modality of treatment of nested variant of urothelial carcinoma is uncertain because nested variant of urothelial carcinoma is rare and there had not been any randomized studies specifically designed for this subtype of bladder tumour [7, 20]. Sternberg and associates [39] stated that traditionally, the standard therapy for patients with locally advanced or metastatic urothelial carcinoma is chemotherapy using methotrexate, vinblastine, doxorubicin, and cisplatin (MVAC) [39]. von der Maase and associates [40] had shown that the gemcitabine-cisplatin regimen has equivalent overall response rates, with less toxicity (range 41% to 57%), with a complete response in 15% to 22%, and a median survival of 12.5 to 14.3 months [40]. Wang and associates [11] stated that even though a number of authors were of the opinion that this subtype of urothelial carcinoma is resistant to radiotherapy and chemotherapy [7, 20, 31], clinical experience with their case would suggest that multimodality therapy including platinum based chemotherapy is beneficial. Wang and associates [11] suggested that multi-institution studies are needed to establish a better therapeutic protocol for these rare cases. Wang and associates [11] concluded that their case report illustrates atypical presentation of bladder cancer in a pancreas and kidney transplant recipient and that their experience should alert physicians and radiologists to the possibility of malignancy in the differential diagnosis and the need for early biopsy to avoid diagnostic confusion with graft rejection.

Wang and associates [11] stated that postoperatively, the patient was treated with four cycles of carboplatin and gemcitabine. She ultimately succumbed to her disease approximately 1 year after diagnosis. Wang and associates [11] iterated that this case should alert physicians and radiologists to be aware of atypical presentation of urothelial carcinoma in bladder-drained pancreas grafts, the aggressiveness of such lesions, and the need for early biopsy to avoid diagnostic confusion with rejection.

Cox and associates [32] reported 23 cases of large nested variant of urothelial carcinoma from the consult files of one of the authors from 2001 to 2010. They reported that the mean patient age was 63.7 years with an age range from 39 years to 89 years, and 86% were men. Out of the 23 cases, 18 of the patients underwent transurethral resection of bladder tumour, 2 underwent nephroureterectomy, and 3 had undergone radical cystectomy. Cox and associates [32] reported that a surface component was present in 19 of the 23 cases, with 16 low-grade papillary urothelial carcinomas, 2 low-grade papillary urothelial carcinoma with less than 5% high-grade urothelial carcinoma, and 1 high-grade papillary urothelial carcinoma. They reported that, out of the 23 cases, twenty had invaded into the muscularis propria. With regard to 21 cases, the invasive component was found to be composed of medium to large nests which varied from rounded circumscribed borders to stromal-tumour interface with a more irregular ragged appearance. Two of the tumours exhibited a verruciform, pushing border into the muscularis propria with the nests having central cyst formation. With regard to the cytological characteristics, the nuclei lacked significant nuclear atypia, where at most occasional scattered slightly enlarged, hyperchromatic nuclei with small-indistinct nucleoli were noted. Four of the cases had focal necrosis and 3 of the cases had more extensive necrosis. Cox and associates [32] also reported that the median mitotic count was 1.5 per 10 high-power fields. The stroma which surrounded the large nests characteristically had a mild-to-moderate fibrous and/or inflammatory reaction; 4 of the cases did not have any stromal reaction, but 2 cases had a moderate-to-marked stromal response. In 7 of the 23 cases, conventional patterns of urothelial invasion were found, 5 of which consisted of ≤5% of the neoplasm. One of the cases had angiolymphatic invasion. Four cases had subsequent radical cystectomy specimens available for review. Two out of the 4 radical cystectomy specimens did not have any residual carcinoma (1 with neoadjuvant radiotherapy); 1 had large nested urothelial carcinoma in the muscularis propria into the perivesical tissue. Cox and associates [32] reported that clinical follow-up was available for 17 of 23 patients with a mean follow-up of 43 months and a follow-up range of 5 months to 9 years. Cox and associates [32] additionally reported the following.

Three of 17 patients developed metastatic disease (2 in the lung, 1 unknown) with 2 of these dead due to disease; another patient died of disease with un known details. Of the aforementioned 3 patients who died of disease, 2 had no and 1 had focal (<5%) conventional invasive urothelial carcinoma on transurethral resection. Cox and associates [32] stipulated the following.

(i) These cases, which posed great diagnostic difficulty both for the contributing pathologists and for the consultant, represent the first formal description of a large nested pattern of urothelial carcinoma.

(ii) This pattern is distinguished from an inverted growth pattern of noninvasive urothelial carcinoma and

from von Brunn nests by either muscularis propria invasion, irregularly infiltrating nests, or a stromal reaction.

(iii) Despite the bland cytological features of these neoplasms, they have well-documented metastatic potential.

Wasco and associates [8] stated that nested variant of urothelial carcinoma is a rare histological variant of urothelial carcinoma which is characterized by deceptively bland histologic features that resemble von Bruun's nests but usually with a poor outcome. They also stated that in their experience, nested variant of urothelial carcinoma is frequently misclassified or underrecognized in view of the fact that its clinico-pathological spectrum is not well defined. Furthermore, its relationship to the usual urothelial carcinoma and response to traditional bladder cancer management are largely unknown. Wasco and associates [8] reported 30 cases of with pure or predominant nested morphology in order to identify its associated histopathological findings, clinical outcome, and immunophenotype. Wasco and associates [8] reported that the ages of the patients ranged from 41 years to 83 years with an average age of 63 years, with a male to female ratio of 2.3 : 1. They also reported that the architectural pattern of the nested component ranged from a predominantly disorderly proliferation of discrete, small, variably sized nests (90%) to focal areas demonstrating confluent nests (40%), cord-like growth (37%), and cystitis cystica-like areas (33%) to tubular growth pattern (13%). The deep tumour-stroma interface was invariably (100%) jagged and infiltrative. Additionally, Wasco and associates [8] stated that despite the overall bland cytology, the tumour nests exhibited focal random cytologic atypia (90%) and focal high-grade cytologic atypia which was centred within the base of the tumour (40%). The tumour stroma ranged from having minimal stromal response to focally desmoplastic and myxoid. They found a component of usual urothelial carcinoma in 63% of cases. Wasco and associates [8] furthermore made the following ensuing reports.

(i) The nested component demonstrated an immunophenotype which was identical to the usual urothelial carcinoma, with CK7, CK20, p63, and CK903 expression in 93%, 68%, 92%, and 92% of cases, respectively.

(ii) At resection, all of the cases except 1 case were demonstrated to be invasive—9% into lamina propria, 4% into muscularis propria, 65% into perivesical fat, and 17% into adjacent organ(s).

(iii) In comparison with pure high-grade urothelial carcinoma, nested variant of urothelial carcinoma was associated with muscleinvasion at transurethral resection (31% versus 70%; $P < 0.0001$), extravesical disease at cystectomy (33% versus 83%, $P < 0.0001$), and metastatic disease (19% versus 67%, $P < 0.0001$).

(iv) Follow-up was available for 29 patients (97%) with a median of 12 months (range, 1 month to 31 months) of follow-up; 3 (10%) died of disease, 16 (55%) were alive with persistent or recurrent disease, and 10 (34%) were alive without disease.

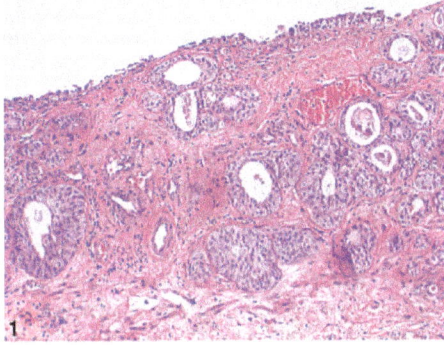

FIGURE 1: Low-power view showing closely packed, irregularly spaced, glandular, and cystic urothelial nests somewhat resembling von Brunn nests. Note that the overlying urothelium appears uninvolved (hematoxylin-eosin, original magnification ×100). Nested variant of urothelial carcinoma taken from Dhall et al. [2]. The figures have been reproduced with the permission of the editor in chief of Archives of Pathology and Laboratory Medicine on behalf of the editorial board of the journal.

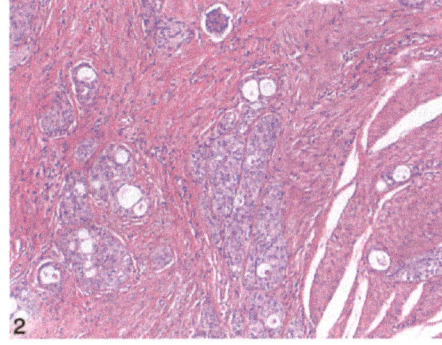

FIGURE 2: Low-power view showing bland tumor cells in the nested pattern infiltrating the muscularis propria (hematoxylin-eosin, original magnification ×100). Nested variant of urothelial carcinoma taken from Dhall et al. [2]. The figures have been reproduced with the permission of the editor in chief of Archives of Pathology and Laboratory Medicine on behalf of the editorial board of the journal.

(v) Response to neoadjuvant chemotherapy was observed in 2 (13%) of 15 patients.

(vi) Nested variant of urothelial carcinoma which was seen either in pure form or with a component of usual urothelial carcinoma had similarly unfavourable outcome ($P = 0.78$).

Wasco and associates [8] concluded that increased awareness and familiarity with the clinicopathologic spectrum of nested variant of urothelial carcinoma is critical for confident recognition and adequate management of this very aggressive variant of urothelial carcinoma.

Dundar and associates [16] reported two cases of nested variant of urothelial carcinoma. In the first case the tumour extended through the bladder wall into the perivesical soft tissue, prostatic urethra, and left seminal vesicle and metastasized to the obturator lymph nodes. In the second case invasion of muscular layer was observed and three recurrences were developed during a follow-up period of 23 months. Dundar and associates [16] stated that both tumours demonstrated high p53 and Ki-67 indices supporting the aggressive nature of such tumours. Details of the two reported cases are as follows.

Case 1. A 70-year-old man presented with symptoms of urinary urgency, increased frequency, and nocturia of one-year duration. He had an ultrasound scan and this revealed a 5 cm diameter polypoid mass in the left posterolateral wall of the bladder. The mass was located at close proximity to the left ureteric orifice and this was associated with left sided hydronephrosis. He underwent transurethral resection of the bladder lesion as well as lesion within the prostatic urethra. Histological examination of the specimen revealed small, closely packed nests of epithelial cells infiltrating the lamina propria and muscularis propria of the bladder wall (Figure 1). The tumour cells were observed to be uniform with only focal moderate atypia. Tumoral invasion was also seen in the

prostatic urethra. He had computed tomography scans of abdomen and thorax as well as scintigraphic examination which demonstrated that there was no metastatic disease. He then underwent radical cystoprostatectomy. Microscopic examination revealed that the tumour had extended through the bladder wall into the perivesical soft tissue, prostatic urethra, and left seminal vesicle. The neoplastic cells characteristically exhibited pale, eosinophilic, or clear cytoplasm and rounded nuclei with inconspicuous nucleoli. The cells were reported to have shown generally mild atypical features but occasionally large atypical cells were observed in the deeply infiltrated areas (Figure 2). Extensive perineural invasion was observed. Additionally, two out of 14 and 2 out of 11 right and left obturator lymph nodes were positive for the tumour, respectively. The iliac lymph nodes were negative for the tumour. He was scheduled to receive systemic chemotherapy which he had not yet received at the time of publication of the paper and therefore there was no follow-up outcome data available.

Case 2. A 56-year-old man had been followed up (for 10 years—since 1996) for a WHO grade 2 papillary urothelial carcinoma which was localized towards the left lateral wall of the urinary bladder. At a routine follow-up cystoscopic examination, two small tumour foci in the dome of the urinary bladder were found which were resected transurethrally. The microscopic features of the tumour were markedly different from those of his previous tumour by the infiltration of neoplastic cells that were arranged in a diffuse pattern of variably sized nests. There was evidence of invasion of lamina propria and muscular layer. There was no evidence of papillary configuration in the tumour. The tumour cells characteristically exhibited pale to eosinophilic cytoplasm with bland nuclear features. The mitotic activity in the tumour was low, and there was no evidence of perineural invasion. The histological findings were reported to be consistent with those of nested variant of urothelial carcinoma. The option of radical cystoprostatectomy was offered to the patient

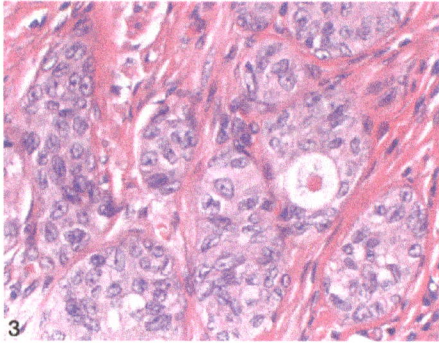

FIGURE 3: On high-power view, the tumour cells show no significant cytologic atypia (hematoxylin-eosin, original magnification ×400). Nested variant of urothelial carcinoma taken from Dhall et al. [2]. The figures have been reproduced with the permission of the editor in chief of Archives of Pathology and Laboratory Medicine on behalf of the editorial board of the journal.

but he refused to undergo cystoprostatectomy. However, during a follow-up period of 23 months, he developed three recurrences of nested variant of urothelial carcinoma.

Immunohistochemical studies of the tumour were undertaken and these showed that the percentages of cells that were positive for Ki-67, p53, and p27 were 20%, 40%, and 40% in Case 1 and 15%, 40%, and 50% in Case 2, respectively (Figure 3). In both Cases 1 and 2, the tumour cells were positive for high-molecular-weight cytokeratin (34βE12) but negative for PSA and low-molecular weight cytokeratin (AE1).

Terada [13] in a report of two cases stated that the nested variant of urothelial carcinoma is characterized by the presence of benign appearing urothelial carcinoma cells in the lamina propria, sparing the surface urothelial involvement, and that the tumour exhibited aggressive clinical course despite having a benign-looking histological appearance. Terada [13] reported two cases one in an 80-year-old woman and the second in a 78-year-old man. Terada [13] reported that in both cases atypical cells forming nests and tubules were observed in the lamina propria without the involvement of surface urothelium. Additionally, Terada [13] reported that one case resembled nephrogenic metaplasia and another resembled proliferated von Brunn's nest or inverted papilloma. Terada [13] reported the results of immunohistochemical studies on both tumours as follows.

(i) Both cases were positive with P53 and high Ki7 labeling, which suggested that both cases were malignant.

(ii) One case was characterized by positive cytokeratins, EMA, p53, Ki-67 (labeling = 15%), CD10, CEA, and MUC1.

(iii) The patients were free of tumour 6 months and at 15 months pursuant to transurethral resection of their bladder tumours.

Cardillo and associates [15] stated that in view of the fact that nested variant of urothelial carcinoma is a recently described rare variant of urothelial carcinoma there had not been any prior report of cytologic findings in urine specimens from patients with nested variant of urothelial carcinoma. Cardillo and associates [15] reviewed urine specimens from patients with histologically confirmed nested variant of urothelial carcinoma. They evaluated urine specimens that were obtained concurrently with or up to 1 month prior to the patient's surgical procedure. They analysed all the specimens for the presence of cells morphologically similar to the nested variant of urothelial carcinoma cells that were observed in the tissue sections. The cells were observed for the ensuing parameters: the number of neoplastic cells; the cellular arrangement, the cell size and shape, cell borders, as well as cytoplasmic, nuclear, and nucleolar characteristics. They included thirteen urine specimens from 7 patients in the study. Cardillo and associates [15] reported that they were able to identify cells that were similar morphologically to cells present in the nests of nested variant of urothelial carcinoma in all cytologic specimens. They iterated that the neoplastic cells for most part were medium sized, round, or polygonal, with abundant, dense, slightly granular basophilic cytoplasm, and well-defined cell borders. The nuclear/cytoplasmic ratio was increased, the nuclear membranes exhibited irregular contours, and the nuclei encompassed coarse chromatin with occasional prominent nucleoli. Cardillo and associates [15] made the following concluding iterations.

(i) The cytologic features of nested variant of urothelial carcinoma are subtle but distinct.

(ii) A primary diagnosis of nested variant of urothelial carcinoma is not recommended in view of the subtleness of the findings.

(iii) However, the presence of cells with the aforedescribed features should warrant a cystoscopic examination with histological confirmation in a patient with a previous history of nested variant of urothelial carcinoma.

De Berardinis and associates in 2012 stated that nested variant of urothelial carcinoma is a rare histological entity, with about 80 reported cases [14]. De Beradinis and associates [14] reported the case of 70-year-old man with haematuria who underwent ultrasound scan and cystoscopy which revealed the presence of carcinoma of the urinary bladder. He underwent transurethral resection of the tumour and histology of the resected tumour revealed a high-grade cancer with lamina propria involvement (G3pT1). He had adjuvant intravesical instillation of Bacillus Calmette-Guérin and at follow-up cystoscopy five months later a recurrent tumour was found in the bladder and this tumour was resected. Histological examination revealed a high-grade (G3) nested variant of transitional cell carcinoma with a deep lamina propria involvement (pT1b). Immunohistochemical examination of the tumour revealed high expression of tumour suppressor gene p53 and immunoreactivity for Ki-67. He then underwent radical cystectomy and histological examination of the specimen revealed a mixed urothelial nested variant tumour which was staged pT2a and grade G3 (poorly differentiated) with lymphatic involvement. Twelve months after the first diagnosis of the bladder cancer, he underwent a cycle of intravenous gemcitabine along with cisplatin. The case was reported just after the operation, therefore, there was no follow-up information on the patient's follow-up outcome. However, De Berardinis and associates [14] were of the opinion that the aggressive behaviour of this neoplasm would suggest that the correct indication for its treatment should be early radical cystectomy with extended lymph adenectomy in order to avoid the progression of the tumour into the urinary bladder wall or metastatic spread. They also stated that it is important to bear in mind that Ki-67 expression that is low in benign lesions and high in nested variant of bladder cancer can be considered a good method to distinguish between the two entities.

Xiao and associates [28] reported 2 cases of nested variant of urothelial carcinoma; the patients in both cases were elderly men, with a predominant involvement of the trigone. Microscopic examination revealed that the tumour cells were arranged in ill-defined nests and had low-grade nuclear features. Both cases had a diffusely infiltrating growth pattern with widespread local disease at cystectomy. Strong immunohistochemical staining for p63 in the neoplastic cells supported the urothelial cell nature of this neoplasm. High p53 and Ki-67 indices of the tumour correlated with the aggressiveness of this subtype of urothelial carcinoma. Details of the two cases were as follows.

Case 1. A 69-year-old man presented with 2 episodes of visible haematuria. He had computed tomography scan which revealed diffuse thickening of the bladder wall and moderate hydronephrosis. There was no evidence of lymphadenopathy or metastatic disease. He did not have urine cytology examination. He underwent cystoscopy and bladder biopsy from the trigone and histological examination of the specimen revealed muscle-invasive urothelial carcinoma involving the trigone. Immunohistochemical staining of the tumour revealed immunoreactivity for high-molecular weight cytokeratin 903 and cytokeratins 7 and 20 and negativity for prostatic specific antigen and prostatic acid phosphatase. He underwent radical cystoprostatectomy. Macroscopic examination revealed that the mucosa of the urinary bladder was oedematous, with focal haemorrhage and necrosis around the trigone. The urinary bladder wall was diffusely thickened and infiltrated by tumour; the trigone of the urinary bladder was most markedly involved, with obstruction of the ureteric orifices (see Figure 5). Microscopic examination revealed that with the exception of the surface mucosa, the bladder wall was extensively infiltrated by neoplastic cells, which were arranged in a diffuse pattern of relatively ill-defined and variably sized nests (see Figures 6 and 7). There was also evidence of focal urothelial carcinoma *in situ* and multiple foci of urothelial dysplasia. The cytologic characteristics of the underlying main neoplasm were markedly distinct from those of the surface urothelial mucosal lesions. The neoplastic cells exhibited clear/pale or amophilic/eosinophilic cytoplasm with poorly defined borders and rounded nuclei with inconspicuous nucleoli. The chromatin was finely granular and distributed in an even fashion. Rarely, the tumour cells exhibited clear and signet ring characteristics. On the whole, there was no evidence of significant nuclear pleomorphism,

and mitosis was rare (see Figure 7). Rarely, large atypical cells were observed in the deeply infiltrated area (muscularis propria and fat). Within the infiltrating tumour, a prominent desmoplastic reaction was conspicuous. The main tumour had extended through the vesical wall into the perivesical soft tissue and this had also involved the prostatic urethra and paraurethral tissues. There was evidence of metastatic carcinoma in the perivesical lymph nodes. Additionally, bilateral obturator and iliac lymph nodes did not contain any metastasis. Nevertheless, metastasis was found in the adjacent obturator adipose tissue. A diagnosis of high-grade nested variant of urothelial carcinoma was made. He subsequently received adjuvant chemotherapy with taxol and carboplatin. He developed bone and soft tissue metastases four months pursuant to resection of his tumour.

Case 2. A 70-year-old man was investigated 3 years earlier when he presented with visible haematuria urinary frequency and occasional straining to void. His repeated urine cytology and intravenous urography were normal and his cystoscopic examination revealed a focal area of localized inflammation on the floor of the urinary bladder lateral to the right ureteric orifice. He was lost to follow-up. However, 3 years later, he presented with recurrent visible haematuria. He had a computed tomography scan which revealed a mild-to-moderate dilation of the distal part of the right ureter and 0.8 cm thickening of the wall of the urinary bladder around the right ureteric orifice. There was no evidence of any significant lymph adenopathy or any other abnormal mass in the pelvis. He underwent transurethral biopsy of the thickened region and histological examination of the specimen revealed infiltration of lamina propria by ill-defined nested neoplastic cells with bland cytologic characteristics (see Figure 9). There was also evidence of perineural invasion by the tumour. The immunohistochemical staining characteristics of the tumour include immunoreactivity for high-molecular cytokeratin 903 and cytokeratin 7 and negativity for prostate specific antigen, prostate acid phosphatase, S100, and chromogranin. He subsequently underwent radical cystoprostatectomy elsewhere. The histology report from the institution where he underwent radical cystoprostatectomy stated that the tumour had extended through the lateral wall of the right trigone with vascular invasion and a focus of urothelial carcinoma *in situ*. The histology report also stated that in addition to the urinary bladder tumour there was focal adenocarcinoma of the prostate gland (Gleason pattern 3 + 3 = 6) which was confined to the left lobe of the prostate gland. The perivesical lymph nodes were negative for metastatic disease. This patient was lost to follow-up two months pursuant to his surgery.

Xiao and associates [28] stated that additional immunohistochemical stainings were done on the tumour specimens of the two patients and these showed that the nested neoplastic cells in both cases were strongly immunoreactive for p63 (a homolog of p53 protein) (Figures 8 and 10); 40% to 50% and 30% to 40% of tumour cells in Case 1 exhibited strong positivity for p53 and Ki-67, respectively, and no staining difference for either p53 or Ki-67 was present between superficial and deep infiltrating tumour cells. Focally positive stains for both p53 and Ki-67 were exhibited in the biopsy specimen of Case 2. The experience learnt from the biological behaviour of both Cases 1 and 2, especially in Case 1, would be indicative of the aggressive nature of nested variant of urothelial carcinoma.

Krishnamoorthy and associates [18] reported the case of a 46-year-old woman who presented with a two-year history of interrupted stream of urine on voiding. She developed acute urinary retention for which she was catheterized. Further evaluation after her catheterization revealed a large urinary bladder tumour. She did not have any history of haematuria or urinary tract infection. Her urine microscopy revealed 15 red blood cells per high power field. She had ultrasound scan of the abdomen which revealed bilateral mild hydroureteronephrosis up to the vesicoureteric junction. A huge heteroechoic pedunculated mass which measured 10 cm in size, with smooth surface and well-defined margin in the bladder, occupying the entire surface of the urinary bladder. She also had a contrast computed tomography scan of the abdomen which revealed normal liver, pancreas, and adrenals. The computed tomography scan also showed bilateral mild hydroureteronephrosis with a 10 mm simple cyst in the interpolar region of the right kidney. There was a large heterodense mass in the urinary bladder which occupied most of the bladder. There were multiple enlarged lymph nodes involving the parailiac right external iliac, left internal iliac, and left inguinal regions, each measuring from 7 mm to 8 mm in size in transverse diameter. She underwent cystoscopy which revealed a solid 10 cm × 10 cm pedunculated lesion arising from the right lateral and anterior wall of the bladder, which was a rounded, mobile, well-circumscribed tumour with a smooth surface. The mucosa over the mass lesion and the adjoining bladder surface appeared intact. The right ureteric orifice was not seen and the left ureteric orifice looked normal. The tumour was bimanually palpable and mobile. She underwent transurethral resection of the tumour and histological examination of the specimen was reported to have shown nested variant of transitional cell carcinoma with marked atypical epithelial proliferation. Microscopic examination of the tumour revealed that the entire tumour was infiltrated by nests of polygonal cells with oval vesicular to hyperchromatic nuclei and eosinophilic to clear cytoplasm. Cystically dilated cells were also seen. The intervening stroma consisted of spindle cells with fusiform nuclei, compressing the cell nests in some areas, forming broad polypoid projections. There were areas of necrosis with acute inflammatory reaction. The metaplastic stromal cells exhibited no increase in mitotic activity. Krishnamoorthy and associates reported this case at a stage when there was no follow-up information regarding the outcome of the patient. Krishnamoorthy and associates [18] stated the following.

(i) Nested variant of urothelial carcinoma can easily be confused with a number of benign lesions; it is very important for the pathologist to consider nested variant of urothelial carcinoma in the differential diagnosis of the lesions that show nested type growth pattern in lesions of the urinary bladder. It is equally important for the treating physician to adopt an aggressive approach towards the management of these lesions.

(ii) The optimal treatment for nested variant of urothelial carcinoma is yet to be determined and this may be because of the rarity of the tumour, very small number of long-term survivors, and the absence of any randomized studies. The aggressive invasive growth and early metastases are the factors that favour radical cystectomy with adjunctive systemic chemotherapy. Nevertheless, a consensus is yet to be arrived at.

(iii) They had reported their case in view of its rarity, its unusual histology, and its prognostic significance emphasizing the need to distinguish it from the classic transitional cell carcinoma.

(iv) The aggressive behaviour of these nested variants underlines the importance of distinguishing them from benign proliferative lesions. Cytologic atypia is not a very good parameter because the mild atypia seen in nested variant of transitional cell carcinoma can be very deceptive, especially at low and medium power magnifications. Though the obvious invasion of the muscularis propria excludes the possibility of a benign lesion, the absence of invasion leads the pathologist onto a diagnostic dilemma.

Ooi and associates [21] reported a rare presentation of nested variant of transitional cell carcinoma in a 74-year-old man who had bilateral hydronephrosis and acute renal failure. At cystoscopy, both ureters were obstructed with the right ureter narrowed along the entire length. Subsequent histopathologic examination from the ureteral resection revealed nested variant of urothelial carcinoma. Bilateral stents were inserted and the patient survived 12 months with a good partial response to chemotherapy. They stated that at the time of the report of their case in 2006, 76 cases of nested variant of urothelial carcinoma had been reported in the literature and at that time their patient was the first, to their knowledge, to present with bilateral hydronephrosis and tumour extension along one ureter. He had extensive liver and bony metastases and he eventually died 12 months pursuant to the establishment of the diagnosis. Ooi and associates [21] stated that even though anecdotal reports of adjunctive chemotherapy with gemcitabine and carboplatin are being done, there are no available randomized studies on the effects of adjunctive chemotherapy in these patients with nested variant of urothelial carcinoma, after cystectomy. Furthermore, Holmäng and Johansson [20] reported that there was no survival advantage with adjunctive radiotherapy in their series of seven patients with T stage in cystectomy specimens ranging from T1 to T4B.

Holmäng and Johansson [20] stipulated that nested variant of transitional cell carcinoma is aggressive and invasive, with a very well-differentiated histology, which is difficult to understand. Nevertheless, it had been postulated that the unusual histology may be due to the peculiarities of the host response mechanisms to carcinogenic stimulus such that the host is able to channel differentiation but cannot control invasion.

Tatsura and associates [12] stated that the nested variant of transitional cell carcinoma has the characteristics of a focus of nests of transitional epithelial cells which infiltrate the lamina propria with apparent involvement of bladder mucosa. They also suggested that immunohistochemical analysis may help in the diagnosis of nested variants of transitional cell carcinoma derived from epithelial cells and that diagnosis and treatment at an early stage should reduce the mortality of patients with nested variant of transitional cell carcinoma.

Murphy and Deana [4] stated that the tumour cells of nested variant of transitional cell carcinoma are organized in nested structures and that many tumour cells are only slightly atypical, but a careful examination revealed that at least some significantly anaplastic cells are identifiable in each case, and the degree of anaplasia has a tendency to parallel the depth of invasion. They additionally stated that the features that identify this lesion as malignant are the tendency for increasing cellular anaplasia in the deeper portions of the lesion, its infiltrative nature, and the presence of muscle invasion. Mai and associates [41] stated that despite the presence of mild or minimal cytological atypia in nested variant of transitional cell carcinoma, these neoplasms are occasionally associated with an aggressive clinical course and even death.

Drew and associates [10] reviewed the clinicopathologic features of 16 nested variants of transitional cell carcinoma over a 13-year period. They reported the following.

(i) Nested variant of transitional cell carcinoma was characterized by the presence of irregular nests and/or tubules of transitional cells infiltrating the lamina propria without surface involvement.

(ii) The neoplastic cells tended to have innocuous features but at least a few cells in every case are cytologically anaplastic.

(iii) There was a marked male predominance.

(iv) Synchronous or metachronous transitional cell carcinomas of more usual histologic make-up may occur.

(v) After a follow-up averaging 16.6 months, only three patients were known to be alive with no evidence of disease.

Drew and associates [10] in 1996 made the ensuing concluding iteration.

Clinicopathologic information from their 16 cases combined with the 8 cases of nested variant of transitional cell carcinoma that were reported before the publication of their paper confirms that nested variant of transitional cell carcinoma is a persistent and aggressive neoplasm that is notable for its innocuous appearance in histologic preparations.

Liedberg and associates [31] reported three cases of the nested variant of urothelial carcinoma that were treated in their institution. They compared their outcome data with those of previously reported cases. They reported that the three patients presented with advanced muscle-invasive nested variant of urothelial carcinoma, of which two had lymph node metastasis at cystoprostatectomy. The

histopathology in the latter two cases showed the same picture in the lymph node as in the primary tumour with nests of tumour cells with mild-to-moderate atypia. In all three cases the tumour involved the ureteric orifice or bladder neck. They concluded the following.

(i) Nested variant of urothelial carcinoma is a rare but an important histopathologic entity.

(ii) Nested variant of urothelial carcinoma has a poor prognosis.

(iii) At an early stage, the tumours might be difficult to differentiate from benign conditions and awareness of this condition is of outermost importance.

Because of the rarity of nested variant of urothelial carcinoma most urologists and pathologists would not have encountered a case of nested variant of urothelial carcinoma before and as a result of this there is the possibility that a case of nested variant of urothelial carcinoma may inadvertently be misdiagnosed. It is therefore pertinent to document iterations of Dhall et al. [2], which summarize the microscopic features of nested variant of urothelial carcinoma as follows.

(i) These tumours are characterized histologically by large numbers of small, closely packed, poorly defined, confluent, and irregular nests of uniform urothelial cells infiltrating the lamina propria, reminiscent of von Brunn nests, and also infiltrating the muscularis propria with retained nested pattern (see Figures 1 and 2).

(ii) These nests exhibit an infiltrative base as described by Volmar et al. [30].

(iii) Small tubules and microcysts may be seen as described by Talbert and Young [3] and Young and Oliva [9].

(iv) The overlying urothelium may be normal in appearance.

(v) The cells comprising nested variant of urothelial carcinoma exhibit no significant cytologic atypia; they are mildly pleomorphic and show slightly increased nuclear-cytoplasmic ratio and occasionally prominent nucleoli (see Figure 3).

(vi) Even though nested variant of urothelial carcinoma cells appears to be histologically bland, a number of authors [4, 10, 20] have observed significant pleomorphism, particularly within regions of muscle invasion.

(vii) Mitotic figures are not readily seen. Mucin is not identified. The surrounding stroma varies from dense and collagenous to loose and myxoid or even oedematous. Lymphatic invasion may be seen [20].

(viii) In view of their deceptively bland appearance, the tumours are sometimes misdiagnosed as benign lesions, especially in the biopsy material leading in some instances to a significant delay in the establishment of diagnosis as stated by Young and Olive [9]. In some instances it is very difficult to establish an unequivocal diagnosis of nested variant of urothelial

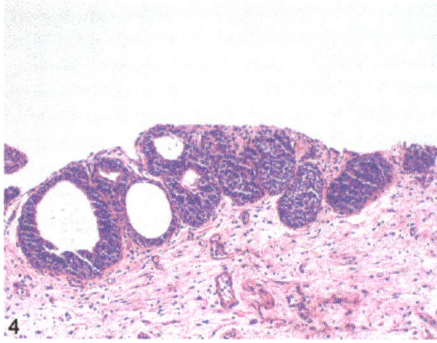

FIGURE 4: von Brunn nests in comparison with nested variant of urothelial carcinoma showing regularly spaced urothelial nests with a relatively flat base (hematoxylin-eosin, original magnification ×200). Nested variant of urothelial carcinoma taken from Dhall et al. [2]. The figures have been reproduced with the permission of the editor in chief of Archives of Pathology and Laboratory Medicine on behalf of the editorial board of the journal.

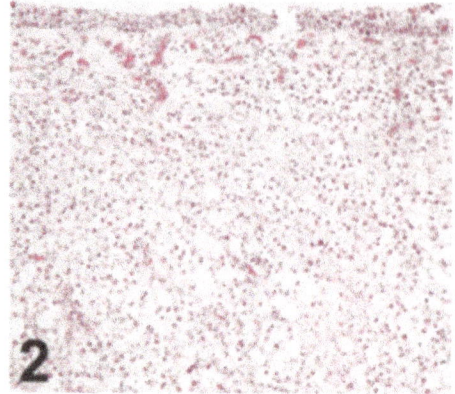

FIGURE 6: The neoplastic cells form ill-defined nests with a diffuse growth pattern. Some tumor cells have clear cytoplasm. The surface mucosa is not involved by the underlying tumor (Case 1) (hematoxylin-eosin, original magnification ×200) Xiao et al. [28].

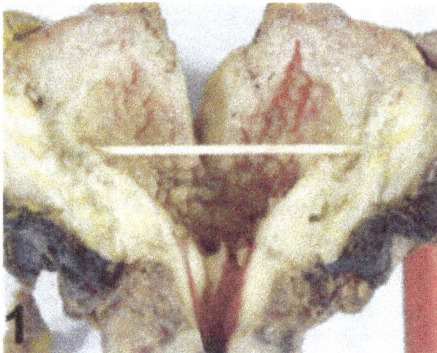

FIGURE 5: Gross photo of Case 1 shows an edematous urinary bladder mucosa and markedly and diffusely thickened bladder wall Xiao et al. [28].

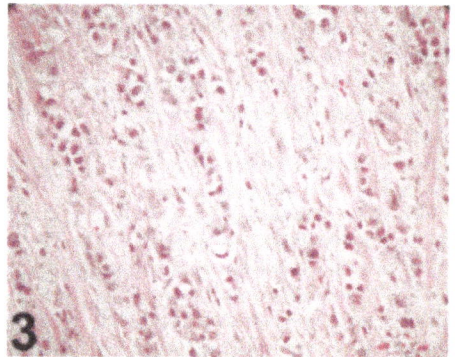

FIGURE 7: The nuclei of the tumor cells are relatively uniform with finely granular chromatin, inconspicuous nucleoli, and rare mitosis (Case 1) (hematoxylin-eosin, original magnification ×400) Xiao et al. [28].

carcinoma in the biopsy material until multiple biopsies are performed.

(ix) Nested variant of urothelial carcinoma must be differentiated from the benign proliferative lesions of the urothelium, such as von Brunn nests, cystitis cystica, cystitis glandularis, nephrogenic adenoma, paraganglioma, and inverted papilloma (see Figure 4 which illustrates von Brunn nests in comparison with nested variant of urothelial carcinoma showing regularly spaced urothelial nests with a relatively flat base).

Dhall and associates [2] stated that the optimal treatment of nested variant of urothelial carcinoma is yet to be determined in view of the rarity of the tumour and in view of absence of randomized studies. They suggested that nested variant of urothelial carcinoma should be approached clinically as a high-grade disease with early cystectomy as an option for pT1 and pT2 tumours [2]. Dhall and associates [2] additionally stated the following that.

(i) Adjuvant chemotherapy and radiation therapy have not been shown by a number of authors to be significantly beneficial in their reported series [12, 20, 28].

(ii) Nested variant of urothelial carcinoma should be kept in mind as a histologically unique variant which should not be confused with von Brunn's nest. Any bladder biopsy with tightly packed nests with any degree of architectural or cytological atypia should be evaluated with caution, and the possibility of nested variant of urothelial carcinoma should be raised in such circumstances.

Linder and associates [22] evaluated the oncological outcomes after radical cystectomy in patients with nested variant of urothelial carcinoma and compared survival to that in patients with pure urothelial carcinoma of the bladder. Linder and associates [22] identified 52 patients with nested variant of urothelial carcinoma of the urinary bladder who were treated with radical cystectomy between 1980 and 2004. The pathological specimens were rereviewed by a single genitourinary pathologist. The patients were matched 1 : 2 by

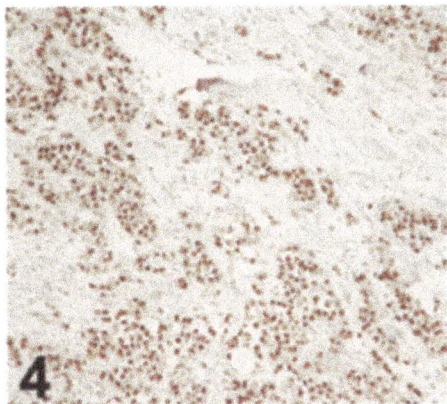

FIGURE 8: The neoplastic cells are strongly immunoreactive for p63 (Case 1) (p63, original magnification ×200) Xiao et al. [28].

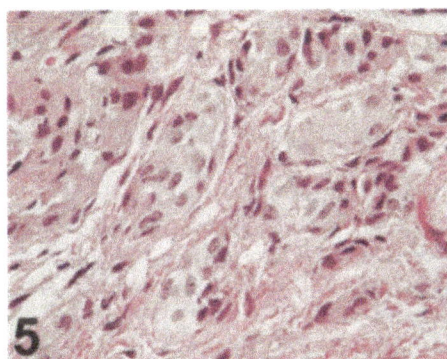

FIGURE 9: The cytologically bland neoplastic cells are arranged in a diffuse pattern of relatively ill-defined and variably sized nests (Case 2) (hematoxylin-eosin, original magnification ×600) Xiao et al. [28].

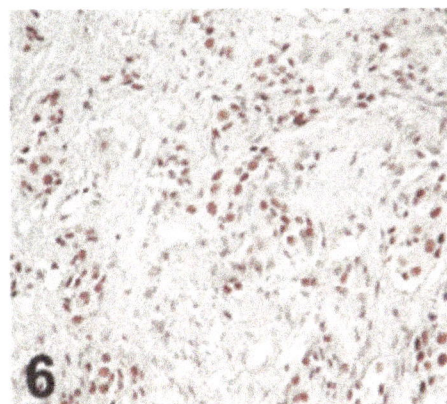

FIGURE 10: The neoplastic cells are strongly immunoreactive for p63 (Case 2) (p63, original magnification ×400) Xiao et al. [28].

age, gender, ECOG (Eastern COOperative Oncology Group) performance status, pathological tumour stage, and nodal status to patients with pure urothelial carcinoma. Survival was estimated using the Kaplan-Meier method and compared with the log rank test. Linder and associates [22] reported that the patients with nested variant of urothelial carcinoma

of the urinary bladder had a median age of 69.5 years (IQR 62, 74) and a median postoperative follow-up of 10.8 years (IQR 9.3, 11.2). They also reported that nested variant cancer was associated with a high rate of adverse pathological features since 36 patients (69%) had pT3-pT4 disease and 10 (19%) had nodal invasion. Eight patients (15%) with nested variant cancer received preoperative chemotherapy. When the patients with the nested variant were matched to a cohort with pure urothelial carcinoma, no significant differences were noted in 10-year local recurrence-free survival (83% versus 80%, $P = 0.46$) or 10-year cancer specific survival (41% versus 46%, $P = 0.75$). Linder and associates [22] concluded that the nested variant of urothelial carcinoma is associated with a high rate of locally advanced disease at radical cystectomy. However, when stage matched to patients with pure urothelial carcinoma, patients with the nested variant did not have an increased rate of recurrence or adverse survival. Linder and associates [22] iterated that further studies are required to validate these findings and guide the optimal multimodal treatment approach to these patients.

Tripodi et al. [23] reported the case of a 49-year-old woman affected by hepatitis C virus who presented with fever, discomfort, urgency, and hypertension. She had a computed tomography scan which showed a sclerosing inflammatory process that involved the connective and adipose tissue of the renal sinus. In absence of renal or pelvic masses felt that an underlying malignancy was excluded and renal abscess or tuberculosis was suspected. Accordingly, nephrectomy and proximal ureterectomy was performed. Tripodi et al. [23] reported the following.

(i) Grossly, the calices, renal pelvis, and pelviureteric junction appeared modestly dilated with whitish, thickened, and uneven mucosa.

(ii) Microscopic examination revealed that the subepithelial connective tissue, the fibromuscular layer, and the renal sinus fat were diffusely infiltrated by small nests of medium to large urothelial cells which were immunohistochemically stained positively with p63 and they had abundant eosinophilic cytoplasm and slightly atypical nuclei.

Tripodi et al. [23] stated the following.

(i) On the basis of morphologic and immunohistochemical features, a diagnosis of nested variant of urothelial carcinoma was made.

(ii) After surgery, the patient recovered from hypertension.

(iii) Pelvic and upper urothelial tract nested variant of urothelial carcinoma was uncommon, and to the best of their knowledge, their case was the second case of nested variant of urothelial carcinoma with renal pelvis involvement.

Cerda et al. [24] submitted an abstract for a poster presentation at the 25th European Congress of Pathology in Lisbon, Portugal (August 31st, to September 4th, 2013).

They reported the case of 2 patients with nested variant of urothelial carcinoma as follows.

Case 1. A 53-year-old man presented with visible haematuria. He had ultrasound scan which showed an exophytic lesion in the urinary bladder. The patient underwent transurethral resection of bladder tumour which was reported on histological examination to be invasive urothelial carcinoma (pT2). He underwent, 2 months later, radical cystoprostatectomy (and the tumour was staged pT3b pN1), radiotherapy, and chemotherapy. The patient died one year later as a result of advanced metastatic disease.

Case 2. An 83-year-old woman who presented with asymptomatic visible haematuria underwent transurethral resection of bladder tumour, which on histological examination was reported to be an invasive urothelial carcinoma (pT2). Because of her advanced stage she did not undergo any surgical procedure. She died 3 years later.

With regard to the results, both tumours were reported to have shown similar histological features; the neoplastic cells were grouped in confluent smalls nests and abortive tubules which were composed of urothelial cells with nuclear atypia infiltrating deeply the wall of the urinary bladder and in Case 1, the perivesical tissue, urethra, and one lymph node were invaded. Immunohistochemistry profile revealed positive staining for CK7, CK20, 34βE12, and p63.

Yildiz et al. [25] reported the case of a 60-year-old man in a Turkish Journal, who presented with visible haematuria. Histologically, the tumour was characterized by irregular nests and small tubules of urothelial carcinoma cells which had infiltrated the lamina propria and deeper layers without involvement of the mucosal layer. Many of the tumour cells were only slightly atypical, but careful examination revealed at least some significantly anaplastic cells; the degree of cellular atypia tended to parallel the depth of invasion. They stated that the tumour tended to be aggressive despite the initial impression of a benign vascular lesion resembling a capillary haemangioma.

Pusztaszeri et al. [26] reported a case of nested variant of urothelial carcinoma of the renal pelvis and ureter which was synchronous with high-grade urothelial papillary carcinoma.

Lau [27] reported the case of a 71-year-old woman who had nested variant of urothelial carcinoma of renal pelvis. Lau [27] stated that the tumour was characterized by a nested pattern of growth and relatively bland cytologic features. The patient presented with a locally advanced disease at the time of nephroureterectomy.

4. Summary

Nested variant of urothelial carcinoma is a rare tumour and to the author's knowledge about 200 cases have so far been reported.

The tumour usually manifests at an advanced stage and tends to exhibit a persistent and progressive clinical course.

Death rate from nested variant of urothelial carcinoma can be up to 25% of cases and persistent or progressive disease has been reported in up to 60% of cases which had led some

authors [10] to conclude that nested variant of urothelial carcinoma has a clinical course which is similar to that of high-grade urothelial carcinomas.

It is important to keep in mind nested variant of urothelial carcinoma as a unique histologic variant which should not be mistaken for florid von Brunn nest.

In cases where bladder biopsy exhibits tightly packed nests with any degree of cytologic atypia or architectural atypia, the biopsy specimens need to be evaluated with care in order to ascertain and exclude the possibility of nested variant of urothelial carcinoma.

Even though reports from case reports had indicated that the prognosis of nested variant of urothelial carcinoma is poor following treatment results of a recent study revealed that there is no significant difference between patients with nested variant of urothelial carcinoma and those with comparatively staged conventional urothelial carcinoma who had undergone cystectomy.

5. Conclusions

Nested variant of urothelial carcinoma is a rare tumour with characteristic histopathologic features which must be carefully identified to establish its diagnosis.

Previous case reports and case series indicated that nested variant of urothelial carcinoma tends to be diagnosed at an advanced stage and is associated with poor prognosis; however, results of a recent study revealed no statistically significant difference between the outcome of patients with nested variant of urothelial carcinoma and patients with conventional urothelial carcinoma of similar stages who had undergone cystectomy.

Correct and early diagnosis of this tumour is essential in order to provide early curative treatment in order to avoid diagnosis at an advanced stage.

There is the need for a multicentre trial to validate this recent finding and to identify treatment protocols that would help improve the outcome of the tumour following treatment.

Conflict of Interests

The author declares that there is no conflict of interests regarding the publication of this paper.

Acknowledgment

The author would like to acknowledge the Editor in Chief and the Editorial Board of Archives of Pathology and Laboratory Medicine for granting him permission to reproduce images from their journal specifically to illustrate features of nested variant of urothelial carcinoma in this paper.

References

[1] J. B. Stern, "Unusual benign bladder tumor of Brunn nest origin," *Urology*, vol. 14, no. 3, pp. 288–289, 1979.

[2] D. Dhall, H. Al-Ahmadie, and S. Olgac, "Nested variant of urothelial carcinoma," *Archives of Pathology and Laboratory*

Medicine, vol. 131, no. 11, pp. 1725–1727, 2007.

[3] M. L. Talbert and R. H. Young, "Carcinomas of the urinary bladder with deceptively benign-appearing foci. A report of three cases," *American Journal of Surgical Pathology*, vol. 13, no. 5, pp. 374–381, 1989.

[4] W. M. Murphy and D. G. Deana, "The nested variant of transitional cell carcinoma: a neoplasm resembling proliferation of Brunn's nests," *Modern Pathology*, vol. 5, no. 3, pp. 240–243, 1992.

[5] R. V. Rouse, "Nested Variant Urothelial (Transitional Cell) Carcinoma Surgical Pathology Criteria," 2012, http://surgpathcriteria.stanford.edu/bladder/tcc-nested-variant-transitional-urothelial-carcinoma/.

[6] R. Parakh, "Bladder urothelial carcinoma—invasive nested variant," 2013, http://pathologyoutlines.com/, http://www.pathologyoutlines.com/topic/bladderurothelialnested.html.

[7] O. Lin, M. Cardillo, G. Dalbagni, I. Linkov, B. Hutchinson, and V. E. Reuter, "Nested variant of urothelial carcinoma: a clinicopathologic and immunohistochemical study of 12 cases," *Modern Pathology*, vol. 16, no. 12, pp. 1289–1298, 2003.

[8] M. J. Wasco, S. Daignault, D. Bradley, and R. B. Shah, "Nested variant of urothelial carcinoma: a clinicopathologic and immunohistochemical study of 30 pure and mixed cases," *Human Pathology*, vol. 41, no. 2, pp. 163–171, 2010.

[9] R. H. Young and E. Oliva, "Transitional cell carcinomas of the urinary bladder that may be underdiagnosed: a report of four invasive cases exemplifying the homology between neoplastic and non-neoplastic transitional cell lesions," *American Journal of Surgical Pathology*, vol. 20, no. 12, pp. 1448–1454, 1996.

[10] P. A. Drew, J. Furman, F. Civantos, and W. M. Murphy, "The nested variant of transitional cell carcinoma: n aggressive neoplasm with innocuous histology," *Modern Pathology*, vol. 9, no. 10, pp. 989–994, 1996.

[11] J. Wang, G. Talmon, S. A. Kazmi, L. E. Siref, and M. C. Morris, "Metastases from nested variant urothelial carcinoma of the urinary bladder in pancreatic allograft mimicking graft rejection," *Journal of Clinical Medicine Research*, vol. 4, no. 2, pp. 145–148, 2012.

[12] H. Tatsura, K. Ogawa, T. Sakata, and T. Okamura, "A nested variant of transitional cell carcinoma of the urinary bladder: a case report," *Japanese Journal of Clinical Oncology*, vol. 31, no. 6, pp. 287–289, 2001.

[13] T. Terada, "Nested variant of urothelial carcinoma of the urinary bladder," *Rare Tumors*, vol. 3, no. 4, article e42, 2011.

[14] E. de Berardinis, G. M. Busetto, R. Giovannone, G. Antonini, M. di Placido, and V. Gentile, "Recurrent transitional cell carcinoma of the bladder: a mixed nested variant case report and literature review," *Canadian Urological Association Journal*, vol. 6, no. 2, pp. e57–e60, 2012.

[15] M. Cardillo, V. E. Reuter, and O. Lin, "Cytologic features of the nested variant of urothelial carcinoma: a study of seven cases," *Cancer*, vol. 99, no. 1, pp. 23–27, 2003.

[16] E. Dundar, M. F. Acikalin, and C. Can, "The nested variant of urothelial carcinoma: an aggressive tumor closely simulating benign lesions," *Pathology and Oncology Research*, vol. 12, no. 2, pp. 105–107, 2006.

[17] C. Badoual, A. M. Bergemer-Fouquet, L. Renjard et al., "A variant of transitional cell carcinoma: the "nested variant of urothelial carcinoma" Report of two cases," *Annales de Pathologie*, vol. 19, no. 2, pp. 119–123, 1999.

[18] S. Krishnamoorthy, A. Korula, and N. Kekre, "The nested variant of transitional cell carcinoma of urinary bladder: an aggressive tumour with a bland morphology," *Indian Journal of Urology*, vol. 22, no. 4, pp. 378–380, 2006.

[19] B. H. Ozdemir, G. Ozdemir, and A. Sertçelik, "The nested variant of the transitional cell bladder carcinoma. A case report and review of the literature," *International Urology and Nephrology*, vol. 32, no. 2, pp. 257–258, 2000.

[20] S. Holmäng and S. L. Johansson, "The nested variant of transitional cell carcinoma—a rare neoplasm with poor prognosis," *Scandinavian Journal of Urology and Nephrology*, vol. 35, no. 2, pp. 102–105, 2001.

[21] S. M. Ooi, J. Vivian, R. Sinniah, and S. Troon, "Nested variant of urothelial carcinoma: a rare presentation," *Urology*, vol. 67, no. 4, pp. 845.e3–845.e5, 2006.

[22] B. J. Linder, I. Frank, J. C. Cheville et al., "Outcomes following radical cystectomy for nested variant of urothelial carcinoma: a matched cohort analysis," *Journal of Urology*, vol. 189, no. 5, pp. 1670–1675, 2012.

[23] S. Tripodi, B. J. Rocca, M. R. Ambrosio, F. Gentile, and M. Cintorino, "Pelvic urothelial carcinoma with nested pattern of growth and an uncommon clinical presentation: a case report," *Analytical and Quantitative Cytology and Histology*, vol. 33, no. 6, pp. 340–344, 2011.

[24] N. Cerda, A. Corominas-Cishek, G. Muñiz et al., "Nested variant of urothelial carcinoma: report of 2 cases," in *Proceedings of the 25th European Congress of Pathology Session Uropathology*, Lisbon, Portugal, August-September 2013, http://www.esp-congress.org/guest/AbstractView?ABSID=6285.

[25] E. Yildiz, H. Özer, and G. Gökçe, "Mesanenin " nested" variant ürotelyal karsinomu: olgu suumu Nestedvariant urothelial carcinoma of the bladder: a case report," *Turkiye Ekopetoloji Dergisi*, vol. 9, no. 1-2, pp. 39–43, 2003.

[26] M. Pusztaszeri, J. Hauser, C. Iselin, J. F. Egger, and M. F. Pelte, "Urothelial carcinoma "nested variant" of renal pelvis and ureter," *Urology*, vol. 69, no. 4, pp. 778.e15–778.e17, 2007.

[27] S. K. Lau, "Nested variant of urothelial carcinoma of the renal pelvis," *Pathology, Research & Practice*, vol. 205, no. 7, pp. 508–512, 2009.

[28] G. Q. Xiao, S. J. Savage, M. E. Gribetz, D. E. Burstein, L. K. Miller, and P. D. Unger, "The nested variant of urothelial carcinoma: clinicopathology of 2 cases," *Archives of Pathology & Laboratory Medicine*, vol. 127, no. 8, pp. e333–e336, 2003.

[29] Q. Huang, P. G. Chu, S. K. Lau, and L. M. Weiss, "Urothelial carcinoma of the urinary bladder with a component of acinar/tubular type differentiation simulating prostatic adenocarcinoma," *Human Pathology*, vol. 35, no. 6, pp. 769–773, 2004.

[30] K. E. Volmar, T. Y. Chan, A. M. de Marzo, and J. I. Epstein, "Florid von Brunn nests mimicking urothelial carcinoma: a morphologic and immunohistochemical comparison to the nested variant of urothelial carcinoma," *American Journal of Surgical Pathology*, vol. 27, no. 9, pp. 1243–1252, 2003.

[31] F. Liedberg, G. Chebil, T. Davidsson, V. Gadaleanu, M. Grabe, and W. Mansson, "The nested variant of urothelial carcinoma: a rare but important bladder neoplasm with aggressive behavior—three case reports and a review of the literature," *Urologic Oncology*, vol. 21, no. 1, pp. 7–9, 2003.

[32] R. Cox and J. I. Epstein, "Large nested variant of urothelial carcinoma: 23 cases mimicking von brunn nests and inverted growth pattern of noninvasive papillary urothelial carcinoma," *American Journal of Surgical Pathology*, vol. 35, no. 9, pp. 1337–1342, 2011.

[33] D. Zani, C. Simeone, A. Antonelli, E. Bettini, A. Moroni, and S. Cosciani Cunico, "Cancer in kidney transplantation," *Urologia Internationalis*, vol. 80, no. 3, pp. 329–331, 2008.

[34] C. M. Vajdic, S. P. McDonald, M. R. E. McCredie et al., "Cancer incidence before and after kidney transplantation," *Journal of the American Medical Association*, vol. 296, no. 23, pp. 2823–2831, 2006.

[35] M. J. Lemmers and J. M. Barry, "De novo carcinoma of the lower urinary tract in renal allograft recipients," *Journal of Urology*, vol. 144, no. 5, pp. 1233–1235, 1990.

[36] R. R. M. Gifford, J. E. Wofford, and W. G. Edwards Jr., "Carcinoma of the bladder in renal transplant patients. A case report and collective review of cases," *Clinical Transplantation*, vol. 12, no. 1, pp. 65–69, 1998.

[37] D. Geetha, B. C. Tong, L. Racusen, J. S. Markowitz, and W. H. Westra, "Bladder carcinoma in a transplant recipient: evidence to implicate the BK human polyomavirus as a causal transforming agent," *Transplantation*, vol. 73, no. 12, pp. 1933–1936, 2002.

[38] World Health Organization Classification of Tumors, "Infiltrating urothelial carcinoma," in *Tumors of the Urinary System and Male Genital Organs*, J. N. Eble, G. Sauter, J. I. Epsteim, and I. A. Sesterhenn, Eds., pp. 93–110, IARC Press, Lyon, France, 2004.

[39] C. N. Sternberg, A. Yagoda, H. I. Scher et al., "Methotrexate, vinblastine, doxorubicin, and cisplatin for advanced transitional cell carcinoma of the urothelium. Efficacy and patterns of response and relapse," *Cancer*, vol. 64, no. 12, pp. 2448–2458, 1989.

[40] H. von der Maase, L. Sengelov, J. T. Roberts et al., "Long-term survival results of a randomized trial comparing gemcitabine plus cisplatin, with methotrexate, vinblastine, doxorubicin, plus cisplatin in patients with bladder cancer," *Journal of Clinical Oncology*, vol. 23, no. 21, pp. 4602–4608, 2005.

[41] K. T. Mai, G. Elmontaser, D. G. Perkins, H. M. Yazdi, W. A. Stinson, and A. Thijssen, "Histopathological and immunohistochemical study of papillary urothelial neoplasms of low malignant potential and grade associated with extensive invasive low-grade urothelial carcinoma," *BJU International*, vol. 94, no. 4, pp. 544–547, 2004.

Complications of Radical Cystectomy and Orthotopic Reconstruction

Wei Shen Tan,[1,2] Benjamin W. Lamb,[2] and John D. Kelly[1,2]

[1]*Division of Surgery and Interventional Science, UCL Medical School, University College London, 74 Huntley Street, London WC1E 6AU, UK*
[2]*Department of Urology, University College London Hospital, 16-18 Westmoreland Street, London W1B 8PH, UK*

Correspondence should be addressed to Wei Shen Tan; tanweishen@hotmail.com

Academic Editor: Fabio Campodonico

Radical cystectomy and orthotopic reconstruction significant morbidity and mortality despite advances in minimal invasive and robotic technology. In this review, we will discuss early and late complications, as well as describe efforts to minimize morbidity and mortality, with a focus on ileal orthotopic bladder substitute (OBS). We summarise efforts to minimize morbidity and mortality including enhanced recovery as well as early and late complications seen after radical cystectomy and OBS. Centralisation of complex cancer services in the UK has led to a fall in mortality and high volume institutions have a significantly lower rate of 30-day mortality compared to low volume institutions. Enhanced recovery pathways have resulted in shorter length of hospital stay and potentially a reduction in morbidity. Early complications of radical cystectomy occur as a direct result of the surgery itself while late complications, which can occur even after 10 years after surgery, are due to urinary diversion. OBS represents the ideal urinary diversion for patients without contraindications. However, all patients with OBS should have regular long term follow-up for oncological surveillance and to identify complications should they arise.

1. Introduction

Radical cystectomy remains the gold standard for treatment of patients with muscle invasive bladder cancer, or recurrent high grade non-muscle invasive bladder cancer. Despite the advent of minimally invasive and robotic technology, radical cystectomy has a significant mortality and morbidity. Ninety-day mortality rates from population studies range from 5.1% to 8.1%, [1, 2] which are high for surgery with curative intent. Morbidity is also significant, with 90-day complication rate between 28%–64%, even in high volume centres [3–5]. The high rates of morbidity and mortality reflect the fact that the majority of patients undergoing this procedure are elderly patients with multiple comorbidities.

In this review, we will discuss early and late complications, as well as describing efforts to minimize morbidity and mortality, with a focus on ileal orthotopic bladder substitute (OBS).

2. Minimizing Morbidity and Mortality

In the United States, an analysis of 35,055 cases from the National Cancer Database reported 30-day and 90-day operative mortality rates of 3.2% and 8.0% for radical cystectomy in low-volume centers and 2.7% and 7.2% in high-volume institutions, respectively [6]. The volume-outcome relationship for radical cystectomy is apparent in the literature, with high concordance between high volume centres showing a reduction in mortality by as much as 37% at 30 days [7]. Within the UK, a restructuring of the organisation of cancer surgery has resulted in the centralization of radical cystectomy surgery [8] which has been associated with a fall in 90-day mortality from 10.3 to 5.1%, with the greatest benefit seen in patients ≥70 years of age [9]. Reduction in mortality within high volume centres is related to a reduction in "failure-to-rescue" events following complex surgery and suggests that the perioperative management of patients undergoing radical cystectomy is critical in improving mortality and morbidity in this group [10].

3. Enhanced Recovery

The enhanced recovery program (ERP) has been shown to reduce the occurrence of adverse events and length of stay for patients undergoing abdominal surgery across a number of disciplines [11]. In some high volume institutions, the introduction of ERP has resulted in a reduction in the median length of stay from 8 to 4 days [12].

Prior to surgery, carbohydrate loading is recommended to minimize the development of insulin resistance and catabolism of protein and fat stores secondary to the physiological stress response seen in patients undergoing surgery [13]. Other features of enhanced recovery used for patients undergoing radical cystectomy include the avoidance of bowel preparation, immediate removal of nasogastric tube after surgery, and the early commencement of oral intake [14].

Postoperative ileus is the most frequent reason for prolonged hospital stay following cystectomy [16]. To reduce the risk of ileus, prokinetics such as metoclopramide should be used postoperatively, and systemic opioid analgesia should be reserved for breakthrough pain. Regular analgesia should consist of acetaminophen and nonsteroidal anti-inflammatories. Additionally, a randomized controlled trial has shown that Alvimopan, a peripherally acting μ receptor opioid antagonist, significantly reduces time to bowel movement in patients undergoing radical cystectomy [17]. In a systemic review and meta-analysis, chewing sugar-free gum has also been shown to reduce time to flatus, bowel movement and hospital length of stay in patients undergoing bowel surgery [18].

4. Early Complications

The modified Memorial Sloan-Kettering Cancer Centre (MSKCC) Clavien system was developed in an effort to standardize the reporting of early complications (Table 1) [4]. The majority of early complications following open radical cystectomy and OBS reconstruction occur as a direct result of the surgery and include gastrointestinal (29%), infection (25%), and wound-related complications (15%) [4]. Multivariate analysis has shown age, prior abdominal or pelvic surgery, ASA > 2 and estimated blood loss as independent predictors of high grade complications [4]. However, high grade complications rates between continent and incontinent diversions were comparable [4, 19].

Intestinal anastomotic leak is rare. However, urinary leakage is more common in the early postoperative period and particular attention should be paid to the constructed diversion to safeguard against this. A prospective randomized controlled trial showed that the use of stents of the ureteroileal anastomosis resulted in a lower rate of urinary leak [20]. Ureteral stents can be externalised for urinary monitoring and easy removal. Alternatively double J stents can be left *in situ* or tied to the urethral catheter for removal after 7–9 days. In our practice, routine daily aspiration and flushing of the pouch with 0.9% saline are essential in the

TABLE 1: Early and late complications of radical cystectomy with OBS reconstruction.

Early complications	Late complications
Genitourinary	Urinary tract infection
Gastrointestinal	Gastrointestinal-bowel obstruction
Infections	Afferent limb stenosis
Wound	Urethral stricture
Cardiac	Stones
Pulmonary	Incontinence/retention
Thromboembolic	Metabolic
Neurological	Orthotopic bladder substitute to vaginal fistula (rare)
Surgical	New malignancy

early postoperative phase to prevent build-up of mucous. Although we routinely use a suprapubic catheter, this is not routine in all centres [21]. Intraoperatively, a passive pelvic drain is typically placed close to the anastomoses and removed when the integrity of the anastomosis is deemed intact. A cystogram typically at three weeks should be performed prior to the removal of the catheter to check for OBS leak.

The majority of urinary leaks can be managed conservatively. If necessary, percutaneous drainage or bilateral nephrostomies to divert urine flow might be necessary in nondraining leaks. The incidence of urinary leak in OBS formation is theoretically higher due to a longer suture line compared to an ileal conduit.

Infection is the second most common perioperative complication. A short course of prophylactic broad spectrum antibiotics such as a second- or third-generation cephalosporins that cover skin, respiratory, urinary, and gastrointestinal organisms is routinely prescribed to reduce the incidence of infection [22]. Adequate analgesia, chest physiotherapy, and early mobilization can help reduce atelectasis and subsequent chest infection. Wound related complications are more common in open cystectomy where a limited laparotomy wound can become infected. Other wound complications include dehiscence or incisional hernia, although these are less frequently observed.

Deep vein thrombosis (DVT) is a recognized serious postoperative complication affecting up to 4.7% of radical cystectomy patients [23]. Analysis from data from the US National Surgical Quality Improvement Programme showed that age, operative time, sepsis, and hospital length of stay are independent predictors for DVT development on multivariate analysis [24]. Fifty-eight percent of patients who developed DVT did so after discharge from hospital [23]. Hence, thromboprophylaxis with low molecular weight heparin is recommended for up to four weeks after cystectomy [22].

5. Late Complications

Patients undergoing OBS may continue to develop complications even up to 10 years after surgery [25]. These complications include urinary tract infection, deterioration in renal function, calculi formation, metabolic complications, voiding dysfunction, and recurrence of disease.

5.1. *Urinary Tract Infection.* The presence of leucocytes and bacteria is commonly seen in urine culture of patients with OBS. This is not surprising given that the intestinal segments which are used to form OBS are heavily colonized by bacteria. Up to 78% of urine cultures in patients with OBS are positive for bacteria [26, 27]. However, despite the bacteria seen, the majority of patients are asymptomatic and have normal inflammatory markers. However, it has been suggested that 58% of patients with asymptomatic bacteriuria will develop a UTI and 18% will present with urosepsis in a 5-year period [27]. It is currently recommended that, in the absence of symptoms of UTI, OBS patients with bacteriuria should not be treated with antibiotics (in order to prevent drug resistance), although there might be a role for prophylactic antibiotics in those with recurrent UTI.

5.2. *Deterioration in Renal Function.* There are two main factors following OBS that are thought to play a role in deterioration of patients' renal function:

(1) Hydronephrosis secondary to ureteroileal strictures.

(2) Reflux of infected urine.

High pressure reflux of infected urine can cause renal function deterioration over time. However, the use of antireflux techniques in ileal OBS is debatable. In a randomized trial, Studer et al. showed that there was no significant difference in serum creatinine, urine infection rates, and bladder capacity between the antireflux nipple valve and a refluxing anastomosis [28]. However, upper tract dilatation due to ureteroileal stenosis was seen in 13.5% of patients with antireflux nipple compared to 3% of patients with the refluxing technique [28]. A recent randomized controlled trial between the T pouch and Studer pouch has shown no difference in postoperative renal function or risk of urinary tract infection at three years' follow-up [29]. However, patients with T pouch had a much higher rate of stenosis at the ureteroileal anastomosis and afferent limb which required surgical intervention.

Most ureteroileal stenoses can be treated endoscopically, normally with balloon dilatation, stenting, or incision, while approximately one in three patients requires open surgery. Another randomized trial comparing ileal or colonic OBS (with or without antireflux technique) and caecal OBS with antireflux implantation showed a fall in glomerular filtration rate (GFR) in all three groups, which were not significantly different after more than 10 years' follow-up [30]. Today, most OBS reconstructions by open or intracorporeal robotic techniques involve refluxing ureteroileal anastomosis [31–33]. As long as the principles of detubularised bowel and a spherical reservoir of sufficient volume are met, intraluminal pressure should be low and refluxing ureters should not compromise renal function. Median follow-up of 10.5 years reports no significant difference in renal function decline between OBS patients with freely refluxing ureteroileal anastamosis and ileal conduit [34].

5.3. *Calculi Formation.* OBS calculi formation has an incidence of 0.5%–8.1% depending on technique used for construction [25, 35]. Stone formation is multifactorial with poor bladder emptying and urinary stasis the main risk factors. Hypocitraturia due to increase in renal calcium and hydrogen ion excretion and hyperoxaluria due to malabsorption predispose to the formation of calcium oxalate and calcium phosphate calculi, respectively. Recurrent proteus infections due to colonization of the OBS with gut bacteria can result in struvite stone formation [26].

Traditionally, OBS were constructed using soluble sutures as the presence of foreign materials was observed to act as a nucleus for stone formation. However, the use of newer titanium stapling devices, which allow for faster and easier bladder reconstruction, have been reported to be resistant to encrustation with a stone rate of 9.2% during a median follow-up of 41 months which is still higher than some conventional series [25, 36]. The majority of stones can be managed via an endoscopic approach although percutaneous and laparoscopic approaches are sometimes necessary [37].

5.4. *Metabolic Complications.* The metabolic consequences of OBS formation are dependent on the type, position, and length of bowel used. They are more commonly seen in OBS than in ileal conduit due to the longer contact time of urine with bowel mucosa. The use of more proximal intestinal segments such as jejunum results in significantly more metabolic abnormalities due to a larger total surface area as a result of more villi. In addition, colonic mucosa has more efficient tight junctions which prevent significant osmotic shifts of water compared to either ilium or jejunum. We will focus on metabolic abnormalities in ileal OBS.

The key driver for metabolic acidosis is the absorption of ammonia (NH_4^-) from urine [38]. As shown in Figure 1, NH_4^- is converted into ammonium (NH_3) and free hydrogen ions (H^+) in the intestinal luminal cells. This results in the accumulation of excess hydrogen ions and metabolic acidosis. In addition, chloride (Cl^-) is absorbed while bicarbonate (HCO_3^-) is secreted.

The presence of hypoosmolar urine in the OBS results in the secretion of sodium (Na^+) from the OBS into the urine in exchange for H^+ ions, further promoting metabolic acidosis. Hyponatremia occurs, which results in aldosterone secretion leading to increased absorption of Na^+ and secretion of potassium (K^+) by the renal collecting tubules. Hypokalaemia is further exacerbated by ileal secretion of K^+. A fluid shift accompanies the movement of solute resulting in a salt depleting, hypovolemic state, which is most apparent during the weaning period from intravenous fluid to oral fluids. The net result is a hypokalaemic hyperchloremic metabolic acidosis [39].

This subclinical acidosis is normally compensated well by patients with normal renal function. However, in severe cases patients might present with fatigue, nausea, and vomiting. The majority of patients with symptomatic acidosis require treatment with sodium bicarbonate (1-2 g three times daily) for the first 6 weeks at least after catheter removal. Patients should also be encouraged to drink a minimum of 2-3 L of fluids per day to prevent dehydration. Other electrolyte

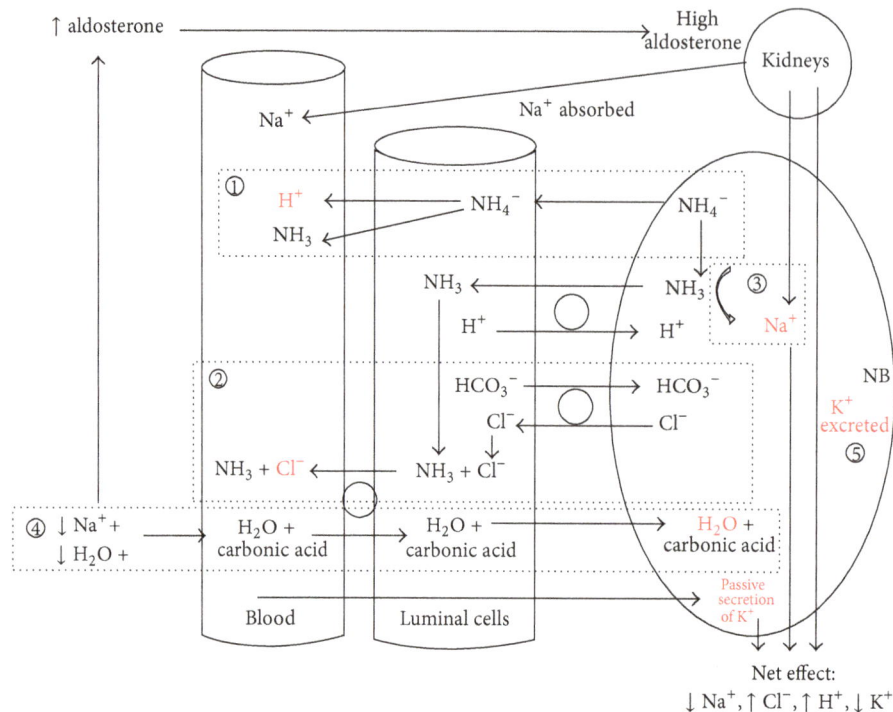

FIGURE 1: Electrolyte abnormalities in patients with ileal and/or colonic OBS. (1) NH_4^- absorption from urine which dissociates to H^+ and NH_3 resulting in metabolic acidosis. (2) Cl^- is exchanged with HCO_3^- and transported into blood. (3) Na^+ is displaced by NH_4^- and not absorbed by bowel resulting in a net loss. (4) There is a net loss of H_2O resulting in dehydration and loss of Na^+ due to NB secretion of Na^+ into urine. (5) Elevated aldosterone levels due to Na^+ loss precipitates K^+ loss from renal tubules. Na^+: sodium; K^+: potassium; NH_4^-: ammonium; NH_3: ammonia; HCO_3^-: bicarbonate; H^+: hydrogen; H_2O: water; Cl^-: chloride; NB: neobladder.

abnormalities can include hypomagnesemia and hypocalcaemia.

Resection up to 60 cm of ilium is generally safe and should not lead to malabsorption although Vitamin B12 deficiency can occur if a longer segment is used, especially if the terminal ileum is utilised, and may require parenteral replacement of Vitamin B12 [40]. Malabsorption of bile salts secondary to resection of the terminal ilium can result in diarrhoea, giving rise to dehydration as well as promoting the formation of oxalate containing renal calculi. Increased reabsorption of urinary ammonia can lead to hyperammonemic encephalopathy and abnormal drug metabolism especially if hepatic function is impaired. Chronic metabolic acidosis promotes the demineralization bone with the release of calcium carbonate and phosphate [41]. Demineralisation leads to osteomalacia and hyperphosphatemia which stimulates urinary phosphate stone formation.

5.5. Incontinence. Many factors influence continence following OBS reconstruction. A functionally intact sphincter that can generate a resistance pressure in excess of intraluminal OBS pressure is essential. Other factors such as patient age, urethral length, sphincter innervation, bladder capacity, the type of bowel segment used, and the ability to completely empty ones bladder emptying can all affect continence. In addition, it is essential to make a distinction between daytime and nocturnal continence, as they have different aetiology.

Analysis of daytime continence rates by Hautmann et al. reports that up to 85–90% of patients report using between one or no pads in a 24-hour period one year after continent diversion [42]. Multivariate analysis has shown that patients aged below 65 years and those treated with radical cystoprostatectomy with nerve sparing techniques had significantly better daytime continence [43]. Other factors include use of colonic segments and decrease in functional urethral length. Continence rates for most patients continue to improve up to 6 to 12 months as the OBS capacity increases. Treatment options for those with persisting severe incontinence may include periurethral collagen injection, a urethral sling, or an artificial urinary sphincter.

It may take patients up to 24 months to regain nocturnal continence as the OBS capacity increases. Analysis of the literature by Hautmann et al. reported that 20% to 30% of patients with OBS reconstruction suffer from nocturnal incontinence [42]. Loss of nocturnal continence is due to the absence of the neurogenic feedback, the sphincter detrusor reflex, and decrease in nocturnal sphincter tone. Multivariate analysis found that large postvoid residual volume, frequency, and amplitude of contractions of the ileal segment were independently associated with nocturnal incontinence [44]. Patients who have nocturnal enuresis are advised to void before going to bed, avoid alcohol and hypnotics in the evening, and set an alarm clock to wake up at least once at night to void. Patients treated with imipramine hydrochloride

TABLE 2: Recommended follow-up regime by European Association of Urology. Adapted from Stenzl et al. [15].

| | Months after cystectomy | | | | | | | | |
	3	6	12	18	24	30	36	48	60
≤pT1									
Ultrasound kidneys	X	—	—	—	—	—	—	—	—
CT chest + CT intravenous urography	—	—	X	—	X	—	X	X	X
Blood test + mid-stream urine culture + urine cytology	X	X	X	—	X	—	X	X	X
pT2									
Ultrasound kidneys	X	—	—	—	—	—	—	—	—
CT chest + CT intravenous urography	—	X	X	X	X	—	X	X	X
Blood test + mid-stream urine culture + urine cytology	X	X	X	—	X	—	X	X	X
≥pT3 +/− N+									
Ultrasound kidneys	X	—	—	—	—	—	—	—	—
CT chest + CT intravenous urography	X	X	X	X	X	X	X	X	X
Blood test + mid stream urine culture + urine cytology	X	X	X	—	X	X	X	X	X

have reported decrease of incontinence rates by 25% [44]. A prospective crossover study showed that oxybutynin and verapamil improved nocturnal incontinence by 70% and 55%, respectively [45].

In summary, continence following OBS construction can be optimised by the use of detubularised ileum, of sufficient length and construction technique to give a large capacity, preservation of urethral sphincter function through nerve sparing techniques, and maximising urethral length.

5.6. Urinary Retention. Voiding in patients with OBS requires both the pelvic floor to relax and a simultaneous increase in intra-abdominal pressure which is best achieved in a sitting position. Occasionally, the use of manual pressure to the suprapubic area and bending forward while sitting may facilitate voiding. Urinary retention is more common in women with 43% of women compared to 20% of men requiring intermittent catheterization [35]. Video urodynamics show that, in women, the OBS falls into the pelvic cavity resulting in mechanical obstruction due to kinking of the OBS-urethral junction [46]. Hence, it has been suggested that in female patients packing of the posterior pelvis coupled with an anterior superior fixation of the OBS might reduce the incidence of urinary retention. Other proposed techniques include sacrocolpopexy with mesh and omental packing between the vagina and bladder [47] or suturing the OBS at the dome to the rectus muscles with posterior packing of the pouch and fixing the peritoneum of the rectum to the vaginal stump [46].

All patients with suspected urinary retention should be evaluated to exclude urethra or ureteroileal anastomosis stricture. The main risk factors for urinary retention after OBS reconstruction are a large capacity OBS due to excessive bowel segment length and nonnerve sparing techniques. Patients are therefore advised to empty their OBS at regular intervals to prevent the development of an atonic pouch.

Treatment for urinary retention is intermittent self-catheterization, and all patients should be counselled about this preoperatively. Alpha blockers are unfortunately not effective [46].

5.7. Long Term Follow-Up. Follow-up should be risk adapted and patients with high risk of recurrence such as extravesical disease, positive lymph node status, positive surgical margins, multifocal tumour, and urethral tumour should be reviewed more regularly [48].

Early follow-up (4 months) is essential to recognize ureteroileal strictures. From 4–60 months oncological surveillance is the primary concern, which is normally performed using CT scans. The majority of tumour recurrences occur within two years of surgery [49]. Although most early recurrences are asymptomatic, symptoms suggesting recurrence include pain, haematuria, urinary retention, flank pain, and palpable mass [49]. Long term follow-up (more than 5 years) is required to identify renal/OBS calculi and recurrence of urethral or upper tract transitional cell carcinoma. In addition to routine blood test such as full blood count, renal function, and electrolyte, live function test and bone profile, bicarbonate, chloride, Vitamin B12, and folate should also be performed.

Urethral recurrence has been observed in 5.6% of patients undergoing RC at a median follow-up of 13.3 months [50]. Common sites of distal recurrence include lung, liver, and bones. Table 2 describes the European Association of Urology (EAU) recommendation for a risk adopted surveillance protocol [15]. MRI is an alternative in patients for whom CT scans are contraindicated due to impaired renal function or contrast allergy. Patients not at high risk and with no clinical suspicion of upper tract recurrence do not routinely need upper tract imaging [48]. The ICUD-EAU Consultation in Bladder Cancer does not recommend the routine use of urinary cytology, urethral washing, and urethroscopy in asymptomatic patients, although they are routinely performed in some centres [48].

6. Conclusion

Radical cystectomy with OBS reconstruction is a challenging procedure that carries a significant risk of short and long term complications. The technique is gaining popularity and should be offered to patients in the absence of absolute contraindications whilst taking into account oncological and patient factors. It is important to manage patient's expectations and ensure that they are committed and fully engaged during the postoperative period. Ileal OBS with freely refluxing ureteroileal anastomosis is most commonly performed and although many techniques exist, no one technique is considered superior. Robotic assisted radical cystectomy is gaining popularity, and although technically challenging intracorporeal OBS reconstruction is routinely performed in select centres. All patients with OBS reconstruction should have regular long term follow-up for oncological surveillance and to identify complications should they arise.

Conflict of Interests

The authors declare that there is no conflict of interests regarding the publication of this paper.

Acknowledgment

The authors are grateful to the UCLH Biomedical Research Centre for funding their work.

References

[1] A. S. Zakaria, F. Santos, A. Dragomir, S. Tanguay, W. Kassouf, and A. G. Aprikian, "Postoperative mortality and complications after radical cystectomy for bladder cancer in Quebec: a population-based analysis during the years 2000–2009," *Canadian Urological Association Journal*, vol. 8, no. 7-8, pp. 259–267, 2014.

[2] L. S. Hounsome, J. Verne, J. S. McGrath, and D. A. Gillatt, "Trends in operative caseload and mortality rates after radical cystectomy for bladder cancer in England for 1998–2010," *European Urology*, vol. 67, no. 6, pp. 1056–1062, 2015.

[3] J. P. Stein, G. Lieskovsky, R. Cote et al., "Radical cystectomy in the treatment of invasive bladder cancer: long-term results in 1,054 patients," *Journal of Clinical Oncology*, vol. 19, no. 3, pp. 666–675, 2001.

[4] A. Shabsigh, R. Korets, K. C. Vora et al., "Defining early morbidity of radical cystectomy for patients with bladder cancer using a standardized reporting methodology," *European Urology*, vol. 55, no. 1, pp. 164–176, 2009.

[5] R. E. Hautmann, R. C. de Petriconi, and B. G. Volkmer, "Lessons learned from 1,000 neobladders: the 90-day complication rate," *The Journal of Urology*, vol. 184, no. 3, pp. 990–994, 2010.

[6] M. E. Nielsen, K. Mallin, M. A. Weaver et al., "Association of hospital volume with conditional 90-day mortality after cystectomy: an analysis of the National Cancer Data Base," *BJU International*, vol. 114, no. 1, pp. 46–55, 2014.

[7] J. F. Finks, N. H. Osborne, and J. D. Birkmeyer, "Trends in hospital volume and operative mortality for high-risk surgery," *The New England Journal of Medicine*, vol. 364, no. 22, pp. 2128–2137, 2011.

[8] T. Powles and J. Kelly, "Innovation: London Cancer—multidisciplinary approach to urological cancer," *Nature Reviews Clinical Oncology*, vol. 10, no. 11, pp. 609–610, 2013.

[9] L. S. Hounsome, J. Verne, J. S. McGrath, and D. A. Gillatt, "Trends in operative caseload and mortality rates after radical cystectomy for bladder cancer in England for 1998–2010," *European Urology*, vol. 67, no. 6, pp. 1056–1062, 2014.

[10] A. A. Ghaferi, J. D. Birkmeyer, and J. B. Dimick, "Variation in hospital mortality associated with inpatient surgery," *The New England Journal of Medicine*, vol. 361, no. 14, pp. 1368–1375, 2009.

[11] H. Kehlet, "Multimodal approach to control postoperative pathophysiology and rehabilitation," *British Journal of Anaesthesia*, vol. 78, no. 5, pp. 606–617, 1997.

[12] S. Daneshmand, H. Ahmadi, A. K. Schuckman et al., "Enhanced recovery protocol after radical cystectomy for bladder cancer," *The Journal of Urology*, vol. 192, no. 1, pp. 50–55, 2014.

[13] A. Thorell, J. Nygren, and O. Ljungqvist, "Insulin resistance: a marker of surgical stress," *Current Opinion in Clinical Nutrition and Metabolic Care*, vol. 2, no. 1, pp. 69–78, 1999.

[14] B. A. Inman, F. Harel, R. Tiguert, L. Lacombe, and Y. Fradet, "Routine nasogastric tubes are not required following cystectomy with urinary diversion: a comparative analysis of 430 patients," *The Journal of Urology*, vol. 170, no. 5, pp. 1888–1891, 2003.

[15] A. Stenzl, N. C. Cowan, M. De Santis et al., "The updated EAU guidelines on muscle-invasive and metastatic bladder cancer," *European Urology*, vol. 55, no. 4, pp. 815–825, 2009.

[16] S. S. Chang, R. G. Baumgartner, N. Wells, M. S. Cookson, and J. A. Smith Jr., "Causes of increased hospital stay after radical cystectomy in a clinical pathway setting," *Journal of Urology*, vol. 167, no. 1, pp. 208–211, 2002.

[17] C. T. Lee, S. S. Chang, A. M. Kamat et al., "Alvimopan accelerates gastrointestinal recovery after radical cystectomy: a multicenter randomized placebo-controlled trial," *European Urology*, vol. 66, no. 2, pp. 265–272, 2014.

[18] E. J. Noble, R. Harris, K. B. Hosie, S. Thomas, and S. J. Lewis, "Gum chewing reduces postoperative ileus? A systematic review and meta-analysis," *International Journal of Surgery*, vol. 7, no. 2, pp. 100–105, 2009.

[19] D. J. Parekh, W. B. Gilbert, M. O. Koch, and J. A. Smith Jr., "Continent urinary reconstruction versus ileal conduit: a contemporary single-institution comparison of perioperative morbidity and mortality," *Urology*, vol. 55, no. 6, pp. 852–855, 2000.

[20] A. Mattei, F. D. Birkhaeuser, C. Baermann, S. H. Warncke, and U. E. Studer, "To stent or not to stent perioperatively the ureteroileal anastomosis of ileal orthotopic bladder substitutes and ileal conduits? Results of a prospective randomized trial," *Journal of Urology*, vol. 179, no. 2, pp. 582–586, 2008.

[21] J. P. Stein and D. G. Skinner, "Surgical Atlas: the orthotopic T-pouch ileal neobladder," *BJU International*, vol. 98, no. 2, pp. 469–482, 2006.

[22] Y. Cerantola, M. Valerio, B. Persson et al., "Guidelines for perioperative care after radical cystectomy for bladder cancer: enhanced recovery after surgery (ERAS) society recommendations," *Clinical Nutrition*, vol. 32, no. 6, pp. 879–887, 2013.

[23] A. J. Sun, H. Djaladat, A. Schuckman, G. Miranda, J. Cai, and S. Daneshmand, "Venous thromboembolism following radical cystectomy: significant predictors, comparison of different anticoagulants and timing of events," *The Journal of Urology*, vol. 193, no. 2, pp. 565–569, 2015.

[24] A. A. Vandlac, N. G. Cowan, Y. Chen et al., "Timing, incidence and risk factors for venous thromboembolism in patients undergoing radical cystectomy for malignancy: a case for extended duration pharmacological prophylaxis," *Journal of Urology*, vol. 191, no. 4, pp. 943–947, 2014.

[25] R. E. Hautmann, R. C. de Petriconi, and B. G. Volkmer, "25 years of experience with 1,000 neobladders: long-term complications," *Journal of Urology*, vol. 185, no. 6, pp. 2207–2212, 2011.

[26] F. Suriano, M. Gallucci, G. P. Flammia et al., "Bacteriuria in patients with an orthotopic ileal neobladder: urinary tract infection or asymptomatic bacteriuria?" *BJU International*, vol. 101, no. 12, pp. 1576–1579, 2008.

[27] D. P. Wood Jr., F. J. Bianco Jr., J. E. Pontes, M. A. Heath, and D. DaJusta, "Incidence and significance of positive urine cultures in patients with an orthotopic neobladder," *Journal of Urology*, vol. 169, no. 6, pp. 2196–2199, 2003.

[28] U. E. Studer, H. Danuser, G. N. Thalmann, J. P. Springer, and W. H. Turner, "Antireflux nipples or afferent tubular segments in 70 patients with ileal low pressure bladder substitutes: long-term results of a prospective randomized trial," *The Journal of Urology*, vol. 156, no. 6, pp. 1913–1917, 1996.

[29] E. C. Skinner, A. S. Fairey, S. Groshen et al., "Randomized trial of studer pouch versus T-pouch orthotopic ileal neobladder in patients with bladder cancer," *The Journal of Urology*, vol. 194, no. 2, pp. 433–440, 2015.

[30] A. Kristjansson, L. Wallin, and W. Mansson, "Renal function up to 16 years after conduit (refluxing or anti-reflux anastomosis) or continent urinary diversion. 1. Glomerular filtration rate and patency of uretero-intestinal anastomosis," *British Journal of Urology*, vol. 76, no. 5, pp. 539–545, 1995.

[31] W. S. Tan, A. Sridhar, M. Goldstraw et al., "Robot-assisted intracorporeal pyramid neobladder," *BJU International*, vol. 116, no. 5, pp. 771–779, 2015.

[32] M. M. Desai, I. S. Gill, A. L. D. C. Abreu et al., "Robotic intracorporeal orthotopic neobladder during radical cystectomy in 132 patients," *The Journal of Urology*, vol. 192, no. 6, pp. 1734–1740, 2014.

[33] R. E. Hautmann, B. G. Volkmer, M. C. Schumacher, J. E. Gschwend, and U. E. Studer, "Long-term results of standard procedures in urology: the ileal neobladder," *World Journal of Urology*, vol. 24, no. 3, pp. 305–314, 2006.

[34] M. S. Eisenberg, R. H. Thompson, I. Frank et al., "Long-term renal function outcomes after radical cystectomy," *The Journal of Urology*, vol. 191, no. 3, pp. 619–625, 2014.

[35] J. P. Stein, M. D. Dunn, M. L. Quek, G. Miranda, and D. G. Skinner, "The orthotopic T pouch ileal neobladder: experience with 209 patients," *Journal of Urology*, vol. 172, no. 2, pp. 584–587, 2004.

[36] M. Ferriero, S. Guaglianone, R. Papalia, G. L. Muto, M. Gallucci, and G. Simone, "Risk assessment of stone formation in stapled orthotopic ileal neobladder," *Journal of Urology*, vol. 193, no. 3, pp. 891–896, 2015.

[37] Z. Okhunov, B. Duty, A. D. Smith, and Z. Okeke, "Management of urolithiasis in patients after urinary diversions," *BJU International*, vol. 108, no. 3, pp. 330–336, 2011.

[38] R. D. Mills and U. E. Studer, "Metabolic consequences of continent urinary diversion," *Journal of Urology*, vol. 161, no. 4, pp. 1057–1066, 1999.

[39] F. Van der Aa, S. Joniau, M. Van Den Branden, and H. Van Poppel, "Metabolic changes after urinary diversion," *Advances in Urology*, vol. 2011, Article ID 764325, 5 pages, 2011.

[40] L. E. Matarese, S. J. O'Keefe, H. M. Kandil, G. Bond, G. Costa, and K. Abu-Elmagd, "Short bowel syndrome: clinical guidelines for nutrition management," *Nutrition in Clinical Practice*, vol. 20, no. 5, pp. 493–502, 2005.

[41] M. Fujisawa, I. Nakamura, N. Yamanaka et al., "Changes in calcium metabolism and bone demineralization after orthotopic intestinal neobladder creation," *Journal of Urology*, vol. 163, no. 4, pp. 1108–1111, 2000.

[42] R. E. Hautmann, H. Abol-Enein, K. Hafez et al., "Urinary diversion," *Urology*, vol. 69, no. 1, supplement, pp. 17–49, 2007.

[43] T. M. Kessler, F. C. Burkhard, P. Perimenis et al., "Attempted nerve sparing surgery and age have a significant effect on urinary continence and erectile function after radical cystoprostatectomy and ileal orthotopic bladder substitution," *Journal of Urology*, vol. 172, no. 4, pp. 1323–1327, 2004.

[44] M. S. El Bahnasawy, Y. Osman, M. A. Gomha, A. A. Shaaban, A. Ashamallah, and M. A. Ghoneim, "Nocturnal enuresis in men with an orthotopic ileal reservoir: urodynamic evaluation," *Journal of Urology*, vol. 164, no. 1, pp. 10–13, 2000.

[45] M. S. El-Bahnasawy, H. Shaaban, M. A. Gomha, and A. Nabeeh, "Clinical and urodynamic efficacy of oxybutynin and verapamil in the treatment of nocturnal enuresis after formation of orthotopic ileal neobladders. A prospective, randomized, crossover study," *Scandinavian Journal of Urology and Nephrology*, vol. 42, no. 4, pp. 344–351, 2008.

[46] B. Ali-El-Dein, M. Gomha, and M. A. Ghoneim, "Critical evaluation of the problem of chronic urinary retention after orthotopic bladder substitution in women," *Journal of Urology*, vol. 168, no. 2, pp. 587–592, 2002.

[47] J. P. Stein, D. A. Ginsberg, and D. G. Skinner, "Indications and technique of the orthotopic neobladder in women," *Urologic Clinics of North America*, vol. 29, no. 3, pp. 725–734, 2002.

[48] G. Gakis, J. Efstathiou, S. P. Lerner et al., "ICUD-EAU international consultation on bladder cancer 2012: radical cystectomy and bladder preservation for muscle-invasive urothelial carcinoma of the bladder," *European Urology*, vol. 63, no. 1, pp. 45–57, 2013.

[49] B. G. Volkmer, R. Kuefer, G. C. Bartsch Jr., K. Gust, and R. E. Hautmann, "Oncological follow up after radical cystectomy for bladder cancer-is there any benefit?" *Journal of Urology*, vol. 181, no. 4, pp. 1587–1593, 2009.

[50] S. A. Boorjian, S. P. Kim, C. J. Weight, J. C. Cheville, P. Thapa, and I. Frank, "Risk factors and outcomes of urethral recurrence following radical cystectomy," *European Urology*, vol. 60, no. 6, pp. 1266–1272, 2011.

3

Frequency of Electrolyte Derangement after Transurethral Resection of Prostate: Need for Postoperative Electrolyte Monitoring

Wajahat Aziz and M. Hammad Ather

Section of Urology, Department of Surgery, Aga Khan University, P.O. Box 3500, Stadium Road, Karachi 74800, Pakistan

Correspondence should be addressed to M. Hammad Ather; hammad.ather@aku.edu

Academic Editor: Nazareno Suardi

Objective. To determine the electrolyte derangement following transurethral resection of prostate (TURP). *Methods.* All patients undergoing TURP from June 2012 to April 2013 were included. Preoperative electrolytes were performed within a week of procedures. Monopolar TURP using 1.5% glycine was performed. Serum Na^+ and K^+ were assessed within 1 hour postoperatively and subsequently if clinically indicated. *Results.* The study included 280 patients. Sixty-six patients (23.6%) had electrolyte derangement after TURP. Patients with deranged electrolytes were older (mean age of 73.41 ± 4.08 yrs. versus 68.93 yrs. ± 10.34) and had a longer mean resection time (42.5 ± 20.04 min versus 28.34 ± 14.64 min). Mean weight of tissue resected (41.49 ± 34.46 g versus 15.33 ± 9.74 g) and volume of irrigant used (23.55 ± 15.20 L versus 12.81 ± 7.57 L) were also significantly higher in patients with deranged electrolytes (all $p = 0.00$). On multivariate logistic regression analysis preoperative sodium level was found to be a significant predictor of postoperative electrolyte derangement (odds ratio 0.267, S.E. = 0.376, and p value = 0.00). *Conclusion.* Electrolyte derangement occurs in older patients, with larger amount of tissue and longer time of resection and higher volume of irrigant, and in those with lower serum preoperative sodium levels.

1. Introduction

Transurethral resection of prostate (TURP) is one of the most common urological procedures performed. Despite introduction of several minimally invasive options like Holmium Laser Enucleation and Holmium Laser Ablation, TURP is still considered the gold standard for surgical management of Benign Prostatic Obstruction (BPO) [1].

Complications after TURP are frequent [2]. Early complications of TURP include bleeding, sepsis, TUR syndrome, incontinence, and urinary retention. The incidence of early complications of TURP has decreased considerably over the past few decades. This is largely attributable to standardization of the procedure, better perioperative management [3], and better anesthetic techniques [4]. Bleeding requiring transfusion, acute kidney injury, and transurethral resection syndrome are the complications of TURP in early postoperative period that greatly influence morbidity of the procedure and may even lead to mortality [5].

Electrolyte imbalance is one of the most worrisome complications of TURP especially due to risk of developing overt TUR syndrome. This syndrome results from the absorption of irrigating fluid through prostatic veins exposed by breaches in the prostatic capsule during TURP. The irrigation fluid used during resection is absorbed via these channels and leads to hypervolemic hyponatremia. Mental confusion, bradycardia, hypotension/hypertension, nausea, vomiting, and visual disturbances associated with hyponatremia are most commonly observed symptoms [6]. These symptoms are mostly the result of brain edema caused by hypervolemic hyponatremic state. Hyperkalemia can also occur after TURP attributable mainly to cell lysis and release of intracellular potassium. Acute kidney injury secondary to obstruction or sepsis can also lead to hyperkalemia in some cases [7].

TUR syndrome has become a rare event in recent years with better appreciation of pathophysiology and advances in technology. Several modifications have led to decreased incidence of this complication. Among these are development of continuous flow resectoscopes, utilization of "nonhemolytic" solutions such as glycine, sorbitol, and mannitol, use of bipolar circuitry, and advances in training techniques [8]. TUR syndrome was found in only 1% of patients in a recent multicenter study [9]. Certain risk factors are known to be associated with increased risk of TUR syndrome including volume and type of irrigant used, resection time, weight of tissue resected, and use of monopolar diathermy [10].

Monitoring of serum electrolytes after TURP is variable in different centers and does not usually take into account the risk factors for developing electrolyte derangement. Major urological associations do not have specific guidelines regarding post-TURP electrolyte monitoring, although such testing is performed routinely in many centers. Routine electrolyte measurement in all patients undergoing TURP irrespective of risk factors for developing TURP syndrome is burdensome for both patient and hospital staff and also incur additional cost. The purpose of the present study is to evaluate the frequency and risk factors for electrolyte derangement after TURP.

2. Material and Methods

Cross-sectional study was conducted at inpatient units of a university hospital. All patients above age 50 years and above undergoing TURP from June 2012 to April 2013 were included. Patients who refuse to participate in the study, who received diuretic intraoperatively or are in immediate postoperative period, and patients with already deranged electrolytes (as per operational definition) or raised serum creatinine (i.e., serum creatinine >1.2) were excluded. Ethical review committee approval was taken before commencement of work on the subject. Preoperative electrolytes done within 1 week before the procedure were recorded. Any one of the six urology consultants carried out TURP or resident under supervision of these consultants using a continuous flow resectoscope with monopolar diathermy and 1.5% glycine as an irrigant. A 3 cc postoperative serum sample was taken within 1 hour of the end of procedure for electrolytes assessment. Serum sodium and potassium were measured using ion selective electrode method. Operative parameters, resection time, volume of irrigant use, weight of tissue resected, volume and type of intravenous fluids, and postoperative clinical symptoms, were recorded. Deranged electrolytes were defined as presence of any or both of serum sodium <130 or >145 mmol/L and serum potassium <3.5 or >5.5 mmol/L.

Data was analyzed using SPSS version 17.0. Results were described in terms of mean and standard deviation for continuous variables. Categorical variables were described in terms of frequency and percentage. The proportion of deranged sodium, potassium, and creatinine after TURP was calculated. Stratification was done with respect to comorbid, current smoking status, and surgeon. Chi square test and Fischer's exact test were applied to determine significance where appropriate. Continuous variables like age, preoperative electrolytes, resection time, volume of irrigation fluid used, and weight of tissue resected were compared using t-test. p value of less than 0.05 was considered significant.

TABLE 1: Baseline characteristics, $n = 280$.

	Median	Std. deviation
Age	73	9.45
Preoperative sodium	142	5.03
Preoperative potassium	4.5	0.46
Preoperative serum creatinine	0.9	0.18
Postoperative sodium	138	5.43
Postoperative potassium	4.3	0.49
Volume of irrigant used	12	10.87
Weight of tissue resected	13	21.76
Resection time	30	17.13

Binary Logistic regression analysis was done to identify risk factors of electrolyte derangement.

3. Results

Two hundred and eighty consecutive patients who underwent TURP were included in the study (Table 1). Mean age of patient was 69.98 years (range 51–90, S.D. 9.45). When patients with electrolyte derangement were compared with those having no electrolyte derangement, the former group was found to be significantly older and had a mean resection time significantly higher than those with no electrolyte derangement. The mean weight of tissue resected and the volume of irrigant used were also significantly higher in patients with postoperative electrolyte derangement (Table 2).

Comorbids including ischemic heart disease (IHD), congestive cardiac failure (CCF), and diabetes mellitus (DM) were not found to be associated with postoperative electrolyte derangement. Hypertensive patients had a higher proportion of electrolyte derangement compared to normotensive (Table 3).

On multivariate logistic regression analysis the only significant factor predicting postoperative electrolyte derangement was preoperative sodium level after controlling for resection time, volume of irrigant used, weight of tissue resected, age, and hypertension (Table 4).

3.1. Discussion. Transurethral resection syndrome (TUR syndrome) is caused by fluid absorption from venous channels in prostatic bed in the presence of continuous irrigation. Absorption of this fluid leads to changes in serum electrolytes and potentially can lead to clinical TUR syndrome. In our study we found a decrease in serum concentration of both sodium and potassium postoperatively. Although the rate of fluid absorption during TURP depends upon a number of factors (Table 5), the average rate is 20 mL/min [11]. We identified an overall decrease in the serum levels of both sodium and potassium, though the overall magnitude of this decrease is subtle (mean decrease of 3.13 mEq/L for sodium and mean decrease of 0.082 for potassium).

Hyperkalemia following TURP is partly explained by cell lysis as happened during resection of tissue. Absorption of fluid into circulation is an alternate mechanism that can cause hyperkalemia after TURP [12]. ECG changes and cardiac

TABLE 2: Comparison of continuous variables between those without electrolyte derangement and those with electrolyte derangement. p value calculated using Student's t-test.

	No electrolyte derangement $n = 214$	Electrolyte derangement $n = 66$	p value
Mean age (years)	68.93 ± 10.35	73.41 ± 4.08	0.00
Mean preoperative serum sodium	141.47 ± 2.70	131.33 ± 2.26	0.00
Mean preoperative serum potassium	4.40 ± 0.42	4.13 ± 0.53	0.00
Mean preoperative serum creatinine	0.9 ± 0.19	0.8 ± 0.19	0.26
Mean postoperative serum sodium	138.19 ± 2.65	128.67 ± 5.78	0.00
Mean postoperative serum potassium	4.31 ± 0.34	4.10 ± 0.81	0.002
Mean resection time (min)	28.34 ± 14.64	42.50 ± 20.04	0.00
Mean volume of irrigant used (liters)	12.81 ± 7.57	23.55 ± 15.20	0.00
Mean weight of tissue resected (grams)	15.33 ± 9.74	41.59 ± 34.45	0.00

TABLE 3: Comparison of categorical variables between those without electrolyte derangement and those with electrolyte derangement. p value calculated using chi square test/Fischer's exact test where applicable.

		No electrolyte derangement, $n = 214$	Electrolyte derangement, $n = 66$	p value
CCF	No	203	62	0.488
	Yes	11	4	
IHD	No	179	61	0.051
	Yes	35	5	
DM	No	164	55	0.249
	Yes	50	11	
HTN	No	108	4	0.00
	Yes	106	62	
Diuretic use	No	208	58	0.006
	Yes	6	8	
Smoker	No	160	49	0.932
	Yes	54	17	
Surgeon	Resident	89	24	0.449
	Consultant	125	42	

CCF: congestive cardiac failure; IHD: ischemic heart disease; HTN: hypertension.

TABLE 4: Logistic regression analysis of predictors of electrolyte derangement.

	Exp(B)	S.E.	p value
Resection time	1.013	0.082	0.873
Volume of irrigant used	0.918	0.116	0.461
Weight of tissue resected	1.249	0.124	0.073
Age	0.934	0.102	0.502
Comorbids	0.035	2.271	0.140
Preoperative sodium	0.267	0.376	0.000
Surgeon	0.103	1.837	0.217

toxicity caused by hyperkalemia usually occur at serum levels above 6 mEq/L. We did not encounter significant rise of serum potassium postoperatively in our series. This is partially explained by hemodilution caused by fluid absorption to offset any changes caused by hemolysis. Also with 1.5% glycine as irrigant, hemolysis is minimal as compared to other hypoosmolar irrigants like water. Singhania and colleagues

compared monopolar versus bipolar saline resection in 60 patients and found no significant changes in potassium levels in either group [13].

When patients with deranged electrolytes were compared with those having no electrolyte derangement, a number of important findings were noted.

First, patients with electrolyte derangement were significantly older than those without electrolyte derangement. Uchida et al. found age of the patient undergoing TURP as a significant risk factor for perioperative blood transfusion and attributed it to more rigid vasculature in elderly, which allows for persistent opening of venous channels [14]. The same mechanism can account for increased fluid absorption and electrolyte derangement in elderly patients.

Second, mean weight of tissue resected was found to be higher in those patients undergoing TURP. The amount of fluid absorption depends mainly on the number and size of venous sinuses opened [15]. The weight of tissue resected serves as a surrogate marker for the number of venous sinuses opened in prostatic bed. To decrease the likelihood

TABLE 5: Factors increasing fluid absorption and electrolyte derangement during TURP.

Factors increasing fluid absorption during TURP	Strategies to minimize fluid absorption
Open prostatic sinuses	
(i) Weight of tissue resected (used as surrogate marker)	(i) Consider open prostatectomy or HoLEP for >80 g prostate
(ii) Capsular breech	(ii) Avoid deep resection
Lengthy resection	
Prostatic sinuses exposed for longer time	Keep resection time under 60 min
High irrigation pressure	
(i) Height of irrigation column	(i) Keep irrigation fluid at height of 60 cm
(ii) Small capacity bladder	(ii) Continuous flow resectoscope
Hypotonic irrigant	(i) Use of isotonic irrigant (ii) Bipolar diathermy

of TUR syndrome, European Urology Association suggests open surgery or transurethral holmium laser enucleation for men with prostates >80 mL [16], whereas TURP is considered the standard procedure for men with prostate 30–80 mL.

Third, increased resection time correlates with electrolyte derangement in our study. Provided that the irrigation fluid column is kept at a constant height, a constant volume of fluid is obtained per minute during resection. However, the amount of fluid absorption not only depends on the duration of exposure of the exposed venous sinuses to the irrigating fluid but also upon the number of prostatic venous sinuses opened and hydrostatic pressure at the prostatic bed. Madsen and Naber demonstrated that hydrostatic pressure at the prostatic bed is an important factor determining fluid absorption during TURP. This hydrostatic pressure depends upon the height of irrigating fluid column and pressure inside bladder during surgery [17]. The ideal height of irrigating fluid is suggested to be 60 cm so that approximately 300 mL of fluid is obtained per minute during resection to maintain good vision. For our study, we fixed the irrigation fluid column height so that other determinants can be assessed. In order to limit the likelihood of a serious electrolyte derangement, it is advocated that resection times should be limited to 1 hour.

Fourth, volume of irrigant used was found to be significantly higher in patients with deranged electrolytes. We used 1.5% glycine in all patients undergoing TURP. So, the type of irrigant used is not a factor in determining fluid absorption in our patients. Volume of irrigant used is consistently found to correlate with the risk of postoperative electrolyte derangement in previous studies [18].

Finally, hypertensive patients were found to be at higher risk of developing postoperative electrolyte derangement. Some antihypertensives, for example, angiotensin converting enzyme inhibitors, are known to inhibit normal regulation of fluid balance and may even cause hyponatremia [19]. On the

other hand although preoperative diuretic use was found to be more common in patients with electrolyte derangement, a conclusive statement cannot be made due to the small number of patients using diuretics preoperatively.

Our sample size calculation was based upon frequency of electrolyte derangement, so logistic regression analysis was not part of initial study protocol. However, on logistic regression analysis, the most significant factor predicting electrolyte derangement was preoperative sodium level with $\text{Exp}(B)$ of 0.267; that is, for each unit rise in preoperative sodium level the odds of electrolyte derangement decrease by approximately 27%. This is an important finding and suggests that low normal values of serum sodium should alert the surgeon to the possibility of postoperative electrolyte derangement.

Few studies have investigated the usefulness of routine electrolyte testing following TURP. Most of them focused on post-TURP Hb monitoring [20]. Emphasis on preoperative optimization and better operative techniques has made transfusion during TURP a rare event. In our study none of the patients had preoperative blood transfusion, so its correlation with electrolyte derangement immediately after TURP could not be assessed. Hakem et al. retrospectively studied 137 patients; they found low postoperative sodium in 2 patients, but there was no TUR syndrome in any patient [7]. They concluded that routine postoperative blood testing following TURP is not required in all cases and recommended blood testing based on clinical need or following technically demanding operations.

Overall 66/280 patients had deranged electrolytes after TURP in our study. None of the patients had clinical TUR syndrome. The significance of mild hyponatremia after TURP is unknown. It may contribute to postoperative nausea, vomiting, and delayed recovery from general anesthesia in at least some patients. In a cross-sectional study patients undergoing TURP, hyponatremia was observed in 28 out of 40 (70%) patients. In this study a value of <135 mEq/L was used to define hyponatremia [6]. Although our clinical laboratory also uses same value as a lower range for normal sodium, we used a threshold of <130 mEq/L as it is more clinically relevant [21].

Several strategies have been proposed to reduce the risk of fluid absorption during TURP, but none is capable of eliminating this complication altogether. It has been suggested to keep resection time below 60 min to minimize fluid absorption; TUR syndrome has been reported after a resection time of only 15 min [22].

Monitoring the extent of fluid absorption during surgery has been suggested to control fluid balance in every patient. The most viable methods to monitor fluid absorption are ethanol monitoring and gravimetric weighing [23]. Newer techniques, such as bipolar resectoscopes and vaporizing the tissue instead of resecting tissue, have reduced fluid absorption and its consequent electrolyte derangement, so routine monitoring of fluid absorption has been largely abandoned outside a study setting. However there is no consensus on routine monitoring of postoperative electrolytes. It has been suggested that with improvements in technology and use of isotonic, nonhemolytic solutions; electrolyte derangement is rare. Particularly with the use of isotonic saline and bipolar resection TURP syndrome is of historical interest only [24].

In light of our findings we suggest a more realistic approach. Electrolyte derangement occurs commonly in patients undergoing TURP, as manifested by a frequency of 16% in our series, though full-blown TUR syndrome is rare. Electrolyte monitoring should be considered in patients having risk factors for increased fluid absorption.

3.2. Conclusion. Electrolyte derangement after TURP is not uncommon. The need for monitoring electrolyte following TURP should be individualized, taking into account the weight of resected tissue, volume of irrigation used, resection time, increasing age, and hypertension. Low normal values of serum sodium should alert the surgeon to the possibility of postoperative electrolyte derangement.

Conflict of Interests

The authors declare that there is no conflict of interests regarding the publication of this paper.

References

[1] T. Lourenco, R. Pickard, L. Vale et al., "Minimally invasive treatments for benign prostatic enlargement: systematic review of randomised controlled trials," *The British Medical Journal*, vol. 337, no. 7676, Article ID a1662, pp. 966–969, 2008.

[2] C. Mamoulakis, D. T. Ubbink, and J. J. M. C. H. de la Rosette, "Bipolar versus monopolar transurethral resection of the prostate: a systematic review and meta-analysis of randomized controlled trials," *European Urology*, vol. 56, no. 5, pp. 798–809, 2009.

[3] M. H. Ather, N. Faruqui, and F. Abid, "Optimization of low pre-operative hemoglobin reduces transfusion requirement in patients undergoing transurethral resection of prostate," *The Journal of the Pakistan Medical Association*, vol. 53, no. 3, pp. 104–106, 2003.

[4] O. Reich, C. Gratzke, A. Bachmann et al., "Morbidity, mortality and early outcome of transurethral resection of the prostate: a prospective multicenter evaluation of 10,654 patients," *The Journal of Urology*, vol. 180, no. 1, pp. 246–249, 2008.

[5] C. Mamoulakis, I. Efthimiou, S. Kazoulis, I. Christoulakis, and F. Sofras, "The modified Clavien classification system: a standardized platform for reporting complications in transurethral resection of the prostate," *World Journal of Urology*, vol. 29, no. 2, pp. 205–210, 2011.

[6] A. Muhammad, A. Shaikh, B. R. Devrajani, Z. Shah, T. Das, and D. Singh, "Serum sodium level in transurethral resection of the prostate (TURP) (a cross sectional descriptive study at two hospitals)," *Medical Channel*, vol. 16, no. 2, pp. 218–220, 2010.

[7] A. R. Hakeem, K. Sairam, and R. O. Plail, "The value of blood tests following transurethral resection of the prostate," *UroToday International Journal*, vol. 2, no. 2, article 5, 2009.

[8] A. Hawary, K. Mukhtar, A. Sinclair, and I. Pearce, "Transurethral resection of the prostate syndrome: almost gone but not forgotten," *Journal of Endourology*, vol. 23, no. 12, pp. 2013–2020, 2009.

[9] M. Suhail, A. Pirzada, and M. Khaskheli, "Comparison of effectiveness of irrigation fluid mannitol 5% with that of glycine 1.5% in preventing post TURP hyponatremia," *MedChannel*, vol. 6, no. 2, pp. 321–325, 2010.

[10] C. Mamoulakis, A. Skolarikos, M. Schulze et al., "Results from an international multicentre double-blind randomized controlled trial on the perioperative efficacy and safety of bipolar vs monopolar transurethral resection of the prostate," *BJU International*, vol. 109, no. 2, pp. 240–248, 2012.

[11] H. Moorthy and S. Philip, "TURP syndrome-current concepts in the pathophysiology and management," *Indian Journal of Urology*, vol. 17, no. 2, pp. 97–102, 2001.

[12] H. K. Moorthy and S. Philip, "Serum electrolytes in TURP syndrome—is the role of potassium under-estimated," *Indian Journal of Anaesthesia*, vol. 46, no. 6, pp. 441–444, 2002.

[13] P. Singhania, D. Nandini, F. Sarita, P. Hemant, and I. Hemalata, "Transurethral resection of prostate: a comparison of standard monopolar versus bipolar saline resection," *International Brazilian Journal of Urology*, vol. 36, no. 2, pp. 183–189, 2010.

[14] T. Uchida, M. Ohori, S. Soh et al., "Factors influencing morbidity in patients undergoing transurethral resection of the prostate," *Urology*, vol. 53, no. 1, pp. 98–105, 1999.

[15] S. Vijayan, "TURP syndrome," *Trends in Anaesthesia and Critical Care*, vol. 1, no. 1, pp. 46–50, 2011.

[16] M. Oelke, A. Bachmann, A. Descazeaud et al., "EAU guidelines on the treatment and follow-up of non-neurogenic male lower urinary tract symptoms including benign prostatic obstruction," *European Urology*, vol. 64, no. 1, pp. 118–140, 2013.

[17] P. O. Madsen and K. G. Naber, "The importance of the pressure in the prostatic fossa and absorption of irrigating fluid during transurethral resection of the prostate," *The Journal of Urology*, vol. 109, no. 3, pp. 446–452, 1973.

[18] K. Gupta, B. Rastogi, M. Jain, P. Gupta, and D. Sharma, "Electrolyte changes: an indirect method to assess irrigation fluid absorption complications during transurethral resection of prostate: a prospective study," *Saudi Journal of Anaesthesia*, vol. 4, no. 3, pp. 142–146, 2010.

[19] S. Chakithandy, R. Evans, and P. Vyakarnam, "Acute severe hyponatraemia and seizures associated with postoperative enalapril administration," *Anaesthesia & Intensive Care*, vol. 37, no. 4, pp. 673–674, 2009.

[20] J. Shah and J. Nethercliffe, "Is routine post-operative haemoglobin measurement required after transurethral resection of the prostate?" *Transfusion Medicine*, vol. 14, no. 5, pp. 343–346, 2004.

[21] K. P. Goh, "Management of hyponatremia," *American Family Physician*, vol. 69, no. 10, pp. 2387–2394, 2004.

[22] B. J. Hurlbert and D. W. Wingard, "Water intoxication after 15 minutes of transurethral resection of the prostate," *Anesthesiology*, vol. 50, no. 4, pp. 355–356, 1979.

[23] L. Salmela, U. Aromaa, T. Lehtonen, P. Peura, and K. T. Olkkola, "The effect of prostatic capsule perforation on the absorption of irrigating fluid during transurethral resection," *British Journal of Urology*, vol. 72, no. 5, pp. 599–604, 1993.

[24] M. M. Issa, M. R. Young, A. R. Bullock, R. Bouet, and J. A. Petros, "Dilutional hyponatremia of TURP syndrome: a historical event in the 21st century," *Urology*, vol. 64, no. 2, pp. 298–301, 2004.

4

Outcomes of Direct Vision Internal Urethrotomy for Bulbar Urethral Strictures: Technique Modification with High Dose Triamcinolone Injection

Rishi Modh, Peter Y. Cai, Alyssa Sheffield, and Lawrence L. Yeung

Department of Urology, University of Florida College of Medicine, Gainesville, FL 32608, USA

Correspondence should be addressed to Peter Y. Cai; peter.yincheng.cai@gmail.com and Lawrence L. Yeung; lyeung@ufl.edu

Academic Editor: Darius J. Bagli

Objective. To evaluate the recurrence rate of bulbar urethral strictures managed with cold knife direct vision internal urethrotomy and high dose corticosteroid injection. *Methods.* 28 patients with bulbar urethral strictures underwent direct vision internal urethrotomy with high dose triamcinolone injection into the periurethral tissue and were followed up for recurrence. *Results.* Our cohort had a mean age of 60 years and average stricture length of 1.85 cm, and 71% underwent multiple previous urethral stricture procedures with an average of 5.7 procedures each. Our technique modification of high dose corticosteroid injection had a recurrence rate of 29% at a mean follow-up of 20 months with a low rate of urinary tract infections. In patients who failed treatment, mean time to stricture recurrence was 7 months. Patients who were successfully treated had significantly better International Prostate Symptom Scores at 6, 9, and 12 months. There was no significant difference in maximum flow velocity on Uroflowmetry at last follow-up but there was significant difference in length of follow-up ($p = 0.02$). *Conclusions.* High dose corticosteroid injection at the time of direct vision internal urethrotomy is a safe and effective procedure to delay anatomical and symptomatic recurrence of bulbar urethral strictures, particularly in those who are poor candidates for urethroplasty.

1. Introduction

Epidemiological data suggests that patients with urethral strictures most commonly present with voiding complaints such as weak stream (49%) and incomplete emptying (27%) and the main causes are idiopathic, iatrogenic (endoscopic procedures, catheterization, prostatectomy, brachytherapy, and hypospadias repair), and traumatic [1, 2]. Management of urethral stricture ranges from commonly performed procedures such as urethral dilation and internal urethrotomy to more definitive reconstructive procedures such as urethroplasty or even urinary diversion in an effort to prevent complications from untreated strictures.

Currently, the most commonly employed procedures for treatment of urethral strictures are dilation and internal urethrotomy [2]. Studies have demonstrated that there is no significant difference between dilation and internal urethrotomy in complications or failure rates [3]. The decision to employ one technique over the other is

often based on clinician preference and location of the stricture.

Although these procedures can be done relatively quickly in an ambulatory setting, one of the major concerns is the high rate of recurrence on long-term follow-up. Historical data shows recurrence rates for 2–4 cm strictures to be 50% within 12 months of urethrotomy [3]. Pansadoro and Emiliozzi demonstrated that, with long-term follow-up, a single urethrotomy had a recurrence rate of 68% [4]. The same group demonstrated that those with longer strictures (>1 cm), a narrow lumen (<15 French), or a history of prior interventions are more likely to recur after urethrotomy.

One proposed solution to decrease stricture recurrence rates is the use of adjunctive corticosteroid injections, which have been used to inhibit scar formation. Corticosteroid injections have been used in other specialties such as in Dermatology for hyperplastic and hypertrophic skin disorders, in Gastroenterology for esophageal strictures, and in Otolaryngology for laryngeal strictures.

Two studies have reported improved patency rates and delayed stricture recurrence with DVIU and steroid injection compared to DVIU alone [5, 6]. These studies utilized periurethral injection of triamcinolone at a dose of 40 mg after urethrotomy. We hypothesized that DVIU of bulbar urethral strictures with higher dose intralesional triamcinolone (320 mg) can significantly delay urethral stricture recurrence.

2. Materials and Methods

We reviewed our Institutional Review Board approved database of patients who underwent DVIU by a single surgeon (L. L. Yeung). All patients who underwent DVIU or dilation and corticosteroid injection for bulbar urethral strictures were included in our study. Patients who did not follow up for at least 6 months, those with penile urethral strictures, or those with multiple strictures were excluded. Every patient was evaluated preoperatively with cystoscopy and retrograde urethrogram to define length and location of stricture and subsequently offered urethroplasty, DVIU with steroid injection, or dilation with steroid injection based on location and length of stricture.

Our follow-up protocol was every 3 months for the first year, every 6 months for the second year, and then yearly with International Prostate Symptom Score (IPSS) and Uroflowmetry and postvoid residual. In order to establish an objective outcome measure, we defined successful treatment as maximum flow velocity greater than 15 mL/sec on Uroflowmetry. Patients who performed clean intermittent self-catheterization preoperatively for incomplete bladder emptying due to myogenic failure were considered a success if they were still able to perform self-catheterization without difficulty on follow-up. For those with equivocal Uroflowmetry rates, cystoscopy was performed to evaluate recurrence. DVIU failure was defined by the need for a subsequent urethral procedure (i.e., urethroplasty, dilation, and DVIU).

Urethrotomy was performed using a Sachse Urethrotome (Karl Storz, USA) by performing radial cuts through the stricture at the 12, 3, 6, and 9 o'clock positions. Urethral dilation was performed using Amplatz Dilators (Cook Medical, USA) to 26 F. A 23 G Williams Cystoscopic Injection Needle (Cook Medical, USA) was used to inject 1 mL (40 mg) triamcinolone at each site every 5–10 mm circumferentially in quadrants along the length of the incised stricture. The Encore 26 Inflator (Boston Scientific, USA) was used to provide positive pressure to aid in the injection of the steroids into the stricture and to provide accurate dose delivery. Although a total of 10 mL of triamcinolone (concentration of 200 mg/5 mL) was available for injection, 8 mL (320 mg) was injected after accounting for waste within the injection needle and tubing from the pressure inflator.

3. Results

In our cohort, we were able to identify twenty-eight patients with a single bulbar urethral stricture who had follow-up of at least 6 months after their initial procedure (Table 1(A)). Since our patients are from a tertiary care center, our cohort

TABLE 1

(A) Patient characteristics	
Number of patients	28
Mean age (range)	60 (24–90)
Mean American Society of Anesthesiologists (ASA) physical status classification	2.6
Mean number of prior procedures (range)	5.7 (0–50)
Percent with prior procedures	71%
Mean stricture length (range)	1.85 (0.5–4 cm)
(B) Stricture etiology	
Radiation	32% (9)
Endoscopic procedure	28% (8)
Pelvic trauma	18% (5)
Catheter trauma	11% (3)
Idiopathic	11% (3)
(C) Overall outcomes	
Number of patients	20
Stricture recurrence	8
Recurrence rate	29%
Patient on Uroflowmetry	14
Patient on cystoscopy	4
Patient on self-catheterization	2
Average follow-up	20 months
Time to recurrence for failures	7 months
(D) Complications	
Clavien Grade II: urinary tract infection	14%

tended to be older with average of 60 years; 71% had prior procedures (urethrotomy, dilation, or urethroplasty) and on average had 5-6 prior procedures. Our cohort was at high risk for recurrence based on these characteristics. Patients with longer (>1 cm) or recurrent strictures included in our study either declined urethroplasty or were not surgical candidates for reconstructive procedures.

As seen in Table 1(B), the majority of the strictures were iatrogenic (32% radiation induced, 28% from prior endoscopic procedures, and 11% from traumatic catheterization). The remaining patients either experienced pelvic trauma or did not have an identifiable cause. Our cohort only experienced a recurrence rate of 29% with 20 months of follow-up (Table 1(C)). Failures tended to recur early with a mean of recurrence of 7 months. While 14% of patients were treated for a lower urinary tract infection (Table 1(D)), no other significant complications were noted.

Our study suggests that patients who failed DVIU treatment had greater number of prior procedures and longer length of strictures, although statistical significance was not achieved in our sample size (Table 2). We were able to collect maximum flow velocity data on 19/20 patients who had successful DVIU treatment and 5/8 patients who failed DVIU treatment. Incomplete data was mainly due to loss of follow-up, presence of suprapubic tubes, and no urge for urination. Overall, no significant difference ($p = 0.34$) in the

Outcomes of Direct Vision Internal Urethrotomy for Bulbar Urethral Strictures: Technique Modification...

39

TABLE 2

	Failure (n = 8)	Success (n = 20)
Comparison between treatment failures and successes		
Any prior procedure	100%	60%
Average number of prior procedures	9.8	4
	p = 0.18	
Average stricture length (cm)	2.2	1.7
	p = 0.16	
Etiology		
Radiation	50%	25%
Endoscopic	13%	35%
Pelvic trauma	25%	15%
Catheter trauma	13%	10%
Unknown	0%	15%
Uroflowmetry results		
Average maximum flow velocity (mL/sec)	13.06	14.90
	p = 0.34	
Average follow-up time (days)	143.80	500.11
	p = 0.02	

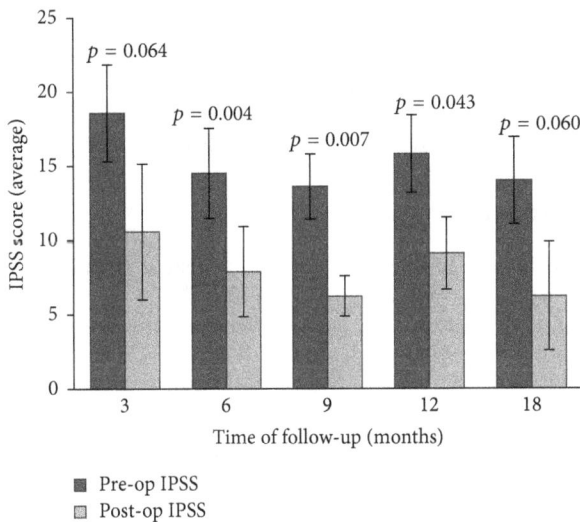

FIGURE 1: Preoperative versus postoperative IPSS at different follow-up times (error bars represent standard error of mean).

last recorded maximum flow velocity was found in patients who were successfully treated (14.90 mL/sec) versus those who failed treatment (13.06 mL/sec). However, there was a significant difference ($p = 0.02$) in follow-up time with those who were successfully treated seen for an average of 500.11 days after treatment while those who failed treatment were seen for an average of 143.80 days after treatment. In addition, analysis of IPSS represented in Figure 1 shows that there was a general trend of decreased IPSS score at all 5 time-points (3, 6, 9, 12, and 18 months) with statistical significance at 6, 9, and 12 months.

4. Discussion

The injection of steroids has also been used to decrease the recurrence of scarring in other fields of medicine. Studies on wound healing of oral mucosa suggest that there is more rapid and scarless healing in mucosal wounds compared to dermal wounds due to differences in expression of extracellular matrix components, immune mediators, and profibrotic mediators, as well as structural differences in blood vessels, mesenchymal stem cells, and fibroblast proliferation rate [7, 8]. Steroids are hypothesized to reduce scar formation by reducing the rate of collagen synthesis in fibroblasts during the wound healing process [9], which may be the mechanism by which steroid injection after urethrotomy delays urethral stricture recurrence. Different doses and methods of delivery have been used for steroids in the management of urethral strictures. Our technique modification uses higher doses of triamcinolone injection after DVIU and an accurate mechanism for delivery. High dose steroids (400 mg) have previously been used in the bladder for treatment of Hunner's ulcer subtype interstitial cystitis with no complications noted [10]. Further randomized studies are needed to determine the ideal dose of steroids.

DVIU is a simple and effective procedure for the management of short urethral strictures. However, stricture recurrence is a significant problem after DVIU particularly for longer and recurrent strictures. We evaluated the efficacy of DVIU with a higher dose of intralesional steroids for all patients who were not able or willing to undergo urethroplasty, regardless of stricture length, prior interventions, or etiology.

Previous studies on intralesional steroid injection after DVIU also demonstrated significantly improved success rates and delayed stricture recurrence compared to DVIU alone. One randomized control trial in fifty male patients showed decreased recurrence rates in the 40 mg triamcinolone group (21.7%) versus control group (50%) after a mean follow-up time of 13.7 ± 5.5 months [5]. Another double-blind, randomized, placebo-controlled study of 70 patients showed that the triamcinolone group versus control group had significantly decreased time to recurrence, 8.08 ± 5.55 months versus 3.6 ± 1.59 months with no evidence of complications from steroid injection [6]. The former study included only patients with bulbar urethral strictures and the later study included 61.42% bulbar and 28.57% penile strictures. Both of these studies only included patients with short strictures and no prior interventions. Another recently published systematic review showed that, in 203 patients across 8 studies, DVIU with corticosteroids were shown to have statistically significant decreased time to recurrence compared to DVIU alone (10.14 versus 5.07 months, $p < 0.00001$) [11].

At our institution, patients identified for our cohort were based on previous evidence endorsing the use of IPSS greater than 15 and maximum flow velocity less than 15 mL/sec as parameters to maximize sensitivity (91%) and specificity (72%) in order to detect the most men with strictures while also excluding a significant portion of those without disease to avoid further invasive testing [12]. Our cohort provides more evidence regarding the efficacy of intralesional steroid injection after DVIU by demonstrating a low recurrence rate (29%) with mean follow-up length of 20 months in patients with a mean of 5.7 prior procedures. In comparison to historical data on patients with no prior intervention, Steenkamp et al. (40% for strictures less than 2 cm, 50% for strictures 2 to 4 cm, and 75% for strictures greater than 4 cm at 12 months) and Pansadoro and Emiliozzi (68% overall and 89% for bulbar urethral strictures at median follow-up of 98 months) showed higher recurrence after single urethrotomy [3, 4]. We are able to demonstrate good efficacy with higher dose steroid injection, especially in patients with long and recurrent strictures. Of the 7 patients, or 25% of the total cohort, who did not have any prior stricture interventions, all of them were successfully treated at a mean follow-up length of 21 months (data not shown).

While our cohort had no significant difference ($p = 0.34$) in the last recorded maximum flow velocity in patients who were successfully treated (14.90 mL/sec) versus those who failed treatment (13.06 mL/sec), there was a significant difference ($p = 0.02$) in follow-up time (500.11 days for successfully treated versus 143.80 days for failed treatment). These results suggest that while final functional outcome may not be improved, successful treatment with DVIU and steroid injection can successfully delay recurrence. We included all Uroflowmetry data collected at clinic in order to minimize selection bias regardless of voiding volume. However, we recognize that a minimum voiding volume of at least 150 mL is often used to avoid inaccurate Uroflowmetry results [13]. In the patients with successful DVIU, patients with maximum flow velocity less than 15 mL/sec ($n = 10$) had an average voiding volume of 109 mL, whereas patients with maximum flow velocity more than 15 mL/sec ($n = 9$) had an average voiding volume of 392 mL ($p = 0.00$). This suggests that one reason why our cohort had no significant difference in maximum flow velocity may be due to low voiding volumes and emphasizes the importance of having patients be informed about needing to perform Uroflowmetry at clinic visits. When considering changes in IPSS scores, DVIU with steroids may help reduce symptoms secondary to urethral strictures at 6, 9, and 12 months but did not have as robust an effect in the subacute period (3 months) and beyond one year. These results altogether support our hypothesis that DVIU with steroids may help delay stricture recurrence and symptoms but does not serve as a permanent solution for urethral strictures.

Some limitations of our study include the retrospective nature of the study and the limited number of patients in our cohort. However, we were able to demonstrate similar efficacy of DVIU with steroid injection as seen in prior studies, despite this study having a more heterogeneous population with strictures at high risk for recurrence. In addition, as mentioned previously, strictures <1 cm have been associated with the highest rate of success [4]. Our study cohort included patients with longer strictures, even up to 4 cm in length, that are often not treated with DVIU. In general, these patients are not recommended to undergo DVIU due to low rates of success previously reported in the literature. However, we encountered patients who were not candidates for reconstructive surgery and after

a patient-centered discussion with the appropriate counseling on the low rates of success for longer strictures, patients who were adamant about pursuing DVIU were granted that option. Another possible limitation is the use of noninvasive techniques (Uroflowmetry and postvoid residual) to monitor stricture recurrence. While performing cystoscopy and/or retrograde urethrography would be more definitive at detecting recurrences, these tests are invasive and patients are subjected to discomfort. Noninvasive methods of stricture surveillance with Uroflowmetry and postvoid residual are widely accepted amongst urologists [14].

5. Conclusions

In our series of patients treated with DVIU and high dose corticosteroid injections, we observed a recurrence rate of only 29% with an average follow-up of 20 month. DVIU with high dose steroids appears to be useful even in those who have had multiple prior interventions and those with longer bulbar urethral strictures. In addition, use of high dose corticosteroids was not associated with any significant adverse side effects. DVIU with high dose corticosteroid injections should be considered in the treatment algorithm of bulbar urethral strictures, particularly for men who are unwilling or unable to undergo urethroplasty. Future randomized control trials are needed to confirm these findings.

Conflict of Interests

The authors have no conflict of interests to disclose.

References

[1] A. R. Mundy and D. E. Andrich, "Urethral strictures," *BJU International*, vol. 107, no. 1, pp. 6–26, 2011.

[2] T. L. Bullock and S. B. Brandes, "Adult anterior urethral strictures: a national practice patterns survey of board certified urologists in the United States," *The Journal of Urology*, vol. 177, no. 2, pp. 685–690, 2007.

[3] J. W. Steenkamp, C. F. Heyns, and M. L. S. de Kock, "Internal urethrotomy versus dilation as treatment for male urethral strictures: a prospective, randomized comparison," *Journal of Urology*, vol. 157, no. 1, pp. 98–101, 1997.

[4] V. Pansadoro and P. Emiliozzi, "Internal urethrotomy in the management of anterior urethral strictures: long-term followup," *The Journal of Urology*, vol. 156, no. 1, pp. 73–75, 1996.

[5] H. Mazdak, M. H. Izadpanahi, A. Ghalamkari et al., "Internal urethrotomy and intraurethral submucosal injection of triamcinolone in short bulbar urethral strictures," *International Urology and Nephrology*, vol. 42, no. 3, pp. 565–568, 2010.

[6] K. T. Tabassi, A. Yarmohamadi, and S. Mohammadi, "Triamcinolone injection following internal urethrotomy for treatment of urethral stricture," *Urology Journal*, vol. 8, no. 2, pp. 132–136, 2011.

[7] J. E. Glim, M. van Egmond, F. B. Niessen, V. Everts, and R. H. J. Beelen, "Detrimental dermal wound healing: what can we learn from the oral mucosa?" *Wound Repair and Regeneration*, vol. 21, no. 5, pp. 648–660, 2013.

[8] J. W. Wong, C. Gallant-Behm, C. Wiebe et al., "Wound healing in oral mucosa results in reduced scar formation as compared

with skin: evidence from the red duroc pig model and humans," *Wound Repair and Regeneration*, vol. 17, no. 5, pp. 717–729, 2009.

[9] S. B. Russell, J. S. Trupin, J. C. Myers et al., "Differential glucocorticoid regulation of collagen mRNAs in human dermal fibroblasts. Keloid-derived and fetal fibroblasts are refractory to down-regulation," *The Journal of Biological Chemistry*, vol. 264, no. 23, pp. 13730–13735, 1989.

[10] M. Cox, J. J. Klutke, and C. G. Klutke, "Assessment of patient outcomes following submucosal injection of triamcinolone for treatment of Hunner's ulcer subtype interstitial cystitis," *The Canadian Journal of Urology*, vol. 16, no. 2, pp. 4536–4540, 2009.

[11] K. Zhang, E. Qi, Y. Zhang, Y. Sa, and Q. Fu, "Efficacy and safety of local steroids for urethra strictures: a systematic review and meta-analysis," *Journal of Endourology*, vol. 28, no. 8, pp. 962–968, 2014.

[12] C. F. Heyns and D. C. Marais, "Prospective evaluation of the American Urological Association symptom index and peak urinary flow rate for the followup of men with known urethral stricture disease," *The Journal of Urology*, vol. 168, no. 5, pp. 2051–2054, 2002.

[13] G. W. Drach, T. N. Layton, and W. J. Binard, "Male peak urinary flow rate: relationships to volume voided and age," *The Journal of Urology*, vol. 122, no. 2, pp. 210–214, 1979.

[14] L. L. Yeung and S. B. Brandes, "Urethroplasty practice and surveillance patterns: a survey of reconstructive urologists," *Urology*, vol. 82, no. 2, pp. 471–475, 2013.

5

Visual Internal Urethrotomy for Adult Male Urethral Stricture Has Poor Long-Term Results

Waleed Al Taweel[1] and Raouf Seyam[1,2]

[1]Department of Urology, King Faisal Hospital and Research Center, Riyadh 11211, Saudi Arabia
[2]Faculty of Medicine, Suez Canal University, Ismailia, Egypt

Correspondence should be addressed to Waleed Al Taweel; drwt1@hotmail.com

Academic Editor: Miroslav L. Djordjevic

Objective. To determine the long-term stricture-free rate after visual internal urethrotomy following initial and follow-up urethrotomies. *Methods.* The records of all male patients who underwent direct visual internal urethrotomy for urethral stricture disease in our hospital between July 2004 and May 2012 were reviewed. The Kaplan-Meier method was used to analyze stricture-free probability after the first, second, third, fourth, and fifth urethrotomies. *Results.* A total of 301 patients were included. The overall stricture-free rate at the 36-month follow-up was 8.3% with a median time to recurrence of 10 months (95% CI of 9.5 to 10.5, range: 2–36). The stricture-free rate after one urethrotomy was 12.1% with a median time to recurrence of eight months (95% CI of 7.1–8.9). After the second urethrotomy, the stricture-free rate was 7.9% with a median time to recurrence of 10 months (95% CI of 9.3 to 10.6). After the third to fifth procedures, the stricture-free rate was 0%. There was no significant difference in the stricture-free rate between single and multiple procedures. *Conclusion.* The long-term stricture-free rate of visual internal urethrotomy is modest even after a single procedure.

1. Introduction

Male urethral stricture continues to be a common and challenging urologic condition. Despite the high failure rate of visual internal urethrotomy (VIU), it remains the most commonly performed procedure for the treatment of urethral strictures [1–7]. Even when VIU is initially performed selectively for short bulbar strictures under optimal conditions, the recurrence rate at 12 months was approximately 40% for strictures shorter than 2 cm. VIU and/or urethral dilation is usually the initial treatment approach offered in most cases of male urethral stricture, with no difference in efficacy between urethral dilation and urethrotomy [8–10]. Repeated urethrotomies were not associated with an improved success rate, and VIU for longer strictures usually failed [11, 12]. Urethral reconstruction is usually offered only after repeated failed transurethral stricture treatments, which in some cases span several years [13]. Unfortunately, repeated transurethral manipulation of bulbar strictures is associated with increased stricture complexity, stricture length, and a marked delay to

curative urethroplasty [14]. Few studies have shown long-term follow-up of patients after VIU [11].

The purposes of this study are to report the overall success rate of VIU and to analyze whether repeated VIUs are associated with a long-term stricture-free rate. This study reflects urologic practice in real-life situations by multiple urologists in a busy tertiary care hospital.

2. Materials and Methods

This is a retrospective study of male patients who presented to the Department of Urology and underwent VIU for urethral stricture disease between July 2004 and May 2012. We evaluated the long-term stricture-free rate after visual internal urethrotomy following initial and subsequent urethrotomies.

We extracted data from medical records and our Integrated Clinical Information System on ascending urethrogram findings, including the site and length of stricture, number of previous urethrotomies, and presence of complex stricture (after urethroplasty or after radiation). All patients with symptoms or signs suggestive of urethral stricture underwent a urethrogram to confirm the diagnosis and determine urethral stricture length. All patients underwent cystourethroscopy before urethrotomy, confirming the diagnosis.

Four urologists performed the urethrotomies using a single incision at the 12 o'clock position or using a modified procedure including multiple radial incisions at the 3, 9, and 12 o'clock positions; the incisions were made with a cold knife or laser. Associated fossa navicularis stricture was treated with meatotomy prior to urethrotomy. Penile urethral strictures were treated with cold knife urethrotomy.

Follow-up data included subjective and objective results and whether subsequent intervention was needed. Symptoms of recurrence included decreased force of the urine stream, feelings of incomplete bladder emptying, or recurrent urinary tract infections. Signs of recurrence were a significant increase in postvoid residual urine on bladder ultrasound or bladder scan, decreased urine flow rate (<15 mL/second), or stricture as determined by diagnostic cystoscopy or retrograde urethrogram. Absence of symptoms or signs of recurrent stricture in any patient at last follow-up defined the success of the procedure. The end point of the follow-up was the last visit that showed failure of treatment or being recurrence-free for 36 months. Only data up to the fifth recurrence after repeated urethrotomy were included.

The Kaplan-Meier method was used to evaluate the stricture-free rate (survival function) after the first, second, third, fourth, and fifth urethrotomies. We used the Statistical Package of Social Science (SPSS, version 20, IBM Corporation, NY, USA). The log-rank test was used to compare survival differences between procedures.

3. Results and Discussion

3.1. Results. The mean age was 37 years (range: 17–82). A total of 446 male patients with urethral stricture disease were identified in the computerized records of the Department of Urology. Sixty-three patients were lost during follow-up. We excluded 82 patients who had complex urethral strictures, strictures longer than 5 cm, or dense palpable spongiofibrosis. This left 301 eligible patients who continued follow-up until the failure of urethrotomy was observed, at which point an alternative management plan was offered to them. We reported the duration of follow-up and time to failure of urethrotomy as the same duration. Further management and follow-up are excluded from this paper.

The stricture characteristics are shown in Table 1. The most common location is bulbar urethral stricture in 227 (75%) patients, penile urethral stricture in 36 (11%) patients, combined penile and bulbar urethral stricture in 24 (8%) patients, and fossa navicularis stricture in 14 (5%) patients. The mean stricture length was 13 mm (range: 4–42). The overall stricture-free rate at the 36-month follow-up was 8.3% with a median time to recurrence of 10 months (95% CI 9.5 to 10.5, range: 2–36). The success rate following single urethrotomy was modest and dropped significantly after repeated urethrotomies (Table 2).

TABLE 1: Stricture characteristics.

Stricture length	Location	Number of patients
<1 cm	Penile	14
	Bulbar	75
	Penile and bulbar	0
	Fossa navicularis	2
1-2 cm	Penile	16
	Bulbar	87
	Penile and bulbar	10
	Fossa navicularis	4
>2 cm	Penile	6
	Bulbar	65
	Penile and bulbar	14
	Fossa navicularis	8

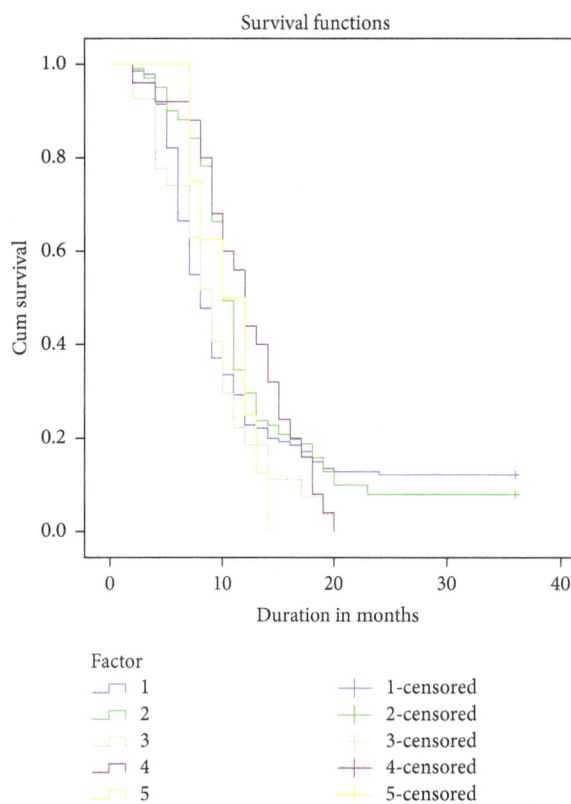

FIGURE 1: Stricture-free probability after the first, second, third, fourth, and fifth urethrotomies (Kaplan-Meier survival analysis).

Most recurrences occurred within the first postoperative year. Survivors or patients without recurrence were only those with a stricture length of <1 cm and in the bulbar urethra. There was no significant difference in the survival analysis of duration to recurrence among patients undergoing single or multiple procedures ($p = 0.181$, Figure 1). There was no significant difference in the outcome based on the length of the stricture or the type of treatment.

3.2. Discussion. Urethral strictures are often treated with urethrotomy, most commonly direct visual internal urethrotomy [15]. With the introduction of lasers, holmium laser

TABLE 2: Urethrotomy and stricture-free rate.

Number of urethrotomies	Stricture-free rate	Median time to failure (months)	Number of stricture-free patients	Total number of patients (%)
First	12.1%	8 (95% CI 7.1 to 8.9)	17	140 (46.5%)
Second	7.9%	10 (95% CI 9.4 to 10.6)	8	101 (33.6%)
Third	0%	9 (95% CI 7.3 to 10.7)	0	27 (9%)
Fourth	0%	12 (95% CI 10.4 to 13.6)	0	25 (8.3%)
Fifth	0%	10 (95% CI 6.3 to 13.7)	0	9 (3%)
Overall	8.3%	10 (95% CI 9.5 to 10.5)	25	301 (100%)

urethrotomy was subsequently used in many centers with equal recurrence outcomes as achieved with VIU [16, 17]. Many urologists prefer VIU over urethral reconstruction because of its ease to perform, low cost, short hospital stay, and perceived low complication rate. They may opt to repeat VIU several times to avoid complex urethral reconstruction, which requires significant surgical experience. This trend continues despite the moderate success rate reported in the selected patients. To reduce the stricture recurrence rate, several investigators evaluated different intralesional adjuvant injections with variable success [18–23]. We set out to report the results of VIU of our patients, including a wider inclusion base and strict criteria of success in a long follow-up period. We felt that these patients constitute a real patient group that tempts urologist to repeatedly administer VIU for the management of their stricture.

Our stricture-free rate of 8.3% at a median of 10 months (range: 2–36) is much lower than that reported by others on long-term follow-up [24]. Heyns et al. found that, after a single dilation or urethrotomy in patients who did not experience restricture within 3 months, the estimated stricture-free rate was 50–60% at 48 months [24]. The higher success rate in that study might be related to the exclusion of patients who failed the treatment in the first three months from the analysis and the shorter stricture length. Another study reported a 32% recurrence-free rate after a median follow-up of 98 months following a single internal urethrotomy. The prognostic characteristics of bulbar urethral strictures associated with good results included single or primary strictures and length shorter than 10 mm [11, 25]. The inclusion of strictures from 1 to 4 cm and the strict success criteria in our study might explain a more realistic success rate of 12.1% after single VIU. Comparison of studies that evaluate the outcome of stricture urethra treatment is greatly affected by the success criteria. This heterogeneity of the definition of success has been clearly shown in a meta-analysis of urethroplasty outcome involving more than 300 articles [26]. We did not separately report the details of the differences in outcome between different stricture lengths, associated location, or type of treatment because there was no significant difference. A focus on these comparisons would have been extremely relevant if we had a significant success rate. However, the overall success rate was poor. Only 25 patients remained stricture-free at 10 months. Compared to the total of 301 patients, subgroup analysis did not show a significant difference because of the small number of successful cases in each comparison cell.

Repeated VIU was associated with more dismal outcomes. This is in accordance with the previously reported data [11, 24, 27]. We found no significant advantage of single versus repeated VIU. We think that the inclusion of long strictures at different sites masks the claimed advantage of single VIU. Our findings stress that an early attempt at urethroplasty is warranted. This is particularly important because repeated urethrotomies have a negative impact on the success of subsequent urethroplasty [28].

Several studies have examined the cost-effectiveness of managing anterior urethral strictures. Urethroplasty as the primary therapy was cost-effective only when the expected success rate of the first VIU was less than 35% [29], whereas VIU became more favorable when the long-term risk of stricture recurrence was less than 60% [30]. If a repeat urethrotomy is required, open urethroplasty is the treatment of choice for recurrent urethral stricture.

4. Conclusions

Visual internal urethrotomy is a simple and popular treatment for male urethral stricture; however, the long-term stricture-free rate is modest even after only a single procedure. Most of the recurrences were found to occur within one year. Thus, definitive curative reconstruction should be planned as early as possible. Repeated visual internal urethrotomies should be considered only in patients who are poor surgical candidates and not because of the convenience of performing a simple procedure.

Conflict of Interests

The authors report no conflict of interests.

References

[1] J. T. Anger, J. C. Buckley, R. A. Santucci, S. P. Elliott, and C. S. Saigal, "Trends in stricture management among male medicare beneficiaries: underuse of urethroplasty?" *Urology*, vol. 77, no. 2, pp. 481–486, 2011.

[2] T. L. Bullock and S. B. Brandes, "Adult anterior urethral strictures: a national practice patterns survey of board certified urologists in the United States," *Journal of Urology*, vol. 177, no. 2, pp. 685–690, 2007.

[3] R. Veeratterapillay and R. S. Pickard, "Long-term effect of urethral dilatation and internal urethrotomy for urethral strictures," *Current Opinion in Urology*, vol. 22, no. 6, pp. 467–473, 2012.

[4] M. A. van Leeuwen, J. J. Brandenburg, E. T. Kok, P. L. M. Vijverberg, and J. L. H. R. Bosch, "Management of adult anterior urethral stricture disease: nationwide survey among urologists in the netherlands," *European Urology*, vol. 60, no. 1, pp. 159–166, 2011.

[5] M. A. Granieri and A. C. Peterson, "The management of bulbar urethral stricture disease before referral for definitive repair: have practice patterns changed?" *Urology*, vol. 84, no. 4, pp. 946–949, 2014.

[6] E. Palminteri, S. Maruccia, E. Berdondini, G. B. Di Pierro, O. Sedigh, and F. Rocco, "Male urethral strictures: a national survey among urologists in Italy," *Urology*, vol. 83, no. 2, pp. 477–482, 2014.

[7] G. G. Ferguson, T. L. Bullock, R. E. Anderson, R. E. Blalock, and S. B. Brandes, "Minimally invasive methods for bulbar urethral strictures: a survey of members of the American Urological Association," *Urology*, vol. 78, no. 3, pp. 701–706, 2011.

[8] J. W. Steenkamp, C. F. Heyns, and M. L. S. De Kock, "Internal urethrotomy versus dilation as treatment for male urethral strictures: a prospective, randomized comparison," *Journal of Urology*, vol. 157, no. 1, pp. 98–101, 1997.

[9] S. S. W. Wong, O. M. Aboumarzouk, R. Narahari, A. O'Riordan, and R. Pickard, "Simple urethral dilatation, endoscopic urethrotomy, and urethroplasty for urethral stricture disease in adult men," *Cochrane Database of Systematic Reviews*, vol. 12, Article ID CD006934, 2012.

[10] J. W. Steenkamp, C. F. Heyns, and M. L. S. de Kock, "Outpatient treatment for male urethral strictures—dilatation versus internal urethrotomy," *South African Journal of Surgery*, vol. 35, no. 3, pp. 125–130, 1997.

[11] V. Pansadoro and P. Emiliozzi, "Internal urethrotomy in the management of anterior urethral strictures: long-term followup," *Journal of Urology*, vol. 156, no. 1, pp. 73–75, 1996.

[12] A. A. Zehri, M. H. Ather, and Q. Afshan, "Predictors of recurrence of urethral stricture disease following optical urethrotomy," *International Journal of Surgery*, vol. 7, no. 4, pp. 361–364, 2009.

[13] C. F. Heyns, J. van der Merwe, J. Basson, and A. van der Merwe, "Treatment of male urethral strictures—possible reasons for the use of repeated dilatation or internal urethrotomy rather than urethroplasty," *South African Journal of Surgery*, vol. 50, no. 3, pp. 82–87, 2012.

[14] S. J. Hudak, T. H. Atkinson, and A. F. Morey, "Repeat transurethral manipulation of bulbar urethral strictures is associated with increased stricture complexity and prolonged disease duration," *Journal of Urology*, vol. 187, no. 5, pp. 1691–1695, 2012.

[15] T. J. Greenwell, C. Castle, D. E. Andrich, J. T. MacDonald, D. L. Nicol, and A. R. Mundy, "Repeat urethrotomy and dilation for the treatment of urethral stricture are neither clinically effective nor cost-effective," *The Journal of Urology*, vol. 172, no. 1, pp. 275–277, 2004.

[16] S. Kamp, T. Knoll, M. M. Osman, K. U. Köhrmann, M. S. Michel, and P. Alken, "Low-power holmium: YAG laser urethrotomy for treatment of urethral strictures: functional outcome and quality of life," *Journal of Endourology*, vol. 20, no. 1, pp. 38–41, 2006.

[17] S. A. Dutkiewicz and M. Wroblewski, "Comparison of treatment results between holmium laser endourethrotomy and optical internal urethrotomy for urethral stricture," *International Urology and Nephrology*, vol. 44, no. 3, pp. 717–724, 2012.

[18] S. Kumar, N. Garg, S. K. Singh, and A. K. Mandal, "Efficacy of optical internal urethrotomy and intralesional injection of Vatsala-Santosh PGI tri-inject (triamcinolone, mitomycin C, and hyaluronidase) in the treatment of anterior urethral stricture," *Advances in Urology*, vol. 2014, Article ID 192710, 4 pages, 2014.

[19] H. Mazdak, I. Meshki, and F. Ghassami, "Effect of mitomycin C on anterior urethral stricture recurrence after internal urethrotomy," *European Urology*, vol. 51, no. 4, pp. 1089–1092, 2007.

[20] E. Hradec, L. Jarolim, and R. Petrik, "Optical internal urethrotomy for strictures of the male urethra. Effect of local steroid injection," *European Urology*, vol. 7, no. 3, pp. 165–168, 1981.

[21] H. Mazdak, M. H. Izadpanahi, A. Ghalamkari et al., "Internal urethrotomy and intraurethral submucosal injection of triamcinolone in short bulbar urethral strictures," *International Urology and Nephrology*, vol. 42, no. 3, pp. 565–568, 2010.

[22] S. Kumar, A. Kapoor, R. Ganesamoni, B. Nanjappa, V. Sharma, and U. K. Mete, "Efficacy of holmium laser urethrotomy in combination with intralesional triamcinolone in the treatment of anterior urethral stricture," *Korean Journal of Urology*, vol. 53, no. 9, pp. 614–618, 2012.

[23] H. M. Kim, D. I. Kang, B. S. Shim, and K. S. Min, "Early experience with hyaluronic acid instillation to assist with visual internal urethrotomy for urethral stricture," *Korean Journal of Urology*, vol. 51, no. 12, pp. 853–857, 2010.

[24] C. F. Heyns, J. W. Steenkamp, M. L. S. De Kock, and P. Whitaker, "Treatment of male urethral strictures: is repeated dilation or internal urethrotomy useful?" *Journal of Urology*, vol. 160, no. 2, pp. 356–358, 1998.

[25] M. Ishigooka, M. Tomaru, T. Hashimoto, I. Sasagawa, T. Nakada, and K. Mitobe, "Recurrence of urethral stricture after single internal urethrotomy," *International Urology and Nephrology*, vol. 27, no. 1, pp. 101–106, 1995.

[26] J. J. Meeks, B. A. Erickson, M. A. Granieri, and C. M. Gonzalez, "Stricture recurrence after urethroplasty: a systematic review," *Journal of Urology*, vol. 182, no. 4, pp. 1266–1270, 2009.

[27] R. Santucci and L. Eisenberg, "Urethrotomy has a much lower success rate than previously reported," *The Journal of Urology*, vol. 183, no. 5, pp. 1859–1862, 2010.

[28] T. M. Kessler, F. Schreiter, G. Kralidis, M. Heitz, R. Olianas, and M. Fisch, "Long-term results of surgery for urethral stricture: a statistical analysis," *Journal of Urology*, vol. 170, no. 3, pp. 840–844, 2003.

[29] J. L. Wright, H. Wessells, A. B. Nathens, and W. Hollingworth, "What is the most cost-effective treatment for 1 to 2-cm bulbar urethral strictures: societal approach using decision analysis," *Urology*, vol. 67, no. 5, pp. 889–893, 2006.

[30] K. F. Rourke and G. H. Jordan, "Primary urethral reconstruction: the cost minimized approach to the bulbous urethral stricture," *Journal of Urology*, vol. 173, no. 4, pp. 1206–1210, 2005.

6

A Randomized Controlled Trial to Compare the Safety and Efficacy of Tadalafil and Tamsulosin in Relieving Double J Stent Related Symptoms

Satinder Pal Aggarwal, Shivam Priyadarshi, Vinay Tomar, S. S. Yadav, Goto Gangkak, Nachiket Vyas, Neeraj Agarwal, and Ujwal Kumar

SMS Medical College and Hospital, Jaipur 302004, India

Correspondence should be addressed to Satinder Pal Aggarwal; satinderpalaggarwal@gmail.com

Academic Editor: Darius J. Bagli

Objectives. To evaluate the safety and efficacy of Tadalafil and Tamsulosin in treating Double J stent related symptoms. *Methods.* In a prospective study, 161 patients with DJ related symptoms were randomized into 3 groups: Group A patients (54), Group B patients (53), and Group C patients (54). They were given Tadalafil, Tamsulosin, and placebo, respectively, at 1st week till removal of DJ stent at 3rd week. All patients completed Ureteral Stent Symptom Questionnaire (USSQ) at 1st week and at 3rd week. The statistical significant difference among groups was determined by the t-test, Kruskal-Wallis test and multivariate analysis were used to assess association of the variables within the three groups, and the level of significance was set at $P < 0.05$. *Results.* Tadalafil and Tamsulosin were comparable in relieving urinary symptoms, general health, and work performance (OR = 0.65, 1.8, and 0.92). But Tadalafil was more effective in relieving body pain, sexual problems, and additional problems than Tamsulosin (OR = 5.95, 19.25, and 2.69) and was statistically significant as $P < 0.05$. *Conclusion.* Tadalafil was as effective as Tamsulosin in relieving urinary symptom but more effective in relieving sexual symptoms and body pain.

1. Introduction

Since its first introduction by Zimskind et al. in 1967, endoscopic stent placement has become an indispensable part of urology [1]. Early era was plagued with frequent stent migration and expulsion. Development of the Double J (DJ) and pigtail stents by Finney and Hepperlen (1978) solved these problems, making ureteral stenting a routine urological procedure [2]. It is employed for relief of ureteral obstruction and ureteral injury and as a ureteral splint in various open, laparoscopic, and endourological procedures.

Despite its usefulness, DJ stent leads to morbid lower urinary tract symptoms (LUTS) such as frequency (50–60%), urgency (57–60%), dysuria (40%), flank pain (19–32%), suprapubic pain (30%), and hematuria (25%), affecting quality of life in approximately 80% of patients [3–5]. More than 80% of patients experience stent related pain affecting daily activities, 32% report sexual dysfunction, and 58% report reduced work capacity [5]. Joshi et al.

had developed a validated self-administered Ureteral Stent Symptom Questionnaire (USSQ), for evaluating stent related symptoms in the clinical and research settings [6]. These symptoms are managed by alpha blockers, anticholinergics, and analgesics [7–18]. Tamsulosin, a selective α-1a/1d blocker, inhibits contraction of the smooth muscles in distal ureter, bladder trigone, and neck, relieving LUTS and flank pain.

PDE-5 receptors are present over lower ureter, trigone, and bladder neck. The role of Tadalafil, PDE-5 inhibitor, in sexual dysfunction, relieving bladder outlet obstruction related lower urinary tract obstruction (LUTS) and lower ureteric stone expulsion, is well studied. The purpose of this study was to evaluate and compare the efficacy and safety of Tadalafil and Tamsulosin.

2. Materials and Methods

This prospective placebo controlled double blind randomized study was conducted among 220 patients (154 men and 66 women) who underwent DJ stenting after uneventful endourological surgeries by a single surgeon from February 2014 to March 2015. The study protocol was approved by the institutional ethics committee and all patients enrolled in this study gave written informed consent.

All patients (aged 18 to 50 years) undergoing unilateral percutaneous nephrolithotomy (PCNL) or ureteroscopic lithotripsy URSL (bilateral normally excreting kidneys) with DJ stenting were evaluated for enrollment in the study. Patients with age less than 18 years and more than 50 years, patients taking nitrate drugs, patients with postoperative residual stone fragments, pregnant women, and patients with bilateral stents, long-term stenting (on regular change), bladder/prostate pathology (leading to irritative bladder symptoms: prostatomegaly, prostatitis, carcinoma prostate, overactive bladder, and neurogenic bladder), history of lower urinary tract surgery, and chronic use of selective alpha-1 blocker and/or anticholinergic agents were excluded from study.

URSL was done with 6.5/8.5 Fr ureteroscope (Wolf) and laser lithotripsy (holmium). PCNL was done using 26 Fr nephroscope (Wolf) and pneumatic lithotripter. The decision for stent placement was taken by operating urologist, depending upon large stone burden, mucosal trauma, and need for ureteral dilation to access tight ureters. 6 Fr and 26 cm long DJ stent composed of polyurethane material was put under fluoroscopy guidance. Postoperative X-ray KUB was done in all patients to rule out residual stone fragment. On day of surgery, injection of ceftazidime 1 gm i/v was given prophylactically to all patients. Foleys catheter was removed on 1st post-op day in both PCNL and URSL patients. Nephrostomy tubes were removed on 2nd post-op day in PCNL patients. Tab levofloxacin 500 mg OD was given for 7 days postoperatively, as per our institutional protocol. Patients were informed about DJ related symptoms and were given USSQ at discharge. They were asked to come after 1 week with completed questionnaire, if they experience symptoms. Scoring at 1st week was done to see the magnitude of DJ related symptoms.

After applying inclusion and exclusion criteria, 161 patients reported DJ related symptoms at 1st week and they were randomized into 3 groups (A, B, and C) in a ratio of 1:1:1 by computer generated module. Group A (54 patients) were put on Tab Tadalafil 5 mg OD, Group B (53 patients) were put on Tab Tamsulosin 0.4 mg OD, and Group C (54 patients) were put on placebo OD. Patients were advised to take analgesics (diclofenac) as per need. Tb Tadalafil 5 mg, Tb Tamsulosin 0.4 mg, and sugar coated placebo tablets were put in 3 identical bottles. Double blinding was done to minimize bias. Nursing staff gave the drug bottle to patient by chit method. All patients were informed about side effects of drugs. They were given USSQ and were asked to come with completed USSQ at 3rd week, before removal of DJ stent. Out of the 158 patients, 2 patients were lost to follow-up, 3 had urinary tract infection (UTI), 1 had hematuria (so early removal of stent), and 2 had stent migration. So data of these 8 patients were not analyzed (Figure 1). Analgesic requirement and side effects of drug during study period in each group were noted.

TABLE 1: Basic parameters of patients.

Variables	Group A Tadalafil	Group B Tamsulosin	Group C Placebo
Patients (n)	52	51	50
Mean age (years)	32.2	34.3	33.4
Sex (M : F)	37:15	35:16	38:12
Average height	5′6″	5′7″	5′6″
Procedures			
PCNL	33	32	33
URSL	19	19	17

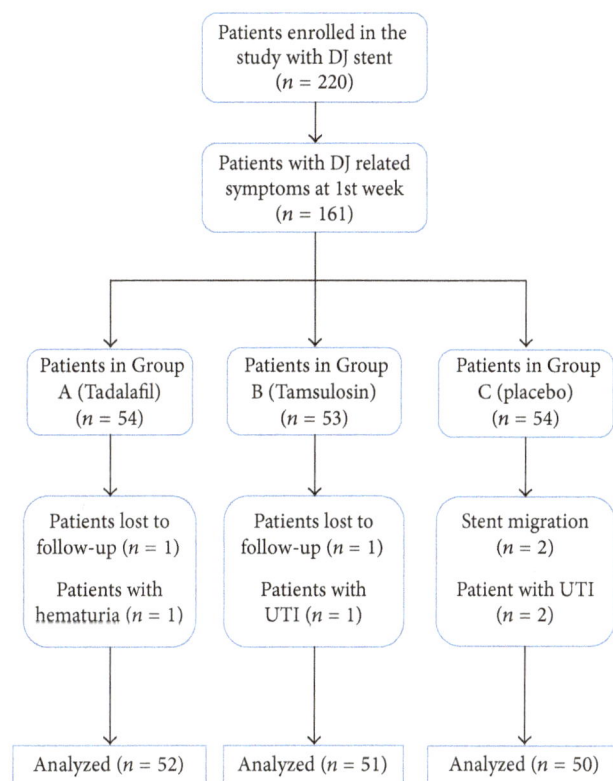

FIGURE 1: Study design.

Data so collected was tabulated in an excel sheet, under the guidance of statistician. Data was analyzed using IBM SPSS Statistics Windows, Version 20.0 (Armonk, NY: IBM Corp.) for the generation of descriptive and inferential statistics. The statistical significant difference among groups was determined by the t-test, Kruskal-Wallis test and multivariate analysis were used to assess association of the variables within the three groups, and the level of significance was set at $P < 0.05$.

3. Results

Out of 220 patients, 161 patients complained of DJ related symptoms (73.2%). Mean age, male to female ratio, average height, and procedures performed were uniform in all 3 groups (Table 1).

TABLE 2: Ureteral stent symptom score at 1st week and 3rd week in three groups.

	Group A (Tadalafil)		t-test	Group B (Tamsulosin)		t-test	Group C (placebo)		t-test
	1st week	3rd week		1st week	3rd week		1st week	3rd week	
Urinary symptoms	40 (12–50)	20.1 (4–24)	**<0.0001**	42.3 (10–51)	21.8 (4.2–28)	**<0.0001**	43 (15–51)	42 (16–49)	0.12
Body pain	20 (4–25)	7.1 (3–14)	**<0.0001**	17 (3–22)	13.4 (3.9–19)	**0.02**	18.8 (12–22)	17 (11–20)	0.06
Sexual health	8 (2–10)	2.9 (1–5)	**<0.0001**	7 (2.3–11)	5.9 (1.6–9)	**0.03**	9 (6–10)	8.2 (4–9)	0.08
General health	23 (13–27)	19.2 (9–22)	**<0.0001**	22 (14–28)	19.6 (7–21)	**<0.0001**	25.6 (11–27)	24.9 (13–25)	0.27
Work performance	14 (4–15)	12.2 (4–14)	**0.03**	12 (3.3–15)	10 (4–13)	**0.02**	15 (12–15)	14 (11–15)	0.27
Additional problems	13 (12–18)	12.4 (3–14)	0.32	12 (3.5–20)	11.8 (3–17)	0.21	16.6 (7–18)	16.3 (8–18)	0.51
Analgesic used Diclofenac (mg)	600[A]			1250[B]			2200[C]		<0.0001[*]

[*]Kruskal-Wallis test; values in the column with different letters indicate significant differences at $P < 0.05$.

TABLE 3: Comparison of mean difference of ureteral stent symptom score at 1st week and 3rd week in three groups.

Characteristics	Mean difference at 1st & 3rd week of three groups			P value
	Group A (Tadalafil)	Group B (Tamsulosin)	Group C (placebo)	
Urinary symptoms	19.9[A]	20.5[A]	1[C]	<0.0001
Body pain	12.9[A]	3.6[B]	1.8[C]	<0.0001
Sexual health	5.1[A]	1.1[B]	0.8[B]	<0.0001
General health	3.8[A]	2.4[B]	0.7[C]	<0.0001
Work performance	1.8[A]	2[A]	1[B]	<0.0001
Additional problems	0.6[A]	0.2[A]	0.3[A]	0.21

[*]Kruskal-Wallis test; values in the column with different letters indicate significant differences at $P < 0.05$.

Both Tadalafil and Tamsulosin led to significant decrease in urinary symptoms, body pain, sexual health, general health, and work performance scores at 3rd week as compared to 1st week score. Placebo does not lead to improvement in symptom score over study period. Also analgesic requirement was significantly less in Tadalafil group as compared to both Tamsulosin and placebo group (Table 2).

For comparing efficacy of Tadalafil with Tamsulosin, mean decrease in symptom score within each group was analyzed using Kruskal-Wallis test (Table 3). Decrease in urinary symptoms, work performance and additional problems were similar in Tadalafil and Tamsulosin group. Improvement in body pain, sexual health, and general health was significantly more in Tadalafil group than both Tamsulosin and placebo group.

When multivariate analysis was applied to assess mean symptom score difference of 1st and 3rd week among three groups, both Tadalafil and Tamsulosin are comparable in relieving urinary symptoms, general health, and work performance (OR = 0.65, 1.8, and 0.92) Table 4. But Tadalafil is more effective in relieving body pain, sexual problems, and additional problems than Tamsulosin (OR = 5.95, 19.25, and 2.69) and was statistically significant as $P < 0.05$. Side effects of Tadalafil and Tamsulosin were minimal. No patient left study due to side effects of drugs.

4. Discussion

DJ stenting is an integral part of today's urology practice. DJ stenting leads to LUTS in 80% of patients, leading to reduced health related quality of life (HrQOL). DJ related symptoms include frequency, urgency, dysuria, hematuria, flank pain, suprapubic pain, and sexual dysfunction [3–5]. Our understanding of pathophysiology of these symptoms is lacking but improving. Bladder mucosal irritation due to contact by the distal curl of the stent, ureteral smooth muscle spasm, and reflux of urine resulting in flank pain are the proposed mechanisms [4]. The USSQ evaluates stent related symptoms in six domains—urinary symptoms, body pain, general health, work performance, sexual performance, and other problems. The urinary symptoms domain has 11 questions. The body pain domain has pain experience, visual analog scale, and six questions. The general health, work performance, and sexual performance domains have six, seven, and four questions, respectively. Each question has 4 to 7 scores. Scores from each question are added to give total score, with higher score indicating more bothersome symptoms [6].

Management of DJ related symptoms is still improving with better understanding of pathophysiology of symptoms. Management is based on preventive and pharmaceutical methods. Preventive strategies include avoiding DJ stenting in uncomplicated cases, appropriate stent length as per patient height, proper positioning, drug eluting stents, and patient counseling regarding symptoms [19–25]. Since the inception of DJ stenting, the quest is still going on for improving DJ design and material to decrease DJ related morbidity. Various modifications in DJ stent design and material have led to reduction in DJ related symptoms [26]. Rane et al. advocated use of appropriate sized DJ, so that bladder curl does not cross the midline to minimize irritation of trigone and thus symptoms [27].

TABLE 4: Multiple regression analysis of mean ureteral stent symptom score at 1st week and 3rd week in three groups.

Variables	Group A Tadalafil	Group B Tamsulosin			Group C Placebo		
	N	N	OR (CI)	P value	N	OR (CI)	P value
Urinary symptoms >20	24	29	0.65 (0.30–1.42)	0.28	0	86.82 (5.09–991.42)	<0.0001
Body pain >10	23	6	5.95 (2.16–16.37)	0.0006	1	40.25 (5.15–314.32)	<0.0001
Sexual health >5	22	2	19.25 (4.21–88.03)	<0.0001	1	35.93 (4.60–280.50)	<0.0001
General health >3	31	22	1.8 (0.86–4.13)	0.12	2	35.43 (7.76–161.84)	<0.0001
Work performance >2	27	27	0.96 (0.44–2.08)	0.92	13	3.07 (1.34–7.08)	0.008
Additional problems >1	19	9	2.69 (1.08–6.71)	0.03	8	3.0227 (1.18–7.77)	0.02

Alpha blockers, anticholinergics, or their combination is prescribed empirically. Alpha blockers result in a significant reduction in the peak contraction pressure, leading to ureteral dilation [28]. Thus, alpha blockers by decreasing muscle spasm and intrarenal urinary reflux may explain the ability to relieve flank pain. Irritative symptoms (frequency, dysuria, and urgency) may improve because of the alpha receptors blockage at the bladder trigone. Deliveliotis et al. were the first to demonstrate that Alfuzosin relieved the stent related symptoms, pain and improved sexual and general health [7]. Beddingfield et al. also concluded in their study that Alfuzosin 10 mg daily improved frequency and flank pain [8]. Similarly, Wang et al. reported that Tamsulosin improved urinary symptoms and flank pain during voiding [9]. More various trials have confirmed the efficacy of alpha blockers in relieving stent related symptoms, making alpha blockers the most commonly prescribed agents [10–13]. Similarly in our study, Tamsulosin was effective in relieving urinary symptoms, body pain, general health, and work performance as compared to placebo. Improvement in general health and work performance can be explained by decreased urinary and body pain symptom score.

Bladder coil of stent may irritate trigone and lead to OAB like symptoms. This hypothesis leads to use of anticholinergics in relieving DJ related symptoms. Lee et al. studied the role of solifenacin in placebo controlled randomized study and found it to be effective [14]. Similarly Park et al. reported efficacy of tolterodine in relieving stent related LUTS in their prospective randomized controlled study [15]. Assuming that both alpha and cholinergic receptors have a role to play in genesis of DJ stent related symptoms, studies have been done comparing combination with monotherapy, proving combination to be better than monotherapy [16–18].

PDE-5 inhibitors are rapidly expanding their therapeutic indications. They are FDA approved for managing erectile dysfunction, prostatomegaly related bladder outlet obstruction, and pulmonary hypertension. They are studied in various randomized trials for medical expulsion therapy for lower ureteric stone expulsion therapy. Tadalafil also relaxes ureter by blocking PDE-5 receptors present on lower ureter, thus reducing spasm and reflux. PDE-5 receptors are also present on bladder trigone and neck; thus by blocking these receptors irritative symptoms might be taken care of. Hajebrahimi et al. conducted a placebo controlled randomized trial to evaluate role of Tadalafil in relieving stent related symptoms. In their study, Tadalafil improved stent associated urinary symptoms, body pain, and sexual matter [29]. We conducted a randomized trial comparing three groups Tadalafil versus Tamsulosin versus placebo in relieving stent related symptoms unlike only couple of studies done in the past (one of which was pilot study and others involve only two groups, i.e., placebo and Tadalafil). So, our study in addition gives comparison in relieving stent related symptoms between Tadalafil and most commonly used alpha blocker Tamsulosin. In our study, Tadalafil was effective in relieving urinary symptoms, body pain, sexual health, general health, and work performance as compared to placebo. In comparison to Tamsulosin, Tadalafil is equally effective in relieving urinary symptoms, general health, and work performance but more effective in relieving body pain, sexual problems, and additional problems. Similar relief in urinary symptoms may be due to similar action of ureteral and trigonal smooth muscle. Increased sexual symptom improvement can be due to resolution of erectile dysfunction and decrease in body pain.

Ours is a single center study; DJ stent was not height specific, use of only single stent design and material which forms limitations of the study. Though the groups were randomized, the effect of same length DJ stent should not have any bearing on the difference in results under each group. Moreover, the average height of patients is also same in all the three groups. To validate the results of our study further large multicentric studies are required.

5. Conclusion

Tadalafil is safe and effective in relieving DJ related symptoms. Tadalafil is as effective as Tamsulosin in relieving urinary symptom but more effective in relieving sexual symptoms and body pain. Therefore Tadalafil could be recommended as preferred drug in sexually active patients undergoing DJ stenting.

Conflict of Interests

The authors declare that there is no conflict of interests regarding the publication of this paper.

Acknowledgments

The authors would like to thank Dr. Ankush Jairath, urologist, Muljibhai Patel Urological Hospital, Nadiad, and Dr. Suresh Goyal, urologist, Dr. SN Medical College, Jodhpur, for reviewing the paper.

References

[1] P. D. Zimskind, T. R. Fetter, and J. L. Wilkerson, "Clinical use of long-term indwelling silicone rubber ureteral splints inserted cystoscopically," *Journal of Urology*, vol. 97, no. 5, pp. 840–844, 1967.

[2] E. Carlos, M. Probst, H. Razvi, and J. D. Denstedt, "Fundamentals of instrumentation and urinary tract drainage," in *Campbell-Walsh Urology*, L. R. Kavoussi, A. W. Partin, and C. A. Peters, Eds., p. 183, Elsevier, Philadelphia, Pa, USA, 10th edition, 2012.

[3] H. B. Joshi, A. Okeke, N. Newns, F. X. Keeley Jr., and A. G. Timoney, "Characterization of urinary symptoms in patients with ureteral stents," *Urology*, vol. 59, no. 4, pp. 511–516, 2002.

[4] R. Thomas, "Indwelling ureteral stents: impact of material and shape on patient comfort," *Journal of Endourology*, vol. 7, no. 2, pp. 137–140, 1993.

[5] H. B. Joshi, A. Stainthorpe, R. P. MacDonagh, F. X. Keeley Jr., and A. G. Timoney, "Indwelling ureteral stents: evaluation of symptoms, quality of life and utility," *Journal of Urology*, vol. 169, no. 3, pp. 1065–1069, 2003.

[6] H. B. Joshi, N. Newns, A. Stainthorpe, R. P. MacDonagh, F. X. Keeley Jr., and A. G. Timoney, "Ureteral stent symptom questionnaire: development and validation of a multidimensional quality of life measure," *The Journal of Urology*, vol. 169, no. 3, pp. 1060–1064, 2003.

[7] C. Deliveliotis, M. Chrisofos, E. Gougousis, A. Papatsoris, A. Dellis, and I. M. Varkarakis, "Is there a role for alpha1-blockers in treating double-J stent-related symptoms?" *Urology*, vol. 67, no. 1, pp. 35–39, 2006.

[8] R. Beddingfield, R. N. Pedro, B. Hinck, C. Kreidberg, K. Feia, and M. Monga, "Alfuzosin to relieve ureteral stent discomfort: a prospective, randomized, placebo controlled study," *The Journal of Urology*, vol. 181, no. 1, pp. 170–176, 2009.

[9] C.-J. Wang, S.-W. Huang, and C.-H. Chang, "Effects of specific α-1A/1D blocker on lower urinary tract symptoms due to double-J stent: a prospectively randomized study," *Urological Research*, vol. 37, no. 3, pp. 147–152, 2009.

[10] R. Damiano, R. Autorino, M. De Sio, A. Giacobbe, I. M. Palumbo, and M. D'Armiento, "Effect of tamsulosin in preventing ureteral stent-related morbidity: a prospective study," *Journal of Endourology*, vol. 22, no. 4, pp. 651–656, 2008.

[11] A. D. Lamb, S. L. Vowler, R. Johnston, N. Dunn, and O. J. Wiseman, "Meta-analysis showing the beneficial effect of α-blockers on ureteric stent discomfort," *BJU International*, vol. 108, no. 11, pp. 1894–1902, 2011.

[12] R. Yakoubi, M. Lemdani, M. Monga, A. Villers, and P. Koenig, "Is there a role for α-blockers in ureteral stent related symptoms? A systematic review and meta-analysis," *Journal of Urology*, vol. 186, no. 3, pp. 928–934, 2011.

[13] A. E. Dellis, F. X. Keeley, V. Manolas, and A. A. Skolarikos, "Role of α-blockers in the treatment of stent-related symptoms: a prospective randomized control study," *Urology*, vol. 83, no. 1, pp. 56–61, 2014.

[14] Y.-J. Lee, K.-H. Huang, H.-J. Yang, H.-C. Chang, J. Chen, and T.-K. Yang, "Solifenacin improves double-J stent-related symptoms in both genders following uncomplicated ureteroscopic lithotripsy," *Urological Research*, vol. 41, no. 3, pp. 247–252, 2013.

[15] S. C. Park, S. W. Jung, J. W. Lee, and J. S. Rim, "The effects of tolterodine extended release and alfuzosin for the treatment of double-J stent-related symptoms," *Journal of Endourology*, vol. 23, no. 11, pp. 1913–1917, 2009.

[16] E. Shalaby, A.-F. Ahmed, A. Maarouf, I. Yahia, M. Ali, and A. Ghobish, "Randomized controlled trial to compare the safety and efficacy of tamsulosin, solifenacin, and combination of both in treatment of double-J stent-related lower urinary symptoms," *Advances in Urology*, vol. 2013, Article ID 752382, 6 pages, 2013.

[17] K. T. Lim, Y. T. Kim, T. Y. Lee, and S. Y. Park, "Effects of tamsulosin, solifenacin, and combination therapy for the treatment of ureteral stent related discomforts," *Korean Journal of Urology*, vol. 52, no. 7, pp. 485–488, 2011.

[18] N. Hao, Y. Tian, W. Liu et al., "Antimuscarinics and α-blockers or α-blockers monotherapy on lower urinary tract symptoms— a meta-analysis," *Urology*, vol. 83, no. 3, pp. 556–562, 2014.

[19] P. G. Borboroglu, C. L. Amling, N. S. Schenkman et al., "Ureteral stenting after ureteroscopy for distal ureteral calculi: a multi-institutional prospective randomized controlled study assessing pain, outcomes and complications," *The Journal of Urology*, vol. 166, no. 5, pp. 1651–1657, 2001.

[20] G. W. Hruby, C. D. Ames, Y. Yan, M. Monga, and J. Landman, "Correlation of ureteric length with anthropometric variables of surface body habitus," *BJU International*, vol. 99, no. 5, pp. 1119–1122, 2007.

[21] D. Yachia, "Recent advances in ureteral stents," *Current Opinion in Urology*, vol. 18, no. 2, pp. 241–246, 2008.

[22] P. A. Cadieux, B. H. Chew, B. E. Knudsen et al., "Triclosan loaded ureteral stents decrease *Proteus mirabilis* 296 infection in a rabbit urinary tract infection model," *Journal of Urology*, vol. 175, no. 6, pp. 2331–2335, 2006.

[23] J. D. Watterson, P. A. Cadieux, D. T. Beiko et al., "Oxalate-degrading enzymes from *Oxalobacter formigenes*: a novel device coating to reduce urinary tract biomaterial-related encrustation," *Journal of Endourology*, vol. 17, no. 5, pp. 269–274, 2003.

[24] P. Zupkas, C. L. Parsons, C. Percival, and M. Monga, "Pentosanpolysulfate coating of silicone reduces encrustation," *Journal of Endourology*, vol. 14, no. 6, pp. 483–488, 2000.

[25] M. Multanen, T. L. J. Tammela, M. Laurila et al., "Biocompatibility, encrustation and biodegradation of ofloxacine and silver nitrate coated poly-L-lactic acid stents in rabbit urethra," *Urological Research*, vol. 30, no. 4, pp. 227–232, 2002.

[26] A. Dellis, H. B. Joshi, A. G. Timoney, and F. X. Keeley Jr., "Relief of stent related symptoms: review of engineering and pharmacological solutions," *The Journal of Urology*, vol. 184, no. 4, pp. 1267–1272, 2010.

[27] A. Rane, A. Saleemi, D. Cahill, S. Sriprasad, N. Shrotri, and R. Tiptaft, "Have stent-related symptoms anything to do with placement technique?" *Journal of Endourology*, vol. 15, no. 7, pp. 741–745, 2001.

[28] K. Davenport, A. G. Timoney, and F. X. Keeley Jr., "Effect of smooth muscle relaxant drugs on proximal human ureteric activity in vivo: a pilot study," *Urological Research*, vol. 35, no. 4, pp. 207–213, 2007.

[29] S. Hajebrahimi, A. Farshi, A. Jabbari, H. S. Bazargani, H. Babaei, and H. Mostafaie, "Does tadalafil alleviate ureteral stent related symptoms? A randomized controlled trial," *European Urology Supplements*, vol. 14, no. 2, 2015.

7

Necrosis of the Ventral Penile Skin Flap: A Complication of Hypospadias Surgery in Children

Ünal Bakal,[1] Musa Abeş,[2] and Mehmet Sarac[1]

[1]*Department of Pediatric Surgery, Faculty of Medicine, Firat University, 23119 Elazig, Turkey*
[2]*Department of Pediatric Surgery, Faculty of Medicine, Adiyaman University, 23119 Elazig, Turkey*

Correspondence should be addressed to Ünal Bakal; unalbakal@hotmail.com

Academic Editor: Fabio Campodonico

Objectives. To review cases of hypospadias that were repaired with TIPU method and consequently resulted in the necrosis of ventral penile skin flaps. *Methods.* Eighty-three patients with hypospadias underwent TIPU procedure by two surgeons. Neourethra in all patients was covered with dartos flap prepared from the preputium or penile shaft. In cases where ventral skin could not be covered primarily, closure was ensured by using preputial Ombredanne or Byars' flaps to repair ventral defects. *Results.* The median age of patients was 4 years. Twenty-five (30.12%) patients that underwent hypospadias repair had urethral opening at the coronal level, 33 (39.75%) at the distal penis, 10 (12.04%) at the midpenis, and 15 (18.07%) at the proximal penis. The ventral skin defect could not be primarily covered in 10 patients with penile shaft hypospadias. Consequently, Byars' method was used in 8 of these patients to cover the defect and the Ombredanne method was used in the remaining 2. Ventral skin flap necrosis developed in 5 patients (4 Byars and 1 Ombredanne). It was medically treated in 4 patients. Urethral fistula developed in the other patient whose necrosis was deeper. The mean hospital stay was 7 days for patients without necrosis, and 14 for those with necrosis. *Conclusion.* We are of the opinion that dartos flaps used in the TIPU method in order to cover neourethra and decrease the incidence of fistula development lead to necrosis in the Ombredanne or Byars' flaps by causing low blood supply to the preputium and thus extend hospital stay.

1. Introduction

In the tubularized incised plate urethroplasty (TIPU) method which uses urethral plates for urethroplasty and the Mathieu procedure which uses proximal parameatal skin flaps, it is sometimes not possible to primarily cover the skin on the ventral surface of the penis after chordee release and urethroplasty. For this purpose, the Ombredanne or Byars' method may be used to transfer preputial skin to the ventral side [1, 2]. In this study, we retrospectively reviewed cases of hypospadias that were repaired with the TIPU method and resulted in the necrosis of ventral penile skin flaps.

2. Material and Method

In our clinic, a total of 111 children received hypospadias repair with different techniques performed by 2 different surgeons between January 2008 and December 2011. We studied 83 of these cases that were repaired with the TIPU method. In all patients, penile skin was degloved to the penoscrotal junction. The dartos flap big enough to fully cover the neourethra was prepared from preputial or penile shaft. Dorsal plication was performed in patients with persisting chordee. Prior to urethroplasty and glanuloplasty, prepitium and penile skin was excluded and a tourniquet was placed on the radix penis. Urethroplasty was performed with 7/0 or 6/0 continuous subcutaneous, and glanuloplasty was performed with 6/0 interrupted polyglactin or polydioxanone sutures. The neourethra was covered with the previously prepared dartos flap. Drainage was done with a nelaton catheter size 6 or 8. It was withdrawn on day 7 on average. In cases where ventral skin could not be covered primarily, closure was ensured by using preputial Ombredanne or Byars' flaps to repair ventral defects. The skin was covered with 6/0 or 7/0 interrupted polyglactin sutures. The dressing was removed between days 3 and 5. Antibiotics were used in all cases

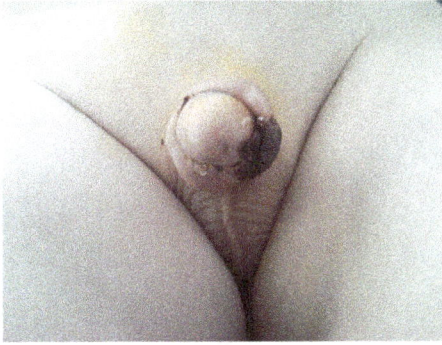

FIGURE 1: Patient in whom ventral penile skin defect was covered with Byars' flap and superficial necrosis developed.

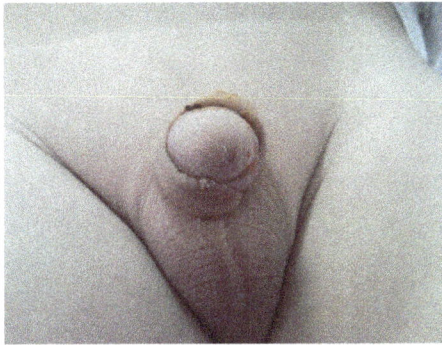

FIGURE 2: Same patient after recovery following medical treatment.

(cefazoline 100 mg/kg/day/3 doses) and oxybutynin was used in some cases (2 mg/kg/2 doses). A rifampicin dressing was used for signs of necrosis in ventral skin.

3. Results

The median age of patients was 4 years (ranging between 1 and 14 years). Twenty-five (30.12%) patients that underwent hypospadias repair had urethral opening at the coronal level, 33 (39.75%) at the distal penis, 10 (12.04%) at the midpenis, and 15 (18.07%) at the proximal penis. The ventral skin defect could not be primarily covered in 10 patients with penile shaft hypospadias. Consequently, Byars' method was used in 8 of these to cover the defect and the Ombredanne method in the remaining 2. Necrosis developed in the skin flap of 5 cases (50%) (4 Byars and 1 Ombredanne). It was superficial and medically treated in 4 (Figures 1 and 2). Urethral fistula developed in the other patient whose necrosis was deeper. The mean hospital stay was 7 days for patients without necrosis and 14 for those with necrosis (between 13 and 15 days).

4. Comment

The tubularized incised plate urethroplasty method is currently the most popular hypospadias treatment worldwide [3]. It may be used to repair all of distal and most of proximal hypospadias cases [3–5]. It may be compared to previous techniques with regard to complications, but cosmetically it

is superior to them [6]. Despite their low incidence rate when compared to other techniques, the most commonly reported complications of the TIPU procedure include formation of fistula 0–39% (mean 5%) and meatal stenosis 0–32% (mean 3%) [3, 6, 7]. In our series, the most common complications were ventral penile skin flap necrosis (6%) and urethral fistula (1,2%).

The causes of skin flap necrosis listed in the literature are hematoma, infections, vascular spasms, and tight dressings [7]. Hematoma and infection were not developed in any of our cases. Tightness of the dressing was equal for all the cases. We are of the opinion that this problem may be related to the dartos flap as skin necrosis was only limited to those that received ventral skin flap and then only to the flap region among our patients, and no other factors existed that might cause necrosis.

In the TIPU procedure, dartos fascia freed from the preputium and the dorsal side of the penis and/or the ventral shaft is used to fully cover the neourethra in order to prevent urethral fistula despite the debated effectiveness of this method [4, 8, 9]. We believe that aggressively freeing the dartos from the preputium and the penile shaft leads to vascular failure in flaps prepared from preputium and dorsal skin, and consequently to necrosis. We attribute the low incidence of fistula formation in our series and the high incidence of ventral skin flap necrosis to the dartos flap. We believe that the dartos used to cover the neourethra prevents fistula but causes necrosis in the preputial ventral skin flaps. Necrosis was superficial in 4 of the 5 cases, who were treated with conservative therapy. Full necrosis and fistula developed only in one patient who recovered in the late stage. We are of the opinion that patients may be followed up with conservative therapy during the early stages for as long as necrosis does not extend, and surgery should be avoided.

5. Conclusion

Particularly in cases where the ventral surface of the penis cannot be covered primarily and preputial skin flaps may be necessary to cover the defect, the dartos flap should not be used aggressively to cover the neourethra; the ventral dartos flap should be used whenever possible instead of preputial and dorsal penile shaft dartos flap; and possible low blood supply to preputial skin flap and ultimately necrosis should be prevented.

Ethical Approval

All persons gave their informed consent prior to their inclusion in the study. This study has been performed in accordance with the ethical standards laid down in the 1964 Declaration of Helsinki and its later amendments.

Conflict of Interests

The authors declare that they have no conflict of interests.

Authors' Contribution

All authors have equally contributed to this study.

References

[1] A. C. Başaklar, *Bebek Ve Çocukların Cerrahi Ve Ürolojik Hastalıkları*, Palme Yayınları, Ankara, Turkey, 2006.

[2] U. Koltuksuz, M. H. Gürsoy, M. Aydınç, M. Mutuş, S. Çetin, and A. Karaman, "An alternative way to cover ventral penile skin defect in Mathieu technique," *European Journal of Pediatric Surgery*, vol. 10, no. 4, pp. 232–234, 2000.

[3] W. T. Snodgrass, "Utilization of urethral plate in hypospadias surgery," *Indian Journal of Urology*, vol. 24, no. 2, pp. 195–199, 2008.

[4] W. T. Snodgrass, N. Bush, and N. Cost, "Tubularized incised plate hypospadias repair for distal hypospadias," *Journal of Pediatric Urology*, vol. 6, no. 4, pp. 408–413, 2010.

[5] W. Snodgrass, M. Koyle, G. Manzoni, R. Hurwitz, A. Caldamone, and R. Ehrlich, "Tubularized incised plate hypospadias repair: results of a multicenter experience," *Journal of Urology*, vol. 156, no. 2, pp. 839–841, 1996.

[6] L. H. P. Braga, A. J. Lorenzo, and J. L. P. Salle, "Tubularized incised plate urethroplasty for distal hypospadias: a literature review," *Indian Journal of Urology*, vol. 24, no. 2, pp. 219–225, 2008.

[7] A. Bhat and A. K. Mandal, "Acute postoperative complications of hypospadias repair," *Indian Journal of Urology*, vol. 24, no. 2, pp. 241–248, 2008.

[8] W. Snodgrass and N. Bush, "Tubularized incised plate proximal hypospadias repair: continued evolution and extended applications," *Journal of Pediatric Urology*, vol. 7, no. 1, pp. 2–9, 2011.

[9] A. Appignani, M. Prestipino, M. Bertozzi, N. Nardi, and F. Falcone, "Double-cross flap protection: new technique for coverage of neourethra in hypospadias repair," *The Journal of Urology*, vol. 182, no. 4, pp. 1521–1527, 2009.

8

Flexible Ureteroscopy Can Be More Efficacious in the Treatment of Proximal Ureteral Stones in Select Patients

Erdal Alkan,[1] **Ali Sarıbacak,**[2] **Ahmet Oguz Ozkanli,**[3] **Mehmet Murad Basar,**[1] **Oguz Acar,**[1] **and Mevlana Derya Balbay**[1]

[1]*Department of Urology, Memorial Şişli Hospital, Şişli, Istanbul, Turkey*
[2]*Department of Urology, Konak Hospital, Izmit, Turkey*
[3]*Department of Anesthesiology, Memorial Şişli Hospital, Şişli, Istanbul, Turkey*

Correspondence should be addressed to Erdal Alkan; eralkan@hotmail.com

Academic Editor: Jason M. Hafron

Purpose. We aimed to compare and evaluate the outcomes and complications of two endoscopic treatment procedures, semirigid ureteroscopy (SR-URS) and flexible ureteroscopy (F-URS), in the treatment of proximal ureteral stones (PUS). *Methods.* SR-URS (group 1) was done on 68 patients whereas 64 patients underwent F-URS (group 2) for the treatment of PUS. Success rate was defined as the absence of stone fragments or presence of asymptomatic insignificant residual fragments < 2 mm. Outcomes and complications were recorded. *Results.* The differences were statistically not significant in age, gender, body mass index (BMI), and stone characteristics between groups. Mean ureteral stone size was 9.1 ± 0.4 mm and 8.9 ± 0.5 mm for groups 1 and 2. Mean operative time was 34.1 ± 1.5 min and 49.4 ± 2.3 min for groups 1 and 2 ($p = 0.001$). SFRs were 76.5% and 87.5% for groups 1 and 2 ($p = 0.078$). Two major complications (ureteral avulsion and ureteral rupture) occurred in group 1. *Conclusion.* F-URS is safer and less invasive than SR-URS in patients with PUS. There is no statistically significant difference in the efficacy of either technique. Nonetheless we recommend F-URS in the management of PUS as a first-line treatment option in select cases of proximal ureteral calculi.

1. Introduction

There are various options in the management of proximal ureteral stones (PUS), which includes medical expulsive therapy (MET), extracorporeal shock wave lithotripsy (ESWL), ureteroscopy (URS; retrograde), percutaneous nephrolithotomy (PCNL), laparoscopy (LAP), and open surgery [1]. Nowadays, ESWL and URS are the most commonly performed treatment options in the management of PUS. Although 2014 update of the European Association of Urology (EAU) urolithiasis guidelines showed that both URS and ESWL should be considered as a first-line therapy for PUS, the optimal treatment of these stones still remains debatable [1]. With the development of endoscopic equipment especially holmium laser and small caliber ureteroscopes, and accumulation of experience, ureteroscopic lithotripsy especially flexible ureteroscopy has been widely used [1, 2].

There are many studies comparing the above-mentioned treatment modalities in the management of PUS [2–6].

However, to our knowledge there is only one study comparing semirigid URS (SR-URS) and flexible URS (F-URS) [7]. We retrospectively compared and evaluated the outcomes and complications of rigid and flexible URS for the treatment of PUS.

2. Materials and Methods

2.1. Patients. Medical reports were retrospectively reviewed for patients with PUS who underwent ureteroscopy (SR-URS or F-URS) between February 2007 and January 2015. All patients were evaluated by CT scan with stone protocol prior to the operation. Each patient was evaluated for body mass index (BMI), stone location, stone number, stone size (assessed by measuring its largest dimension in CT imaging), stone burden (cumulative stone length of the stones), operative time, hospital stay, stone free rates (SFR), and perioperative complications. Inclusion criteria included adult patients (≥20 years) and patient having PUS with or without small renal stones (≤10 mm). Nevertheless all stones regardless of their size within the proximal ureter were included. Exclusion criteria included acute urinary tract infection, operation history of ipsilateral ureter or kidney, congenital ureteropelvic junction obstruction, coexisting ureteral disorders (including tumor or stricture), and patients with simultaneous middle or lower ureteral stones. Patients who had internal stent preoperatively were also excluded. Additionally, when the renal stones were larger than 10 mm, these patients were also excluded regardless of proximal ureteric stone size. Ureteroscopy was indicated and preferred by these patients due to failed ESWL, obesity, and patient preference. Patients with PUS ≤ 5 mm were treated with medical expulsive therapy for 3 weeks in each group. At the end of this period, an ureteroscopic lithotripsy was planned since spontaneous passage of the stones did not occur.

The patients were divided into two groups: patients who underwent SR-URS and F-URS were included in group 1 ($n = 68$) and group 2 ($n = 64$), respectively. F-URS had been mainly preferred in the following conditions due to institutional policy: (1) PUS together with concomitant renal stone, (2) patients with grade 3 or 4 hydroureteronephrosis, and (3) less than 5 cm distance from ureteropelvic junction to the ureteral stone. Patients with PUS only were treated with semirigid ureteroscopy when the ureteric stone was located further than 5 cm from the ureteropelvic junction. This area can be easily reached with semirigid ureteroscopy which limits the use of more expensive flexible ureteroscopy and extends its life span. Stone clearance was assessed intraoperatively and checked with CT or urinary US at postoperative 3 months. Success rate was defined as the absence of stone fragments or presence of asymptomatic insignificant residual fragments <2 mm. Perioperative complications were recorded according to the Clavien-Dindo classification system [8]. All procedures were performed by three experienced surgeons with similar indication and the same surgical techniques.

2.2. Techniques

2.2.1. Rigid Ureteroscopic Lithotripsy. Using a urological guide wire, a 7.5 F semirigid ureteroscope (Karl Storz, Germany) was inserted into the ureter. A stone cone (Stone Cone Nitinol Retrieval Coil, 3.0 F × 115 cm × 7 mm coil; Boston Scientific, Natick, MA, USA) was advanced beyond the stone and fragmented into small pieces by holmium laser (Sphinx, Lisa Laser, 30 watts, Katlenburg-Lindau, Germany) using 365 μm (PercuFib, Lisa Laser, Katlenburg-Lindau, Germany) laser fibers. Larger stone fragments were removed by endoscopic forceps. At the end of the procedure, a 4.8 F 26 cm internal stent was inserted based on surgeon's decision. When the stone was pushed back to the kidney, the procedure was completed using flexible ureteroscope, and rigid ureteroscopy was accepted as unsuccessful. These patients were not included in group 2. In case semirigid ureteroscope could not be advanced up to the proximal ureter due to ureteral stricture, an internal stent was inserted into the ureter and the intervention was delayed at least 15 days. This procedure was also accepted as unsuccessful.

2.2.2. Flexible Ureteroscopic Lithotripsy. An access sheath (Flexor ureteral access sheath 12/14 F 35 cm; FUS, Cook Medical, Bloomington, IN, USA) was introduced into the proximal ureter over a 0.038-inch safety hydrophilic guide wire (Sensor, Microvasive, Boston Scientific Corp, Natick, MA, USA). URF P-5 flexible ureteroscope (Olympus, Tokyo, Japan) and Cobra Flexible Dual-Channel Ureteroscope (Richard Wolf, Knittlingen, Germany) were used in all cases according to their availability. The stone was fragmented with holmium laser (Sphinx, Lisa Laser, 30 watts, Katlenburg-Lindau, Germany) in combination with 200 μm or 272 μm (LithoFib and FlexiFib, Lisa Laser, Katlenburg-Lindau, Germany) laser fibers in the proximal ureter. In case the stone was pushed back to the collecting system, the stone was fragmented in the kidney. When required, a nitinol basket (Ngage nitinol stone extractor 2,2 F 115 cm basket; Cook Medical Bloomington, IN, USA) was used for the removal of stone fragments. Endoscopically, intraoperative success was defined as extraction of all stone fragments or laser lithotripsy of all stones to less than 2 mm fragments. Moreover, in cases of coexistent renal stones, these stones were also fragmented, simultaneously. After breaking up or removing the stone, a 4.8 F 26 cm internal stent was left in place based on surgeon's discretion. In cases where the ureteral access sheath or flexible ureteroscope could not be advanced up to the proximal ureter, an internal stent was inserted into the ureter; the procedure was called unsuccessful and the intervention was delayed for at least 15 days.

2.3. Statistical Analysis. Statistical analysis was performed using the Statistical Package for Social Sciences version 16.0 software (SPSS Inc., Chicago, IL). The measurement data were expressed as mean ± standard error. Student's t-test and chi-square test were used for statistical analysis. A value of $p < 0.05$ was considered as statistically significant.

3. Results

One hundred and thirty-two patients (86 men and 46 women) were included in this study. Patients' demographics data and stone characteristics are listed in Table 1. Both groups were similar regarding age, gender, BMI, and stone characteristics (Table 1). There were 15 (23%; 15/64) patients with PUS together with renal stones in group 2, all of which were treated with flexible ureteroscope in the same session. Mean renal stone number, renal stone size, and renal stone burden were 1.5 ± 0.2 (1–3), 6.6 ± 0.4 (4–10) mm, and 9.3 ± 1.0 (5–18) mm, respectively, in group 2.

Treatment outcomes are shown in detail in Table 2. A ureteral access sheath was used in 55 (86%; 55/64) patients in group 2. Flexible ureteroscope could have been advanced up into the collecting system without placing access sheath in 5 (8%; 5/64) patients. On the other hand neither flexible ureteroscope nor access sheath could have been advanced up to the proximal ureter in 4 (6%; 4/64) patients. Internal stent placements were left in place in these cases, and the ureteroscopic interventions were successfully completed with flexible ureteroscope 15 days later.

TABLE 1: Patients' demographics data and stone characteristics.

	Group 1 (R-URS)	Group 2 (F-URS)	p value
Gender (M/F)	41/27	45/19	0.554
Mean patient age (year)	38.2 ± 1.3	39.9 ± 1.3	0.991
(Range)	(21–74)	(21–75)	
Mean BMI (kg/mm^2)	27.1 ± 0.4	27.8 ± 0.5	0.136
(Range)	(21–41)	(22–45)	
Mean ureteral stone number (n)	1.1 ± 0.1	1.0 ± 0.1	0.353
(Range)	(1-2)	(1–5)	
Mean ureteral stone size (mm)	9.1 ± 0.4	8.9 ± 0.5	0.599
(Range)	(5–20)	(5–20)	
Mean ureteral stone burden (mm)	9.8 ± 0.4	9.2 ± 0.4	0.607
(Range)	(5–22)	(6–23)	
Laterality (R/L)	30/38	28/36	0.553

TABLE 2: Operative and postoperative data.

	Group 1 (R-URS)	Group 2 (F-URS)	p value
Mean operative time (min)	34.1 ± 1.5	49.4 ± 2.3	**0.001**
(Range)	(10–75)	(20–90)	
Mean hospital stay (hour)	28.0 ± 1.9	24.5 ± 1.1	**0.001**
(Range)	(12–96)	(12–72)	
Use of basket catheter (n)	52/68	30/64	**0.001**
Use of internal stent (n)	32/68	39/64	0.077
Mean internal stenting time (day)	23.2 ± 2.6	27.3 ± 2.3	0.598
(Range)	(7–90)	(3–90)	
SFR	76.5%	87.5%	0.078

SFR in group 1 was 76.5%. Rigid ureteroscope could have not been advanced up to the proximal ureter in 5 (7%; 5/68) patients. Internal stents were left in place in these cases, and the procedures were completed with flexible ureteroscope after 15 days. Ureteral stones were pushed back to the renal collecting system during the procedure in 8 (12%; 8/68) patients (5 stones during ureteroscopy, 3 stones during lithotripsy), and lithotripsy was completed using flexible ureteroscope. Residual stone fragments larger than 2 mm, most of which were located in the lower calyces on postoperative imaging studies, were detected in 3 (9%; 3/68) patients.

SFR in group 2 was 87.5%, which was not statistically significant compared to that of group 1 ($\chi^2 = 0.696$; $p = 0.078$). Since neither flexible ureteroscope nor access sheath could have been advanced up to the proximal ureter in 4 (6%; 4/64) patients due to ureteral pathology such as a narrow ureteric lumen and ureteral structures, the procedures were postponed for 15 days. The residual fragments greater than 2 mm remained in 4 (6%; 4/64) patients with PUS and concomitant renal stones in this group, mainly due to intrarenal hemorrhage. There was grade 3 or 4 hydronephrosis in these patients.

Complications were summarized in Table 3. Two major intraoperative complications (ureteral avulsion and ureteral perforation) were seen in group 1 (3%; 2/68). Ureteral avulsion, at the level of ureterovesical junction was seen in

TABLE 3: Intraoperative and postoperative complications.

	Group 1 (R-URS)	Group 2 (F-URS)	p value
Intraoperative	9 (13%)	7 (11%)	0.446
(i) Ureteral avulsion	1	—	
(ii) Ureteral perforation	1	—	
(iii) Minor ureteral trauma	6	3	
(iv) Minor hemorrhage	1	4	
Postoperative	6 (9%)	7 (11%)	0.453
(i) Urinary tract infection	2	1	
(ii) Renal colic	4	6	

a female patient with a PUS 13 mm in size. Ureteral avulsion occurred when reentrance into the ureter was attempted after overdistention of the bladder as a result of prolonged fragmentation. Extravesical ureteroneocystostomy by Lich-Gregoir technique was successfully performed. The patient was discharged uneventfully at postoperative day 4. Another major intraoperative complication was ureteral rupture, seen in a female with a PUS of 10 mm. Ureteral perforation occurred and was repaired by open ureteroureteral anastomosis. The patient was discharged uneventfully at postoperative day 4.

Some minor intraoperative complications including minor ureteral trauma were seen in 6 (9%; 6/68) and 3 (5%; 3/64) patients in groups 1 and 2, respectively. Procedures were not cancelled but internal stents were left in place after the operation in all. Likewise, intraoperative minor hemorrhage was seen in 1 (1%; 1/68) and 4 (6%; 4/64) patients in groups 1 and 2, respectively. None of the patients were given blood transfusions.

Two different postoperative complications (urinary tract infections, and renal colic) were detected (Table 3). Urinary tract infections (Clavien 2) were observed in 2 (3%; 2/68) patients and in 1 (2%; 1/64) patient in groups 1 and 2 and were treated with appropriate antibiotics without hospitalization. Postoperative renal colic after discharge were seen in 4 (6%; 4/68) and 5 (8%; 5/64) patients in groups 1 and 2. Out of these 10 patients, 8 (Clavien 2) were treated with parenteral medications in the emergency setting in both groups (three in group 1; five in group 2). The remaining two patients were treated with internal stent placement (Clavien 3b) due to pain related to hydronephrosis (one in group 1; one in group 2).

4. Discussion

The primary goal of complete stone clearance for the management of PUS is to preserve renal function, prevent further stone growth, cure infection, and relieve obstruction [9]. MET is an important treatment option in ureteral stones especially when the stone size is smaller than 5 mm. Since the spontaneous passage rate is only 22%, the majority of PUS need intervention, which depend on various factors including stone size, duration, pain, cost, occurrence of obstruction, and availability of instrument [10, 11]. Currently, the majority of PUS has been treated with ESWL or URS. Nowadays, while ESWL is used in the small (<2 cm) nonimpacted stones, URS is performed in more complicated conditions such as patient with larger and impacted stones [5, 6]. Both procedures have some advantages and disadvantages. ESWL has several advantages including being noninvasive, being safe, not requiring any anesthesia, requiring surgical skills, and being performed as an outpatient setting. On the other hand, URS has a lower retreatment rate and provides immediate stone-free status. But URS requires anesthesia and surgical skills are an invasive procedure and have more complications [3, 5].

Nowadays, ureteroscopic lithotripsy (semirigid or flexible) has been usually performed in the management of PUS. The most important advantage of F-URS compared to SR-URS in treating PUS is to treat coexisting renal stones together with PUS. Multiple stones are detected in 20–25% patients with urolithiasis [12]. In our study, renal stones coexisting with PUS were found in 15 (23%) patients in group 2, and these patients were simultaneously treated with flexible ureteroscope.

There are different success rates of ureteroscopy in the treatment of PUS. Some studies have demonstrated that SFRs of SR-URS have ranged from 51% to 100% in the management of PUS [1, 6, 7, 13–15]. Moufid and colleagues in a retrospective study reported their experience in the management of PUS on 30 patients treated with semirigid

ureteroscopic lithotripsy and found that SFRs were 63% [13]. In their study, mean operative time and mean ureteral stone size were 52 ± 17 minutes and 29 ± 1.8 mm, respectively. In our study, rigid ureteroscope was used in 68 patients. In this group (group 1), SFRs, mean operative time, and mean stone size were 76.5%, 34.1 ± 1.5 minutes, and 9.1 ± 0.4 mm, respectively, similar to the literature.

The most important handicap in treating PUS with rigid ureteroscope is pushing the whole stone or stone fragments back into the renal collecting system, which is accepted as a failure and ratio of which between 12% and 25% [4, 16, 17]. In our series, although a stone cone was routinely used in all procedures in group 1, the stones or their fragments were pushed back into the kidney in 8 (12%; 8/68) patients which was due to incomplete blockade of stone cone. We observed that combining F-URS with rigid one resulted in difficulty in the management of PUS because of hemorrhage secondary to high pressure irrigant flow during previous R-URS, which was a contradictory finding in some published series [15, 18]. In our study, hemorrhage, which may blur the vision intraoperatively, was detected in all patients who have been converted to F-URS in group 1. Therefore, when there is a risk of pushing stones or their fragments back, it is better to carry out the procedure with the use of a flexible ureteroscope at the outset, which also prevents bleeding from a previous R-URS.

Flexible ureteroscopic lithotripsy has been performed much more commonly in the treatment of upper urinary system stones lately. In cases where flexible ureteroscope is used in the management of PUS, it has been demonstrated that SFRs are between 79% and 89% [5, 15]. Karadag and colleagues reported their experience in the management of PUS on 61 patients assigned to flexible ureteroscopic lithotripsy and found that SFRs, mean operative time, and mean stone size were 93.4%, 84.1 ± 16.7 minutes, and 11 ± 2.2 mm [7]. In our study, F-URS was performed in 64 patients (group 2). SFRs, mean operative time, and mean stone size were 87.5%, 49.4 ± 2.3 minutes, and 8.9 ± 0.5 mm, respectively.

We have shown that SR-URS was associated with longer hospital stay ($p = 0.001$) and excessive basket catheter use ($p = 0.001$). Longer hospital stays in SR-URS group were due to subsequent open surgery as a result of the major complication. On the other hand, we observed that mean operative time in F-URS group was longer than that of SR-URS group ($p = 0.001$). We think that longer operative times in F-URS group were due to extra time spent for the treatment of coexisting renal stones. However, use of internal stent ($p = 0.077$) and mean internal stenting time ($p = 0.598$) were similar in both groups.

The overall complication rate after URS was reported to be 9–25% [1, 19]. In our series, while intraoperative complication rates were 13% in group 1 and 11% in group 2 ($p = 0.446$; $\chi^2 = 0.163$), postoperative complication rates in groups 1 and 2 were 9% and 11%, respectively ($p = 0.453$; $\chi^2 = 0.166$). Ureteral perforation and avulsion are the most serious complications encountered during URS [1, 17, 20]. The incidences of ureteral avulsion and perforation were reported to be 0.1% and 1.7%, respectively in one series [1]. Although complication rates in our study were statistically similar in each group, major complications such as ureteral avulsion and perforation occurred only in group 1. Ureteral avulsion occurred in one patient when reentering into the ureter after overdistention of the bladder as a result of prolonged procedure. This patient was successfully treated with open extravesical ureteroneocystostomy. Ureteral perforation occurred in another patient during stone fragmentation by holmium laser and was treated with open surgery. Both patients in group 1 were discharged from hospital uneventfully at postoperative day 4. Therefore, when rigid ureteroscope is to be used in the treatment of PUS, it should be kept in mind that serious complications may occur.

In times of austerity, cost effectiveness is one of the most important issues in the management of stone disease. The durability and fragility of the rigid ureteroscopes are better than those of the flexible ones. Lifespan of flexible ureteroscopes is limited and the most common cause of scopes' failure is thermal laser damage [21]. 50 consecutive uses from a single flexible ureteroscope were reported by Traxer et al. [21]. In another study by Gurbuz et al., it was reported that the basic cost of flexible ureteroscope per case was $118 [22]. On the other hand, the other ancillary equipments such as fine laser fibers ($24/case), ureteral access sheaths ($231/case), and stone retrieval nitinol baskets ($611/case) that are used F-URS necessitates an extra cost compared to SR-URS [22]. Nonetheless Gurbuz et al. reported that cost for standard F-URS per case was $543 [22]. Due to this reason, when planning to use F-URS for the treatment of PUS, cost issue mentioned above should also be considered.

There are some limitations of our series. Firstly, the present study is limited by both its retrospective nature and being conducted at a single center. Secondly, the small number of patients is another limitation. Randomized prospective and larger series with longer follow-up are necessary to confirm the effectiveness of SR-URS or F-URS. Despite these limitations, to our knowledge, it is the second study to compare the results of SR-URS and F-URS in the management of PUS.

5. Conclusions

Our data showed that F-URS is safer and less invasive than SR-URS in patients with PUS. Despite the fact that there is no statistically significant difference in the efficacy of either technique, there was a trend towards the better performance of F-URS. Therefore, we recommend F-URS in the management of PUS as a first-line treatment option in select cases of proximal ureteral calculi.

Conflict of Interests

The authors confirm that the paper has not been submitted elsewhere and there is no conflict of interests. There are no competing financial interests in relation to the work.

Acknowledgment

The preliminary results of this study were presented at the poster session at the 32nd World Congress of Endourology and ESWL.

References

[1] C. Türk, T. Knoll, A. Petrik, K. Sarica, M. Straub, and C. Seitz, *Guidelines on Urolithiasis*, EAU, 2014, http://www.uroweb.org/gls/pdf.

[2] Y.-H. Lee, J.-Y. Tsai, B.-P. Jiaan, T. Wu, and C.-C. Yu, "Prospective randomized trial comparing shock wave lithotripsy and ureteroscopic lithotripsy for management of large upper third ureteral stones," *Urology*, vol. 67, no. 3, pp. 480–484, 2006.

[3] G. Nabi, P. Downey, F. Keeley, G. Watson, and S. McClinton, "Extracorporeal shock wave lithotripsy (ESWL) versus ureteroscopic management for ureteric calculi," *Cochrane Database of Systematic Reviews*, vol. 24, no. 1, Article ID CD006029, 2007.

[4] Y.-Q. Fang, J.-G. Qiu, D.-J. Wang, H.-L. Zhan, and J. Situ, "Comparative study on ureteroscopic lithotripsy and laparoscopic ureterolithotomy for treatment of unilateral upper ureteral stones," *Acta Cirurgica Brasileira*, vol. 27, no. 3, pp. 266–270, 2012.

[5] U. Ozturk, N. C. Şener, H. N. Goktug, A. Gucuk, I. Nalbant, and M. A. Imamoglu, "The comparison of laparoscopy, shock wave lithotripsy and retrograde intrarenal surgery for large proximal ureteral stones," *Journal of the Canadian Urological Association*, vol. 7, no. 11-12, pp. E673–E676, 2013.

[6] Y. Liu, Z. Zhou, A. Xia, H. Dai, L. Guo, and J. Zheng, "Clinical observation of different minimally invasive surgeries for the treatment of impacted upper ureteral calculi," *Pakistan Journal of Medical Sciences*, vol. 29, no. 6, pp. 1358–1362, 2013.

[7] M. A. Karadag, A. Demir, K. Cecen et al., "Flexible ureterorenoscopy versus semirigid ureteroscopy for the treatment of proximal ureteral stones: a retrospective comparative analysis of 124 patients," *Urology Journal*, vol. 11, no. 5, pp. 1867–1872, 2014.

[8] D. Dindo, N. Demartines, and P.-A. Clavien, "Classification of surgical complications: a new proposal with evaluation in a cohort of 6336 patients and results of a survey," *Annals of Surgery*, vol. 240, no. 2, pp. 205–213, 2004.

[9] J. S. Wolf Jr., "Treatment selection and outcomes: Ureteral calculi," *Urologic Clinics of North America*, vol. 34, no. 3, pp. 421–430, 2007.

[10] R. M. Morse and M. I. Resnick, "Ureteral calculi: natural history and treatment in an era of advanced technology," *Journal of Urology*, vol. 145, no. 2, pp. 263–265, 1991.

[11] M. R. Nikoobakht, A. Emamzadeh, A. R. Abedi, K. Moradi, and A. Mehrsai, "Transureteral lithotripsy versus extracorporeal shock wave lithotripsy in management of upper ureteral calculi: a comparative study," *Urology Journal*, vol. 4, no. 4, pp. 207–211, 2007.

[12] T. Abe, K. Akakura, M. Kawaguchi et al., "Outcomes of shockwave lithotripsy for upper urinary-tract stones: a large-scale study at a single institution," *Journal of Endourology*, vol. 19, no. 7, pp. 768–773, 2005.

[13] K. Moufid, N. Abbaka, D. Touiti, L. Adermouch, M. Amine, and M. Lezrek, "Large impacted upper ureteral calculi: a comparative study between retrograde ureterolithotripsy and percutaneous antegrade ureterolithotripsy in the modified lateral position," *Urology Annals*, vol. 5, no. 3, pp. 140–146, 2013.

[14] H. Zhu, X. Ye, X. Xiao, X. Chen, Q. Zhang, and H. Wang, "Retrograde, antegrade, and laparoscopic approaches to the management of large upper ureteral stones after shockwave lithotripsy failure: a four-year retrospective study," *Journal of Endourology*, vol. 28, no. 1, pp. 100–103, 2014.

[15] D.-Y. Liu, H.-C. He, J. Wang et al., "Ureteroscopic lithotripsy using holmium laser for 187 patients with proximal ureteral stones," *Chinese Medical Journal*, vol. 125, no. 9, pp. 1542–1546, 2012.

[16] G. K. Chow, M. L. Blute, D. E. Patterson, and J. W. Segura, "Ureteroscopy: update on current practice and long term complications," *The Journal of Urology*, vol. 165, no. 2, p. 71, 2001.

[17] F. Yencilek, K. Sarica, S. Erturhan, F. Yagci, and A. Erbagci, "Treatment of ureteral calculi with semirigid ureteroscopy: where should we stop?" *Urologia Internationalis*, vol. 84, no. 3, pp. 260–264, 2010.

[18] K. Shigemura, T. Yasufuku, M. Yamashita, S. Arakawa, and M. Fujisawa, "Efficacy of combining flexible and rigid ureteroscopy for transurethral lithotripsy," *Kobe Journal of Medical Sciences*, vol. 56, no. 1, pp. E24–E28, 2010.

[19] P. Geavlete, D. Georgescu, G. Nita, V. Mirciulescu, and V. Cauni, "Complications of 2735 retrograde semirigid ureteroscopy procedures: a single-center experience," *Journal of Endourology*, vol. 20, no. 3, pp. 179–185, 2006.

[20] R. F. Youssef, A. R. El-Nahas, A. M. El-Assmy et al., "Shock wave lithotripsy versus semirigid ureteroscopy for proximal ureteral calculi (<20 mm): a comparative matched-pair study," *Urology*, vol. 73, no. 6, pp. 1184–1187, 2009.

[21] O. Traxer, F. Dubosq, K. Jamali, B. Gattegno, and P. Thibault, "New-generation flexible ureterorenoscopes are more durable than previous ones," *Urology*, vol. 68, no. 2, pp. 276–279, 2006.

[22] C. Gurbuz, G. Atiş, O. Arikan et al., "The cost analysis of flexible ureteroscopic lithotripsy in 302 cases," *Urolithiasis*, vol. 42, no. 2, pp. 155–158, 2014.

9

The Role of Interferon in the Management of BCG Refractory Nonmuscle Invasive Bladder Cancer

Andres F. Correa, Katherine Theisen, Matthew Ferroni, Jodi K. Maranchie, Ronald Hrebinko, Benjamin J. Davies, and Jeffrey R. Gingrich

Department of Urology, University of Pittsburgh Medical Center, 3471 5th Avenue, Suite 700 Kaufmann Building, Pittsburgh, PA 15213, USA

Correspondence should be addressed to Andres F. Correa; correaaf@upmc.edu

Academic Editor: Felix Chun

Background. Thirty to forty percent of patients with high grade nonmuscle invasive bladder cancer (NMIBC) fail to respond to intravesical therapy with bacillus Calmette-Guerin (BCG). Interferon-α2B plus BCG has been shown to be effective in a subset of patients with NMIBC BCG refractory disease. Here we present a contemporary series on the effectiveness and safety of intravesical BCG plus interferon-α2B therapy in patients with BCG refractory NMIBC. *Methods.* From January of 2005 to April of 2014 we retrospectively found 44 patients who underwent induction with combination IFN/BCG for the management of BCG refractory NMIBC. A chart review was performed to assess initial pathological stage/grade, pathological stage/grade at the time of induction, time to IFN/BCG failure, pathological stage/grade at failure, postfailure therapy, and current disease state. *Results.* Of the 44 patients who met criteria for the analysis. High risk disease was found in 88.6% of patients at induction. The 12-month and 24-month recurrence-free survival were 38.6% and 18.2%, respectively. 25 (56.8%) ultimately had disease recurrence. Radical cystectomy was performed in 16 (36.4%) patients. *Conclusion.* Combination BCG plus interferon-α2B remains a reasonably safe alternative treatment for select patients with BCG refractory disease prior to proceeding to radical cystectomy.

1. Introduction

In 2014, approximately 75,000 new cases of bladder cancer will be diagnosed in the USA [1]. At diagnosis, roughly 80% of bladder tumors will be classified as nonmuscle invasive. Nonmuscle invasive bladder cancer is prone to recur and, worse, progress to muscle invasive disease. Bacillus Calmette-Guerin (BCG) is the only intravesical agent proven to reduce rates of recurrence and to delay progression in intermediate and high risk nonmuscle invasive bladder cancer (NMIBC) [2]. The approximately 30% to 40% of patients who will fail BCG therapy represent a frequent dilemma to the treating physician. Although 50% of patients who did not respond to initial therapy will respond to a second induction regimen [3], failure of reinduction with BCG is associated with recurrence and progression with a 30% chance of developing muscle invasive disease [4]. Early radical cystectomy has been shown to improve survival in this patient population [5–7]; however, it carries a significant degree of morbidity, mortality, and

life-style changes. Sadly, there remains no reliable gold standard salvage intravesical therapy for this cohort of patients.

While the etiology of BCG failure remains unclear, there are various factors that may explain this phenomenon. Intravesical BCG acts as an immune modulator which elicits a TH1-type response in the bladder. When an appropriate TH1-type response is triggered, chemokine signaling elicits the recruitment of monocytic and granulocytic lymphocytes capable of eliminating bladder tumor cells [8]. Failure to elicit this immune response leads to BCG failure. This occurs when an insufficient BCG concentration is used or a predominant TH2-type immune response is elicited.

Interferon-α (IFN-α) is a pleiotropic immune modulator that has demonstrated antiproliferative activity in several preclinical studies. While the results of interferon-α2β (IFN-α2β) as intravesical monotherapy has proven to be inferior to standard therapies [9], *in vitro* studies have shown that the addition of IFN-α2β to BCG potentiates the TH1-type response [10]. O'Donnell and colleagues proposed the addition of IFN-$\alpha 2\beta$ to a BCG regimen with the hope it would synergistically elicit an appropriate host response in patients who have failed induction BCG therapy. In the original study consisting of 40 patients, a good response to combination therapy was observed with 12-month and 24-month disease-free rates of 63% and 53%, respectively [10]. This data was further explored in a multicenter randomized trial by Joudi et al. [11] which included 1,007 patients and reported a lower 2-year disease-free rate of only 45% after combination therapy in patients who had failed BCG induction therapy. Consequently, newer salvage intravesical treatments with chemoagents, thermochemotherapy, and electromotive therapy have been introduced to try to improve on these results for patients following BCG failure.

Herein we review our single institution contemporary experience of combination BCG plus IFN-$\alpha 2\beta$ as salvage intravesical therapy for patients with NMIBC who failed BCG therapy and, secondly, perform a literature review of the newly introduced salvage intravesical therapies to place in perspective the current role of IFN-$\alpha 2\beta$ in the salvage treatment of BCG refractory NMIBC.

2. Methods

We retrospectively reviewed the charts of patients who underwent treatment with combination therapy, BCG plus IFN-$\alpha 2\beta$ for the treatment of BCG refractory NMIBC from January of 2005 to April of 2014. BCG refractory status was defined as worsening or nonimproving disease despite full induction or maintenance course of BCG therapy. All patients were treated per O'Donnell et al.'s intravesical protocol which constitutes 6 weekly installations of 1/3 BCG dose plus 50 million units of interferon-$\alpha 2\beta$ diluted in 50 cc of buffered saline [12]. If induction was successful patients were continued in a maintenance protocol with instillations at 3, 6, 12, 18, 24, and 30 months, respectively. Patients were surveyed at 3-month intervals during the 1st year, 6 months during the 2nd year, and annually thereafter. Failure was determined when a bladder recurrence was noted during the surveillance period. Patients that failed were again offered a bladder extirpation procedure. BCG naïve or intolerant patients along with patients presenting upper tract disease who received combination therapy were excluded from the analysis.

Charts were reviewed to assess initial pathological stage/grade, pathological stage/grade at the time of induction, time to IFN/BCG failure, pathological stage/grade at failure, postfailure therapy, and current disease state. Pearson chi-square tests were performed to analyze patient and/or tumor characteristics associated with failure of combination therapy. Analyses were performed using SigmaXL software (SigmaXL, Toronto, Ontario, Canada) with p values < 0.05 being considered statistically significant.

3. Results

The initial search revealed 50 patients who underwent intravesical combination therapy with BCG plus INF-$\alpha 2\beta$

TABLE 1: Patient and tumor characteristics at the time of BCG/IFN induction.

Number of patients	44	
Median age (range)	63.5	(38–92)
Male	35	79.5%
Female	7	20.5%
Median ASA	3	(2–4)
Median # of BCG inductions	1	(0–10)
<2 BCG	20	45.5%
BCG = 2	9	20.5%
>2 BCG	13	29.5%
Time to BCG failure		
<6 months	20	45.5%
6–12 months	12	27.3%
12–24 months	6	13.6%
>24 months	10	22.7%
Pathology at induction		
pTis	15	34.1%
pTa	16	36.4%
pT1	13	29.5%
Grade at induction		
LG	5	11.4%
HG	39	88.6%
Failure of combination INF/BCG		
Yes	25	56.8%
No	19	43.2%
Recurrence-free at 12 months	17	38.6%
Recurrence-free at 24 months	8	18.2%
Radical cystectomy	16	36.4%
Disease-free at 12 months	38	86.4%
Disease-free at 24 months	27	61.4%
Metastatic disease	2	4.5%
Deceased at follow-up	2	4.5%
Median follow-up	28.47	(5.3–115.3)

for treatment of urothelial carcinoma, though 4 patients were noted to be BCG naïve and 2 were found to have an upper tract disease and therefore excluded. Therefore, 44 patients met inclusion criteria for analysis of which 35 (79%) were male, as shown in Table 1. Thirty-one (70%) patients underwent combination therapy with the goal of bladder preservation rather than cystectomy. The remainder 13 (30%) patients had severe comorbidities prohibiting radical cystectomy. Median age at time of diagnosis was 63 years (38–92). The median ASA class for the overall cohort was 3 (2–4), while the ASA class for the bladder sparing group was 2 (2–3). The most common stage at induction was pTa (50%) followed by pT1 (45.5%), with 88.6% of tumors displaying high grade disease. Patients who had failed BCG within 6 months were common, accounting for 43% of the entire cohort. Of the patients that failed BCG within 6 months, 9 (47.3%) failed within 3 months and 16 (89.4%) received a second BCG induction prior to combination therapy. All patients but 7 (16%) patients tolerated induction therapy with

TABLE 2: Patient and pathological tumor characteristics between BCG/IFN failures and nonfailures.

	Failures		Nonfailures		p value
No	25	56.8%	19	43.2%	
Male	18	40.9%	17	38.6%	0.15
Female	7	15.9%	2	4.5%	0.15
Time to BCG failure					
<6 months	16	36.4%	4	9.1%	0.0046
6–12 months	6	13.6%	6	13.6%	0.5
12–24 months	1	2.3%	5	11.4%	0.84
>24 months	6	13.6%	4	9.1%	0.21
Pathology at induction					
Tis	7	15.9%	8	18.2%	0.33
Ta	10	22.7%	5	11.4%	0.27
T1	8	18.2%	6	13.6%	0.44
Grade at induction					
HG	22	50.0%	17	38.6%	0.93
LG	3	6.8%	2	4.5%	0.93
Tumor size					
<1 cm	7	15.9%	6	13.6%	0.79
1–5 cm	16	36.4%	12	27.3%	0.95
>5 cm	2	4.5%	1	2.3%	0.72
Multifocality					
Yes	11	25.0%	6	13.6%	0.4
Hx smoking	16	36.4%	12	27.3%	0.95

28 (63.6%) patients continuing on maintenance therapy. Six (14%) patients did require treatment for a UTI during the induction phase. One patient developed a postinstallation fever requiring admission and treatment with antituberculin agent.

Of the 44 patients, 19 (43.2%) were recurrence-free with median follow-up of 28 months. However, 12-month and 24-month recurrence-free rates for the cohort were only 38.6% and 18.2%, respectively. Sixteen (36.3%) patients underwent salvage cystectomy following failure. Two (4.5%) patients developed metastatic disease and there were 2 (4.5%) cancer specific deaths. The bladder preservation rate in the cohort was 61.3%, with 12-month and 24-month disease-free rates for the cohort of 86.4% and 61.4%, respectively.

A comparison of the clinical and pathological patient characteristics between failures and nonfailures is shown in Table 2. Early BCG monotherapy failure (<6 months) was significantly associated with failure of combination therapy. Larger tumors and multifocal disease were more frequent in the failure group but this difference was not found to be statistically significant.

Twenty-five (56.8%) patients experienced a recurrence at follow-up. Median time to recurrence was 7.2 months. The most common stages at recurrence were pTa and pT1 diseases which accounted for 40% and 44% tumors resected at failure. High grade disease was seen in 92% of recurrences. The incidence of upstaging and upgrading in the failure

group was 36% and 12%, respectively. Three (12.0%) patients were found to have muscle invasive disease at time of recurrence. Sixteen patients underwent salvage cystectomy. Of the remaining 9 patients that refused radical cystectomy, 7 underwent salvage intravesical therapy (1 repeat BCG, 4 MMC, 1 additional BCG/INF, and 1 enrolled in a clinical trial utilizing investigational Mycobacteria cell wall DNA complex), 1 was managed with systemic therapy, and 1 refused further treatment.

At radical cystectomy 8 (50.0%) patients were found to have pT1 disease. One patient was found to have pT0 disease. Advanced stage was found in 5 (20%) patients. Of these, four presented with pT2 disease and one with pT3 disease. Micropapillary features were seen in 3 (60%) specimens showing advance stage. Four of the five patients who showed progression to an advanced stage at cystectomy had failed BCG monotherapy within 6 months. Positive lymph nodes were found in 2 (13.3%) of the 16 patients that underwent radical cystectomy. Of the patients treated with salvage cystectomy, 2 (8%) patients went on to develop metastatic disease.

At a median follow-up of 19 months following cystectomy, 5 (31%) developed postcystectomy related complications. Two patients developed hernias (1 incisional and 1 parastomal), 1 developed recurrent pyelonephritis, 1 developed left ureteroenteric anastomotic stricture, and 1 developed a urethrovesical anastomotic contracture following orthotopic neobladder diversion.

4. Discussion

Intravesical immunotherapy with BCG has been shown to be the most effective treatment for high risk NMIBC with response rates in order of 55% to 65% [20, 21]. Consequently, 30% to 40% of patients with high grade NMIBC will ultimately fail BCG therapy [8]. Recently, there have been several reports advocating for early cystectomy due to higher risk of progression to advance disease and improve cancer specific survival in this subgroup of patients [5, 7]. Early cystectomy is not an option in a significant portion of this population due to patient's unwillingness to undergo major surgery, and there is potential for significant morbidity and mortality due to comorbidity competing risks. To date there is no current gold standard intravesical salvage therapy for this patient subgroup. The goal of this study is to assess the disease recurrence rate following combination therapy at our institution and to determine a population in which combination therapy would be beneficial.

At our institution, the standard of care is to offer radical cystectomy to patients with BCG refractory or resistant disease. Combination therapy with BCG plus interferon is offered to those patients who desire continued bladder preservation strategies or/and to patients that have severe medical comorbidities in whom radical cystectomy is prohibited. The cohort for this study was made mainly of patients wishing for a bladder preservation protocol with a median age of 62 years and ASA class of 2. All salvage cystectomies were performed in the bladder preservation cohort.

The postcystectomy complication rate was 31% consistent with that reported in the literature [13, 22]. Patients that underwent intravesical combination therapy tolerated the regimen well with 84% completing an induction phase and 64% continuing with maintenance therapy. The likely reason for this high tolerance was the exclusion of patients intolerant to BCG from the analysis and the BCG dose reduction to 1/3 of total dose.

O'Donnell and colleagues presented the initial report on the use of combination BCG plus interferon for patients who had failed BCG monotherapy. The results were encouraging with 12- and 24-month disease-free survival of 63% and 53%, respectively [12]. A multicenter randomized trial followed, consisting of 1007 patients with included BCG naïve and BCG refractory disease treated with combination therapy. At 24-month median follow-up, 59% and 45% remained recurrence-free in the BCG naïve and BCG refractory groups, respectively [11]. Lamm and colleagues also reported their experience in a series of 32 patients of which 20 had failed prior BCG therapy. At median follow-up of 22 months the disease-free survival was calculated at 50% [23].

Our series presents even lower 12-month and 24-month recurrence-free survival rates of 38.6% and 18.2. Comparing tumor pathological characteristics at induction the current series presents with a higher number of high risk malignancies with 88.6% of tumors harboring high grade features (T1, Tis, and grade 3) compared to 78% and 44% in the aforementioned series. Progression to advanced stage disease (pT2 or greater) was seen in 5 (6.8%) patients, which is comparable to the reports by O'Donnell and Lam et al. [12, 14] where the reported incidence ranged from 3% to 12.5%. A concerning finding was the presence of micropapillary features in roughly 20% of patients who underwent salvage cystectomy. At median follow-up of 28 months the bladder preservation rate was 61.3% comparable to the literature ranging from 55% to 75% [12, 23].

Our results are in line with those reported by Rosevear and colleagues, [15] where failure of induction BCG monotherapy within 6 months was associated with failure of combination BCG plus interferon therapy. Not only was BCG failure <6 months associated with failure of combination therapy but also 73.3% of patients undergoing cystectomy had failed BGC monotherapy within 6 months as well. 66.7% of the patients who developed disease progression or advanced disease were again noted to fail BCG monotherapy within 6 months. While patients with large tumors and multifocal disease at induction were more common in the failure group a statistically significant association was not seen. Timing of initial induction BCG monotherapy failure appears to be a significant predictor of salvage combination therapy failure and disease progression. Consequently, patients who fail BCG within 6 months should be even more strongly counseled towards early radical cystectomy.

Valrubicin was approved by the FDA in 1998 following a phase III study [16] for patients with BCG refractory carcinoma *in situ* (CIS). In the pivotal trial the disease-free status at 12 months was 10%, inferior to the results reported by O'Donnell and colleagues with combination BCG plus interferon. This low event-free survival (EFS) was recently validated in a retrospective study by Cookson et al. [17], where the 12-month EFS following valrubicin instillation was calculated at 16.4%. Valrubicin was seldom used during the current study period due to the low number of patients with CIS in the recurrence specimen and the fact that the medication was off the market for half of the study period (2004–2009).

Over the last 10 years several novel intravesical therapies have been proposed for the management of BCG refractory NMIBC. These can be categorized as chemotherapy, immunotherapy, and device assisted therapy. A direct visual comparison between the different treatment modalities can be seen in Table 3.

Gemcitabine is a nucleoside analogue that causes defective DNA replication, leading to tumor cell apoptosis. In a phase II trial Dalbagni et al. [18] followed up 30 BCG failure patients after administering 2 cycles of intravesical gemcitabine and cisplatin (2000 mg/100 mL) for 3 consecutive weeks. At a median follow-up of 19 months the initial CR was 50% with 12-month recurrence-free rate of 21%. Most recently Mohanty et al. [19] treated 35 patients, following BCG failure, with 2000 mg of intravesical gemcitabine weekly for 6 weeks. At median follow-up of 18 months, 60% showed no recurrence, 31% recurred with similar stage/grade, and 9% progressed to muscle invasive disease. Di Lorenzo et al. [24] randomized 80 high risk patients who had failed initial treatment with BCG to gemcitabine (2000 mg/50 mL) or a BCG (81 mg) group. At median follow-up of 15 months 52.5% and 87.5% of the patients experienced a recurrence in the gemcitabine and BCG groups, respectively. Twenty-one (33%) and 13 (37.5%) suffered disease progression requiring radical cystectomy.

Docetaxel is a semisynthetic microtubule inhibitor. Barlow and colleagues [25] treated 33 patients with BCG refractory disease with a 6-week induction course of docetaxel. The median follow-up was 20 months and the 12-month and 24-month recurrence-free survival was calculated at 45% and 32%, respectively.

Thermochemotherapy (TC) including the Synergo system incorporates a combination of intravesical mitomycin-C (MMC) and bladder wall hyperthermia using thermocouple catheter and microwave equipment. The technology is based on the finding that inducing bladder wall to temperatures of 42°C improves the absorption of sequentially administered intravesical MMC. Nativ et al. [26] reported the results of 110 patients with BCG refractory high risk NMIBC using the Synergo system. The protocol consisted of weekly TC therapy for 6–8 weeks followed by six sessions every 6–8 weeks. The reported 12-month and 24-month disease-free survival was 85% and 56%, respectively.

Finally electromotive drug administration (EMDA) has shown promise in the treatment of high risk NMIBC. The concept behind this technology is to create a current gradient between the intravesical chemotherapy agent and the bladder wall; in order, to improve the transmembrane transport of the chemotherapeutic agent. Di Stasi and colleagues [27] performed a prospective trial in 108 BCG naïve patients randomizing them to EMDA + MMC versus passive MMC versus standard BCG. Complete response rates at 3 months

TABLE 3: Studies of intravesical treatments used in patients with bacillus Calmette-Guerin failure.

Study	Treatment modality	n	Follow-up	Recurrence-free survival	Progression, %	Cystectomy rate, %	High risk* disease, %
UMPC series	BCG plus IFN-$\alpha 2\beta$	44	28 months	39% and 18% at 12 months and 24 months	12	36	86
O'Donnell et al. [12]	BCG plus IFN-$\alpha 2\beta$	40	30 months	63% and 53% at 12 months and 24 months	12	55	78
Stein et al. [13]	BCG plus IFN-$\alpha 2\beta$	32	22 months	53% at median follow-up	16	22	44
Joudi et al. [11]	BCG plus IFN-$\alpha 2\beta$	1,007	24 months	45% at 24 months	—	—	70
Lam et al. [14]	IV gemcitabine	30	19 months	21% at median follow-up	3.5	37	100
Rosevear et al. [15]	IV gemcitabine	35	18 months	60% at median follow-up	8.75	—	62
Dinney et al. [16]	IV gemcitabine	80	15.5 months	19% at median follow-up	33	33	87
Cookson et al. [17]	IV docetaxel	33	29 months	32–45% at median follow-up	—	—	76
Dalbagni et al. [18]	Thermochemotherapy	111	16 months	85% and 56% at 12 months and 24 months	3	—	26
Mohanty et al. [19]	Electromotive	108	6 months	CR 53% and 58% at 3 months and 6 months	—	—	100

*High risk: CIS, T1, or grade ≥3.

and 6 months were 53%, 28%, and 56% and 58%, 31%, and 64% for the EMDA + MCC, passive MMC, and standard BCG groups, respectively. Median time to recurrence was 35, 19.5, and 26 months, respectively. The authors concluded that EMDA + MMC is comparable to standard BCG therapy in patients with high risk NMIBC.

As shown in Table 3 all proposed intravesical salvage treatments for BCG failure NMIBC have similar recurrence and progression rates and the differences mainly accounted for by the different patient populations. At the moment, combination immunotherapy of BCG plus interferon has the largest volume of data for its use in this cohort of patients. While some chemotherapy and device assisted intravesical therapies show promise in small cohort studies, the institution of these therapies requires further investigation and may require investment into technology with limited in-clinic use.

5. Conclusion

Herein, we present our contemporary experience with combination BCG plus interferon-$\alpha 2\beta$ as salvage intravesical therapy for patients with BCG refractory NMIBC. BCG plus interferon therapy appears to be effective in a subset of patients which needs to be clarified through further investigation. It is an overall well-tolerated therapy with acceptable recurrence- and progression-free rates compared to other salvage regimens. While no standardized criteria and regimen have been established for the management of this patient population, results from this study confirm, as prior series suggested, that salvage intravesical therapy should not be

offered to patients who fail BCG induction therapy within 6 months.

Conflict of Interests

The authors declare that there is no conflict of interests regarding the publication of this paper.

References

[1] American Cancer Society, *What Are the Key Statistics about Bladder Cancer?* American Cancer Society, 2014.

[2] H. W. Herr, D. D. Wartinger, W. R. Fair, and H. F. Oettgen, "Bacillus Calmette-Guerin therapy for superficial bladder cancer: a 10-year followup," *The Journal of Urology*, vol. 147, no. 4, pp. 1020–1023, 1992.

[3] M. Babjuk, M. Burger, R. Zigeuner et al., "EAU guidelines on non-muscle-invasive urothelial carcinoma of the bladder: update 2013," *European Urology*, vol. 64, no. 4, pp. 639–653, 2013.

[4] W. J. Catalona, M. A. Hudson, D. P. Gillen, G. L. Andriole, and T. L. Ratliff, "Risks and benefits of repeated courses of intravesical bacillus Calmette-Guerin therapy for superficial bladder cancer," *The Journal of Urology*, vol. 137, no. 2, pp. 220–224, 1987.

[5] G. V. Raj, H. Herr, A. M. Serio et al., "Treatment paradigm shift may improve survival of patients with high risk superficial bladder cancer," *The Journal of Urology*, vol. 177, no. 4, pp. 1283–1286, 2007.

[6] F. J. Bianco Jr., D. Justa, D. J. Grignon, W. A. Sakr, J. E. Pontes, and D. P. Wood Jr., "Management of clinical T1 bladder transitional cell carcinoma by radical cystectomy," *Urologic Oncology:*

Seminars and Original Investigations, vol. 22, no. 4, pp. 290–294, 2004.

[7] R. E. Hautmann, B. G. Volkmer, and K. Gust, "Quantification of the survival benefit of early versus deferred cystectomy in high-risk non-muscle invasive bladder cancer (T1 G3)," *World Journal of Urology*, vol. 27, no. 3, pp. 347–351, 2009.

[8] A. R. Zlotta, N. E. Fleshner, and M. A. Jewett, "The management of BCG failure in non-muscle-invasive bladder cancer: an update," *Canadian Urological Association Journal*, vol. 3, pp. S199–S205, 2009.

[9] P.-U. Malmström, "A randomized comparative dose-ranging study of interferon-α and mitomycin-C as an internal control in primary or recurrent superficial transitional cell carcinoma of the bladder," *BJU International*, vol. 89, no. 7, pp. 681–686, 2002.

[10] Y. Luo, X. Chen, T. M. Downs, W. C. DeWolf, and M. A. O'Donnell, "IFN-α 2B enhances Th1 cytokine responses in bladder cancer patients receiving *Mycobacterium bovis* bacillus Calmette-Guerin immunotherapy," *Journal of Immunology*, vol. 162, no. 4, pp. 2399–2405, 1999.

[11] F. N. Joudi, B. J. Smith, and M. A. O'Donnell, "Final results from a national multicenter phase II trial of combination bacillus Calmette-Guérin plus interferon α-2B for reducing recurrence of superficial bladder cancer," *Urologic Oncology: Seminars and Original Investigations*, vol. 24, no. 4, pp. 344–348, 2006.

[12] M. A. O'Donnell, J. Krohn, and W. C. DeWolf, "Salvage intravesical therapy with interferon-α 2B plus low dose bacillus Calmette-Guerin is effective in patients with superficial bladder cancer in whom bacillus Calmette-Guerin alone previously failed," *The Journal of Urology*, vol. 166, no. 4, pp. 1300–1304, 2001.

[13] J. P. Stein, G. Lieskovsky, R. Cote et al., "Radical cystectomy in the treatment of invasive bladder cancer: long-term results in 1,054 patients," *Journal of Clinical Oncology*, vol. 19, no. 3, pp. 666–675, 2001.

[14] J. S. Lam, M. C. Benson, M. A. O'Donnell et al., "Bacillus Calmete-Guérin plus interferon-α2B intravesical therapy maintains an extended treatment plan for superficial bladder cancer with minimal toxicity," *Urologic Oncology: Seminars and Original Investigations*, vol. 21, no. 5, pp. 354–360, 2003.

[15] H. M. Rosevear, A. J. Lightfoot, K. K. Birusingh, J. L. Maymí, K. G. Nepple, and M. A. O'Donnell, "Factors affecting response to bacillus Calmette-Guérin plus interferon for urothelial carcinoma in situ," *Journal of Urology*, vol. 186, no. 3, pp. 817–823, 2011.

[16] C. P. N. Dinney, R. E. Greenberg, and G. D. Steinberg, "Intravesical valrubicin in patients with bladder carcinoma in situ and contraindication to or failure after bacillus Calmette-Guérin," *Urologic Oncology: Seminars and Original Investigations*, vol. 31, no. 8, pp. 1635–1642, 2013.

[17] M. S. Cookson, S. S. Chang, C. Lihou et al., "Use of intravesical valrubicin in clinical practice for treatment of nonmuscle-invasive bladder cancer, including carcinoma in situ of the bladder," *Therapeutic Advances in Urology*, vol. 6, no. 5, pp. 181–191, 2014.

[18] G. Dalbagni, P. Russo, B. Bochner et al., "Phase II trial of intravesical gemcitabine in bacille Calmette- Guérin-refractory transitional cell carcinoma of the bladder," *Journal of Clinical Oncology*, vol. 24, no. 18, pp. 2729–2734, 2006.

[19] N. K. Mohanty, R. L. Nayak, P. Vasudeva, and R. P. Arora, "Intravesicle gemcitabine in management of BCG refractory superficial TCC of urinary bladder-our experience," *Urologic Oncology: Seminars and Original Investigations*, vol. 26, no. 6, pp. 616–619, 2008.

[20] H. W. Herr, C. M. Pinsky, W. F. Whitmore Jr., P. C. Sogani, H. F. Oettgen, and M. R. Melamed, "Long-term effect of intravesical bacillus Calmette-Guerin on flat carcinoma in situ of the bladder," *The Journal of Urology*, vol. 135, no. 2, pp. 265–267, 1986.

[21] R. B. Nadler, W. J. Catalona, M. A. Hudson, and T. L. Ratliff, "Durability of the tumor-free response for intravesical bacillus Calmette-Guerin therapy," *Journal of Urology*, vol. 152, no. 2, pp. 367–373, 1994.

[22] M. Buscarini, E. Pasin, and J. P. Stein, "Complications of radical cystectomy," *Minerva Urologica e Nefrologica*, vol. 59, no. 1, pp. 67–87, 2007.

[23] D. Lamm, M. Brausi, M. A. O'Donnell, and J. A. Witjes, "Interferon alfa in the treatment paradigm for non-muscle-invasive bladder cancer," *Urologic Oncology: Seminars and Original Investigations*, vol. 32, no. 1, pp. 35.e21–35.e30, 2014.

[24] G. Di Lorenzo, S. Perdonà, R. Damiano et al., "Gemcitabine versus bacille Calmette-Guérin after initial bacille Calmette-Guérin failure in non-muscle-invasive bladder cancer: a multicenter prospective randomized trial," *Cancer*, vol. 116, no. 8, pp. 1893–1900, 2010.

[25] L. J. Barlow, J. M. McKiernan, and M. C. Benson, "The novel use of intravesical docetaxel for the treatment of non-muscle invasive bladder cancer refractory to BCG therapy: a single institution experience," *World Journal of Urology*, vol. 27, no. 3, pp. 331–335, 2009.

[26] O. Nativ, J. A. Witjes, K. Hendricksen et al., "Combined thermo-chemotherapy for recurrent bladder cancer after bacillus Calmette-Guerin," *The Journal of Urology*, vol. 182, no. 4, pp. 1313–1317, 2009.

[27] S. M. Di Stasi, A. Giannantoni, R. L. Stephen et al., "Intravesical electromotive mitomycin C versus passive transport mitomycin C for high risk superficial bladder cancer: a prospective randomized study," *The Journal of Urology*, vol. 170, no. 3, pp. 777–782, 2003.

10

Posterior Urethral Strictures

Joel Gelman and Eric S. Wisenbaugh

University of California, Irvine, 333 City Boulevard West, Suite 1240, Orange, CA 92868, USA

Correspondence should be addressed to Eric S. Wisenbaugh; eric.wisenbaugh@gmail.com

Academic Editor: Francisco E. Martins

Pelvic fracture urethral injuries are typically partial and more often complete disruptions of the most proximal bulbar and distal membranous urethra. Emergency management includes suprapubic tube placement. Subsequent primary realignment to place a urethral catheter remains a controversial topic, but what is not controversial is that when there is the development of a stricture (which is usually obliterative with a distraction defect) after suprapubic tube placement or urethral catheter removal, the standard of care is delayed urethral reconstruction with excision and primary anastomosis. This paper reviews the management of patients who suffer pelvic fracture urethral injuries and the techniques of preoperative urethral imaging and subsequent posterior urethroplasty.

1. Introduction

Pelvic fracture trauma in males, often secondary to motor vehicle trauma or pelvic crush injuries, can be associated with injuries to the posterior urethra, especially where there is pubic symphysis diastasis or there are displaced inferomedial pubic bone fractures [1]. The term "prostatomembranous disruption" is often used to describe these injuries, and this terminology suggests that the transection occurs at the junction of the prostatic and membranous portions of the posterior urethra. However, more recent studies, including an autopsy review of male patients who sustained pelvic fracture related urethral injuries and died of associated multiple trauma, revealed that the injuries are generally membranous and distal to the urogenital diaphragm [2]. There can be proximal or distal extension, but the injury generally remains distal to the verumontanum of the prostate. As long as the bladder neck remains intact, continence should be maintained in these patients after repair. Additionally, in many patients, there also remains a significant rhabdosphincter contribution, as demonstrated by video-urodynamic testing after reconstruction [3].

The classic sign of urethral injury in a patient with a pelvic fracture is blood at the urethral meatus, but other symptoms such as bladder distension, inability to void, and perineal hematoma should raise a high index of suspicion as well. Older texts emphasize the finding of a high riding prostate on digital rectal examination, but this is not a reliable finding on physical exam.

2. Initial Evaluation and Management

A retrograde urethrogram (RUG) is indicated when a urethral injury is suspected and will typically reveal significant extravasation due to a partial tear or, more often, a complete disruption (Figure 1). Initial management should be placement of a suprapubic tube as the most effective and immediate way to drain the bladder. The ideal suprapubic tube is no less than 16 French in size and positioned in the midline 2-finger breadth above the pubic symphysis. Subsequently, options include primary realignment or suprapubic diversion for several months followed by posterior urethroplasty.

The purpose of primary realignment is to approximate the severed ends of the urethra to potentially avoid subsequent stricture formation. Historically, this was performed through an open approach with an attempt at immediate repair. This procedure was mostly abandoned due to the prohibitively high rates of erectile dysfunction and incontinence that resulted compared to those who underwent delayed repair [4]. The advancement of endoscopic technology, however, has allowed primary endoscopic realignment (PER) of

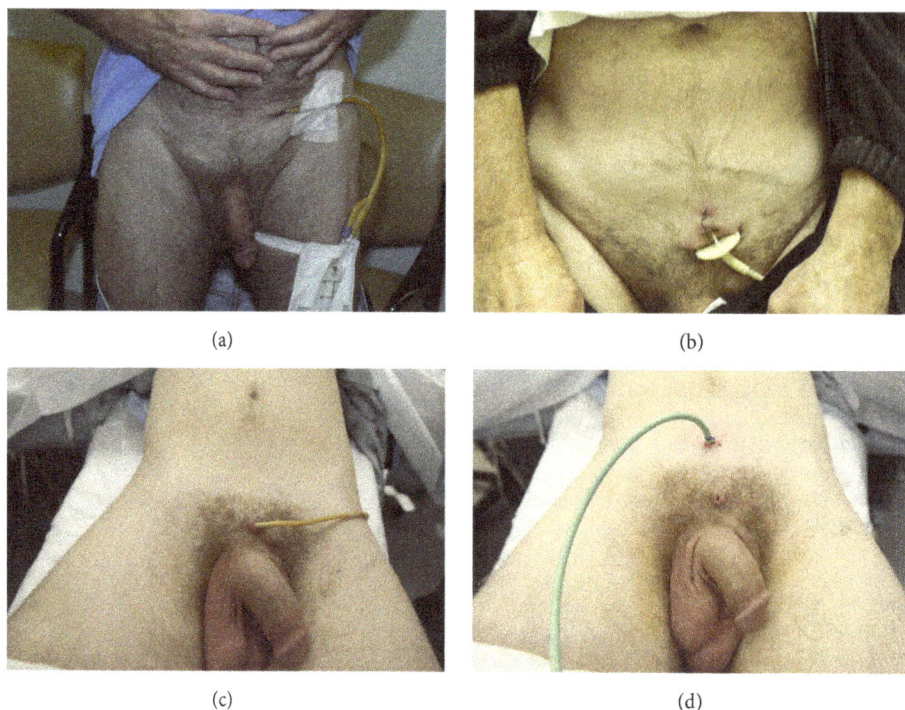

FIGURE 1: (a) Laterally placed suprapubic tube. (b) Small "pigtail" catheter of inadequate caliber. (c) Suprapubic tube placed below the ideal location. (d) Suprapubic tube repositioned midline 2-finger breadth above the midline pubic symphysis.

the urethra without the potentially damaging extensive manipulation that was required for immediate open repair and is now attempted routinely in some centers.

Stricture formation can potentially be avoided with this approach. However stricture rates remain high after PER and it is essential that these patients be followed in the long term. A recent meta-analysis reported a 49% rate of stricture formation after PER, yet this is likely an underestimate as the literature consists of mostly small case series that are retrospective and have variable follow-up that does not always include cystoscopy to confirm patency [5].

While sometimes successful, PER can have unintended consequences when strictures are not treated appropriately. In a recent study, the mean time to definitive resolution of stenosis was dramatically longer in patients who underwent PER (122 months versus 6 months) because they underwent multiple endoscopic interventions without resolution of their stenosis [6]. Repeated, not only are unsuccessful interventions costly to the healthcare system, but they can also expose the patient to painful self-dilations or office dilations as well as the potential for acute urinary retention requiring emergency management.

The purpose of limiting the immediate management to placement of a suprapubic tube is to allow a successful, definitive repair once the tissues have had time to heal, typically after 3 months. Placement of a suprapubic tube can easily be accomplished in any trauma center without the need for immediate reconstructive expertise, and the patient can subsequently be referred for further management. In this

situation, posterior urethroplasty is highly successful, with a patency rate of 97.6% at our own institution.

Although the benefits of primary realignment are the subject of controversy, it should be emphasized that when a stricture develops after primary realignment, the subsequent management is not controversial. The best approach is suprapubic tube urinary diversion for several months followed by urethral reconstruction. Management with dilations, urethrotomies, and/or self-catheterization should not be advised in an attempt to avoid open surgery as these options manage a chronic problem whereas a properly performed urethroplasty is almost always curative.

3. Preoperative Planning

3.1. Three-Month Delay. We wait 3 months from the time of injury or catheter removal in cases of failed primary realignment before performing urethroplasty to allow time for the initial extravasation to heal, hematoma to resolve, and the extent of the injury to become clearly defined. It has been shown that, after manipulation, several months of "urethral rest" is required before anterior urethral strictures become clearly defined [7]. When there is a pelvic fracture associated injury to the posterior urethra, initial imaging reveals extravasation, whereas imaging 3 months after injury typically confirms no extravasation and clear delineation of the location and length of the defect. Recent publications indicate that the delay is often a minimum of 3–6 months. However, the interval between initial injury and urethroplasty can exceed one year when there are associated injuries [8–12].

3.2. Suprapubic Tubes.

3.2. Suprapubic Tubes. Although the ideal suprapubic tube is at least 16 Fr, midline, and well above the midline pubic symphysis, patients are often initially managed with tubes that are far lateral to the midline or just above the symphysis. In some cases, very small caliber "pigtail" catheters are placed (Figure 1). Small caliber pigtail catheters are especially prone to encrustation and ultimately urinary retention. Moreover, catheters placed just above the symphysis are more uncomfortable than catheters placed in a higher position away from the bone. When patients are referred for posterior urethral reconstruction and have tubes of inadequate caliber, or if the tube is not in the ideal position, it is our preference to percutaneously place a new 16 Fr tube. This is generally done as soon as possible when the caliber is small and in no less than 1 month prior to urethroplasty so there will be an established stable tract at the time of surgery.

The main benefit of having the suprapubic tube midline in the ideal location with an established tract is that this facilitates the surgery and prevents the need for a temporary vesicostomy. During posterior urethroplasty with the patient in the lithotomy position, after perineal exposure is achieved and the urethra is transected, a metal sound is generally advanced through the established tract, and perineal dissection proceeds towards the tip of the sound until the sound can be seen and advanced into the perineum. When the caliber of the tract is inadequate, sounds will not advance without dilation at the time of the surgery. This can be associated with bleeding and compromise of the tract. When the tube is just above the bone, a very acute angle is needed to advance the sound through the bladder neck. Moreover, when the tract is lateral to the midline, the rigid sound cannot be reliably advanced medially towards the midline bladder neck and then distally along the posterior urethra. One option is to create a temporary vesicostomy. However, this adds considerable time and morbidity to the reconstructive surgery and therefore this is not our preference.

3.3. Preoperative Urethral Imaging and Cystoscopy. Prior to definitive urethral reconstruction, urethroscopy, antegrade cystoscopy, and simultaneous antegrade cystourethrogram and retrograde urethrogram (RUG) provide a definitive diagnosis of the exact length and location of the defect. One common imaging technique is for the bladder to be filled with contrast by gravity through the suprapubic tube and for a RUG to be performed as the patient is asked to Valsalva and attempt to void. This attempt to void can open the bladder neck and allow filling of the posterior urethra proximal to the obliteration, and the length of the defect will be determined (Figure 2(a)). However, in many cases, the patient cannot relax to void when the urethra is obliterated and contrast is being injected through the penis. When the bladder neck is intact, the appearance will be as shown (Figure 2(b)). The distance between the bladder and the distal end of the defect is not the length of the distraction defect because the prostatic urethra is not visualized. In a recent study where the goal was to determine if the type of urethroplasty could be predicted based on certain features from the preoperative imaging, 38% of the 100 study patients evaluated with a Valsalva cystourethrogram and RUG were excluded because there was no visualization of the urethra below the bladder neck [7].

Our preferred approach is to first perform antegrade cystoscopy with the patient prepped and draped in the oblique position after a 14 × 17 scout film is obtained to confirm proper position and penetration. Antegrade cystoscopy is important to inspect for bladder stones that may need to be removed preoperatively and also provides assessment of the bladder neck. An open bladder neck at rest suggests that there may be an increased incidence of incontinence subsequent to urethral reconstruction. Iselin and Webster identified 15 patients who sustained pelvic fracture urethral injuries and had an open bladder neck at rest [13]. Six were continent and 8 were incontinent after urethroplasty. However, MacDiarmid et al. identified 4 patients that had an open bladder neck at rest and all of these patients were continent after surgery [14]. Although some surgeons occasionally perform bladder neck reconstruction at the time of posterior urethroplasty [15], most do not feel this is necessary given the observation that an open bladder neck at rest does not reliably predict postoperative incontinence. When we observe an open bladder neck at rest, the patient is counseled that there may be an increased incidence of postoperative incontinence, but this finding does not influence our management.

3.4. Preoperative Urethral Evaluation: Urethral Imaging. Once the scope is advanced through the bladder neck, the location of the proximal aspect of the injury is noted, and this is almost always distal to the verumontanum of the prostate within the membranous urethra. With the tip of the scope at the level of the obliteration, full-strength contrast is injected, which will then backfill the posterior urethra and bladder. Simultaneously, a RUG is performed. Our preferred technique for performing a RUG is to place a gauze around the coronal sulcus to place the penis on stretch and inject contrast through a cone-shaped Taylor adaptor (Cook Urological) connected to a 60 cc syringe filled with full-strength contrast (Figure 3). Many published textbooks advocate the advancement of a catheter into the fossa navicularis and inflation of the balloon with 1–3 cc of contrast to form a seal. However, the balloon caliber of catheters of several different sizes when inflated with only 2 cc of fluid or air is approximately 59 French and the normal caliber of the adult anterior urethra is approximately 30 French except at the level of the urethral meatus and fossa navicularis where the caliber is approximately 24 French (Figure 4(a)). Therefore, the balloon will dilate the normal distal anterior urethra, which can be associated with considerable pain and even stricture disease of the fossa navicularis. We have seen patients referred for strictures initially limited to the bulbar urethra who then developed narrow caliber fossa strictures after undergoing painful urethral imaging where the technique included balloon inflation within the fossa navicularis (Figure 4(b)).

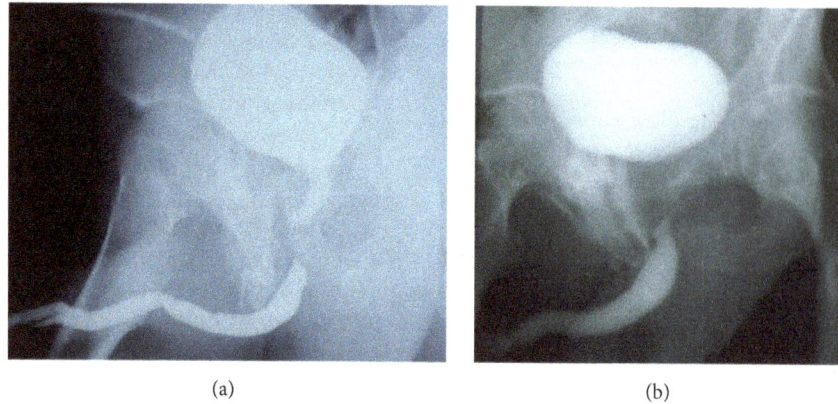

FIGURE 2: (a) After the bladder is filled with contrast through the suprapubic tube, a RUG is performed as the patient is asked to attempt to void. If the bladder neck opens, contrast fills the prostatic urethra, and the membranous urethral defect is seen. (b) When the bladder neck does not open, the length of the defect cannot be determined accurately.

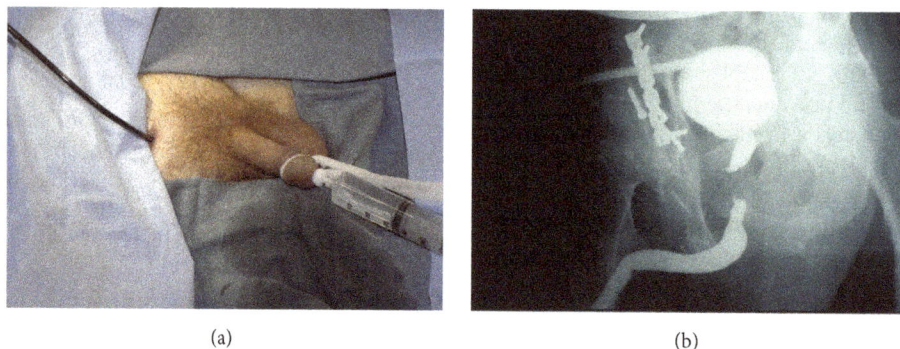

FIGURE 3: (a) A RUG is performed as contrast is simultaneously injected into the posterior urethra through the flexible cystoscope, with the tip in the distal prostatic urethra. (b) Imaging accurately demonstrating the length and location of the defect.

Simultaneous antegrade and retrograde imaging and endoscopy performed with proper technique will clearly define the exact length and location of the defect. Other imaging modalities that can be used include MRI and ultrasound [16]. However, we have never found an indication to perform these additional tests. Fluoroscopy offers the advantage of dynamic real time imaging. However, disadvantages include a reduced field of view and decreased resolution compared to conventional radiographs. We prefer flat plate imaging using digital cassettes that can be digitized and stored electronically and also printed on 14 × 17 film. Although magnification and positioning can influence the scale, we have observed that the length of the obliteration measured directly on the film very accurately corresponds to the length of the defect at the time of surgery. Most defects are 1 to 3 cm in length.

Defining the exact location of a stricture is also critical to management. Although pelvic fracture trauma typically injures the posterior urethra, if there is also straddle trauma at the time of the pelvic fracture, the injury can be to the bulbar urethra, which changes the treatment strategy. For example, a man who sustained pelvic fracture trauma during a race car accident was found to have significant extravasation on a RUG on the day of the injury and managed with a laterally placed suprapubic tube. Delayed imaging and antegrade

cystoscopy confirmed a proximal bulbar urethral defect and a normal membranous urethra (Figure 5). Although both traumatic proximal bulbar and membranous disruptions are managed with excision and primary anastomosis, bulbar urethroplasty does not require antegrade access to facilitate identification of the patent proximal segment. If the injury was membranous, then a new midline suprapubic tube would have been placed to facilitate subsequent antegrade access to the proximal segment at the time of posterior urethroplasty. However, since antegrade access is not required for bulbar urethroplasty, the placement of a new midline tube was not required.

3.5. Preoperative Vascular Evaluation. The anterior urethra has a dual blood supply, with an additional minor contribution provided by perforating vessels between the corpora cavernosa and the corpus spongiosum. The bulbar arteries enter the corpus spongiosum at the level of the most proximal bulbar urethra and provide antegrade flow to the corpus spongiosum of the anterior urethra. In addition, the dorsal arteries course within the neurovascular structures along the dorsal aspect of the penis superficial to the corporal bodies and supply the glans penis, which is the distal expansion of

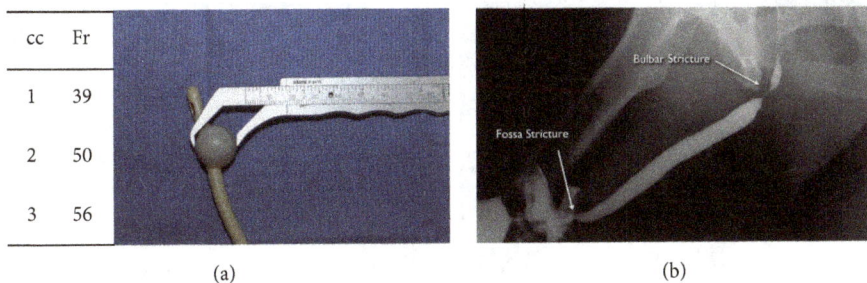

FIGURE 4: (a) Catheter balloon inflation with only 1–3 cc of air or fluid is associated with balloon inflation well beyond the normal caliber of the normal fossa navicularis. (b) Repeat RUG demonstrating, in addition to the previously seen bulbar stricture, a new fossa navicularis stricture that developed after a RUG was performed using fossa balloon inflation technique.

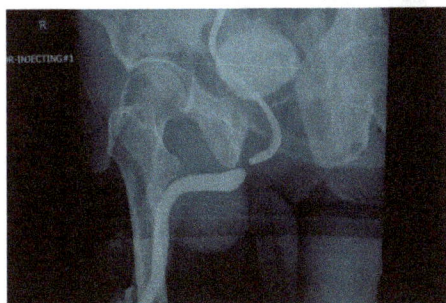

FIGURE 5: Simultaneous antegrade and retrograde urethral imaging demonstrating a bulbar urethral obliteration, further confirmed with antegrade cystoscopy.

the corpus spongiosum. This provides a secondary blood supply to the anterior urethra as the blood courses in retrograde fashion along the corpus spongiosum. When the urethra is completely transected at the departure of the anterior urethra, any patent bulbar arteries are ligated or cauterized. The anterior urethra then survives as a flap based on the retrograde dorsal artery contribution in addition to perforating vessels. Although unpublished, it has been observed by several reconstructive urologists that, in rare cases, long segment bulbar strictures developed as an ischemic complication of posterior urethroplasty. The mechanism of the ischemic stenosis was presumed to be compromised of the bulbar artery supply during surgery in patients who suffered perineal trauma that compromised dorsal artery supply. We have observed cases of ischemic stenosis in patients with hypospadias who developed discreet bulbar strictures and were treated with a urethral stent [17]. Prior to stent placement, these patients were noted on urethroscopy to have a normal caliber anterior urethra distal to the bulbar stricture. Subsequent to stent placement, they developed severe panurethral disease. This makes sense anatomically as hypospadias and corrective surgery are associated with a compromise of the corpus spongiosum distally and the associated retrograde blood supply to the more proximal anterior urethra. These patients were likely "bulbar dependent," and stent expansion compromised the antegrade bulbar artery flow distal to the stent. Therefore, in addition to antegrade cystoscopy and contrast imaging, we perform a preoperative vascular evaluation to

identify patients who have severe arterial inflow compromise to both dorsal arteries and perform penile revascularization prior to urethral reconstruction in selected cases. Penile revascularization provides a microvascular anastomosis of the inferior epigastric artery to the dorsal artery of the penis (Figure 6).

Erectile dysfunction and pudendal vascular injuries are highly associated with pelvic fracture urethral disruptions. A recent meta-analysis revealed that 34% of all patients with pelvic fracture urethral injury developed erectile dysfunction, even prior to any treatment other than suprapubic tube placemat [18]. In a study by Shenfeld et al., 25 patients who sustained traumatic posterior urethral disruptions were evaluated with nocturnal penile tumescence testing [19]. Eighteen patients (72%) were found to have erectile dysfunction, and these patients underwent a penile duplex with pharmacologic erection that revealed arterial inflow impairment in 5/18 patients. The remaining patients were considered to have a neurogenic etiology of their erectile dysfunction. Davics et al. performed a penile duplex testing on 56 men who sustained posterior urethral disruptions and identified 25 men with vascular compromise. These patients underwent arteriogram. Twenty-one had reconstitution of one or both pudendals, and 4 did not. These 4 patients underwent revascularization prior to urethral reconstruction, and no patient developed ischemic stenosis after surgery [20]. A limitation of this study is that it is not known if any of these patients would have developed stenosis if reconstruction had been performed without prior revascularization. This is an area of controversy. However, we believe vascular testing and revascularization in selected cases are justified based on the anatomic principals and the available data. Moreover, revascularization will often successfully treat the erectile dysfunction associated with pelvic fracture injuries [21].

3.6. Posterior Urethral Reconstruction: Preparation and Patient Positioning. Prior to definitive repair, patients are placed in high lithotomy during a physical examination to assess hip flexion and ability to tolerate this position. Some patients may have unresolved back or other orthopedic problems, which may then be exacerbated by prolonged lithotomy positioning. In our series of 85 patients, the longest delay was 19 months. This patient had severe compromise of hip flexion

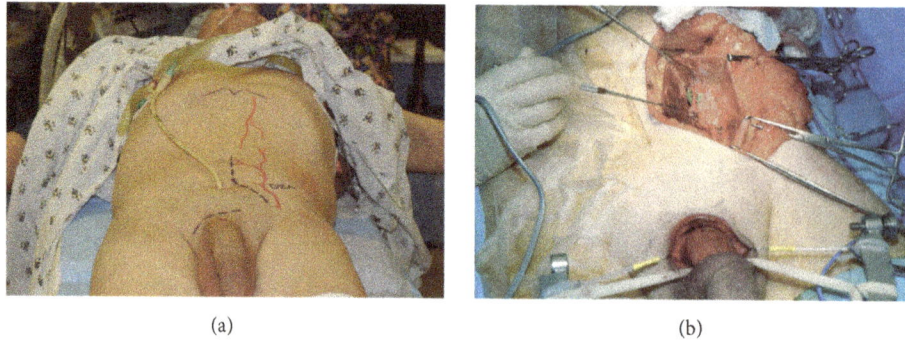

FIGURE 6: Inferior epigastric artery to dorsal artery penile revascularization, shown subsequent to skin marking (a) and during surgery (b).

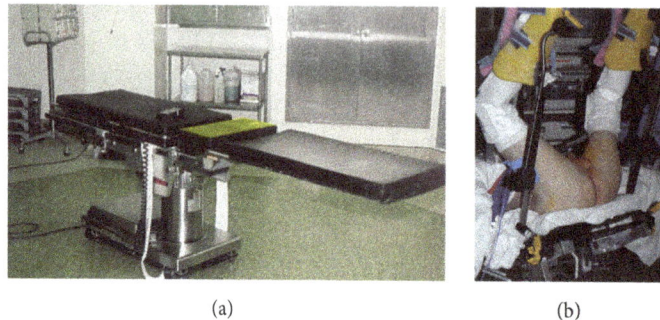

FIGURE 7: (a) Modified Skytron Custom 6000 Surgical Table with pelvic tilt mechanism (highlighted in yellow). (b) Patient positioned in exaggerated lithotomy.

that persisted more than 12 months after the injury. With ongoing physical therapy, mobility returned to normal, and positioning was safely accomplished without compromise. A urine culture is sent the week prior to surgery. The specimen is obtained by clamping the suprapubic tube and then unclamping the tube 20 minutes later over a specimen container. The sample is then obtained directly from the suprapubic tube and not the drainage bag. Any mixed growth is separately cultured. Patients are admitted the day prior to surgery for dual coverage antibiotics. Our protocol is to administer piperacillin/tazobactam and tobramycin but adjust the antibiotics if indicated based on the culture result. To date, no patient suffered the complication of a perineal infection, which can be associated with urethral compromise and stricture development.

Although some reconstructive urologists prefer a low lithotomy position, we prefer the exposure of exaggerated lithotomy. However, this position can be associated with severe complications including neuropraxia, compartment syndrome, and rhabdomyolysis [22–24]. Fortunately, neuropraxia is usually not permanent. Sensory deficits are more common than motor impairment, and the risk of a positioning complication is related to the time in lithotomy. One form of exaggerated lithotomy, often used for perineal prostatectomy, places hips under considerable flexion so that the thighs are parallel to the back and the floor. In a study by Holzbeierlein et al., of 111 men who underwent a radical perineal prostatectomy in this extreme lithotomy position with a mean duration of less than 3 hours, 23 (21%) suffered

a positioning complication. Of these 23 patients, 17 had symptoms at the time of discharge, and 6 required physical therapy support for ambulation [25].

We use Skytron Custom 6000 Table modified by Jordan to offer an electronic pelvic tilt mechanism to cradle the pelvis as an alternative to raising the buttocks and placing a beanbag support (Figure 7(a)). In addition, stirrups are modified to provide additional extension so that hip and knee flexion is reduced. Foam padding is placed along the dorsal feet and anterior legs to evenly distribute the pressure (Figure 7(b)). We previously used gel pads but found that use of the softer foam pads reduced the incidence of temporary (24–28 hours) dorsal foot numbness. Extreme flexion of the hips and knees is avoided, and the boots are tilted so that there is no pressure on the calves.

3.7. Posterior Urethral Reconstruction: Surgical Technique

3.7.1. Exposure. A midline perineal incision is one option. We prefer an inverted "Y" shaped lambda incision to obtain generous exposure (Figure 8(a)). This is carried medial to the ischial tuberosities posteriorly and along the median scrotal raphe. Dissection then proceeds sharply through the subcutaneous fat longitudinally along the midline until the bulbospongiosus muscle is encountered. The Jordan-Simpson perineal retractor is used to facilitate exposure as shown (Figure 8(b)). Although other retractors are commercially available such as the Lone Star retractor, advantages of the Jordan retractor include the fixation of the ring and

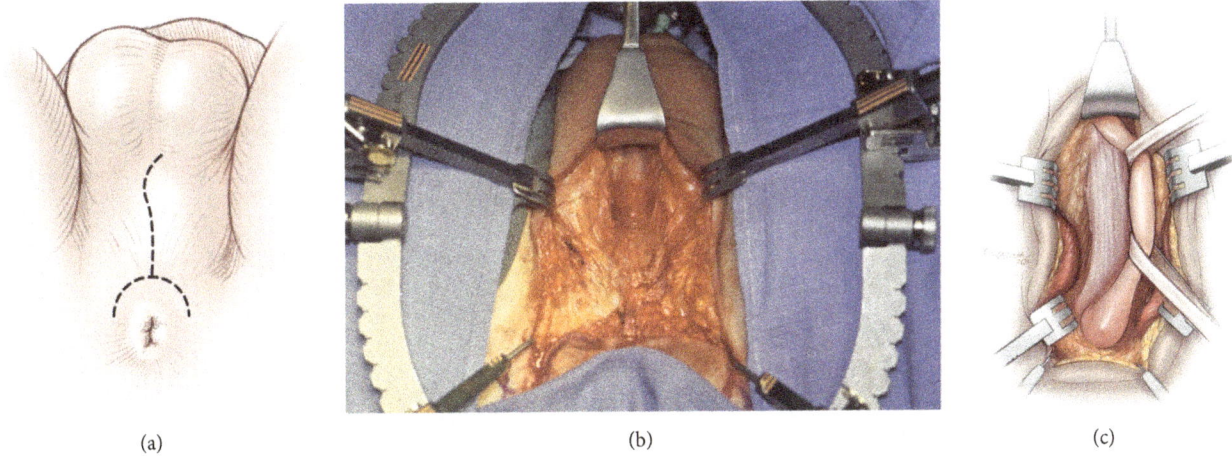

(a)   (b)   (c)

FIGURE 8: (a) Lambda incision with the patient in the exaggerated lithotomy position. (b) Jordan-Simpson perineal retractor is used to facilitate exposure of the corpus spongiosum. (c) The corpus spongiosum is circumferentially mobilized along the bulbar urethra.

the ability to use a variety of different specialized blades in addition to the hooks used in the Lone Star system. In addition, tilt ratchets facilitate lateral retraction to facilitate exposure. The bulbospongiosus muscle is then divided and retracted laterally to expose the bulb. The bulb is detached from the perineal body and we find that the use of a bipolar cautery facilitates this dissection and maintains hemostasis to the extent that suction is seldom required. The urethra is then circumferentially mobilized from the penoscrotal junction distally to the departure of the anterior urethra proximally (Figure 8(c)). This is done sharply without the use of right angle clamps, which can tear the corpus spongiosum. The bulbar arteries are transected and cauterized if patent.

Several recent papers describe bulbar artery sparing anastomotic anterior urethroplasty [26, 27]. Although the use of artery sparing surgery during posterior urethral reconstruction has not been published, an abstract recently presented described the successful use of this technique in 9 patients [28]. Intraoperative ultrasound was performed, and the artery with the strongest signal was preserved. No patient developed a recurrent stricture with a mean follow-up of 10 months. This may possibly represent a future modification of operative technique.

3.7.2. Proximal Exposure and Scar Excision. Once the urethra has been adequately mobilized, it is transected at the distal aspect of the defect, which can be accurately located intraoperatively with the use of a 16 Fr catheter or bougie á boule. Subsequently, unless preoperative imaging suggests very short segment obliteration, we routinely separate the corporal bodies at the level of the triangular ligament and retract them laterally to improve proximal exposure and facilitate excision of the scar tissue, which is generally whitish in color and firm.

The suprapubic tube is then removed and a curved metal sound is advanced through the established tract into the bladder and then through the bladder neck, guided by feel, until the impulse of the tip of the sound can be palpated in the perineum as the sound is manipulated. This guides the dissection in the appropriate direction towards the patent proximal urethra. One option is to advance a Van Buren sound. Although these instruments are often readily available and familiar to most urologists, the fact that the instrument is curved only at the tip and tapered to a more pointed tip relative to the shaft of the instrument renders these instruments poorly suited to use in posterior urethroplasty, especially when an exaggerated lithotomy position is used. However, the semicircular Haygrove sound is designed to best follow the path from the suprapubic access to the membranous urethra (Figures 9(a) and 9(b)). The tip is curved and smooth, and the caliber is not greater than 16–18 Fr and, therefore, no tract dilation is required if the indwelling suprapubic tube was 16 Fr.

There are cases, however, when the tip of the sound may not be palpable. This may be due to the presence of very dense scar or malposition of the sound. This presents a significant challenge because if dissection proceeds in the wrong direction, what is entered may be the bladder or the posterior urethra proximal to the distal aspect of the patent urethra. This could essentially "bypass" the bladder neck and may lead to severe postoperative incontinence. This is a major limitation of using a solid sound that is guided blindly. A flexible cystoscope can be used in these cases, but since the active scope deflection is limited only to the tip of the scope, it may be difficult to advance the tip of the scope to the proper position, especially when the patient is in high lithotomy and the surgeon is positioned at the level of the perineum. To prevent the possibility of false passages, some surgeons perform rigid antegrade cystoscopy before the patient is prepped and draped in the exaggerated lithotomy position, advance the scope through the bladder neck and prostatic urethra, and then palpate the perineum to determine if the tip of the scope is palpable or not [29]. When the tip of the scope is not palpable, or if the suprapubic tube is laterally located, a temporary vesicostomy is created prior to lithotomy positioning and then taken down subsequent to the completion of the repair (Figure 9(c)). It was determined that the creation

(a)

(b)   (c)

(d)   (e)

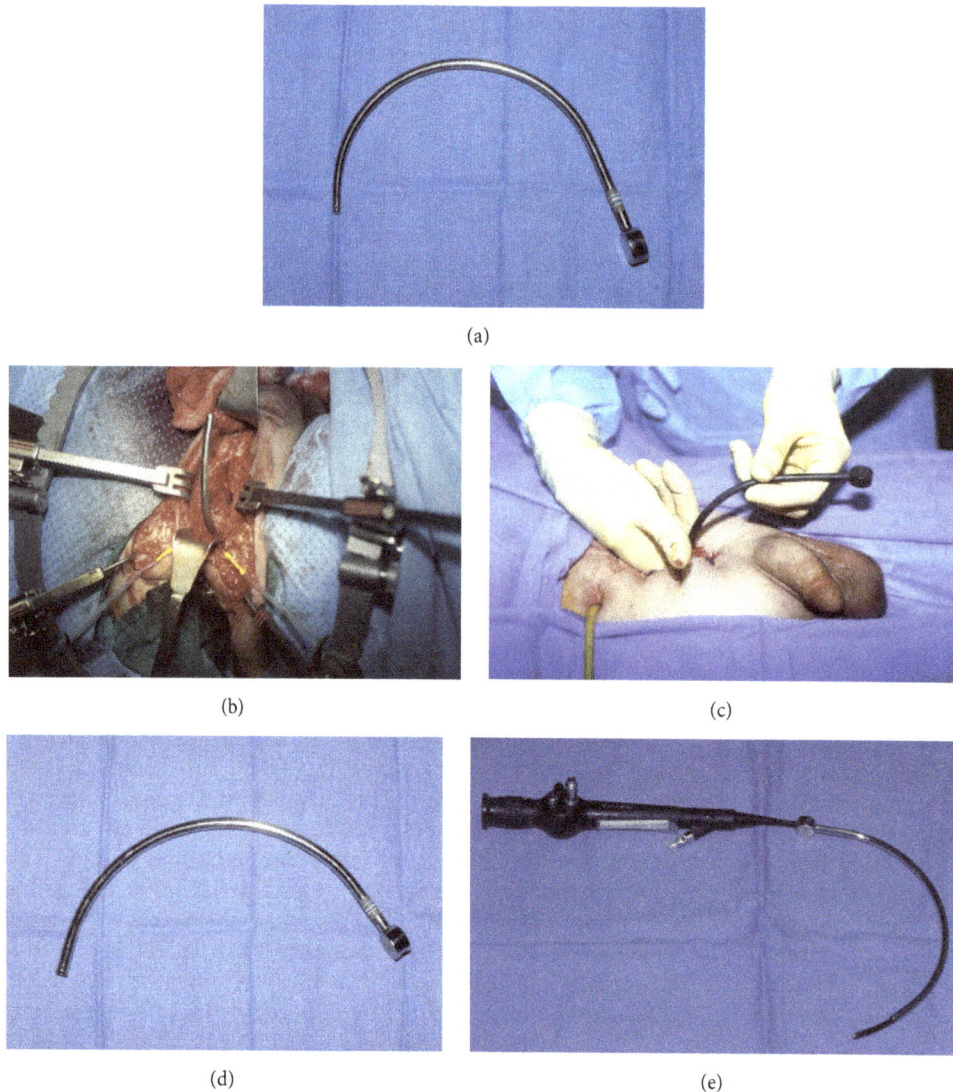

FIGURE 9: (a) Solid Haygrove sound. (b) After dissection of the obliterative scar, the tip of the sound (placed through the suprapubic tract) can then be advanced through the patent proximal urethra into the perineum. (c) Temporary vesicostomy in a patient with a laterally placed suprapubic tube. (d) Gelman visualizing posterior urethral sound. (e) Flexible scope advanced through the hollow visualizing sound.

of the vesicostomy allows the surgeon to palpably identify the bladder neck before instrumentation of the posterior urethra and that this maneuver eliminates the occurrence of false passages and the misanastomosis of the anterior urethra to sites other than the apical prostatic urethra. While this maneuver can be effective, it adds considerable time and morbidity to the surgery.

It is for this reason that we prefer to always proceed with a midline suprapubic tube, even if this requires placement of a new tube no less than 1 month prior to urethroplasty to allow time for the tract to mature and use a new visualizing sound (Gelman Urethral Sound, CS Surgical) (Figure 9(d)). This sound has a contour similar to the Haygrove sound but is hollow, allowing a flexible cystoscopy to be advanced through the sound (Figure 9(e)). The tip of the sound and/or the tip of the cystoscope can then be directed to the obliteration under direct vision. An additional advantage is that the light from

the scope can be seen to further guide the dissection. Prior to the development of the visualizing sound, 2/9 patients at our institution required a temporary vesicostomy at the time of reconstruction. Subsequently, 76 patients (ages 4–77 years) underwent reconstruction (including 6 pediatric patients and 14 patients who had unsuccessful procedures prior to referral), and 0/76 patients required a temporary vesicostomy. In every case, the sound could be directed to the proper position under direct vision. It is our experience that the visualizing posterior urethral sound greatly facilitates the reliable identification and dissection of the proximal segment during posterior urethral reconstruction. With the use of this device, the open dissection can be limited to the perineal exploration, even in pediatric and difficult cases. One disadvantage of the sound is that the outside diameter (OD) is greater than the OD of the solid Haygrove sound, and the solid sound can be manipulated more easily.

Therefore, we continue to use the solid sound when the tip can be readily palpated in the perineum. Although the larger diameter hollow sound will not advance as easily through the suprapubic tract when 16–18 Fr indwelling tubes are used prior to surgery, the tip of the flexible cystoscope can be first advanced into the bladder, and the sound can then be advanced over the scope using the scope as the equivalent of a guide wire.

The most complex portion of posterior urethral reconstruction is the proximal exposure and dissection subsequent to transection of the urethra. One option is to sharply incise scar tissue, advance a nasal speculum through the scar, and place "J" shaped sutures through the speculum to initiate the anastomosis [30]. It is our preference to excise the scar tissue until normal healthy tissue is encountered. Supple tissue more readily everts, bringing the mucosa forward from deep within the pelvis during the placement of the first several sutures, and this facilitates the placement of subsequent sutures. Our objective is to achieve the proximal preplacement of 10-12 3-0 absorbable monofilament sutures. We alternate using violet PDS and clear Monocryl to help maintain orientation at the time of the completion of the anastomosis.

3.7.3. Infrapubectomy. In cases where the scar is especially dense and the defect is long, it is possible that the tip of the sound will not be palpable, and the light of the cystoscope will not be seen even when using the visualizing sound. In these cases, scar tissue just below the midline symphysis is excised sharply in a 1-2 cm diameter area. As the dissection extends deep into the pelvis, infrapubectomy is often required to facilitate the proximal scar excision. The corporal bodies, which have already been separated, are retracted laterally exposing the dorsal vein, which is then mobilized and ligated to expose the midline symphysis pubis. Periosteal elevators are then used to sweep the medial crura laterally and free the undersurface of the bone from adherent tissue. Kerrison rongeurs provide controlled bone removal, which widens the exposure and facilitates further proximal dissection. Moreover, the separation of the corpora and infrapubectomy provide a more direct route for the urethra to course, and this facilitates a tension-free repair.

3.7.4. Additional Maneuvers. Some authors have reported that, in addition to distal mobilization, crural separation, and infrapubectomy, supracrural corporal rerouting was required to achieve an acceptable amount of tension in selected cases [31]. This technique appears to be associated with a high rate of restenosis. In a recently published combined series of 142 cases, 4 underwent rerouting and 3 of these patients (75%) developed restenosis [12]. Other surgeons never find supracrural rerouting to be a beneficial maneuver. It is often stated that the objective is a "tension-free" anastomosis. This is not necessary as there is normally a certain amount of innate tension along the corpus spongiosum. It is for this reason that when the urethra is transected, there is generally some retraction of the distal segment. Our goal is not a tension-free anastomosis, but rather an anastomosis without unacceptable tension that would lead to tethering of the penis

during erections or separation of the anastomosis. To date, we have never encountered a case where supracrural rerouting was required.

Another option in complex cases where there is a large defect is a transpubic approach [32–34]. This is a technique we have never found necessary, and more recent reports confirm that infrapubectomy generally provides adequate proximal exposure in complex cases [35].

Another tool that has been reported to bridge longer defects is the use of tissue transfer with flaps or grafts [31]. This appears to have been performed mostly in older series, and recent reports do not support the use of or need for tissue transfer. It is fortunate that excision and primary anastomosis can reliably be achieved during posterior urethral reconstruction given that tube flaps and grafts are generally associated with a high failure rate, and the tissues surrounding the membranous urethra deep within the pelvis proximal to the triangular ligament do not represent an excellent bed for graft spread fixation.

3.7.5. Anastomosis. Once the proximal sutures are placed along a widely patent proximal segment surrounded by pink healthy mucosa proximally, and flexible cystoscopy further confirms that the opening is distal to the verumontanum at the appropriate location, the distal segment is dorsally spatulated and calibrated using bougie á boule. The caliber should be greater than 30 Fr. The anastomosis is then completed as a stenting catheter is placed. It is our preference to use a 14 Fr soft silicone catheter. A small round drain is placed deep adjacent to the corpus spongiosum deep to the bulbospongiosus muscle, which is then reapproximated along the ventral midline, and a second flat 7 mm drain is placed superficial to the muscle. The incision is then closed in 2 layers with absorbable suture and a clear dressing is placed. No compressive dressing is required.

3.8. Postoperative Care. Our protocol is to maintain the stenting urethral catheter and the suprapubic tube urinary diversion for 3 weeks and then perform a VCUG by removing the stenting catheter, filling the bladder with contrast by gravity installation and then obtaining a film during urination. In the rare case of extravasation, a new stenting catheter is replaced and a repeat study is performed the following week. Other surgeons favor catheter removal without postoperative imaging [36]. In most cases, the force of stream will be excellent, and the suprapubic tube is then removed. If the stream is weak, the tube is plugged and the patient is instructed to unplug the tube at home, if unable to urinate, to check residuals by unplugging the tube after micturition. One possible reason for voiding difficulty is neurogenic bladder dysfunction related to the initial injury, especially if there is associated back trauma. Several months after tube removal, flexible urethroscopy is performed to definitively confirm wide patency of the repair. Patients are then encouraged to have a baseline flow rate and postvoid residual assessment and then to have this repeated annually. There is currently a lack of consensus regarding appropriate follow-up after surgery.

3.9. Outcomes. In our series of 85 patients, prior to referral, 17 underwent failed endoscopic treatment and 17 underwent failed open surgery. At the time of surgery, 19 patients underwent infrapubectomy, and no patient required supracrural rerouting. No patient required transfusion, and the only persistent neuropraxia was in one patient who had persistent tingling of the toes that resolved after several months. At the time of urethroscopy 4 months after surgery, 2 patients were noted to have medium caliber narrowing. One of these patients underwent dilation 2 years after surgery and the other was observed and never required treatment. This corresponds to a success rate of 97.6% success, using the strict definition of maintaining durable wide patency of the repair and with no further treatment required.

Other series report a similar success rate for adults, adolescents, and children, and this indicates that a stricture recurrence after a properly performed posterior urethroplasty should be a rare event [35, 37]. Of the patients who presented to our center after failed surgery, the recurrence was often within days or weeks, suggesting that these were technical failures, likely due to inadequate scar excision. Further suggesting that technical inexperience of the surgeon is likely the most common cause of failure is the fact that these patients usually have a successful outcome with the same technique of excisional repair when the revision surgery is performed by a specialist in urethral reconstruction. Published papers from referral centers confirm that when open repair fails, excision and primary anastomosis still remains the procedure of choice, and when properly performed, it offers a very high success rate [38, 39]. In conclusion, delayed posterior urethral disruption injuries are highly amenable to successful reconstruction with excisional posterior urethroplasty via a perineal approach.

Conflict of Interests

The authors declare that there is no conflict of interests regarding the publication of this paper.

References

[1] A. M. Basta, C. C. Blackmore, and H. Wessells, "Predicting urethral injury from pelvic fracture patterns in male patients with blunt traum," *Journal of Urology*, vol. 177, no. 2, pp. 571–575, 2007.

[2] V. B. Mouraviev and R. A. Santucci, "Cadaveric anatomy of pelvic fracture urethral distraction injury: most injuries are distal to the external urinary sphincter," *Journal of Urology*, vol. 173, no. 3, pp. 869–872, 2005.

[3] J. M. Whitson, J. W. McAninch, E. A. Tanagho, M. J. Metro, and N. U. Rahman, "Mechanism of continence after repair of posterior urethral disruption: evidence of rhabdosphincter activity," *Journal of Urology*, vol. 179, no. 3, pp. 1035–1039, 2008.

[4] K. S. Coffield and W. L. Weems, "Experience with management of posterior urethral injury associated with pelvic fracture," *The Journal of Urology*, vol. 117, no. 6, pp. 722–724, 1977.

[5] J. N. Warner and R. A. Santucci, "The management of the acute setting of pelvic fracture urethral injury (realignment vs.

[6] suprapubic cystostomy alone)," *Arab Journal of Urology*, vol. 13, no. 1, pp. 7–12, 2015.

[6] T. J. Tausch and A. F. Morey, "The case against primary endoscopic realignment of pelvic fracture urethral injuries," *Arab Journal of Urology*, vol. 13, no. 1, pp. 13–16, 2015.

[7] R. P. Terlecki, M. C. Steele, C. Valadez, and A. F. Morey, "Urethral rest: role and rationale in preparation for anterior urethroplasty," *Urology*, vol. 77, no. 6, pp. 1477–1481, 2011.

[8] D. E. Andrich, K. J. O'Malley, D. J. Summerton, T. J. Greenwell, and A. R. Mundy, "The type of urethroplasty for a pelvic fracture urethral distraction defect cannot be predicted preoperatively," *Journal of Urology*, vol. 170, no. 2, pp. 464–467, 2003.

[9] H. M. Tunç, A. H. Tefekli, T. Kaplancan, and T. Esen, "Delayed repair of post-traumatic posterior urethral distraction injuries: long-term results," *Urology*, vol. 55, no. 6, pp. 837–841, 2000.

[10] M. M. Koraitim, "On the art of anastomotic posterior urethroplasty: a 27-year experience," *Journal of Urology*, vol. 173, no. 1, pp. 135–139, 2005.

[11] Q. Fu, J. Zhang, Y.-L. Sa, S.-B. Jin, and Y.-M. Xu, "Transperineal bulboprostatic anastomosis in patients with simple traumatic posterior urethral strictures: a retrospective study from a referral urethral center," *Urology*, vol. 74, no. 5, pp. 1132–1136, 2009.

[12] W. S. Kizer, N. A. Armenakas, S. B. Brandes, A. G. Cavalcanti, R. A. Santucci, and A. F. Morey, "Simplified reconstruction of posterior urethral disruption defects: limited role of supracrural rerouting," *Journal of Urology*, vol. 177, no. 4, pp. 1378–1382, 2007.

[13] C. E. Iselin and G. D. Webster, "The significance of the open bladder neck associated with pelvic fracture urethral distraction defects," *Journal of Urology*, vol. 162, no. 2, pp. 347–351, 1999.

[14] S. MacDiarmid, D. Rosario, and C. R. Chapple, "The importance of accurate assessment and conservative management of the open bladder neck in patients with post-pelvic fracture membranous urethral distraction defects," *British Journal of Urology*, vol. 75, no. 1, pp. 65–67, 1995.

[15] M. M. Koraitim, "Assessment and management of an open bladder neck at posterior urethroplasty," *Urology*, vol. 76, no. 2, pp. 476–479, 2010.

[16] M. M. Oh, M. H. Jin, D. J. Sung, D. K. Yoon, J. J. Kim, and D. G. Moon, "Magnetic resonance urethrography to assess obliterative posterior urethral stricture: comparison to conventional retrograde urethrography with voiding cystourethrography," *Journal of Urology*, vol. 183, no. 2, pp. 603–607, 2010.

[17] E. Rodriguez Jr. and J. Gelman, "Pan-urethral strictures can develop as a complication of UroLume placement for bulbar stricture disease in patients with hypospadias," *Urology*, vol. 67, no. 6, pp. 1290–e11, 2006.

[18] S. D. Blaschko, M. T. Sanford, B. J. Schlomer et al., "The incidence of erectile dysfunction after pelvic fracture urethral injury: a systematic review and meta-analysis," *Arab Journal of Urology*, vol. 13, no. 1, pp. 68–74, 2015.

[19] O. Z. Shenfeld, D. Kiselgorf, O. N. Gofrit, A. G. Verstandig, E. H. Landau, and D. Pode, "The incidence and causes of erectile dysfunction after pelvic fractures associated with posterior urethral disruption," *Journal of Urology*, vol. 169, no. 6, pp. 2173–2176, 2003.

[20] T. O. Davies, L. B. Colen, N. Cowan, and G. H. Jordan, "Preoperative vascular evaluation of patients with pelvic fracture urethral distraction defects (PFUDD)," *The Journal of Urology*, vol. 181, supplement, p. 29, 2009.

[21] J. M. Zuckerman, K. A. McCammon, B. E. Tisdale et al., "Outcome of penile revascularization for arteriogenic erectile dysfunction after pelvic fracture urethral injuries," *Urology*, vol. 80, no. 6, pp. 1369–1373, 2012.

[22] K. W. Angermeier and G. H. Jordan, "Complications of the exaggerated lithotomy position: a review of 177 cases," *The Journal of Urology*, vol. 151, no. 4, pp. 866–868, 1994.

[23] S. A. Bildsten, R. R. Dmochowski, M. R. Spindel, and J. R. Auman, "The risk of rhabdomyolysis and acute renal failure with the patient in the exaggerated lithotomy position," *Journal of Urology*, vol. 152, no. 6, pp. 1970–1972, 1994.

[24] J. G. Anema, A. F. Morey, J. W. McAninch, L. A. Mario, and H. Wessells, "Complications related to the high lithotomy position during urethral reconstruction," *The Journal of Urology*, vol. 164, no. 2, pp. 360–363, 2000.

[25] J. M. Holzbeierlein, P. Langenstroer, H. J. Porter, and J. B. Thrasher, "Case selection and outcome of radical perineal prostatectomy in localized prostate cancer," *International Brazilian Journal of Urology*, vol. 29, no. 4, pp. 291–299, 2003.

[26] G. H. Jordan, E. A. Eltahawy, and R. Virasoro, "The technique of vessel sparing excision and primary anastomosis for proximal bulbous urethral reconstruction," *The Journal of Urology*, vol. 177, no. 5, pp. 1799–1802, 2007.

[27] D. E. Andrich and A. R. Mundy, "Non-transecting anastomotic bulbar urethroplasty: a preliminary report," *British Journal of Andrology*, vol. 109, no. 7, pp. 1090–1094, 2012.

[28] R. Gomez, P. Marchetti, and G. Catalan, "1226 bulbar artery sparing during reconstruction of pelvic fracture urethral distraction defects," *The Journal of Urology*, vol. 183, no. 4, supplement, pp. e474–e475, 2010.

[29] G. H. Jordan and K. McCammon, "Surgery of the penis and urethra," in *Campbell-Walsh Urology*, A. J. Wein, L. R. Kavoussi, A. C. Novick, A. W. Partin, and C. A. Peters, Eds., pp. 956–1000, WB Saunders, Philadelphia, Pa, USA, 10th edition, 2012.

[30] L. K. Carr and G. D. Webster, "Posterior urethral reconstruction," *Urology Clinics of North America*, vol. 5, pp. 125–137, 1997.

[31] G. D. Webster and S. Sihelnik, "The management of strictures of the membranous urethra," *Journal of Urology*, vol. 134, no. 3, pp. 469–473, 1985.

[32] K. Waterhouse, J. I. Abrahams, H. Gruber, R. E. Hackett, U. B. Patil, and B. K. Peng, "The transpubic approach to the lower urinary tract," *Journal of Urology*, vol. 109, no. 3, pp. 486–490, 1973.

[33] M. M. Koraitim, "The lessons of 145 posttraumatic posterior urethral strictures treated in 17 years," *The Journal of Urology*, vol. 153, no. 1, pp. 63–66, 1995.

[34] A. Pratap, C. S. Agrawal, A. Tiwari, B. K. Bhattarai, R. K. Pandit, and N. Anchal, "Complex posterior urethral disruptions: management by combined abdominal transpubic perineal urethroplasty," *The Journal of Urology*, vol. 175, no. 5, pp. 1751–1754, 2006.

[35] M. M. Koraitim, "Transpubic urethroplasty revisited: total, superior, or inferior pubectomy?" *Urology*, vol. 75, no. 3, pp. 691–694, 2010.

[36] R. P. Terlecki, M. C. Steele, C. Valadez, and A. F. Morey, "Low yield of early postoperative imaging after anastomotic urethroplasty," *Urology*, vol. 78, no. 2, pp. 450–453, 2011.

[37] O. Z. Shenfeld, J. Gdor, R. Katz, O. N. Gofrit, D. Pode, and E. H. Landau, "Urethroplasty, by perineal approach, for bulbar and membranous urethral strictures in children and adolescents," *Urology*, vol. 71, no. 3, pp. 430–433, 2008.

[38] M. R. Cooperberg, J. W. McAninch, N. F. Alsikafi, and S. P. Elliott, "Urethral reconstruction for traumatic posterior urethral disruption: outcomes of a 25-year experience," *Journal of Urology*, vol. 178, no. 5, pp. 2006–2010, 2007.

[39] O. Z. Shenfeld, O. N. Gofrit, Y. Gdor, E. H. Landau, and D. Pode, "Anastomotic urethroplasty for failed previously treated membranous urethral rupture," *Urology*, vol. 63, no. 5, pp. 837–840, 2004.

11

Surgical Repair of Bulbar Urethral Strictures: Advantages of Ventral, Dorsal, and Lateral Approaches and When to Choose Them

Krishnan Venkatesan,[1] Stephen Blakely,[2,3] and Dmitriy Nikolavsky[2]

[1]Department of Urology, MedStar Washington Hospital Center, 110 Irving Street NW, Suite 3B-19, Washington, DC 20010, USA
[2]Department of Urology, State University of New York Upstate Medical University, 750 East Adams Street, Syracuse, NY 13210, USA
[3]Division of Urology, University of Colorado, 12605 E. 16th Avenue, Aurora, CO 80045, USA

Correspondence should be addressed to Dmitriy Nikolavsky; nikolavd@upstate.edu

Academic Editor: Francisco E. Martins

Objectives. To review the available literature describing the three most common approaches for buccal mucosal graft (BMG) augmentation during reconstruction of bulbar urethral strictures. Due to its excellent histological properties, buccal mucosa graft is now routinely used in urethral reconstruction. The best approach for the placement of such a graft remains controversial. *Methods*. PubMed search was conducted for available English literature describing outcomes of bulbar urethroplasty augmentation techniques using dorsal, ventral, and lateral approaches. Prospective and retrospective studies as well as meta-analyses and latest systematic reviews were included. *Results*. Most of the studies reviewed are of retrospective nature and majority described dorsal or ventral approaches. Medium- and long-term outcomes of all three approaches were comparable ranging between 80 and 88%. *Conclusion*. Various techniques of BMG augmentation urethroplasty have been described for repairs of bulbar urethral strictures. In this review, we describe and compare the three most common "competing" approaches for bulbar urethroplasty with utilization of BMG.

1. Introduction

Buccal mucosa graft (BMG) is now routinely used in urethral reconstruction since its popularization by Burger et al. in 1992 in pediatric reconstruction [1] and subsequently by El-Kasaby et al. in 1993 for adult urethroplasty [2]. Its use in urethroplasty is arguably the gold standard for treatment of medium- and long-length strictures [3]. The first use of buccal mucosa in urethral reconstruction is attributed to Professor Sapezhko who by 1894 had performed 4 operations on humans [4, 5]. In 1941, Humby, a British surgeon, described using buccal mucosa in hypospadias repair [6]. The excellent histological properties of buccal mucosa were subsequently described by Duckett et al. [7]. In comparison to skin, buccal mucosa holds the distinct advantage of being hairless and accustomed to a moist environment. Moreover, it has a thicker epithelial layer, thinner lamina propria, and a greater density of capillaries with an abundance of Type IV collagen.

All these qualities are thought to improve graft inosculation and survival after transplantation.

Various techniques of BMG augmentation urethroplasty have been described for repairs of bulbar urethral strictures. In this review, we describe and compare the three most common "competing" approaches for bulbar urethroplasty with utilization of BMG.

2. Technique

2.1. Indications. Before describing the approach to bulbar stricture in detail, it is important to reiterate the indications for the use of oral mucosa in urethral reconstruction. The authors follow a traditional algorithm, where bulbar strictures <2 cm in length can mostly be treated with excision and primary anastomosis, whereby strictures longer than 2 cm may require adjunct maneuvers and the use of graft tissue to augment the caliber of the urethra. These maneuvers may include augmented anastomotic urethroplasty typically used for strictures between 2 and 5 cm in length or, for longer strictures, "pure" urethral augmentation in order to establish a larger gauge urethra. The choice of where and how to augment the urethra is discussed here in further detail.

2.2. Dorsal Onlay. This technique was first described by Barbagli et al. in 1998 and involved circumferential bulbar urethral dissection, dorsal stricturotomy followed by augmentation of the stricturotomy by a penile skin graft (in the first 31 patients) or by BMG (in the last 6 patients) [8]. The key step of the procedure was "quilting" or spread-fixation of the graft on the tunica albuginea overlying the corpora cavernosa prior to suturing the edges of urethral mucosa to the edges of the graft. Even spread-fixation has a range of implementation techniques; some surgeons prefer a "traditional" manner of suturing through the graft to the underlying tunica albuginea, while others advocate for use of a biologic "glue." The advantage of suture quilting the graft includes microfenestration of the graft resulting from the surgical needle, which may aid in allowing any trapped blood to escape, preventing hematoma under the graft, and increasing the likelihood of proper buccal mucosa engraftment. This maneuver is critical in fostering sufficient graft apposition to the well-vascularized tissue of the corpora cavernosa and minimizing the risks of graft contracture and pseudodiverticula formation.

One of the advantages of the dorsal approach is that it yields a relatively bloodless operation. This is because the bulbar urethra is eccentrically located in the corpus spongiosum, with only thin dorsal coverage by corpus spongiosum that requires incision. Another advantage of the dorsal approach is its versatility and applicability for strictures of any length and location. The dorsal stricturotomy in the bulbous urethra can be extended proximally towards the membranous urethra or distally into penile urethra if required by intraoperative findings without dramatically altering the plan for reconstruction. In the event that complete or near-complete obliteration is identified after committing to dorsal stricturotomy, several solutions are described. These include (a) excision of the obstructed segment and conversion to augmented anastomotic urethroplasty [9], (b) removal of ventral mucosal strip and addition of ventral BMG onlay [10], and (c) ventral stricturotomy and addition of elliptical ventral inlay [11].

One of the disadvantages of the original dorsal approach is the need to circumferentially mobilize the urethra. Kulkarni et al. addressed this with their modification where mobilization is undertaken unilaterally and carried just across the midline dorsally, preserving the lateral blood supply on the contralateral side [12].

There have been numerous studies examining the success of BMG bulbar urethroplasty over the last two decades, with a wide range of follow-up and varying definitions of success. The Société Internationale d'Urologie (SIU) with the International Consultation on Urological Disease (ICUD) published a systematic review of 66 studies, describing outcomes of a total of 934 patients after dorsal onlay urethroplasty with average follow-up of 42 months and mean success rates of 88.3% [13]. Soon after, Barbagli et al. published a long-term

retrospective paper on the deterioration rate of augmentation urethroplasty [14]. In this study, only patients with follow-up of greater than 6 years were included, totaling 81 patients after dorsal onlay BMG urethroplasty. At a median follow-up of 111 months, the authors reported an 80.2% success rate, defined as requiring absolutely no further instrumentation including dilation. This compared to 81.5% and 83.3% for ventral and lateral onlay techniques, respectively, with similar lengths of follow-up. The overall conclusion drawn from these reviews is that no significant difference exists in recurrence rates between dorsal, ventral, and lateral approaches to bulbar urethroplasty [13, 14].

2.3. Ventral Onlay. The ventral "patch" onlay urethroplasty came to the forefront of urethral reconstruction in 1996 when, encouraged by the use of BMG in complex pediatric hypospadias repair, Morey and McAninch applied the graft to repair strictures of the bulbar urethra [15]. The authors describe direct saggittal ventral urethrotomy through the diseased bulbar urethra, followed by sewing of the graft to each edge of the native urethral mucosa. Subsequently, the corpus spongiosum is closed over the graft in a second layer and the bulbospongiosus muscle over this. While there is no separate tissue to which the graft can be "quilted," the spongiosal closure typically incorporates a small "bite" of the graft, to increase proper apposition to the spongiosum that will provide its blood supply. The technique was introduced contemporarily with Barbagli's dorsal onlay technique, and the advantages and superiority of each have been the subject of intense debate ever since.

Proponents of the ventral onlay cite a straightforward approach, not requiring extensive circumferential mobilization and the technical demand of dorsal graft placement. This allows urologists who treat strictures only occasionally to still feel comfortable in performing urethroplasty for strictures that may not be amenable to excision and primary anastomosis. Moreover, the argument may be made that the thicker, ventrally placed corpus spongiosum provides a more robust vascular bed for buccal mucosa engraftment. Another anatomic consideration is specific location of the bulbar stricture. Patterson and Chapple, in a comparison of surgical techniques, note that, for very proximal bulbar strictures, ventral onlay poses a clear advantage in exposure and technique and is the appropriate choice [16]. Palminteri et al. also contend that ventral placement of BMG in bulbar urethroplasty has no significant impact on sexual quality of life and in fact improved most measures of sexual life, aside from postejaculatory dribbling [17]. An additional benefit is that the ventral approach is amenable to use in complex situations, including recurrent stricture [18], after radiation [19], and with adjunct maneuvers such as gracilis muscle flap coverage in particularly high risk, long segment strictures [20]. The ventral approach has also been used as a direct route to the dorsal aspect of the urethra, allowing preservation of bilateral vascular supports to the urethra [21].

Opponents of the ventral technique point to the need to make incision through the thicker ventral corpus spongiosum in order to reach the eccentrically located bulbar urethra, resulting in a bloodier operation. There is also a concern about increased risk of sacculation, diverticulum, or pouch formation, as well as more frequent irritative voiding symptoms and urine infection [22]. In their review of 11 series, Patterson and Chapple note several groups with higher incidence of sacculation or diverticulum formation with resultant worse postvoid dribbling in ventral onlays. They go on, however, to document that an equal number of series found no significant anatomic or clinical difference in these findings in comparing ventral or dorsal onlay [16]. What is ultimately evident is that, in experienced hands and with meticulous technique, these issues can be minimized; furthermore, the issue of sacculation seems dramatically higher in older series based on the use of skin, versus the more modern use of BMG [3].

This being said, there are certain disadvantages to the ventral approach. Several authors [23, 24] have noted finite incidence of urethrocutaneous fistulae after ventral stricture repair with BMG, which is essentially unheard of in the dorsal approach. Reiterating an advantage of the dorsal approach mentioned earlier here, the ventral approach is less versatile, as it does not lend itself to extension of the urethrotomy distally into the penis should intraoperative findings require it.

While the global definition of success varies, a common criterion in most if not all series is the patency rate. The International Consultation on Urological Disease (ICUD) reviewed techniques in management of anterior strictures and found the success rate of ventral onlay to range from 43 to 100%. The authors summarize these series, generating a total number of 563 patients treated at a mean follow-up of 34.4 months, yielding a mean success rate of 88.8%, comparable with dorsal onlay urethroplasty. A number of smaller series, including a recent prospective randomized study, have compared dorsal and ventral techniques and reached a similar conclusion to the ICUD group: that there is no significant difference in success rates based on graft placement [13, 25, 26].

2.4. Lateral Onlay. Lateral onlay BMG augmentation urethroplasty is described but not well established in the literature. It is utilized infrequently and this is reflected by its limited description in the literature. The procedure resembles the ventral onlay technique described above; however, the urethrotomy is made laterally after unilateral urethral mobilization. The graft is similarly sutured in place and the spongiosum is closed over the graft.

As described above, the various locations of the urethrotomy in substitution urethroplasty afford different benefits and can also result in varying consequences. The lateral urethrotomy was described by Barbagli et al. in 2005 [27]. This actually preceded the description of the modified dorsal onlay technique where dissection remains unilateral. In a similar vein to the one-sided dissection technique described by Kulkarni et al. [12], it was felt that eliminating circumferential dissection would help preserve the contralateral urethral blood supply. Furthermore, avoiding urethrotomy through the robust ventral spongiosum may decrease intraoperative blood loss.

While the advantages of one-sided dissection are shared with the modern dorsal onlay technique, several advantages are lost with a lateral onlay procedure. There is a stronger potential for sacculation and diverticulum formation. Additionally, the corpora cavernosa, which are used as a structured vascular bed in dorsal onlay urethroplasty, are not utilized in the same manner in the lateral technique. And while it may seem easier to carry lateral urethrotomy as compared to a dorsal urethrotomy proximally into the membranous urethra, there is no actual data to support the use of lateral onlay in this setting.

In both lateral and ventral onlay, the spongiosum is closed over the BMG. However, in the case of lateral closure, the spongiosum can be rotated dorsally to protect the suture line. Unfortunately, the lateral spongiosal tissue is not as thick and vascular and accordingly may serve as a lower-quality bed for buccal mucosa engraftment. Like ventral grafting, lateral onlay urethroplasty should not be utilized in repair of pendulous urethral strictures. Aside from the similar concerns for sacculation, there is also a conceptual concern for lateral curvature. This is not specifically documented in the literature, likely because it is a technique already not employed in this arena.

One study describes outcomes in 6 patients undergoing lateral onlay urethroplasty. The nonreintervention rate at a mean of 42 months was 83%. Keeping in mind the context of a small sample size and the retrospective nature of the analysis, the lateral technique was comparable to dorsal (85%) and ventral (83%) onlay techniques [27].

The lateral approach offers few advantages, and those too are largely outweighed by its own disadvantages and the advantages of the dorsal and ventral approaches. This technique should be used sparingly and reserved for special circumstances when intraoperative limitations compromise the ability to complete dorsal mobilization.

3. Complications

The complications of bulbar urethral augmentation relate ostensibly more to the surgery itself, rather than any specific technique, although, as discussed in each of the sections above, particular techniques may predispose patients to specific postoperative concerns. Complications can include wound and/or urine infection, urethrocutaneous fistula, perineal hematoma, blood loss requiring transfusion, or nerve injuries related to positioning. The overall incidence is low, and, in their series comparing these 3 approaches, Barbagli et al. noted no such complications amongst 50 patients [27].

4. Conclusion

Because the ventral, dorsal, or lateral placement of BMG is typically determined based on location and length of stricture and surgeon preference, comparative studies are limited. This review outlines the best available evidence supporting each technique. Aside from one randomized trial and one systematic review, the remainder of the studies referenced in this paper are retrospective reviews. While the best data suggest that patency outcomes are similar for each technique, appropriate patient selection is paramount to utilize the strengths of a given technique and avoid its shortcoming.

Conflict of Interests

The authors declare that there is no conflict of interests regarding the publication of this paper.

References

[1] R. A. Burger, S. C. Muller, H. El-Damanhoury, A. Tschakaloff, H. Riedmiller, and R. Hohenfellner, "The buccal mucosal graft for urethral reconstruction: a preliminary report," *Journal of Urology*, vol. 147, no. 3, pp. 662–664, 1992.

[2] A. W. El-Kasaby, M. Fath-Alla, A. M. Noweir et al., "The use of buccal mucosa patch graft in the management of anterior urethral strictures," *Journal of Urology*, vol. 149, no. 2, pp. 276–278, 1993.

[3] S. Bhargava and C. R. Chapple, "Buccal mucosal urethroplasty: is it the new gold standard?" *BJU International*, vol. 93, no. 9, pp. 1191–1193, 2004.

[4] I. Korneyev, D. Ilyin, D. Schultheiss, and C. Chapple, "The first oral mucosal graft urethroplasty was carried out in the 19th century: the pioneering experience of Kirill Sapezhko (1857–1928)," *European Urology*, vol. 62, no. 4, pp. 624–627, 2012.

[5] K. M. Sapezhko, "On treatments of urethral defects by the way of mucosal transplantation," *Khirurgicheskaya Letopis*, vol. 4, pp. 775–783, 1894.

[6] G. Humby and T. T. Higgins, "A one-stage operation for hypospadias," *British Journal of Surgery*, vol. 29, no. 113, pp. 84–92, 1941.

[7] J. W. Duckett, D. Coplen, D. Ewalt, and L. S. Baskin, "Buccal mucosal urethral replacement," *The Journal of Urology*, vol. 153, no. 5, pp. 1660–1663, 1995.

[8] G. Barbagli, E. Palminteri, and M. Rizzo, "Dorsal onlay graft urethroplasty using penile skin or buccal mucosa in adult bulbourethral strictures," *Journal of Urology*, vol. 160, no. 4, pp. 1307–1309, 1998.

[9] C. E. Iselin and G. D. Webster, "Dorsal onlay urethroplasty for urethral stricture repair," *World Journal of Urology*, vol. 16, no. 3, pp. 181–185, 1998.

[10] J. Gelman and J. A. Siegel, "Ventral and dorsal buccal grafting for 1-stage repair of complex anterior urethral strictures," *Urology*, vol. 83, no. 6, pp. 1418–1422, 2014.

[11] R. C. Kovell and R. P. Terlecki, "Ventral inlay buccal mucosal graft urethroplasty: a novel surgical technique for the management of urethral stricture disease," *Korean Journal of Urology*, vol. 56, no. 2, pp. 164–167, 2015.

[12] S. Kulkarni, G. Barbagli, S. Sansalone, and M. Lazzeri, "One-sided anterior urethroplasty: a new dorsal onlay graft technique," *BJU International*, vol. 104, no. 8, pp. 1150–1155, 2009.

[13] C. Chapple, D. Andrich, A. Atala et al., "SIU/ICUD consultation on urethral strictures: the management of anterior urethral stricture disease using substitution urethroplasty," *Urology*, vol. 83, supplement 3, pp. S31–S47, 2014.

[14] G. Barbagli, S. B. Kulkarni, N. Fossati et al., "Long-term followup and deterioration rate of anterior substitution urethroplasty," *Journal of Urology*, vol. 192, no. 3, pp. 808–813, 2014.

[15] A. F. Morey and J. W. McAninch, "When and how to use buccal mucosal grafts in adult bulbar urethroplasty," *Urology*, vol. 48, no. 2, pp. 194–198, 1996.

[16] J. M. Patterson and C. R. Chapple, "Surgical techniques in substitution urethroplasty using buccal mucosa for the treatment of anterior urethral strictures," *European Urology*, vol. 53, no. 6, pp. 1162–1171, 2008.

[17] E. Palminteri, E. Berdondini, C. De Nunzio et al., "The impact of ventral oral graft bulbar urethroplasty on sexual life," *Urology*, vol. 81, no. 4, pp. 891–898, 2013.

[18] T. Heinke, E. W. Gerharz, R. Bonfig, and H. Riedmiller, "Ventral onlay urethroplasty using buccal mucosa for complex stricture repair," *Urology*, vol. 61, no. 5, pp. 1004–1007, 2003.

[19] S. A. Ahyai, M. Schmid, M. Kuhl et al., "Outcomes of ventral onlay buccal mucosa graft urethroplasty in patients after radiotherapy," *The Journal of Urology*, vol. 194, no. 2, pp. 441–446, 2015.

[20] D. A. Palmer, J. C. Buckley, L. N. Zinman, and A. J. Vanni, "Urethroplasty for high risk, long segment urethral strictures with ventral buccal mucosa graft and gracilis muscle flap," *Journal of Urology*, vol. 193, no. 3, pp. 902–905, 2014.

[21] V. L. N. M. Pisapati, S. Paturi, S. Bethu et al., "Dorsal buccal mucosal graft urethroplasty for anterior urethral stricture by Asopa technique," *European Urology*, vol. 56, no. 1, pp. 201–206, 2009.

[22] D. E. Andrich, C. J. Leach, and A. R. Mundy, "The Barbagli procedure gives the best results for patch urethroplasty of the bulbar urethra," *BJU International*, vol. 88, no. 4, pp. 385–389, 2001.

[23] D. Dubey, A. Kumar, A. Mandhani, A. Srivastava, R. Kapoor, and M. Bhandari, "Buccal mucosal urethroplasty: a versatile technique for all urethral segments," *BJU International*, vol. 95, no. 4, pp. 625–629, 2005.

[24] J. Fichtner, D. Filipas, M. Fisch, R. Hohenfellner, and J. W. Thüroff, "Long-term outcome of ventral buccal mucosa onlay graft urethroplasty for urethral stricture repair," *Urology*, vol. 64, no. 4, pp. 648–650, 2004.

[25] J. Hosscini, A. Kaviani, M. Hosseini, M. M. Mazloomfard, and A. Razi, "Dorsal versus ventral oral mucosal graft urethroplasty," *Urology Journal*, vol. 8, no. 1, pp. 48–53, 2011.

[26] P. Vasudeva, B. Nanda, A. Kumar, N. Kumar, H. Singh, and R. Kumar, "Dorsal versus ventral onlay buccal mucosal graft urethroplasty for long-segment bulbar urethral stricture: a prospective randomized study," *International Journal of Urolog*, vol. 22, no. 10, pp. 967–971, 2015.

[27] G. Barbagli, E. Palminterim, G. Guazzoni, F. Montorsi, D. Turini, and M. Lazzeri, "Bulbar urethroplasty using buccal mucosa grafts placed on the ventral, dorsal or lateral surface of the urethra: are results affected by the surgical technique?" *Journal of Urology*, vol. 174, no. 3, pp. 957–958, 2005.

12

Anastomotic Repair versus Free Graft Urethroplasty for Bulbar Strictures: A Focus on the Impact on Sexual Function

Matthias Beysens,[1] Enzo Palminteri,[2] Willem Oosterlinck,[1] Anne-Françoise Spinoit,[1] Piet Hoebeke,[1] Philippe François,[3] Karel Decaestecker,[1] and Nicolaas Lumen[1]

[1]*Department of Urology, Ghent University Hospital, 9000 Ghent, Belgium*
[2]*Center for Urethral and Genital Surgery, 52100 Arezzo, Italy*
[3]*Department of Urology, CH Mouscron, 7700 Mouscron, Belgium*

Correspondence should be addressed to Nicolaas Lumen; nicolaas.lumen@uzgent.be

Academic Editor: Francisco E. Martins

Objectives. To evaluate alterations in sexual function and genital sensitivity after anastomotic repair (AR) and free graft urethroplasty (FGU) for bulbar urethral strictures. *Methods.* Patients treated with AR ($n = 31$) or FGU ($n = 16$) were prospectively evaluated before, 6 weeks and 6 months after urethroplasty. Evaluation included International Prostate Symptom Score (IPSS), 5-Item International Index of Erectile Function (IIEF-5), Ejaculation/Orgasm Score (EOS), and 3 questions on genital sensitivity. *Results.* At 6 weeks, there was a significant decline of IIEF-5 for AR (-4.8; $p = 0.005$), whereas there was no significant change for FGU ($+0.9$; $p = 0.115$). After 6 months, differences with baseline were not significant overall and among subgroups. At 6 weeks, there was a significant decline in EOS for AR (-1.4; $p = 0.022$). In the FGU group there was no significant change ($+0.6$; $p = 0.12$). Overall and among subgroups, EOS normalized at 6 months. After 6 weeks and 6 months, respectively, 62.2 and 52% of patients reported alterations in penile sensitivity with no significant differences among subgroups. *Conclusions.* AR is associated with a transient decline in erectile and ejaculatory function. This was not observed with FGU. Bulbar AR and FGU are likely to alter genital sensitivity.

1. Introduction

Although a short bulbar stricture can be treated by dilation or endoscopic urethrotomy, longer or recurrent strictures are best treated by urethroplasty as it provides the best chance of success [1–3]. Anastomotic repair (AR) and free graft urethroplasty (FGU) are established treatments for bulbar strictures with the choice of technique mainly depending on stricture length [1, 3, 4]. The main goal of urethroplasty is to restore urethral patency, and, as a consequence, most papers have focused on this criterion to evaluate success of urethroplasty [1, 3, 5]. In the past decade, there is an upcoming concern that especially bulbar urethroplasty might affect sexual functioning [6–8]. The aim of this paper is to evaluate and compare sexual function after AR and FGU for bulbar strictures in a prospective fashion.

2. Materials and Methods

2.1. Patient Recruitment. Out of 258 male patients who underwent urethroplasty between October 2010 and February 2014, 90 patients with a bulbar stricture only were planned to be treated with AR or FGU and eligible to participate in this prospective study. Only native Dutch speaking patients who signed the informed consent (Institutional Review Board Approval EC UZG 2008/234) and who filled in the preoperative questionnaires and at least one postoperative questionnaire (at 6 weeks and/or 6 months) were included in this analysis. Finally, 47 patients were included for further analysis and divided into two groups: AR ($n = 31$) versus FGU ($n = 16$) (Figure 1). Prepuce and oral mucosa was used as graft in, respectively, 12 and 4 patients. Stricture location and stricture length were evaluated by retrograde

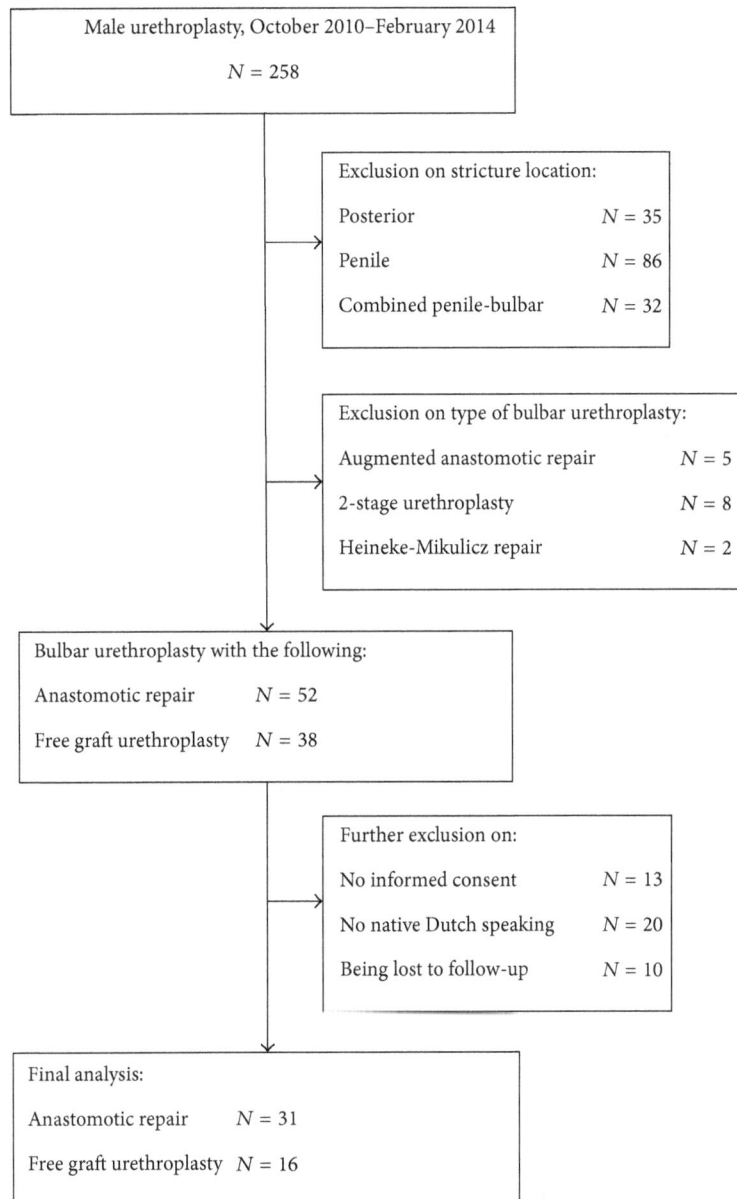

Male urethroplasty, October 2010–February 2014

$N = 258$

Exclusion on stricture location:

Posterior $N = 35$

Penile $N = 86$

Combined penile-bulbar $N = 32$

Exclusion on type of bulbar urethroplasty:

Augmented anastomotic repair $N = 5$

2-stage urethroplasty $N = 8$

Heineke-Mikulicz repair $N = 2$

Bulbar urethroplasty with the following:

Anastomotic repair $N = 52$

Free graft urethroplasty $N = 38$

Further exclusion on:

No informed consent $N = 13$

No native Dutch speaking $N = 20$

Being lost to follow-up $N = 10$

Final analysis:

Anastomotic repair $N = 31$

Free graft urethroplasty $N = 16$

FIGURE 1: Flowchart of patient inclusion.

urethrography. This study included the following evaluations:

(i) urinary symptoms: maximum urinary flow (Q_{max}) and the International Prostate Symptom Score (IPSS) questionnaire; the IPSS ranges from 0 (no lower urinary tract symptoms) to 35 (severe lower urinary tract symptoms);

(ii) erectile function: the abridged 5-item version of the International Index of Erectile Function (IIEF-5) [9]; this score ranges from 1 (no sexual intercourse) to 25 (no erectile dysfunction);

(iii) ejaculation/orgasm: the sum of questions 9 and 10 from IIEF (long version) [10]; this Ejaculation/Orgasm Score (EOS) ranges from 2 (no ejaculation/orgasm) to 10 (normal ejaculation and orgasm);

(iv) postoperative genital sensitivity: a nonvalidated in-house questionnaire containing 3 dichotomous questions on glans tumescence, alterations in genital sensitivity, and cold feeling in the glans; further analysis of glans tumescence was only done in patients reporting normal erectile function (IIEF-5 $\geq$ 20) in order to avoid contamination of diminished glans tumescence due to globally diminished penile tumescence.

Patients were evaluated preoperatively, after 6 weeks and 6 months. In the first six months, no phosphodiesterase-5 inhibitors were prescribed to stimulate sexual rehabilitation. In case of suspicion of stricture recurrence ($Q_{max} < 15$ mL/s and/or IPSS > 19), retrograde urethrography and urethroscopy were done. A functional definition of failure

TABLE 1: Patients' characteristics (SD = standard deviation; FGU = free graft urethroplasty; AR = anastomotic repair; DVIU = direct vision internal urethrotomy; Q_{max} = maximum urinary flow; IPSS = International Prostate Symptom Score; IIEF = International Index of Erectile Function; EOS = Ejaculation/Orgasm Score).

		All ($n = 47$)	FGU ($n = 16$)	AR ($n = 31$)	p value
Age (years)	Mean (SD)	40 (16)	48 (18)	37 (13)	*0.018*
Follow-up (months)	Mean (SD)	23.3 (10.9)	25.2 (12.5)	22.2 (10)	0.376
Stricture length (cm)	Mean (SD)	3 (2.4)	5.4 (2.6)	1.8 (0.8)	*<0.001*
Stricture etiology					
Traumatic	Number (%)	4 (8.5)	0 (0)	4 (12.9)	
Inflammatory	Number (%)	1 (2.1)	0 (0)	1 (3.2)	0.071
Iatrogenic	Number (%)	14 (29.8)	8 (50)	6 (19.4)	
Idiopathic	Number (%)	28 (59.6)	8 (50)	20 (64.5)	
Previous interventions					
None	Number (%)	4 (8.5)	2 (12.5)	2 (6.5)	
DVIU/dilation(s)	Number (%)	34 (72.3)	11 (68.8)	23 (74.2)	0.877
Urethroplasty(ies)	Number (%)	9 (19.1)	3 (18.8)	6 (19.4)	
Preop Q_{max} (mL/s)	Mean (SD)	6.3 (4.6)	6.9 (4)	6 (5)	0.629
Preop IPSS (.../35)	Mean (SD)	22 (8)	23 (7)	21 (8)	0.368
Preop IIEF-5 (.../25)	Mean (SD)	20 (7)	18 (8)	22 (6)	0.202
Preop EOS (.../10)	Mean (SD)	8 (3)	7 (4)	9 (3)	0.135
Suprapubic catheter					
Yes	Number (%)	8 (17)	2 (12.5)	6 (19.4)	0.697
No	Number (%)	39 (83)	14 (87.5)	25 (80.6)	

was used which includes the need for any additional urethral manipulation (including dilation) [11].

2.2. Surgical Technique. Patients were operated on in a single center (GUH) by two surgeons (Nicolaas Lumen and Willem Oosterlinck). AR was preferred whenever a tension-free anastomosis could be made (stricture length < 3 cm on urethrography and/or peroperative findings). For longer strictures, FGU was performed. For both techniques, a midline perineal incision is made; the bulbospongiosus muscle is incised at the midline and dissected away from the corpus spongiosum. In case of AR, the corpus spongiosum is circumferentially freed at the level of the stricture. The corpus spongiosum and urethra are transected at this site. The fibrotic urethra and spongiosus edges are resected until healthy urethra is present at both the distal and proximal ends. The urethra is then spatulated in order to obtain a broad oblique anastomosis, which is finalized by 8–10 interrupted resorbable 4.0 sutures. In case of FGU, the stricture is opened ventrally on the tip of the catheter. The stricture length is measured and a graft is taken accordingly. The graft is sutured into the urethra in a ventral onlay fashion. The corpus spongiosum is closed over the graft for vascular supply and mechanical support (spongioplasty). The urethral catheter is maintained for 14 days and a voiding cystourethrogram is made upon removal.

2.3. Statistical Analysis. Descriptive statistics were performed to evaluate the whole population and both subgroups. To

compare both groups, continuous variables were evaluated by independent-samples t-test or the Welch modified t-test for, respectively, equal and unequal distributions. Categorical variables were evaluated by chi-square or Fischer's exact test. The 2-year recurrence-free survival was estimated by Kaplan-Meier statistics and groups were compared by log rank statistics. To evaluate changes in IPSS, IIEF-5 score, and EOS between baseline and at 6 weeks and 6 months, mean differences were calculated by paired-samples t-test.

3. Results

Patients treated by AR were significantly younger (37 versus 48 years; $p = 0.018$) and strictures were shorter with AR compared to FGU (1.8 versus 5.4 cm; $p < 0.001$). Both groups were comparable for follow-up duration, stricture etiology, previous interventions, and presence of suprapubic catheter and for preoperative urinary flow, IPSS, IIEF-5, and EOS (Table 1). After a mean follow-up of 23 months, 6 patients (12.8%) suffered a recurrence: 3 (9.7%) patients treated with AR and 3 (18.8%) patients treated with FGU ($p = 0.395$). Estimated 2-year recurrence-free survival rate was 93% and 72%, respectively, for AR and FGU ($p = 0.347$). Overall and in both groups, there was a significant improvement of the urinary flow at latest follow-up. Accordingly, there was a significant improvement in IPSS after 6 weeks and 6 months overall and in both groups (Table 2; Figure 2(a)).

Thirty-three patients, respectively, 19 and 14 patients in the AR- and FGU-group, reported to have sexual intercourse

TABLE 2: Mean paired differences (Δ) of the maximum urinary flow (Q_{max}) and International Prostate Symptom Score (IPSS). The standard deviation is provided between brackets (FGU = free graft urethroplasty; AR = anastomotic repair).

	ΔQ_{max} (mL/s)	p value	ΔIPSS (6 weeks versus preop)	p value	ΔIPSS (6 months versus preop)	p value
All	+19.8 (13.9)	<0.001	−17 (8)	<0.001	−20 (9)	<0.001
FGU	+13.8 (11.7)	0.007	−16 (10)	<0.001	−21 (8)	<0.001
AR	+22.3 (14.3)	<0.001	−17 (7)	<0.001	−20 (9)	<0.001

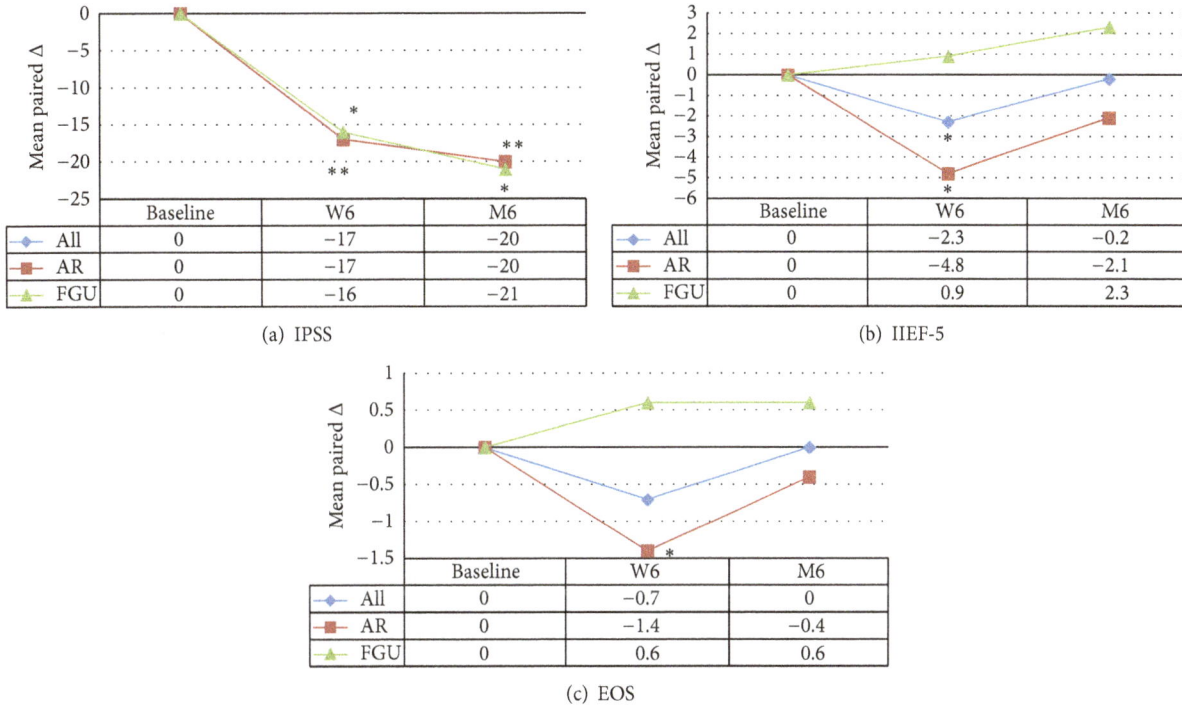

(a) IPSS

	Baseline	W6	M6
All	0	−17	−20
AR	0	−17	−20
FGU	0	−16	−21

(b) IIEF-5

	Baseline	W6	M6
All	0	−2.3	−0.2
AR	0	−4.8	−2.1
FGU	0	0.9	2.3

(c) EOS

	Baseline	W6	M6
All	0	−0.7	0
AR	0	−1.4	−0.4
FGU	0	0.6	0.6

FIGURE 2: Evolution of International Prostate Symptom Score (a), International Index of Erectile Function-5 (b), and Ejaculation/Orgasm Score (c) for all patients and subdivided for anastomotic repair (AR) and free graft urethroplasty (FGU) ($^*p < 0.05$).

and filled in the IIEF-5 (Table 3; Figure 2(b)). Overall, there was a significant decline in IIEF-5 score after 6 weeks (−2.3; $p = 0.026$). This decline remained significant for AR (−4.8; $p = 0.005$). However, for FGU, there was no significant change in IIEF-5 score (+0.9; $p = 0.115$). After 6 months, there were no longer significant changes in IIEF-5 score overall (−0.2; $p = 0.907$), for AR (−2.1; $p = 0.263$) and for FGU (+2.3; $p = 0.313$).

Thirty-seven patients, respectively, 23 and 14 patients in the AR- and FGU-group, tried to have ejaculation/orgasm (by masturbation or sexual intercourse) and completed the EOS (Table 3; Figure 2(c)). Overall, there was no significant postoperative change in EOS at 6 weeks (−0.7; $p = 0.111$). However, in the AR-group there was a significant decline in EOS (−1.4; $p = 0.022$). This was not the case in the FGU-group (+0.6; $p = 0.12$). After 6 months, EOS returned to baseline. The decline for AR (−0.4; $p = 0.431$) was no longer significant.

At 6 weeks and 6 months, respectively, 45 and 25 patients filled in the questionnaire on genital sensitivity and on cold feeling in the glans. At 6 weeks, 28 patients (62.2%) reported

to have altered genital sensitivity. This proportion was not significantly different between AR and FGU (66.7 versus 53.3%; $p = 0.517$). Only one patient, treated by AR, had a cold feeling in the glans. At 6 months, 13 patients (52%) reported to have altered genital sensitivity. Again, this proportion was not significantly different with AR compared to FGU (58.8% versus 37.5%; $p = 0.411$). At 6 months, no one reported a cold feeling in the glans. Of 20 patients with IIEF-5 $\geq$ 20 at 6 weeks 1/10 (10%) and 4/10 (40%) of patients in, respectively, the AR- and FGU-groups reported no glans tumescence ($p = 0.303$). At 6 months, 1/6 (16.7%) and 3/5 (60%) patients with IIEF-5 $\geq$ 20, respectively, treated by AR and FGU reported no glans tumescence ($p = 0.242$). Of the 4 patients treated with oral mucosa, 2 had altered genital sensitivity and no glans tumescence at 6 weeks and 6 months.

4. Discussion

Although this series is a prospective study, no randomization was done between AR and FGU because the use of AR is limited by the stricture length. The limit for AR is usually

TABLE 3: Mean paired differences (Δ) of the 5-Item International Index of Erectile Function (IIEF-5) and Ejaculation/Orgasm Score (EOS). The standard deviation is provided between brackets (FGU = free graft urethroplasty; AR = anastomotic repair).

		ΔIIEF-5 (6 weeks versus preop)	p value		ΔIIEF-5 (6 months versus preop)	p value
All	n = 33	−2.3 (5.8)	0.026	n = 18	−0.2 (6)	0.907
FGU	n = 14	+0.9 (2)	0.115	n = 8	+2.3 (5.8)	0.313
AR	n = 19	−4.8 (6.5)	0.005	n = 10	−2.1 (5.6)	0.263
		ΔEOS (6 weeks versus preop)	p value		ΔEOS (6 months versus preop)	p value
All	n = 37	−0.7 (2.5)	0.111	n = 22	0 (1.9)	1
FGU	n = 14	+0.6 (1.3)	0.12	n = 8	+0.6 (2.2)	0.448
AR	n = 23	−1.4 (2.8)	0.022	n = 14	−0.4 (1.6)	0.431

set at 2-3 cm [4, 12]. This also explains why strictures treated with AR were significantly shorter compared to FGU in this series. Another difference between both groups was younger patient's age with AR. For this observation, we have the following explanation: patients treated with AR have shorter strictures (cf. supra) and short bulbar strictures are predominantly idiopathic/congenital in origin and thus occurring at a younger age [13]. Despite these differences in age and stricture length between AR and FGU, preoperative erectile and orgasmic function was not significantly different between these groups. It has been reported that longer stricture length and more advanced patient age are more likely to be associated with postoperative erectile dysfunction (ED) [14–16]. The observed difference in patient age and stricture length would thus be in favor of AR in terms of postoperative erectile function. This has not been observed in this series, on the contrary.

The success rate of 90.3% for AR in this series is in line with the 93.8% composite success rate reported by the SIU/ICUD consultation [1]. For longer strictures at the bulbar urethra, FGU is the preferred technique of substitution urethroplasty as flaps are associated with more morbidity [3]. Our 81.2% success rate of ventral FGU is again in line with the overall 88.8% success rate reported by the SIU/ICUD consultation [3]. Because of its excellent success rate, the SIU/ICUD consultation recommends AR as optimal treatment for short bulbar strictures [1]. This recommendation is questioned because of a potential higher risk of sexual dysfunction related to AR [17].

An increasing number of papers report on sexual dysfunction after urethroplasty [6–8, 18]. Although the results are far from uniform, there is a trend for a higher incidence of sexual dysfunction after AR compared to FGU. Palminteri et al. found that 35% and 65% of patients treated by FGU reported improvement in erectile and ejaculatory function [8]. This is in line with our results revealing a trend to improvement in erectile and orgasmic function in the FGU-group. Al-Qudah and Santucci reported ED as late complication in 17% of patients after AR but no ED after FGU [18]. In their prospective study, Erickson et al. found the highest incidence of ED (50%) in the group treated by AR, compared to FGU, where only 26% of patients suffered

from ED. However, these differences were not statistically significant [7]. In their logistic regression model, Xie et al. reported that the method of treatment is a significant factor to predict for postoperative ED, with the highest risk of ED for AR [6].

Other authors did not find a significant decline in erectile function [19, 20] nor did they find a difference between AR and FGU [15, 16, 21, 22]. These contradictory results can be explained by several factors. First, timing of evaluation seems to be very important. Erickson et al. found a significant worse erectile function when evaluation is done <1 year after urethroplasty [15]. Xie et al. found a significant decline of erectile function with AR after 3 months but a normalization after 6 months [6]. This was also noted by Mundy, who found ED in 53% and 33% of patients after AR and FGU, respectively, at a 3-month follow-up. This decreased to 5% and 0.9% after longer follow-up [23]. In the AR-group, we also found a transient decline in erectile function after 6 weeks with recuperation after 6 months. Therefore, it is likely that if erectile function is at earliest assessed >3 months after urethroplasty [19, 22], a transient decline in erectile function might have been missed. Secondly, the evaluation tool to assess erectile function might be important. The IIEF-5 is a validated questionnaire to assess erectile function and was therefore used in this series. Other authors, however, used an in-house questionnaire with dichotomous answers (erectile dysfunction present or absent) [16, 19, 22]. Other factors that might be important to explain contradictory findings among studies are retrospective evaluation (with risk of recall bias) [9, 16, 19, 22] and small patient groups [21].

We speculate that the observed transient decline in erectile function with AR might be related to the following:

(i) more extensive and circumferential dissection of the corpus spongiosum containing the bulbar urethra; proximal dissection and mobilization of the corpus spongiosum nearby the urogenital diaphragm and in the intracrural space might provoke neuropraxia and/or thermal damage (coagulation) of erectile nerves penetrating the corporal bodies at that location (Figure 3); this hypothesis is supported by neuroanatomical findings reported by Yucel and Baskin [24] and Akman et al. [25];

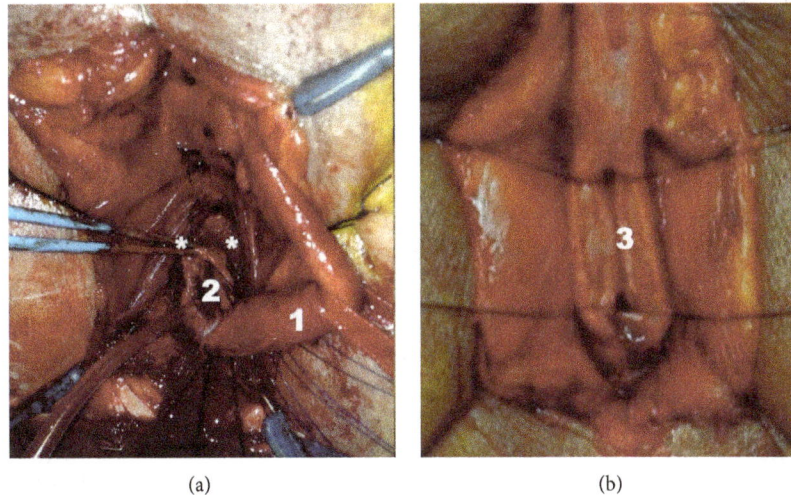

(a)   (b)

FIGURE 3: Peroperative photographs of AR (a) and FGU (b): a more extensive dissection with AR can be appreciated; 1: circumferentially mobilized bulbar urethra; 2: transected urethra; *: region where erectile nerves are expected; and 3: ventrally opened bulbar urethra.

(ii) complete transection of the corpus spongiosum that might be associated with a higher risk of bleeding and with postoperative haematoma and inflammation; this needs some time to recover; this might withhold patients to have satisfactory sexual activity or might provoke psychological problems.

In this series, ventral FGU was performed, with no significant decrease in sexual functioning at 6 weeks and 6 months. It would be interesting to know whether dorsal FGU affects sexual functioning. One would expect a higher incidence of sexual dysfunction if the hypothesis of more extensive and circumferential dissection of the bulbar corpus spongiosum is (in part) responsible for sexual dysfunction.

In this series, a transient decline in EOS was seen with AR, whereas there was no significant difference observed with FGU. Erickson et al. found an improvement of ejaculatory function after urethroplasty (mix of AR and FGU) [15], but a later prospective study failed to show any significant changes in ejaculatory function after urethroplasty (also mix of AR and FGU) [26]. Improvement of ejaculatory function after urethroplasty might be related to desobstruction of the urethra [26]. However this cannot explain the transient decline in ejaculatory function after AR that was seen in our series. Barbagli et al. also reported postoperative ejaculatory dysfunction in 23.3% of patients treated with AR [19]. We hypothesize that the higher rate of ejaculatory dysfunction associated with AR is because of the more extensive detachment of the bulbospongiosus muscle in AR needed for a full mobilization of the bulbar urethra. This detachment can indeed interfere with ejaculatory function. Timing of questioning might again be important: recovery of postoperative ejaculatory dysfunction can be expected once the bulbospongiosus muscle has recovered from the surgical trauma. This cannot be expected after 6 weeks but can be expected after 6 months. Another explanation is that ejaculatory and orgasmic dysfunction is related to ED, which was also more frequent after AR.

In this series, postoperative changes in genital sensitivity were present in approximately 2 out of 3 and 1 out of 2 patients after, respectively, 6 weeks and 6 months. Changes in genital sensitivity were not significantly different among subgroups. Palminteri et al. found a change in genital sensitivity after FGU in 50% of patients [8]. This is in line with our findings, but substantially higher than the 18.3% reported rate by Barbagli et al. [19]. However, this was a retrospective series with a possible risk of underreporting. In the same series [19], only one patient (1.6%) reported a cold glans, which is in concordance with the finding in our series. Postoperative changes in genital sensitivity might be explained by postoperative haematoma formation, oedema, and inflammation. Furthermore, in the majority of patients treated by FGU, a preputial skin graft was used. These factors might certainly explain the high rate of early (6 weeks) changes in genital sensitivity. However, even after 6 months, changes in genital sensitivity were still frequently reported, and this occurs also in patients treated with oral mucosa. This might be explained by damage to some sensory branches of the perineal nerves that supply the ventral surface of the penis [24]. By transecting the entire corpus spongiosum, one would expect a higher rate of impaired glans tumescence after AR. This was not observed in this series. However, interpretation of the results is hampered by the small number of patients.

This series again underlines the concern of possible alterations in sexual functioning and genital sensitivity after bulbar urethroplasty. Therefore it should be part of the evaluation of patients treated by urethroplasty. Jackson et al. recently validated patient reported outcome measures (PROMs) for urethroplasty [27]. However, this PROM lacks a section on sexual functioning.

Furthermore, it would be interesting to evaluate whether modifications in urethroplasty techniques such as muscle- and nerve-sparing bulbar urethroplasty [28] and vessel-sparing anastomotic repair [29] will be associated with less sexual dysfunction.

Important limitations of the present series are the small sample size and the missing data in the postoperative questionnaires.

5. Conclusions

AR is associated with a transient decline in erectile and ejaculatory function. This was not observed with FGU. Bulbar urethroplasty is likely to provoke changes in genital sensitivity. Further prospective studies with validated and internationally accepted patient reported outcome measures (PROMs) are needed for further confirmation.

Conflict of Interests

The authors have no conflict of interests.

References

[1] A. F. Morey, N. Watkin, O. Shenfeld, E. Eltahawy, and C. Giudice, "SIU/ICUD consultation on urethral strictures: anterior urethra—primary anastomosis," *Urology*, vol. 83, no. 3, pp. S23–S26, 2014.

[2] J. C. Buckley, C. Heyns, P. Gilling, and J. Carney, "SIU/ICUD consultation on urethral strictures: dilation, internal urethrotomy, and stenting of male anterior urethral strictures," *Urology*, vol. 83, no. 3, pp. S18–S22, 2014.

[3] C. Chapple, D. Andrich, A. Atala et al., "SIU/ICUD consultation on urethral strictures: the management of anterior urethral stricture disease using substitution urethroplasty," *Urology*, vol. 83, no. 3, pp. S31–S47, 2014.

[4] N. Lumen, P. Hoebeke, and W. Oosterlinck, "Urethroplasty for urethral strictures: quality assessment of an in-home algorithm," *International Journal of Urology*, vol. 17, no. 2, pp. 167–174, 2010.

[5] J. J. Meeks, B. A. Erickson, M. A. Granieri, and C. M. Gonzalez, "Stricture recurrence after urethroplasty: a systematic review," *The Journal of Urology*, vol. 182, no. 4, pp. 1266–1270, 2009.

[6] H. Xie, Y.-M. Xu, X.-L. Xu, Y.-L. Sa, D.-L. Wu, and X.-C. Zhang, "Evaluation of erectile function after urethral reconstruction: a prospective study," *Asian Journal of Andrology*, vol. 11, no. 2, pp. 209–214, 2009.

[7] B. A. Erickson, M. A. Granieri, J. J. Meeks, J. P. Cashy, and C. M. Gonzalez, "Prospective analysis of erectile dysfunction after anterior urethroplasty: incidence and recovery of function," *The Journal of Urology*, vol. 183, no. 2, pp. 657–661, 2010.

[8] E. Palminteri, E. Berdondini, C. De Nunzio et al., "The impact of ventral oral graft bulbar urethroplasty on sexual life," *Urology*, vol. 81, no. 4, pp. 891–898, 2013.

[9] R. C. Rosen, J. C. Cappelleri, M. D. Smith, J. Lipsky, and B. M. Peñ, "Development and evaluation of an abridged, 5-item version of the International Index of Erectile Function (IIEF-5) as a diagnostic tool for erectile dysfunction," *International Journal of Impotence Research*, vol. 11, no. 6, pp. 319–326, 1999.

[10] R. C. Rosen, A. Riley, G. Wagner, I. H. Osterloh, J. Kirkpatrick, and A. Mishra, "The international index of erectile function (IIEF): A multidimensional scale for assessment of erectile dysfunction," *Urology*, vol. 49, no. 6, pp. 822–830, 1997.

[11] B. A. Erickson, S. P. Elliott, B. B. Voelzke et al., "Multi-institutional 1-year bulbar urethroplasty outcomes using a standardized prospective cystoscopic follow-up protocol," *Urology*, vol. 84, no. 1, pp. 213–216, 2014.

[12] D. E. Andrich and A. R. Mundy, "What is the best technique for urethroplasty?" *European Urology*, vol. 54, no. 5, pp. 1031–1041, 2008.

[13] N. Lumen, P. Hoebeke, P. Willemsen, B. De Troyer, R. Pieters, and W. Oosterlinck, "Etiology of urethral stricture disease in the 21st century," *The Journal of Urology*, vol. 182, no. 3, pp. 983–987, 2009.

[14] J. Carlton, M. Patel, and A. F. Morey, "Erectile function after urethral reconstruction," *Asian Journal of Andrology*, vol. 10, no. 1, pp. 75–78, 2008.

[15] B. A. Erickson, J. S. Wysock, K. T. McVary, and C. M. Gonzalez, "Erectile function, sexual drive, and ejaculatory function after reconstructive surgery for anterior urethral stricture disease," *BJU International*, vol. 99, no. 3, pp. 607–611, 2007.

[16] J. W. Coursey, A. F. Morey, J. W. McAninch et al., "Erectile function after anterior urethroplasty," *The Journal of Urology*, vol. 166, no. 6, pp. 2273–2276, 2001.

[17] E. Palminteri, G. Franco, E. Berdondini, F. Fusco, A. de Cillis, and V. Gentile, "Anterior urethroplasty and effects on sexual life: which is the best technique?" *Minerva Urologica e Nefrologica*, vol. 62, no. 4, pp. 371–376, 2010.

[18] H. S. Al-Qudah and R. A. Santucci, "Extended complications of urethroplasty," *International Brazilian Journal of Urology*, vol. 31, pp. 315–325, 2005.

[19] G. Barbagli, M. De Angelis, G. Romano, and M. Lazzeri, "Long-term followup of bulbar end-to-end anastomosis: a retrospective analysis of 153 patients in a single center experience," *The Journal of Urology*, vol. 178, no. 6, pp. 2470–2473, 2007.

[20] E. K. Johnson and J. M. Latini, "The impact of urethroplasty on voiding symptoms and sexual function," *Urology*, vol. 78, no. 1, pp. 198–201, 2011.

[21] J. T. Anger, N. D. Sherman, and G. D. Webster, "The effect of bulbar urethroplasty on erectile function," *The Journal of Urology*, vol. 178, no. 3, pp. 1009–1011, 2007.

[22] T. O. Ekerhult, K. Lindqvist, R. Peeker, and L. Grenabo, "Low risk of sexual dysfunction after transection and nontransection urethroplasty for bulbar urethral stricture," *The Journal of Urology*, vol. 190, no. 2, pp. 635–638, 2013.

[23] A. R. Mundy, "Results and complications of urethroplasty and its future," *British Journal of Urology*, vol. 71, no. 3, pp. 322–325, 1993.

[24] S. Yucel and L. S. Baskin, "Neuroanatomy of the male urethra and perineum," *BJU International*, vol. 92, no. 6, pp. 624–630, 2003.

[25] Y. Akman, W. Liu, Y. W. Li, and L. S. Baskin, "Penile anatomy under the pubic arch: reconstructive implications," *The Journal of Urology*, vol. 166, no. 1, pp. 225–230, 2001.

[26] B. A. Erickson, M. A. Granieri, J. J. Meeks, K. T. McVary, and C. M. Gonzalez, "Prospective analysis of ejaculatory function after anterior urethral reconstruction," *The Journal of Urology*, vol. 184, no. 1, pp. 238–242, 2010.

[27] M. J. Jackson, J. Sciberras, A. Mangera et al., "Defining a patient-reported outcome measure for urethral stricture surgery," *European Urology*, vol. 60, no. 1, pp. 60–68, 2011.

[28] G. Barbagli, S. de Stefani, F. Annino, C. de Carne, and G. Bianchi, "Muscle- and nerve-sparing bulbar urethroplasty: a new technique," *European Urology*, vol. 54, no. 2, pp. 335–343, 2008.

[29] U. Gur and G. H. Jordan, "Vessel-sparing excision and primary anastomosis (for proximal bulbar urethral strictures)," *BJU International*, vol. 101, no. 9, pp. 1183–1195, 2008.

13

Management of Long-Segment and Panurethral Stricture Disease

Francisco E. Martins,[1,2] **Sanjay B. Kulkarni,**[3] **Pankaj Joshi,**[3]
Jonathan Warner,[4] **and Natalia Martins**[2]

[1]*Department of Urology, Hospital Santa Maria, University of Lisbon, School of Medicine, 1600-161 Lisbon, Portugal*
[2]*ULSNA-Hospital de Portalegre, 7300-074 Portalegre, Portugal*
[3]*Kulkarni Reconstructive Urology Center, Pune 411038, India*
[4]*City of Hope Medical Center, Duarte, CA 91010, USA*

Correspondence should be addressed to Francisco E. Martins; faemartins@gmail.com

Academic Editor: Kostis Gyftopoulos

Long-segment urethral stricture or panurethral stricture disease, involving the different anatomic segments of anterior urethra, is a relatively less common lesion of the anterior urethra compared to bulbar stricture. However, it is a particularly difficult surgical challenge for the reconstructive urologist. The etiology varies according to age and geographic location, lichen sclerosus being the most prevalent in some regions of the globe. Other common and significant causes are previous endoscopic urethral manipulations (urethral catheterization, cystourethroscopy, and transurethral resection), previous urethral surgery, trauma, inflammation, and idiopathic. The iatrogenic causes are the most predominant in the Western or industrialized countries, and lichen sclerosus is the most common in India. Several surgical procedures and their modifications, including those performed in one or more stages and with the use of adjunct tissue transfer maneuvers, have been developed and used worldwide, with varying long-term success. A one-stage, minimally invasive technique approached through a single perineal incision has gained widespread popularity for its effectiveness and reproducibility. Nonetheless, for a successful result, the reconstructive urologist should be experienced and familiar with the different treatment modalities currently available and select the best procedure for the individual patient.

1. Introduction

Management of long-segment urethral stricture remains a challenge in reconstructive urology. The surgical treatment of urethral strictures varies according to etiology, location, length, and density of the lesion and fibrosis involving surrounding tissues [1–3]. Treatment of strictures involving the bulbar urethra is relatively well defined and, in most cases, is amenable to excision and end-to-end anastomosis or a short patch onlay substitution urethroplasty [4]. However, long-segment urethral stricture or panurethral stricture disease is less common and the literature on the subject is not abundant.

In the treatment of this condition, several issues must be factored in, such as cause of the stricture, previous urethral surgeries, the quality of the urethral plate, availability of different autologous tissues to be used as flaps or grafts,

experience, expertise, and preference of the treating urologist, including his familiarity with tissue transfer techniques [5]. Lichen sclerosus (LS), also known as balanitis xerotica obliterans (BXO), raises specific problems related to treatment, prognosis, and prolonged follow-up [6–10]. The complexity of this condition may require a different dynamic treatment paradigm. However, although a multistage reconstruction may be used by some surgeons in certain situations due to hostile urethral tissues, in the majority of cases, LS is amenable to a single-stage reconstruction with highly favorable results. Additionally, reconstruction of long-segment urethral strictures is not only about restoring voiding function but also preserving sexual function in all its aspects, such as erection, ejaculation, and orgasm as well as guaranteeing good penile cosmesis.

Current surgical options employed are associated with reasonable success rates and may include a single- or a multiple-stage reconstruction, with the use of a flap, a graft, or a combination of both, and lastly, in extreme circumstances a perineal urethrostomy may offer the best solution for the patient who does not wish to go the extra (long) mile.

2. Materials and Methods

A review of the international literature was conducted using MEDLINE/PubMed database and Google Search, using keywords as "complex urethral stricture," "long segment urethral stricture," "panurethral," "lichen sclerosus," "oral mucosa," and "urethroplasty." We included in the review only articles published in the English language from 1990 to 2015.

3. Epidemiology, Etiology, and Pathogenesis

Generally speaking, male urethral stricture is a common disease worldwide and has been so for centuries. The first known description of urethral dilatation is credited to Shusruta more than 600 years BC [11]. In the 19th century, expert opinion estimated an incidence of 15–20% in the adult male population [12]. In the 21st century in the UK NHS more than 16,000 men required hospital admission annually due to urethral stricture and more than 12,000 of these admissions ended up necessitating surgical treatment with more than £10,000 million [12]. The estimated prevalence in the UK averages 10/100,000 young males doubling this figure by the age of 55 years and rising to over 100/100,000 in males over 65 years. In the USA male urethral stricture accounted for about 5,000 inpatient visits and 1.5 million office visits annually between 1992 and 2000. The incidence was estimated to be approximately 0.6% in susceptible populations [13]. The estimated costs to the medical system for male urethral disease in the USA surpassed US$ 190 million in 2000 [13]. However, there are no direct measures to assess the true incidence of urethral stricture disease worldwide, much less so for panurethral stricture disease in particular. A recent study, including 268 patients, reported panurethral or multifocal anterior urethral stricture in a total of 36 patients (13.4%). However, in a more recent retrospective analysis of all strictures that had been treated surgically at a single institution, the vast majority of strictures were anterior (92.2%) with panurethral strictures totalling 4.9% [14].

Urethral stricture disease can have a profound impact on quality of life, including sexual life, as a result of a number of complications associated with urinary obstruction, such as infection, bladder calculi, urethral diverticulum, fistulation, sepsis, and ultimately chronic renal failure.

The etiology of long-segment or panurethral strictures may vary in industrialized and developing countries. Today, in industrialized countries, most urethral strictures in general have iatrogenic or idiopathic origin [2, 3]. Iatrogenic causes include urethral catheterization, cystourethroscopy, transurethral resection, and previous urethral surgeries. Other causes include idiopathic, trauma, infection/inflammation, and lichen sclerosus. In the developing world, the most common cause of panurethral stricture is genital lichen sclerosus (LS) [6]. Although less frequent, gonorrhea still remains an important cause of long-segment strictures in the developing world.

The pathogenesis of long-segment or panurethral stricture disease has not been widely studied. Historically, and although it is an important cause in some regions of the developing world, infection was blamed as the main cause of urethral stricture [15]. However, it must follow a similar pathogenic process as other types of urethral stricture, that is, injury to the epithelium of the urethra and underlying corpus spongiosum, ultimately leading to fibrosis during the healing process. Excepting a traumatic cause when the urethral lumen is obliterated, corpus spongiosum deep to the urethral epithelium is replaced by dense fibrous tissue and the normal urethral pseudostratified columnar epithelium being replaced by squamous metaplasia [16–18]. Metaplastic change can also occur proximal to a stricture, due to chronic distension under pressure of voiding [12]. Small tears occurring repeatedly in the metaplastic tissue result in focal urinary extravasation, which in turn leads to a fibrotic reaction within the spongiosum. Initially, this fibrosis can be asymptomatic, but, over time, the scar or fibrotic plaque produced can enhance the narrowing of the urethral lumen, resulting in symptomatic urinary obstruction.

The pathology of a urethral stricture is characterized by changes in the extracellular matrix of the spongiosal tissue and replacement of the normal connective tissue by dense fibrosis associated with a decrease in the ratio of type III to type I collagen and a significant decrease in the smooth muscle and nitric oxide content in the strictured urethral tissue [19, 20].

The pathology of lichen sclerosus in inducing urethral stricture is different. LS is a chronic, progressive, inflammatory process which in the male can involve foreskin, glans, and anterior urethra. The etiology is for the most part unclear, although it has been associated with an autoimmune reaction and a genetic pattern. However, an infectious cause has been suggested [21]. This is an atrophic rather than a proliferative process that usually originates in the foreskin or glans as diffuse or patchy plaques of white discoloration giving the glans a characteristically mottled appearance (Figure 1). It can progress further to include the meatus, fossa navicularis, penile urethra, and eventually the bulbar urethra, resulting in a long-segment or panurethral stricture disease [7, 8]. It remains unclear whether LS-induced urethral strictures develop as a consequence of extension of glandular disease into the penile urethra or whether they result from chronically obstructed voiding or instrumentation, or both [22]. Long-segment urethral strictures, as any anterior urethral stricture, typically occur following trauma or infection, but mostly from iatrogenic causes, especially urethral catheterization, dilatation, and endoscopic manipulation, or may be idiopathic. Nonetheless, LS has been reported as the most frequent cause of this type of stricture, especially in India [6, 8, 9].

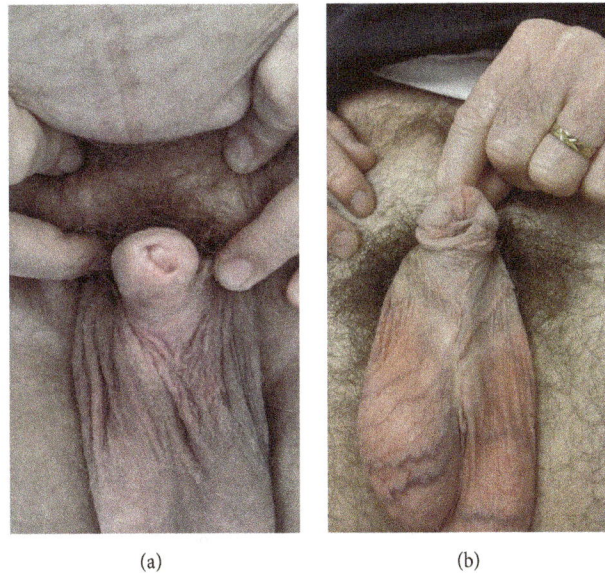

FIGURE 1: Lichen sclerosus of the glans and prepuce (a) and hypospadias cripple (b). Both patients with panurethral stricture.

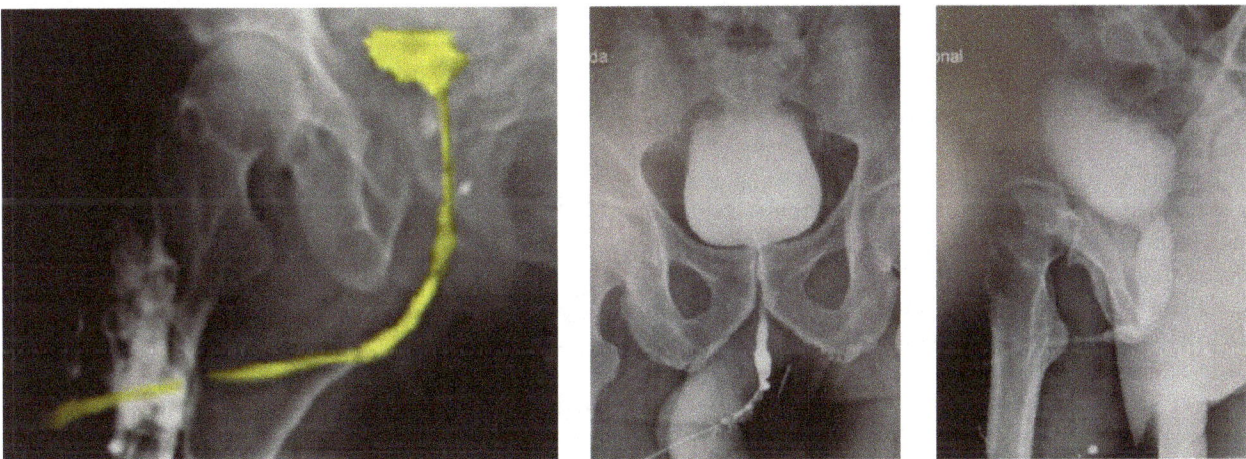

FIGURE 2: Retrograde and voiding urethrogram of panurethral stricture disease.

4. Diagnostic Evaluation

A critical initial pitfall in the diagnostic evaluation is not to fully understand and properly diagnose the stricture as being panurethral. Symptomatic stricture disease typically presents with progressive obstructive voiding complaints, such as a weak stream, frequency, incomplete emptying, terminal dribbling and straining, or complications of an obstructive voiding syndrome, such as recurrent tract infections, epididymitis, haematuria, and bladder stones. Symptomatic evaluation should be best formalized using a validated questionnaire, such as the AUA symptom index [24, 25].

Physical examination may be vague and uneventful in some cases. Nonetheless, the penis should always be carefully examined for scars related to previous surgery, penile malformations, signs of LS, or associated penile cancer. Careful attention should also be drawn to palpation of the spongiosum and genital area in general. The mouth should also be carefully inspected, particularly if an oral mucosa graft is planned.

Uroflowmetry, ultrasonography, and cystourethroscopy may be important adjuncts in the diagnosis of panurethral stricture disease, but the most critical is retrograde urethrography (RUG) and voiding cystourethrography (VCUG). The latter tests determine the location, length, and severity of the stricture in great detail (Figure 2). Endoscopy can give an idea of the elasticity and appearance of the urethra, especially following previous urethroplasty(ies). Ultrasonography can be used to determine the length and degree of fibrosis and eventually influence the operative approach [26]. Although ultrasonography seems to provide important additional information during preoperative evaluation, it has not gained the expected widespread popularity. This may be due to its relatively limited usefulness in the more proximal bulbar urethra, where the distance between the ultrasound probe and the target area surpasses its resolution accuracy.

It is of paramount importance that these imaging modalities ensure that all diseased portions of the urethra are included in the repair. Often, the narrowing of the lumen can be fairly uniform, with spots of more severe reduction in caliber. Thus, a panurethral stricture can be erroneously interpreted as just a short stricture and the other less severe areas underestimated as being of "normal" caliber. To avoid this diagnostic error, some authors have suggested that if the urethral lumen does not expand to $\geq 8\,mm$ in diameter on imaging, then it is probably stenosed. Sometimes, it may be necessary to proceed to a full examination under anesthesia with endoscopy and bougienage and retrograde urethral imaging [27].

5. Surgical Reconstruction

In rare instances, where symptoms are not particularly troublesome, surgical treatment may not be necessary. In the majority of patients, both urethral dilatation and direct vision internal urethrotomy are inappropriate and, therefore, have no place in the treatment of panurethral stricture disease. At the other extreme end of the spectrum of this disease, typically patients who have undergone multiple failed surgical attempts, particularly when associated with significant comorbidity, might prefer a definitive perineal urethrostomy or even opt a simple suprapubic cystostomy catheter.

Panurethral stricture disease is definitely a complex subset of urethral stricture disease. Defining "panurethral" has been a matter of debate. This has implications in the interpretation of the literature as there is no homogeneity in the study populations. In a recent multi-institution study including 466 patients, long-segment or panurethral stricture was defined as any single stricture or multifocal diseased areas of the penile and bulbar (anterior) urethra measuring $\geq 8\,cm$ in length [23]. Several surgical reconstructive procedures have been described to address this full-length anterior urethral strictures (Table 1). When planning the surgical treatment of panurethral stricture disease, some surgeons have concerns of whether to select a one- or two-stage operation and, if a one-stage operation is chosen, whether adequate transfer tissue for reconstruction is available. Panurethral stricture disease associated with LS has been successfully treated with a single-stage repair and OM onlay grafting. Indeed, the authors' experience has clearly shown that it should be preferred over a multistage approach, which in their opinion has no role in the surgical treatment of genitourethral LS [6, 23]. The main arguments are the high failure rate; the fact that genitourethral LS is a penile skin disease and, lastly, that staged operations will allow ingrowth of the disease into the urethra. In less common instances, where there is significant urethral narrowing with an unsalvageable plate, after multiple failed previous repairs, or if the stricture disease is associated with infection, abscess or calculi, a two-stage marsupializing procedure, like the Johanson procedure, may be preferable. In the majority of cases, substitution urethroplasty is the rule. Substitution urethroplasty can be performed using a flap, a graft, or sometimes a combination of both.

TABLE 1: Options for surgical reconstruction of long-segment and panurethral strictures.

Flaps
Circular fasciocutaneous penile flap (McAninch flap)
Q-flap and variants (Quartey and Jordan)
Biaxial epilated scrotal flap (Gil-Vernet)
Grafts
Oral mucosa (cheek, tongue, and lower lip)—Kulkarni technique
Postauricular skin (Wolf)
Penile and preputial skin
Bladder mucosa
Colonic mucosa
Combination of flaps and grafts
Staged procedures
Johanson technique and variants
Schreiter's mesh graft technique
Tunica albuginea (Monseur) urethroplasty
Perineal urethrostomy

5.1. Flaps. Several flaps have been described and used in panurethral stricture reconstruction. In 1993, McAninch described the *circular fasciocutaneous penile flap* for the reconstruction of extensive urethral stricture [28]. Circular fasciocutaneous penile flap originates on the distal penis and uses Buck's fascia as the major vascular supply. He reported his results with the use of this flap for 1-stage reconstruction of complex anterior urethral strictures involving long penile and also bulbar urethral strictures in 66 men [29]. The stricture length measured up to 24 cm (average 9.08 cm). The flap was used as an onlay procedure and tubularized flap for urethral substitution. In some cases, additional adjunctive tissue transfer and proximal graft placement were required. Initial success rate was 79%, rising up to 95% after an additional procedure. Recurrent strictures occurred usually at the proximal and distal anastomotic sites. The penile circular fasciocutaneous flap reliably provided 12–15 cm of length for reconstruction in most patients, although approximately 90% had been previously circumcised. The less favorable results were seen in patients after flap tubularization for urethral replacement. The McAninch technique is worldwide considered as a reliable surgical option for panurethral strictures and numerous publications are available in the literature about its use. A major advantage of the McAninch flap is its versatility, as it can be utilized in all areas of the urethra, from the membranous area to the external meatus [29, 30]. Because of compartment syndrome noted in 2 different cases due to prolonged exaggerated lithotomy position that usually occurs if the patient remains in this position more than 5 hours, the authors begin the operation with flap harvesting with the patient in the supine position, thereby reducing exposure to the lithotomy position by 2-3 hours.

The *Q-flap* is a modification of the McAninch circular penile fasciocutaneous skin flap. It is so called because it incorporates an additional midline ventral longitudinal penile extension, thus resembling the letter Q. Similar "hockey-stick" flap configurations have also been described by Quartey [31]. Morey et al. reported their experience with the Q-flap in 15 patients with a mean stricture length of 15.5 cm (range 12–21) who underwent single-stage urethral reconstruction. All patients had a prepuce and the flap was harvested with the patient initially supine to avoid compartment syndrome [32]. The flap is outlined with the penis on stretch and the penis degloved, meticulously preserving the blood supply on the tunica dartos pedicle. The Q-flap is sewn into place after ventral urethrotomy as an onlay flap with running 4-0 absorbable suture, similar to the McAninch flap procedure. The fossa navicularis is typically reconstructed through a glans-wings or a glans-preserving technique. Once the pendulous portion of the onlay flap is sewn in, the patient is repositioned into the lithotomy position and the flap is transferred to the perineum through a scrotal tunnel wide enough to accommodate loose passage of the flap. The potential major advantage of these flap procedures is to allow a single-stage reconstruction of long-segment and complex strictures and to avoid the need for additional, morbid, time-consuming tissue transfer techniques.

These two procedures are extremely labor-intensive and are among the most difficult and tedious in reconstructive urology. A common complication with the above two flaps, particularly with unexperienced surgeons, is necrosis of penile skin proximal to the flap [29, 30]. In some instances, this penile skin necrosis may lead to wound infection and ultimately to disruption of the flap and necrosis.

In 1997, Gil-Vernet et al. described another type of flap for urethroplasty, the *biaxial epilated scrotal flap* [33]. They used this flap, which measured up to 20 × 2.5 cm, to reconstruct the entire anterior urethra from the bulbomembranous urethra to the external meatus. This flap consists of scrotal skin, dartos, external spermatic fascia, cremasteric fibers and fascia, internal spermatic fascia, and scrotal septum. Tunica vaginalis is not included. Vascular anastomoses between cremasteric (deep) and scrotal (superficial) blood supply plexuses are included in the flap and hence biaxial flap. The authors used this technique in 37 men including 10 with panurethral stricture disease. Two of these 10 patients failed due to graft shrinkage, necessitating perineal urethrostomy. There were also problems with incorrect scrotal skin epilation leading to sclerosis, vascular lesions, and penile ventral curvature. Nonetheless, the authors considered this flap technique ideal for urethral reconstruction from the penoscrotal angle to the prostatic apex. Because of anatomical proximity, good tissue availability, and potentially good tolerance to contact with urine due to abundance of sebaceous glands, this is always the authors' first option for bulbomembranous urethroplasty. They also believe that scrotal skin flap is less likely to develop lichen sclerosus as compared to penile skin. Despite all the potential advantages mentioned by the authors, epilation, deepithelialization, and flap mobilization may not be so straightforward. Epilation is an extremely time-consuming process. Although flaps with their own blood supply would be more appropriate in severely fibrotic urethral beds, such as after previously failed urethroplasties, several problems with postvoid dribbling of urine, ejaculatory dysfunction,

and flap outpouching or pseudodiverticulum formation are truly troublesome and impact on quality of life [30]. It should be kept in mind that, in general, the use of skin flaps for urethral reconstruction is more technically demanding than substitution urethroplasty. In a study by McAninch and Morey, for patients with an average stricture length of 9 cm, the initial overall success rate of the fasciocutaneous flap reconstruction was 79%. Recurrent stricture rate was noted in 13% of onlay grafts and in 58% of tubularized repairs [29].

5.2. Grafts. The use of grafts in urethral reconstruction has become a more popularized surgical option worldwide. Theoretically, grafts in general are inherently less reliable because they need to be vascularized. However, they are quick and relatively easier to harvest and deploy. There are several studies of both flaps and grafts showing similar restricture rates [34]. Therefore, in the authors' opinion, a graft should be the procedure of choice due to its simplicity and speed by which it can be harvested and deployed, since the restricture rate is similar. There may be specific indications favoring a flap rather than a graft: revision surgery following multiple failed attempts, any cause of local devascularization such as irradiation or severe peripheral vascular insufficiency, and local infection, all of which hamper the ability of a graft to take. In summary, a graft repair is preferred due to the reasons mentioned above. Both grafts and flaps contract, although full-thickness flaps tend to contract less than split-thickness flaps and grafts, and patch grafts do better than tubed grafts, which may imply a two-stage procedure if a circumferential reconstruction of the urethra is necessary.

The widespread popularity of *oral mucosa* in urethral reconstruction has similarly allowed the introduction of new techniques in long segment and panurethral stricture repair. In 2000, Kulkarni et al. first described the use of long oral mucosa grafts to repair the entire anterior urethra through a simple perineal incision in a single stage, thus preserving the penile components, their anatomy, function, and cosmesis [35] (Figure 3). In 2009, the same authors described a modification of their original technique, suggesting a minimally invasive procedure with dissection of the urethra from the corpora cavernosa along one side only, thus preserving the entire neurovascular supply to the urethra [36] (Figure 4). Buccal mucosa graft urethroplasty has been used for long anterior urethral strictures by several authors following the initial report by Kulkarni et al. in 2000 [37–40]. All these authors have reported favorable results at short- and medium-term follow-up with acceptable complication rates. In 2004, Gupta et al. described a technique of dorsal graft placement by ventral sagittal urethrotomy and minimal-access perineal approach and used this technique in patients with anterior urethral stricture, including 2 with panurethral stricture disease [40]. In the Kulkarni technique, the whole anterior urethra is repaired by a single perineal incision, single technique, and single substitute material (Figure 4). In a retrospective study including 117 patients with panurethral stricture disease treated from June 1998 to December 2010, the overall success rate was 83.7%. Mean stricture length was 14 cm and median follow-up was 59 months. Most recurrent

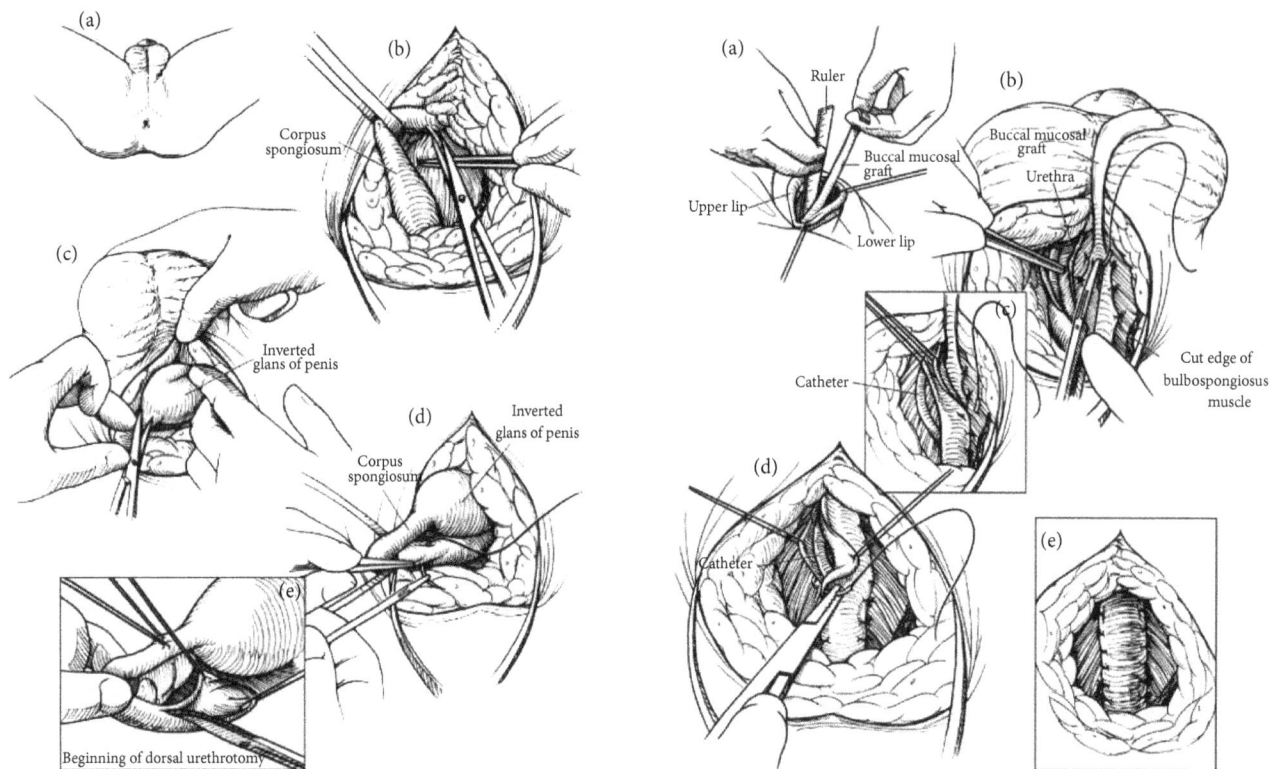

(a) A midline perineal incision bifurcated posteriorly which is used for its excellent access to the proximal bulbar urethra

(b) Full mobilization of the anterior urethra through the perineum as for a total urethrectomy. A Gelpi retractor which is used

(c) The glans penis which is inverted and delivered to the perineal wound for dissection of the distalmost segment of the urethra

(d) Placement of stay sutures in preparation for dorsal external urethrotomy

(e) Dorsal external urethrotomy which is begun in the proximal bulbar urethra

(a) Harvesting of buccal mucosa graft involving lower lip and both inner cheeks

(b) The urethra which is fully mobilized and rotated 180° for external urethrotomy along its dorsal surface. A single strip of BM which is spread and sutured to the tunica albuginea of the corpora cavernosa. Quilting sutures which are applied along the graft

(c) The right urethral margin which is sutured to the ipsilateral side of the patch

(d) Suturing of the left side of the urethra-graft anastomosis

(e) Suturing which is completed and the grafted area which is covered by urethral plate

FIGURE 3: Schematic representation of the Kulkarni operation.

strictures occurred at the proximal anastomotic site and none of these was a full-length recurrence [6]. The major advantage of this technique is that it is minimally invasive and performed in one stage. It also avoids the psychological trauma of 2 (or more) operations and the need of living for 6 months with bifid scrotum after staged procedures. Additionally, because it is a one-side dissection the risk of injury to the neurovascular bundles to the penis and urethra is minimal. This procedure is carried out through the perineum, avoiding a penile scar, and does not lead to a hypospadiac meatus.

More recently, some authors have described the use of *lingual mucosa* in urethroplasty [41–45]. The graft characteristics of lingual mucosa are similar to those of buccal mucosa (cheek and lip) [41, 42]. Lingual mucosal graft was used as the sole graft in 18 men with long anterior urethral strictures by Das et al. [41]. Most cases were etiologically associated with LS or infection. Overall success rate was 83.3%. However, separate results regarding panurethral strictures were not

given. A particular advantage of lingual mucosa is that it can be harvested in continuity across the midline with the opposite side of the tongue, allowing a graft of sufficient length for panurethral strictures.

Prepuce and penile skin in the form of flaps or grafts are recognized alternatives for this type of reconstruction and are mentioned in the Table 1. In experienced hands, oral mucosal grafts measuring 10×1.5 cm can routinely be harvested from each inner cheek. If necessary, lingual grafts can be harvested in addition. A great number of our patients who have LS have scarred prepuce and glans and already had circumcision. In LS, no form of genital skin can or should be used. Preputial/distal penile skin graft was described for dorsal onlay anterior urethroplasty. In most studies, panurethral stricture patients were a minority [46, 47]. Most failures occurred if the skin graft was placed onto the penile urethra. Although previous circumcision did not preclude the use of penile skin, buccal mucosa was recommended as the best choice if the shaft skin was not abundant [46].

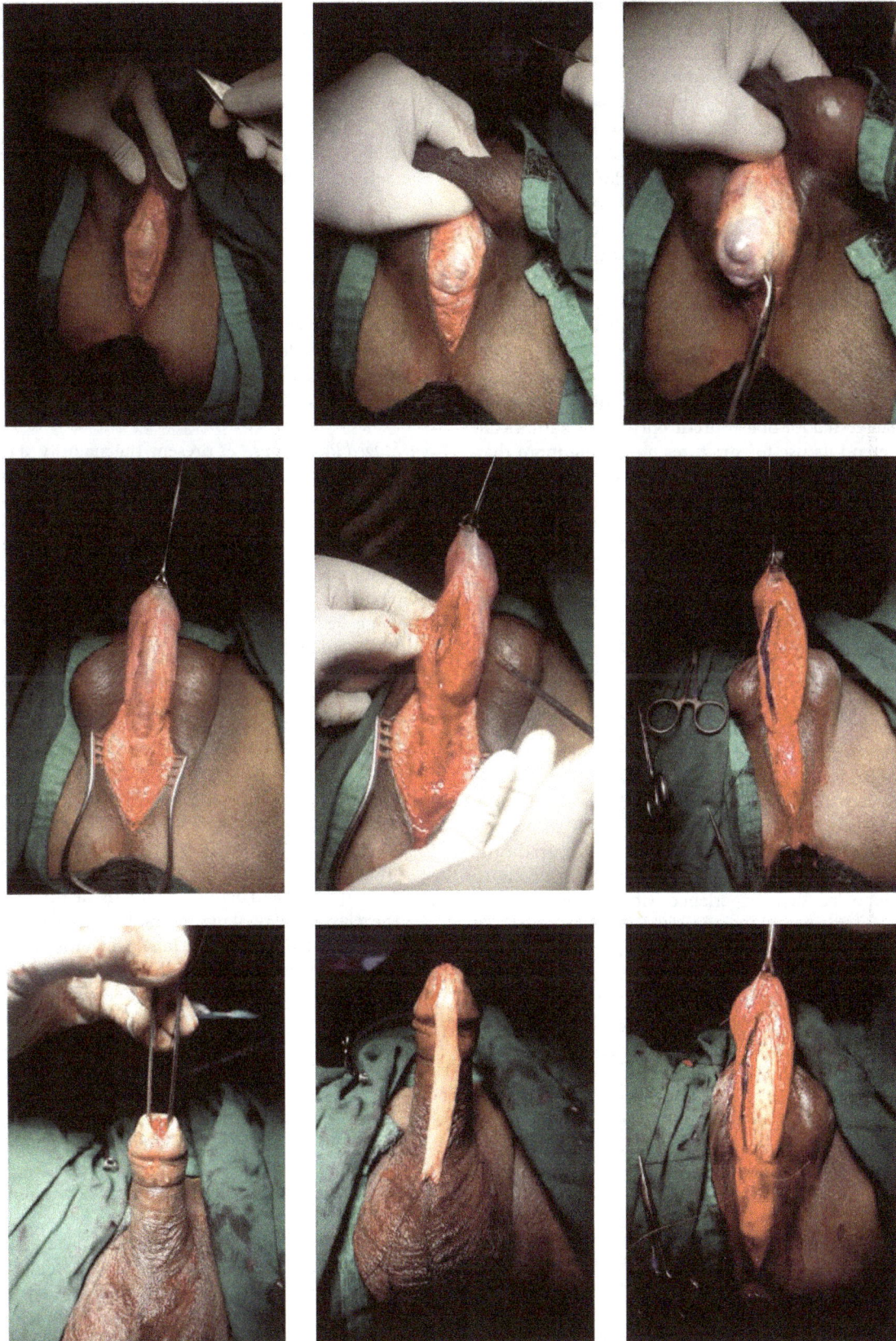

FIGURE 4: Kulkarni operation.

Postauricular skin has also been used as a good alternative for men with panurethral strictures with high success rate [48–50]. Postauricular skin is thin and has a dense subdermal plexus, and, therefore, graft take and functional outcomes are superior to other nongenital skin grafts. However, Andrich and Mundy cautioned that no skin graft should be used for urethroplasty in LS patients. LS is a skin disease and can also affect any skin graft in due course [49].

Another subject of controversy is the location for graft placement. Ventral graft placement, particularly in the pendulous urethra, is usually associated with poorer results. In the bulbar urethra, similar results can be expected, as long as ventral grafting is not used for long and complex strictures. A flap or a two-stage procedure is advocated by some authors for these strictures [46]. Dorsal graft placement usually produces the best outcomes and, therefore, is the method of choice in panurethral strictures [6, 23, 51–53]. Although doubled-sided dorsal plus ventral oral mucosa grafting has also been suggested for bulbar urethroplasty, the authors did not recommend its use for strictures measuring more than 4 cm in length [54]. Therefore, this technique is not indicated in long-segment or panurethral stricture disease.

Colonic mucosa has been employed for the reconstruction of panurethral stricture disease [55]. This graft is harvested from sigmoid colon using a laparoscopic approach or by a lower abdominal paramedian incision. Full-thickness grafts of 12 to 15 cm in length of sigmoid colon mucosa can be obtained and the colon continuity is immediately restored by an end-to-end anastomosis. An unstretched colonic mucosa graft is trimmed and sized to an appropriate individual need (ranging from 15 to 22 cm in length and 3 cm in width) and is tubularized over a 16 to 18 Fr fenestrated or fluted silicone catheter with interrupted 5-0 absorbable suture to create a neourethra. An end-to-end anastomosis is performed between the neourethra and the proximal end of the native urethra. The distal end of the neourethra is pulled through the glans tunnel to form the neomeatus. Xu et al. reported their experience with 35 patients who underwent colonic mucosal graft urethroplasty for complex, long-segment urethral strictures, ranging from 11 to 21 cm in length (mean 15.1). Five (14.2%) of these patients developed recurrent strictures. However, 3 of the recurrences were not related to the urethroplasty. Therefore, they concluded that tubularized urethroplasty using colonic mucosa grafts was successful and had a lower recurrence rate than patch urethroplasty. Nonetheless, this procedure needs further investigation and confirmation and, therefore, should be reserved as an alternative in complex patients where other options are not available or possible.

5.3. Combination of Flaps and Grafts. The exclusive use of long flaps for complex or panurethral strictures may be a technically challenging ordeal and are usually associated with long operating times and morbidity due to positioning and the surgical procedure itself. Furthermore, sufficient length of skin flaps may not be available, particularly in circumcised men or if LS is present. In such cases, a reasonable treatment option is to combine a shorter flap with a graft, and the graft

placed proximally in the bulbar urethra [51]. A penile circular fasciocutaneous flap combined with an oral mucosa graft placed proximally was used by Wessells et al. in 7 patients with a mean stricture length of 18.3 cm [56]. The mean flap length was 12.6 cm (range 10–15) and mean graft length was 6.2 cm (range 3–9). The overall success rate was 88% at 16 months follow-up. Unfortunately, the authors did not mention results specific to panurethral strictures separately. The authors emphasized the importance of avoiding tubed reconstructions as these are associated with high risk of restricture and other flap-related complications.

Oral mucosa has become the graft material of choice for substitution urethroplasty, but at times it may be insufficient to completely reconstruct a long-segment or panurethral stricture. The combined use of oral mucosa and a genital skin flap has proved to be a reliable and durable alternative for single-stage reconstruction of long-segment or panurethral stricture disease [51].

5.4. Staged Procedures. At present, the majority of uncomplicated anterior urethral strictures can be successfully managed with a single-stage procedure. However, complex strictures associated with adverse local conditions, such as extensive scarred tissue formation of the urethra, infection, fistulation, prior multiple failed urethral reconstruction attempts, totally obliterated residual urethra, graft or flap-related factors, or following heavy irradiation, represent a challenge and are more appropriately treated with a staged procedure. A staged reconstruction may also be indicated in some long urethral strictures. All these situations are associated with unhealthy, poorly vascularized, and inelastic urethral and neighbouring tissues for urethral reconstruction. Although LS can be managed with a single-stage reconstruction, in some cases a staged procedure may be a reasonable option, as it may have a beneficial impact on the natural history of the disease [57–60]. A perineal urethrostomy for urinary diversion avoids continuous extravasation into the corpus spongiosum and promotes quicker and better urethral tissue healing.

The classical two-stage method was developed in the 1950s by Johanson [61]. The Johanson procedure is based on marsupialization of the strictured urethra, followed by a second surgical stage approximately 4–6 months after the first stage has healed (Figures 5 and 6). In the past, scrotal or perineal skin was used for urethral reconstruction. The great achievement of Johanson's technique was its use in all types of strictures, apart from initiating an era of urethral reconstructive surgery. The drawbacks of this technique resulted from the use of hair-growing scrotal and perineal skin, which lead to chronic urinary tract infection, abscesses, lithogenesis, fistulation, sacculation, and diverticula formation in the reconstructed urethra.

In the 1980s, Schreiter reported a two-stage mesh graft procedure in an attempt to avoid the use of scrotal or perineal skin by using a hairless skin graft which is transferred to a two-stage procedure [62, 63]. Although this technique can be employed in every type of stricture, apparently its best indication is in complex strictures, especially associated with severe tissue scarring and absence of healthy penile skin for urethral reconstruction.

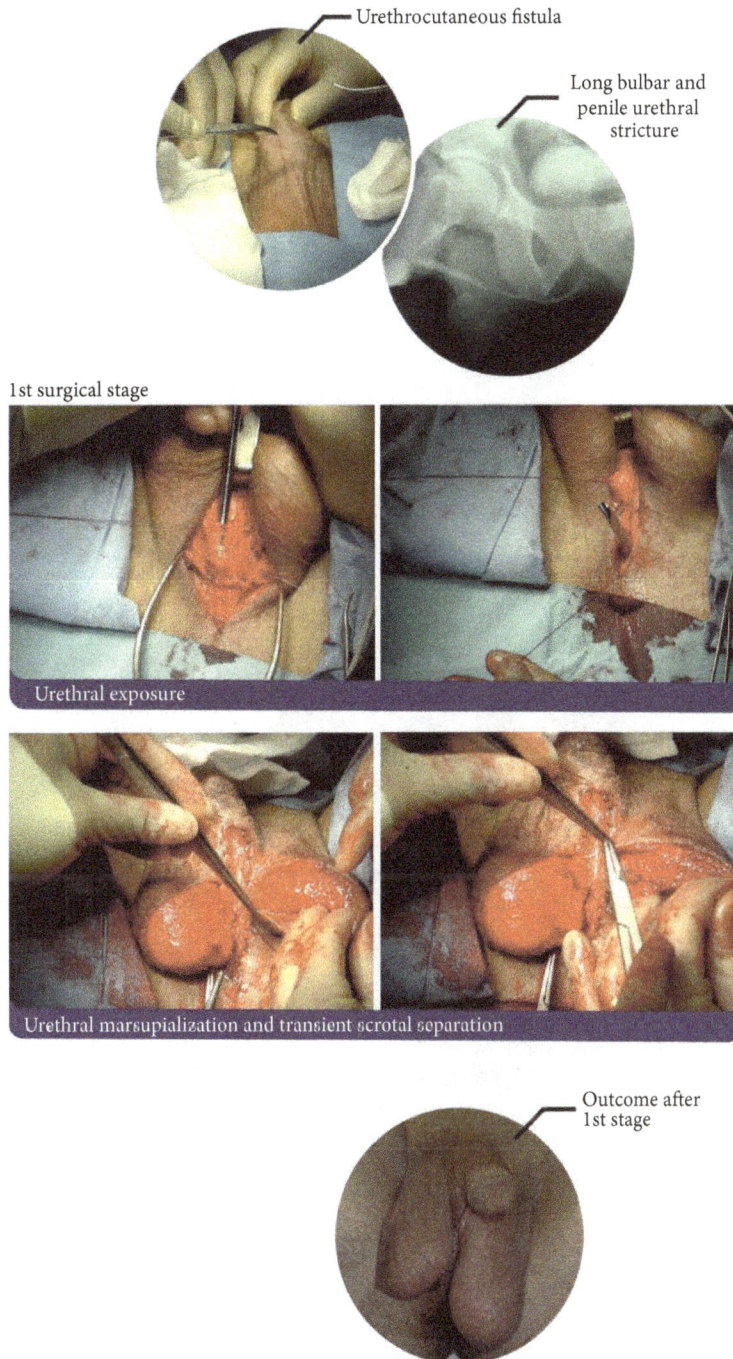

FIGURE 5: First stage of Johanson reconstruction with OMG inlay of panurethral stricture.

More recently, other authors have reported on a two-stage Johanson-type urethroplasty with oral mucosa grafting for anterior urethral strictures. For penile urethral strictures, Patterson and Chapple favor a two-stage procedure with dorsal onlay oral mucosa grafting after complete excision of the scarred urethra [64].

Staged reconstructions are associated with significant inconvenience to some patients, exposing them to an increased risk of morbidity due to multiple general anesthetics. Additionally, revision is common after two-stage

operations and in one series half of the patients ended up needing a three-stage repair [65].

5.5. *Tunica Albuginea (Monseur) Urethroplasty.* In 1969, Monseur described a procedure by which a neourethra was created and its lumen continuity was maintained by the tunica albuginea through a supraurethral or subcavernosal groove without the need of a graft or flap [66]. Recently, there has been some renewed interest in this technique and various

Outcome after 4 months

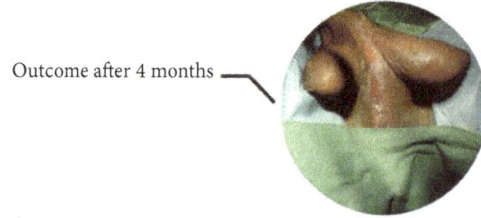

2nd surgical stage

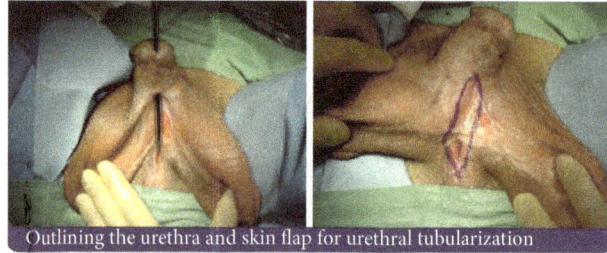

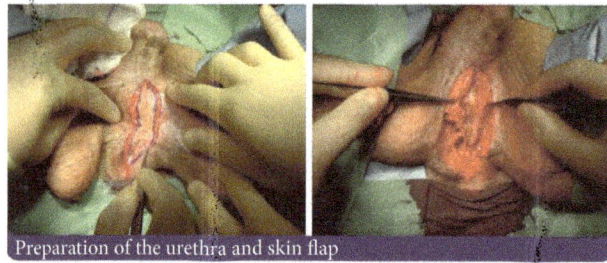

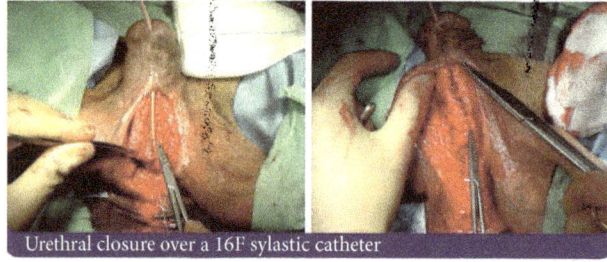

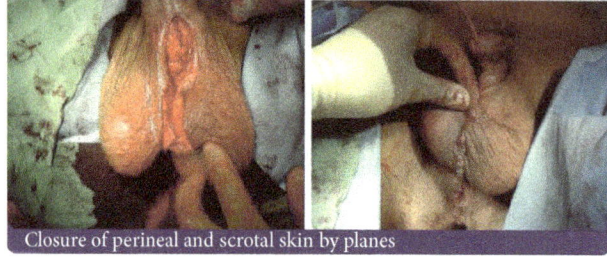

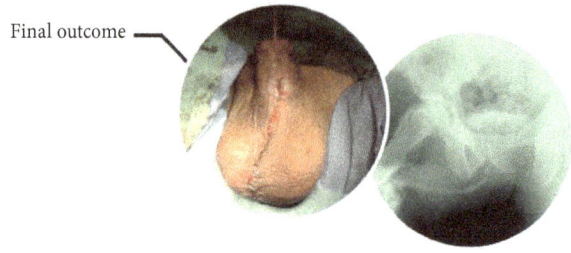

Outlining the urethra and skin flap for urethral tubularization

Preparation of the urethra and skin flap

Urethral closure over a 16F sylastic catheter

Closure of perineal and scrotal skin by planes

Final outcome

FIGURE 6: Second stage and closure.

reports have been published on the use of Monseur's tunica albuginea urethroplasty for short- and long-segment urethral strictures with acceptable success rates [67, 68]. The authors reported on the utility of this technique in cases where oral mucosa urethroplasty is not feasible due to lack of healthy oral mucosa associated with tobacco chewing or need of very long grafts to bridge panurethral strictures [69]. The authors described some similarity with the tubularized incised plate (TIP) urethroplasty described by Snodgrass and Bush, where the tunica exposed after incision of the urethral dorsal plate forms the roof of the neourethra and has stood the test of time for that purpose [70]. The authors argue that flap procedures are considered extremely labor-intensive, tedious, and among the most difficult in reconstructive urology [32]. Oral mucosa graft procedures, although very successful in medium-sized strictures, may not be feasible in very long strictures. Because some studies have shown that, even in dorsal onlay grafting, oral mucosa and penile skin grafts have shown similar results, while both proving superior to flaps, these authors concluded that it is not the type of graft, but rather the site of graft that is ultimately responsible for the success of the procedure [71]. Other studies have reported that a ventral onlay graft has a significant disadvantage over a dorsal onlay. It is claimed that complications are decreased if the graft is placed dorsally over the urethral groove [72]. Based on the concept advocated by Monseur, Barbagli et al. introduced the dorsally placed (onlay) graft technique and postulated that dorsal graft placement is superior as it allows better mechanical support for the graft and a richer and predictable vascular blood supply for the graft from the underlying corpora cavernosa [73, 74]. So if it is assumed that dorsal onlay grafts yield results better than ventral, then it must be the site of graft placement rather than the type of graft material that is ultimately responsible for the better success rates [75]. Lastly, the authors claim that Monseur's tunica albuginea urethroplasty is easy to perform, with short learning curve, without graft morbidity, requiring less time and resources, and success rates are comparable to oral mucosa urethroplasty. Tunica albuginea appears to be sufficient to allow regrowth of urethral epithelium and a patent distensible lumen if proved by urethrosccopic biopsy. However, we think that further studies are necessary.

6. Success and Complications

Generally, urethroplasty has excellent success rates and far exceed those found with direct vision internal urethrotomy. Serious complications following urethroplasty are relatively uncommon, 3% of them occurring in the early postoperative period and 18% in a late follow-up period [76]. Most reports in the literature contain heterogeneous data, that is, different types of strictures treated by different modalities and surgeons. When complications are mentioned, they are mixed for all the procedures. Another pitfall found in the literature is in comparing success rates in different series, as these have variable definitions of treatment failure. Therefore, consensus in reconstructive urology needs to be established in the future.

TABLE 2: Major and minor complications of "panurethroplasty"*.

Major	Minor
Early	Early
Hematuria	Oral numbness
RUG leak	Drooling when eating or Speaking
Oral discomfort	Speech impairment
Wound dehiscence	Perineal hypoesthesia
Wound tightness	Scrotal hyperesthesia
Epididymitis	Stensen's duct squirting
Penile ecchymosis	Penile pain
Penile swelling	Penile shortening
Penile skin ischemia/necrosis	Postvoid dribbling
UTI	Stress incontinence
Wound infection	Urine splaying
Late	Late
Rectal injury	Recurrent stricture
Urosepsis	Sexual dysfunction
	Chordee
	Fistulation

*Generally, similar and common to any urethroplasty.

Generally, complications of urethroplasty are directly related to location of stricture, length of stricture, operative technique, and type of transfer tissue employed (Table 2). Complications after urethroplasty can be divided into major and minor groups, occurring early or late. Most minor complications are usually mild and temporary and may be amenable to simple corrective procedures. Major complications are usually severe and complicated and result in failure of urethroplasty. In this review we will focus on complications associated with the reconstructive procedures of long-segment anterior urethral or panurethral strictures (Table 3).

Oral mucosal grafts are now considered the standard substitution material for urethral surgery. Surgical procedures involving oral mucosa onlay have better success rates and less morbidity compared with fasciocutaneous flaps [23, 46, 73, 74, 76]. One report has mentioned complication rates of fasciocutaneous flaps between 3% and 56% [77]. In a multi-institutional study, Warner et al. reported on the complication rates of different surgical techniques to repair long-segment and panurethral strictures [23]. The complication rate was higher in the fasciocutaneous cohort compared with those without a flap (32% versus 14%, resp.; $P = 0.02$). In this review, a 2-stage Johanson urethroplasty was not as successful as the buccal mucosal graft procedure (BMG) (64% versus 82.5%, resp.). It was found that 2-stage Johanson urethroplasties performed with skin had a higher failure rate than those performed with a BMG (66.7% recurrence rate versus 28.3%, resp.). Meticulous follow-up of patients after long-segment or "panurethroplasty" may show an important percentage of early and late complications. Perineal neuralgia or neuropraxia is a well-known

TABLE 3: Complications by most common techniques for pan-urethroplasty.

Type of surgery	Early	Late	Recurrence
FC flap	Transient pain and numbness Fistula (resolved)	Fistula	37.5%
OMG	UTI Penile edema Bleeding	Chordee Fistula ED Oral and lip discomfort numbness Cold glans	17.5%
Second-stage Johanson	Wound dehiscence UTI Scrotal abscess Penile numbness Epididymitis	ED Graft contracture Fistula Chordee Cold glans	35.7%
PU and definitive 1st-stage Johanson	Wound dehiscence UTI Transient pain and numbness	Chordee Fistula	24.1%
FC flap + graft	Wound hematoma PE Penile skin ischemia	Fistula Chordee	23.5%

FC: fasciocutaneous; OMG: oral mucosal graft; UTI: urinary tract infection; ED: erectile dysfunction; PU: perineal urethrostomy; PE: pulmonary embolism. Adapted from [23].

complication of bulbar and posterior urethroplasty, or any surgery performed in the exaggerated lithotomy position (i.e., radical perineal prostatectomy and urorectal fistula repair) [78–80]. The most common position-related complications of complex urethroplasty include superficial peroneal nerve neuropraxia, rhabdomyolysis, and lower extremity compartment syndrome. Although several causes of neuropraxia have been identified, the mechanical nerve compression seems to be the most common. It usually resolves spontaneously within 6–8 weeks. Recent studies have reported much lower position-related complication rates not exceeding 3% due to shortening of overall lithotomy position and meticulous protocol of patient protection during this type of surgery. In the authors' personal series, the severe neuropraxia rate has been in accordance with these reports.

Although most complications are minor, with little impact, and easily corrected, they seem to occur in a higher number than previously published (40%) [76]. These complications are important to the patient and should be discussed in the counseling before surgery.

7. Impact on Sexual Function

Impairment of male sexual function (penile sensation, erectile, and ejaculatory dysfunctions) are usually underreported. However, this scenario has been changed recently. In 2001, Coursey et al. reported a study on erectile function after anterior urethroplasty based on a questionnaire evaluation of erectile dysfunction. ED occurred in 19% of patients after OMG and 27% after anastomotic urethroplasty. Although he postulated that men with a long stricture might be at increased risk for transient erectile changes, the overall postoperative sexual dysfunction rate was no higher than circumcision [81]. Based on validated inventory questionnaires, such as the International Index of Erectile Function (IIEF-5) or

the O'Leary Brief Male Sexual Function Inventory (BMSFI), the majority of the studies published recently have not shown that urethral reconstructive surgery impairs erectile function and sexual drive. Ejaculatory function was even improved in the younger ages [82–86]. Although erectile dysfunction has been associated with urethroplasty operations, its incidence is largely unknown. A 1% incidence of de novo erectile dysfunction after anterior urethroplasty was found in a meta-analysis study by Blaschko et al. However, in most cases the erectile dysfunction was transient and resolved within the first 12 months [85]. Another study reported an incidence of transient erectile dysfunction after anterior urethroplasty in approximately 40%, although recovery was observed in most by 6 months [83]. In 2006, the same authors had described a relationship between older age and a higher incidence of erectile dysfunction after surgery. Nonetheless, overall, men had not reported a decline in erectile dysfunction or sexual drive after urethroplasty [82]. In 2015, Xu et al. published a study dealing specifically with the impact of erectile dysfunction on complex panurethral stricture disease. They concluded that the surgical reconstruction with the use of grafts (buccal, lingual, and colonic mucosa) had limited effect on erectile function. The only adverse factor was extension of the stricture to posterior urethra, in which case an impairment was observed [86]. Ejaculatory dysfunction was reported in patients after ventrally placed flaps or grafts, possibly due to urethrocele formation [87]. However, no ejaculatory dysfunction has been reported in patients after dorsal onlays [77, 87].

8. Conclusion

One-stage repairs with BMG offer an excellent option for patients with long-segment and panurethral stricture disease. In cases with obliterative or absent urethral plate, a 2-stage

Johanson urethroplasty with BMG offers a viable alternative. In cases of LS, 1-stage BMG has better outcomes than a 2-stage repair. If BMGs are not available, FC flaps offer similar success; however, these are associated with higher rates of complications. Skin grafts should be avoided, unless no alternatives exist. Finally, the valuable role of PU cannot be understated in the setting of multiple failed urethroplasties.

The options currently available to reconstruct the urethra are in permanent development and attention should be focused on both old and new concepts. No surgical technique should compromise penile length, cause chordee, and affect cosmesis. Oral morbidity should be given attention after OMG to avoid permanent late sequelae in mouth function. Critical attention should also be given to sexual function as any urethral reconstructive method can eventually cause its occurrence.

Conflict of Interests

The authors declare that there is no conflict of interests regarding the publication of this paper.

References

[1] A. C. Peterson and G. D. Webster, "Management of urethral stricture disease: developing options for surgical intervention," *BJU International*, vol. 94, no. 7, pp. 971–976, 2004.

[2] A. S. Fenton, A. F. Morey, R. Aviles, and C. R. Garcia, "Anterior urethral strictures: etiology and characteristics," *Urology*, vol. 65, no. 6, pp. 1055–1058, 2005.

[3] N. Lumen, P. Hoebeke, P. Willemsen, B. De Troyer, R. Pieters, and W. Oosterlinck, "Etiology of urethral stricture disease in the 21st century," *Journal of Urology*, vol. 182, no. 3, pp. 983–987, 2009.

[4] E. A. Eltahawy, R. Virasoro, S. M. Schlossberg, K. A. McCammon, and G. H. Jordan, "Long-term follow-up for excision and primary anastomosis for anterior urethral strictures," *Journal of Urology*, vol. 177, no. 5, pp. 1803–1806, 2007.

[5] A. Goel, A. Goel, A. Jain, and B. P. Singh, "Management of panurethral strictures," *Indian Journal of Urology*, vol. 27, no. 3, pp. 378–384, 2011.

[6] S. B. Kulkarni, P. M. Joshi, and K. Venkatesan, "Management of panurethral stricture disease in India," *Journal of Urology*, vol. 188, no. 3, pp. 824–830, 2012.

[7] I. Depasquale, A. J. Park, and A. Bracka, "The treatment of balanitis xerotica obliterans," *BJU International*, vol. 86, no. 4, pp. 459–465, 2000.

[8] G. Barbagli, F. Mirri, M. Gallucci, S. Sansalone, G. Romano, and M. Lazzeri, "Histological evidence of urethral involvement in male patients with genital lichen sclerosus: a preliminary report," *Journal of Urology*, vol. 185, no. 6, pp. 2171–2176, 2011.

[9] S. B. Kulkarni, G. Barbagli, D. Kirpekar, F. Mirri, and M. Lazzeri, "Lichen sclerosus of the male genitalia and urethra: surgical options and results in a multicenter international experience with 215 patients," *European Urology*, vol. 55, no. 4, pp. 945–956, 2009.

[10] E. Palminteri, E. Berdondini, M. Lazzeri, F. Mirri, and G. Barbagli, "Resurfacing and reconstruction of the glans penis," *European Urology*, vol. 52, no. 3, pp. 893–900, 2007.

[11] S. Das, "Shusruta of India, the pioneer in the treatment of urethral stricture," *Surgery Gynecology and Obstetrics*, vol. 157, no. 6, pp. 581–582, 1983.

[12] A. R. Mundy and D. E. Andrich, "Urethral strictures," *BJU International*, vol. 107, no. 1, pp. 6–26, 2011.

[13] R. A. Santucci, G. F. Joyce, and M. Wise, "Male urethral stricture disease," *Journal of Urology*, vol. 177, no. 5, pp. 1667–1674, 2007.

[14] E. Palminteri, E. Berdondini, P. Verze, C. De Nunzio, A. Vitarelli, and L. Carmignani, "Contemporary urethral stricture characteristics in the developed world," *Urology*, vol. 81, no. 1, pp. 191–197, 2013.

[15] M. Wassermann and N. Hakke, "Uréthite chronique et rétrécissments, nouvelle contribution a l'anatomie pathologique des rétrécissments de l'uréthre," *Annales des Maladies des Organes Génito-Urinaires*, vol. 12, pp. 241–263, 1884.

[16] D. E. Beard and W. E. Goodyear, "Urethral stricture: a pathological study," *The Journal of Urology*, vol. 59, pp. 619–626, 1948.

[17] R. M. Chambers and B. Baitera, "The anatomy of the urethral stricture," *British Journal of Urology*, vol. 49, no. 6, pp. 545–551, 1977.

[18] B. N. Breyer, J. W. McAninch, J. M. Whitson et al., "Multivariate analysis of risk factors for long-term urethroplasty outcome," *Journal of Urology*, vol. 183, no. 2, pp. 613–617, 2010.

[19] L. S. Baskin, S. C. Constantinescu, P. S. Howard et al., "Biochemical characterization and quantitation of the collagenous components of urethral stricture tissue," *Journal of Urology*, vol. 150, no. 2, pp. 642–647, 1993.

[20] A. G. Cavalcanti, S. Yucel, D. Y. Deng, J. W. McAninch, and L. S. Baskin, "The distribution of neuronal and inducible nitric oxide synthase in urethral stricture formation," *Journal of Urology*, vol. 171, no. 5, pp. 1943–1947, 2004.

[21] G. Kaya, M. Berset, C. Prins, P. Chavaz, and J.-H. Saurat, "Chronic borreliosis presenting with morphea- and lichen sclerosus et atrophicus-like cutaneous lesions: a case report," *Dermatology*, vol. 202, no. 4, pp. 373–375, 2001.

[22] E. Palminteri, "Penile urethroplasty," in *Atlas of Penile Reconstructive Surgery*, E. Austoni, Ed., pp. 137–148, Pacini Editore Medicine SpA, 2010.

[23] J. N. Warner, I. Malkawi, M. Dhradkeh et al., "A multiinstitutional evaluation of the management and outcomes of long-segment urethral strictures," *Urology*, vol. 85, no. 6, pp. 1483–1488, 2015.

[24] M. J. Barry, F. J. Foweler, M. P. O'Leary, R. C. Bruskewitz, H. L. Holtgrewe, and W. K. Mebust, "Correlation of the American Urological Association symptom index with self-administered versions of the Marsden-Iversen, Boyarsky and Maine Medical Assessment Program symptom indexes. Measurement Committee of the American Urological Association," *The Journal of Urology*, vol. 148, no. 5, pp. 1558–1564, 1992.

[25] M. J. Jackson, J. N'Dow, and R. Pickard, "The importance of patient-reported outcome measures in reconstructive urology," *Current Opinion in Urology*, vol. 20, no. 6, pp. 495–499, 2010.

[26] J. C. Buckley, A. K. Wu, and J. W. McAninch, "Impact of urethral ultrasonography on decision-making in anterior urethroplasty," *BJU International*, vol. 109, no. 3, pp. 438–442, 2012.

[27] S. B. Brandes, "Panurethral strictures," in *Urethral Reconstructive Surgery*, S. B. Brandes, Ed., Current Clinical Urology, pp. 165–170, Humana Press, 2008.

[28] J. W. McAninch, "Reconstruction of extensive urethral strictures: circular fasciocutaneous penile flap," *The Journal of Urology*, vol. 149, no. 3, pp. 488–491, 1993.

[29] J. W. McAninch and A. F. Morey, "Penile circular fasciocutaneous skin flap in 1-stage reconstruction of complex anterior urethral strictures," *Journal of Urology*, vol. 159, no. 4, pp. 1209–1213, 1998.

[30] D. Dubey, A. Kumar, P. Bansal et al., "Substitution urethroplasty for anterior urethral strictures: a critical appraisal of various techniques," *BJU International*, vol. 91, no. 3, pp. 215–218, 2003.

[31] J. K. M. Quartey, "Quartey flap reconstruction of urethral strictures," in *Traumatic and Reconstructive Urology*, J. W. McAninch, Ed., WB Saunders, Philadelphia, Pa, USA, 1996.

[32] A. F. Morey, L. K. Tran, and L. M. Zinman, "Q-flap reconstruction of panurethral strictures," *BJU International*, vol. 86, no. 9, pp. 1039–1042, 2000.

[33] J. Gil-Vernet, O. Arango, A. Gil-Vernet, J. Gil-Vernet Jr., and A. Gelabert-Mas, "A new biaxial epilated scrotal flap for reconstructive urethral surgery," *Journal of Urology*, vol. 158, no. 2, pp. 412–420, 1997.

[34] H. Wessells and J. W. McAninch, "Current controversies in anterior urethral stricture repair: free-graft versus pedicled skin-flap reconstruction," *World Journal of Urology*, vol. 16, no. 3, pp. 175–180, 1998.

[35] S. B. Kulkarni, J. S. Kulkarni, and D. V. Kirpekar, "A new technique for urethroplasty for balanitis xerotica obliterans," *The Journal of Urology*, vol. 163, article 352, abstract V 31, 2000.

[36] S. Kulkarni, G. Barbagli, S. Sansalone, and M. Lazzeri, "One-sided anterior urethroplasty: a new dorsal onlay graft technique," *BJU International*, vol. 104, no. 8, pp. 1150–1155, 2009.

[37] D. Dubey, A. Kumar, A. Mandhani, A. Srivastava, R. Kapoor, and M. Bhandari, "Buccal mucosal urethroplasty: a versatile technique for all urethral segments," *BJU International*, vol. 95, no. 4, pp. 625–629, 2005.

[38] Y.-M. Xu, Y.-L. Sa, Q. Fu, J. Zhang, J.-M. Si, and Z.-S. Liu, "Oral mucosal grafts urethroplasty for the treatment of long segmented anterior urethral strictures," *World Journal of Urology*, vol. 27, no. 4, pp. 565–571, 2009.

[39] B. Datta, M. P. Rao, R. L. Acharya et al., "Dorsal onlay buccal mucosal graft urethroplasty in long anterior urethral stricture," *International Brazilian Journal of Urology*, vol. 33, no. 2, pp. 181–187, 2007.

[40] N. P. Gupta, M. S. Ansari, P. N. Dogra, and S. Tandon, "Dorsal buccal mucosal graft urethroplasty by a ventral sagittal urethrotomy and minimal-access perineal approach for anterior urethral stricture," *BJU International*, vol. 93, no. 9, pp. 1287–1290, 2004.

[41] S. K. Das, A. Kumar, G. K. Sharma et al., "Lingual mucosal graft urethroplasty for anterior urethral strictures," *Urology*, vol. 73, no. 1, pp. 105–108, 2009.

[42] G. Barbagli, M. De Angelis, G. Romano, P. G. Ciabatti, and M. Lazzeri, "The use of lingual mucosal graft in adult anterior urethroplasty: surgical steps and short-term outcome," *European Urology*, vol. 54, no. 3, pp. 671–676, 2008.

[43] A. Simonato, A. Gregori, C. Ambruosi et al., "Lingual mucosal graft urethroplasty for anterior urethral reconstruction," *European Urology*, vol. 54, no. 1, pp. 79–87, 2008.

[44] A. Srivastava, A. Dutta, and D. K. Jain, "Initial experience with lingual mucosal graft urethroplasty for anterior urethral strictures," *Medical Journal Armed Forces India*, vol. 69, no. 1, pp. 16–20, 2013.

[45] N. Lumen, S. Vierstraete-Verlinde, W. Oosterlinck et al., "Buccal versus lingual mucosa graft anterior urethroplasty: a prospective comparison of surgical outcome and donor site morbidity," *The Journal of Urology*, 2015.

[46] H. Wessells and J. W. Mcaninch, "Use of free grafts in urethral stricture reconstruction," *Journal of Urology*, vol. 155, no. 6, pp. 1912–1915, 1996.

[47] S. S. Bapat, A. S. Padhye, P. B. Yadav, and A. A. Bhave, "Preputial skin free graft as dorsal onlay urethroplasty: our experience of 73 patients," *Indian Journal of Urology*, vol. 23, no. 4, pp. 366–368, 2007.

[48] B. Manoj, N. Sanjeev, P. N. Pandurang, M. Jaideep, and M. Ravi, "Postauricular skin as an alternative to oral mucosa for anterior onlay graft urethroplasty: a preliminary experience in patients with oral mucosa changes," *Urology*, vol. 74, no. 2, pp. 345–348, 2009.

[49] D. E. Andrich and A. R. Mundy, "Surgical treatment of urethral stricture disease," *Contemporary Urology*, vol. 13, pp. 32–44, 2001.

[50] T. Nitkunan, N. Johal, K. O'Malley, and P. Cuckow, "Secondary hypospadias repair in two stages," *Journal of Pediatric Urology*, vol. 2, no. 6, pp. 559–563, 2006.

[51] R. K. Berglund and K. W. Angermeier, "Combined buccal mucosa graft and genital skin flap for reconstruction of extensive anterior urethral strictures," *Urology*, vol. 68, no. 4, pp. 707–710, 2006.

[52] W. B. Zimmerman and R. A. Santucci, "Buccal mucosa urethroplasty for adult urethral strictures," *Indian Journal of Urology*, vol. 27, no. 3, pp. 364–370, 2011.

[53] G. Barbagli, S. Sansalone, R. Djinovic, G. Romano, and M. Lazzeri, "Current controversies in reconstructive surgery of the anterior urethra: a clinical overview," *The International Brazilian Journal of Urology*, vol. 38, no. 3, pp. 307–316, 2012.

[54] E. Palminteri, N. Lumen, E. Berdondini et al., "Two-sided dorsal plus ventral oral graft bulbar urethroplasty: long-term results and predictive factors," *Urology*, vol. 85, no. 4, pp. 942–947, 2015.

[55] Y.-M. Xu, Y. Qiao, Y.-L. Sa, J. Zhang, Q. Fu, and L.-J. Song, "Urethral reconstruction using colonic mucosa graft for complex strictures," *Journal of Urology*, vol. 182, no. 3, pp. 1040–1043, 2009.

[56] H. Wessells, A. F. Morey, and J. W. McAninch, "Single stage reconstruction of complex anterior urethral strictures: combined tissue transfer techniques," *Journal of Urology*, vol. 157, no. 4, pp. 1271–1274, 1997.

[57] G. Barbagli, M. Lazzeri, E. Palminteri, and D. Turini, "Lichen sclerosis of male genitalia involving anterior urethra," *The Lancet*, vol. 354, no. 9176, p. 429, 1999.

[58] I. Depasquale, A. J. Park, and A. Bracka, "The treatment of balanitis xerotica obliterans," *BJU International*, vol. 86, no. 4, pp. 459–465, 2000.

[59] D. E. Andrich and A. R. Mundy, "Substitution urethroplasty with buccal mucosal-free grafts," *Journal of Urology*, vol. 165, no. 4, pp. 1131–1133, 2001.

[60] G. Barbagli, E. Palminteri, and M. Lazzeri, "Lichen sclerosus of male genitalia," *Contemporary Urology*, vol. 13, pp. 47–58, 2001.

[61] B. Johanson, "Reconstruction of the male urethra in strictures," *Acta Chirurgica Scandinavica*, vol. 167, supplement, article 1, 1953.

[62] F. Schreiter and F. Noll, "Meshgraft urethroplasty," *World Journal of Urology*, vol. 5, no. 1, pp. 41–46, 1987.

[63] F. Schreiter and F. Noll, "Mesh graft urethroplasty using split thickness skin graft or foreskin," *The Journal of Urology*, vol. 142, no. 5, pp. 1223–1226, 1989.

[64] J. M. Patterson and C. R. Chapple, "Surgical techniques in substitution urethroplasty using buccal mucosa for the treatment

of anterior urethral strictures," *European Urology*, vol. 53, no. 6, pp. 1162–1171, 2008.

[65] D. E. Andrich, T. J. Greenwell, and A. R. Mundy, "The problems of penile urethroplasty with particular reference to 2-stage reconstructions," *Journal of Urology*, vol. 170, no. 1, pp. 87–89, 2003.

[66] J. Monseur, "A new procedure for urethroplasty for urethral stricture: reconstruction of the urethral canal by means of suburethral strips and the subcavernous groove," *Journal d'Urologie et de Nephrologie*, vol. 75, no. 3, pp. 201–209, 1969.

[67] R. K. Mathur, A. Himanshu, and O. Sudarshan, "Technique of anterior urethra urethroplasty using tunica albuginea of corpora cavernosa," *International Journal of Urology*, vol. 14, no. 3, pp. 209–213, 2007.

[68] R. K. Mathur, A. K. Sharma, and S. Odiya, "Tunica albuginea urethroplasty for anterior urethral strictures: a urethroscopic analysis," *International Journal of Urology*, vol. 16, no. 9, pp. 751–755, 2009.

[69] R. K. Mathur and A. Sharma, "Tunica albuginea urethroplasty for panurethral strictures," *Urology Journal*, vol. 7, no. 2, pp. 120–124, 2010.

[70] W. Snodgrass and N. Bush, "Tubularized incised plate proximal hypospadias repair: continued evolution and extended applications," *Journal of Pediatric Urology*, vol. 7, no. 1, pp. 2–9, 2011.

[71] G. Barbagli, G. Morgia, and M. Lazzeri, "Retrospective outcome analysis of one-stage penile urethroplasty using a flap or graft in a homogeneous series of patients," *BJU International*, vol. 102, no. 7, pp. 853–860, 2008.

[72] C. E. Iselin and G. D. Webster, "Dorsal onlay graft urethroplasty for repair of bulbar urethral stricture," *Journal of Urology*, vol. 161, no. 3, pp. 815–818, 1999.

[73] G. Barbagli, E. Palminteri, and M. Rizzo, "Dorsal onlay graft urethroplasty using penile skin or buccal mucosa in adult bulbourethral strictures," *Journal of Urology*, vol. 160, no. 4, pp. 1307–1309, 1998.

[74] D. E. Andrich, C. J. Leach, and A. R. Mundy, "The Barbagli procedure gives the best results for patch urethroplasty of the bulbar urethra," *BJU International*, vol. 88, no. 4, pp. 385–389, 2001.

[75] A. K. Sharma, C. S. Ratkal, M. Shivlingaiah, G. N. Girish, R. P. Sanjay, and G. K. Venkatesh, "Analysis of short-term results of monsieur's tunica albuginea urethroplasty as a definitive procedure for pan-anterior urethral stricture," *Urology Annals*, vol. 5, no. 4, pp. 228–231, 2013.

[76] H. S. Al-Qudah and R. A. Santucci, "Extended complications of urethroplasty," *The International Brazilian Journal of Urology*, vol. 31, no. 4, pp. 315–325, 2005.

[77] G. Barbagli, C. Selli, A. Tosto, and E. Palminteri, "Dorsal free graft urethroplasty," *Journal of Urology*, vol. 155, no. 1, pp. 123–126, 1996.

[78] J. G. Anema, A. F. Morey, J. W. Mcaninch, L. A. Mario, and H. Wessells, "Complications related to the high lithotomy position during urethral reconstruction," *Journal of Urology*, vol. 164, no. 2, pp. 360–363, 2000.

[79] D. T. Price, J. Vieweg, F. Roland et al., "Transient lower extremity neurapraxia associated with radical perineal prostatectomy: a complication of the exaggerated lithotomy position," *Journal of Urology*, vol. 160, no. 4, pp. 1376–1378, 1998.

[80] K. W. Angermeier and G. H. Jordan, "Complications of the exaggerated lithotomy position: a review of 177 cases," *The Journal of Urology*, vol. 151, no. 4, pp. 866–868, 1994.

[81] J. W. Coursey, A. F. Morey, J. W. McAninch et al., "Erectile function after anterior urethroplasty," *Journal of Urology*, vol. 166, no. 6, pp. 2273–2276, 2001.

[82] B. A. Erickson, J. S. Wysock, K. T. McVary, and C. M. Gonzalez, "Erectile function, sexual drive, and ejaculatory function after reconstructive surgery for anterior urethral stricture disease," *BJU International*, vol. 99, no. 3, pp. 607–611, 2007.

[83] B. A. Erickson, M. A. Granieri, J. J. Meeks, J. P. Cashy, and C. M. Gonzalez, "Prospective analysis of erectile dysfunction after anterior urethroplasty: incidence and recovery of function," *Journal of Urology*, vol. 183, no. 2, pp. 657–661, 2010.

[84] U. P. Singh, R. Maheshwari, V. Kumar, A. Srivastava, and R. Kapoor, "Impact on sexual function after reconstructive surgery for anterior urethral stricture disease," *Indian Journal of Urology*, vol. 26, no. 2, pp. 188–192, 2010.

[85] S. D. Blaschko, M. T. Sanford, N. M. Cinman, J. W. McAninch, and B. N. Breyer, "*De novo* erectile dysfunction after anterior urethroplasty: a systematic review and meta-analysis," *BJU International*, vol. 112, no. 5, pp. 655–663, 2013.

[86] Y. Xu, Q. Fu, Y. Sa, Y. Qiao, and H. Xie, "The relationship between erectile function and complex panurethral stricture: a preliminary investigative and descriptive study," *Asian Journal of Andrology*, vol. 17, no. 2, pp. 315–318, 2015.

[87] M. Bhandari, D. Dubey, and B. S. Verma, "Dorsal or ventral placement of the preputial/penile skin onlay flap for anterior urethral strictures: does it make a difference?" *BJU International*, vol. 88, no. 1, pp. 39–43, 2001.

14

Acridine Orange and Flow Cytometry: Which Is Better to Measure the Effect of Varicocele on Sperm DNA Integrity?

Essam-Elden M. Mohammed,[1] Eman Mosad,[2] Asmaa M. Zahran,[2] Diaa A. Hameed,[3] Emad A. Taha,[4] and Mohamed A. Mohamed[5]

[1]*Dermatology and Andrology Department, Faculty of Medicine, Al-Azhar University, Assiut, Egypt*
[2]*Clinical Pathology Department, South Egypt Cancer Institute, Assiut University, Assiut, Egypt*
[3]*Urology Department, Faculty of Medicine, Assiut University, Assiut, Egypt*
[4]*Dermatology and Andrology Department, Faculty of Medicine, Assiut University, Assiut, Egypt*
[5]*Gynaecology and Obstetric Department, Faculty of Medicine, Al-Azhar University, Assiut, Egypt*

Correspondence should be addressed to Essam-Elden M. Mohammed; dessam73@yahoo.com

Academic Editor: Mohammad H. Ather

We evaluated the effect of varicocelectomy on semen parameters and levels of sperm DNA damage in infertile men. A total of 75 infertile men with varicocele and 40 fertile men (controls) were included in this study. Semen analysis and sperm DNA damage expressed as the DNA fragmentation index using acridine orange staining and chromatin condensation test by flow cytometry were assessed before and 6 months after varicocelectomy. The patients were also followed up for 1 year for pregnancy outcome. Semen parameters were significantly lower in varicocele patients compared to controls ($P < 0.05$). Mean percentages of sperm DNA fragmentation and sperm DNA chromatin condensation in patients were significantly higher than those in controls ($P < 0.05$). After varicocelectomy, sperm DNA fragmentation improved significantly, whereas sperm chromatin condensation was not significantly changed. In 15 out of 75 varicocele patients, clinical pregnancy was diagnosed; those with positive pregnancy outcome had significant improvement in sperm count, progressive sperm motility, and sperm DNA fragmentation, but there was no significant difference in sperm DNA condensation compared to negative pregnancy outcome patients. We concluded from this study that acridine orange stain is more reliable method than flow cytometry in the evaluation of sperm DNA integrity after varicocelectomy.

1. Introduction

Sperm DNA integrity is important for the transmission of genetic code, and it is considered as a marker of integrity of spermatogenesis and male fertility potential [1]. About 10% of the spermatozoa from fertile men and 20–25% of the spermatozoa from infertile men have measurable levels of DNA damage [2]. High levels of sperm DNA fragmentation (DFI) have been significantly associated with a bad pregnancy outcome [3–5].

Sperm DNA damage may be associated with many environmental conditions such as some medications, pollution, smoking, pesticides, chemicals, high temperature, and various pathologic cases such as cryptorchidism, fever, aging, infection, chemotherapy, cancer, and varicocele [6, 7].

The prognostic value of sperm DNA fragmentation is becoming better than the routine semen parameters, although the cut-off values of it are not established yet [8].

In this study, we evaluate the effect of varicocele on semen parameters and levels of sperm DNA integrity in infertile men with varicocele before and after varicocelectomy by acridine orange staining and flow cytometry.

2. Materials and Methods

From January 2012 to March 2015, a total of 75 men with at least 1-year history of infertility, a palpable varicocele, oligo, atheno, or teratozoospermia were selected from our andrology clinic. After the ethical committee approval, all the patients accepted to participate in the study and signed an informed consent. Forty healthy fertile volunteers (control group) were also included in this prospective study.

Patients were subjected to complete history taking and thorough general and local examination. Varicocele was detected clinically and confirmed by scrotal ultrasound (Fukuda Denshi Tellus UF-850XTD, Tokyo, Japan) equipped with color flow imaging when at least 1 scrotal vein had a maximum diameter of at least 3 mm and retrograde flow was observed at rest or after Valsalva maneuver. Grade 1 varicocele was diagnosed when reflux was measured at less than 1 second, grade II was diagnosed when reflux lasted 1-2 seconds, and grade III was diagnosed when reflux was noted at more than 2 seconds as described by Cornud et al. [9].

Semen samples were obtained by masturbation and collected in a sterile plastic container before and 3 months after subinguinal varicocelectomy with loop magnification that was done by either of the 3 surgeons with at least 7 years of experience. They were allowed to liquefy for 30 min at 37°C, after which an analysis was performed to measure the following parameters: sperm concentration/mL, percentage of sperm motility, percentage of abnormal sperm morphology evaluated according to WHO guidelines [10].

2.1. Acridine Orange (AO) Assay. The AO assay measures the ability of sperm nuclear DNA to denature by acid which forms metachromatic shift of AO fluorescence from green (native DNA) to red (denatured DNA). The fluorochrome AO intercalates in double-stranded DNA as a monomer which binds to single-stranded DNA. The monomeric AO bound to native DNA fluoresce green, whereas the aggregated AO on denatured DNA fluoresces red [11].

The AO assay may be used for fluorescence microscopy or by flow cytometry. To perform this assay for fluorescent microscopy, thick semen layers are fixed in fixative (methanol : acetic acid 3 : 1) for 2 hours. The slides are stained for 5 minutes and rinsed with water. The slides were washed with distilled water then covered with glass cover and examined under a ZEISS mot plus (Germany) fluorescent microscope at the excitation wavelength of 450–490 nm. An average of 200 sperm cells was evaluated on each slide by the same examiner. Spermatozoa which show green fluorescence were considered as normal DNA content, whereas sperms displaying a spectrum of yellow-orange to red fluorescence were considered to be with damaged DNA (Figure 1). The ratio between (yellow to red)/(green+yellow to red) fluorescence was considered as DFI percentages and the percentage of sample showing a ratio <1 was calculated in the group.

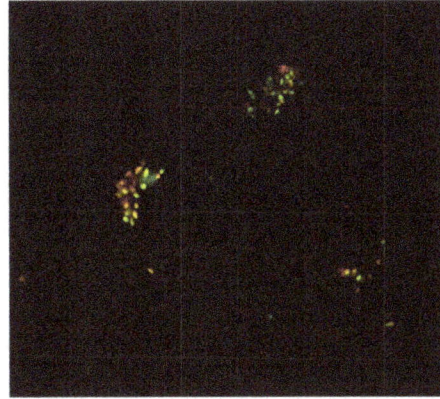

FIGURE 1: Fluorescence microscopy of acridine orange destained cells shows that spermatozoa displaying green fluorescence were considered to be with normal DNA content, whereas sperms displaying a spectrum of yellow-orange to red fluorescence were considered to be with damaged DNA. Original magnification ×200.

2.2. Flow Cytometric Detection of Sperm DNA Chromatin Condensation. Flow cytometric detection of sperm DNA chromatin damage was made according to the method as described by Martinez-Soto et al. [12]. It depends on the fluorescence emission from sperm cells stained with propidium iodide (PI) that binds to DNA. The semen sample were diluted with phosphate buffered saline (PBS) to 2×10^6 sperm/mL. Fifty μL of semen sample was directly stained with 50 μg/mL PI, using the cycle test kit (Becton Dickinson, USA); PI was mixed with the semen and analyzed immediately by FACSCalibur flow cytometry with CellQuest software (Becton Dickinson Biosciences, USA). Ten thousand events were measured for each specimen; this permitted state of condensation of the sperm chromatin was analyzed, as the DNA condensation is directly related to PI uptake. The geometric mean fluorescence intensity (GMFI) was used to measure the degree of sperm DNA staining with PI. The sperm with altered nuclear condensation (DNA decondensation and fragmentation) takes more stains (Figure 2). These tests were performed on patients before and 3 months after varicocelectomy.

3. Statistical Analysis

The SPSS program, version 16.0.1 (SPSS Inc., Chicago, IL), was used in statistical analysis. The data were expressed as mean ± SE and the differences were evaluated by paired t-test. Relationships between values were studied by Spearman correlation test. $P < 0.05$ was set as statistically significant.

4. Results

Varicocele was detected by physical examination and confirmed by Doppler ultrasound in the 75 patients who entered the study. The mean age was 31 years (range: 20–57) for patients and 30.2 years (range: 21–37) for controls. The main sperm characteristics of control and patients are shown in

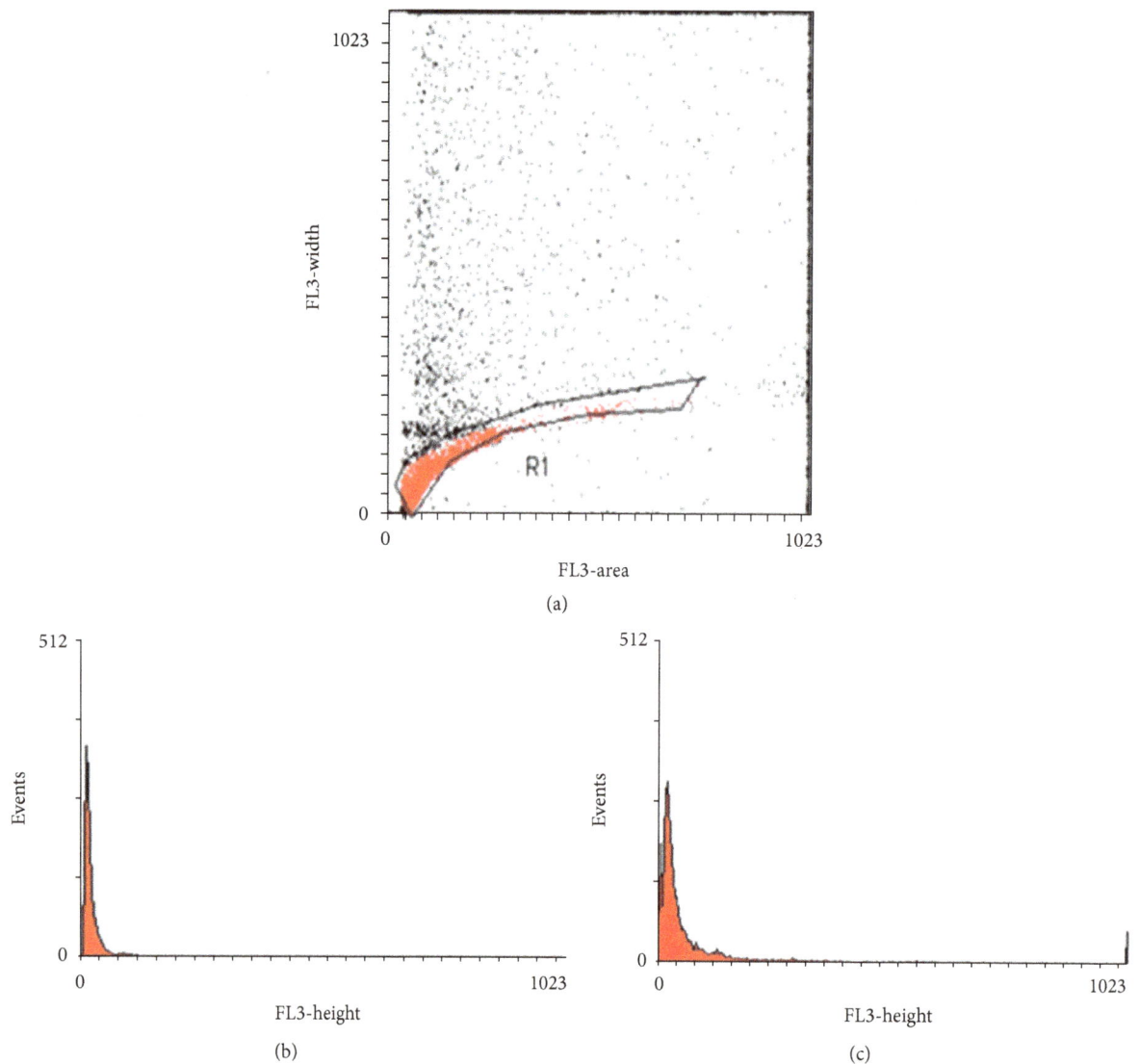

FIGURE 2: Flow cytometric detection of sperm DNA chromatin condensation. (a) Dot plot histogram (FL3A versus FL3W) obtained after propidium iodide staining of spermatozoa. Cells gated in R1 region were analyzed, while debris and aggregates were excluded from the analysis. The fluorescence intensity of cells (spermatozoa) was measured in R1 gate. (b) Histogram of fluorescence intensity of spermatozoa from normal control person. (c) Histogram of fluorescence intensity of spermatozoa from infertile person with varicocele.

Table 1. All patients had an abnormality in one or more of these parameters. There was a significant decrease in sperm concentration and percentage of progressive sperm motility and normal sperm morphology in varicocele patients compared to the controls (Table 1).

Comparisons of DFI results and GMFI between controls and patients with varicocele are shown in Table 1. The mean values for DFI and GMFI of sperm DNA chromatin condensation in the control group were lower.

In patients with varicocele, DFI and GMFI had no correlation with sperm concentration, but they were negatively correlated with progressive motility and normal sperm morphology.

Sperm DNA fragmentation by acridine orange and sperm count changed significantly after varicocelectomy, but no significant changes were detected regarding sperm motility,

morphology, and DNA chromatin condensation by flow cytometry (Table 2). In 15 out of 75 varicocele patients (20%), clinical pregnancy (confirmed by ultrasound detection of fetal pulse) was achieved. Those with positive pregnancy outcome showed significant improvement in sperm count and sperm motility compared with negative pregnancy group ($P < 0.05$). Also, those with positive pregnancy outcome had significantly lower DNA fragmentation % by acridine orange, but there is no significant difference in sperm DNA condensation by flow cytometry on comparing them to others who failed to make their partners conceive (Table 3).

5. Discussion

As it is well known [13–15], our study showed that the mean semen parameters were significantly lower in varicocele

TABLE 1: Clinical and laboratory data of studied groups (mean ± SD).

Variables	Varicocele group ($n = 75$)	Fertile group ($n = 40$)	P value
Sperm count (mil/mL)	26.2 ± 2.7*	74.2 ± 19.2	0.005
Motility A + B (%)	27.8 ± 16.5*	62.5 ± 11.9	0.02
Normal forms (%)	59.8 ± 13.6*	71.03 ± 8.2	0.02
Sperm DFI (%) by acridine orange	32.4 ± 7.4*	18.2 ± 4.8	0.003
GMFI of sperm DNA chromatin condensation by flow cytometry (%)	25.4 ± 8.8*	12.8 ± 2.2	0.005
Mean age (years)	31 ± 8.2	30.2 ± 2	NS

*Significant $P < 0.05$.
GMFI: the geometric mean fluorescence intensity.
DFI: DNA fragmentation index.

TABLE 2: Pre- and postvaricocelectomy semen parameters, sperm DFI, and GMFI of sperm DNA chromatin condensation by flow cytometry.

Variables	Before varicocelectomy	After varicocelectomy	P value
Sperm count (mil/mL)	26.2 ± 2.7*	51 ± 4.2	0.05
Motility A + B (%)	27.8 ± 16.5	32 ± 7	NS
Normal forms (%)	59.8 ± 13.6	65.03 ± 8.0	NS
Sperm DFI (%) by acridine orange	32.4 ± 7.4*	20 ± 4.1	0.05
GMFI of sperm DNA chromatin condensation by flow cytometry (%)	25.4 ± 8.8	22 ± 4.1	NS

*Significant $P < 0.05$.

TABLE 3: Comparison between those who achieved clinical pregnancy and those who failed after varicocelectomy.

Variables	Positive pregnancy after varicocelectomy ($n = 15$)	No pregnancy after varicocelectomy ($n = 60$)	P value
Sperm count (mil/mL)	59.4 ± 5.3*	41 ± 4.2	0.04
Motility A + B (%)	40.2 ± 17.5*	22.4 ± 8.4	0.03
Normal forms (%)	67.02 ± 15.4	63.46 ± 11.0	NS
Sperm DFI (%) by acridine orange	16.4 ± 6.4*	24.2 ± 4.1	0.04
GMFI of sperm DNA chromatin condensation by flow cytometry (%)	20.3 ± 6.8	23.5 ± 5.4	NS

*Significant $P < 0.05$.

patients than in control group. The low sperm count may be due to the high apoptosis in the germ cell that occurs in varicocele, while the decreased motility may be due to the abnormal morphology of the sperm which affects its motility, the increased oxygen concentration of free radicals, or the antisperm antibodies [15].

Also, a large scale study by the WHO showed that infertile men with varicocele have lower sperm concentration significantly compared to idiopathic infertility, but it did not give any evidence regarding motility and morphology of the sperm [16]. Poor chromatin condensation has been correlated with numerous reproductive outcomes [17, 18]. So DFI provides additional information about sperm quality and conception outcome [18, 19].

In our study, there was a high percentage of sperm with damaged DNA among patients with varicocele detected by AO and flow cytometry; this was well documented in the previous studies [20, 21]. Having a higher percentage of sperm with damaged DNA assessed by AO staining suggests that increased DFI is one of the possible causes of infertility and can contribute to the higher prevalence of infertility among patients with varicocele [15, 22].

Several factors associated with varicocele may lead to DNA damage including heat, stress [23], exposure to toxic agents [24], testicular hypoxia [25], androgen deprivation [26], and increased oxidative stress [27].

The high percentage of sperm DFI in varicocele patients may be caused by an impaired chromatin condensation [28] Also, the nature of the nuclear damage could be related to a strong and prolonged exposure to DNA nuclear-damaging factors. Not only the DNA, but also the proteins of the nuclear matrix could lead to an advanced lytic stage [27].

Our results demonstrated that those with positive pregnancy outcome after varicocelectomy had significantly lower sperm DFI with acridine orange test than others who failed. A prospective study of infertile, oligospermic men with clinical varicocele who underwent surgical repair showed a significant improvement in postvaricocelectomy semen parameters and DFI [29]. A lower DFI was associated with higher spontaneous and ART pregnancy rates. Similarly, a positive effect of subinguinal microsurgical clinical varicocele repair on sperm DNA integrity and chromatin compaction (reflected by a significant decrease in sperm DFI and high DNA stainability, resp.) was reported in another prospective study [19]. In a study by [7, 18], the probability of fertilization in natural conception and in intrauterine insemination was found to be close to zero if the proportion of sperm cells with DNA damage exceeds 30% as detected by SCSA proposing the threshold for DFI >30% in infertile men for poor ART outcome. In our study, we found that after varicocelectomy sperm count improved significantly, while the morphology and motility improvements did not reach statistical significance. Likewise, sperm DNA fragmentation by acridine orange not only improved significantly after varicocelectomy, but also correlated with positive pregnancy outcome, while the improvement measured by chromatin condensation by flow cytometry neither reached statistical significance nor correlated with positive pregnancy outcome.

After varicocelectomy, flow cytometry showed that the DFI was 22.5% of sperm DNA, which may be an accepted threshold for a successful ART outcome. This is comparable to the work of Pasqualotto et al. [5] who reported (27–30%) DNA damage as a threshold for successful pregnancy.

In conclusion, the current study demonstrated an increase in sperm DFI in infertile patients with varicocele. After varicocelectomy, acridine orange test yielded significant results compared to flow cytometry that correlated with pregnancy outcome which suggests that it may be used as cheap and simple DNA integrity evaluation test for diagnostic and prognostic purpose in basic andrology laboratories.

Conflict of Interests

The authors declare that there is no conflict of interests that could be perceived as prejudicing the impartiality of the research reported.

References

[1] M. Benchaib, V. Braun, J. Lornage et al., "Sperm DNA fragmentation decreases the pregnancy rate in an assisted reproductive technique," *Human Reproduction*, vol. 18, no. 5, pp. 1023–1028, 2003.

[2] R. Smith, H. Kaune, D. Parodi et al., "Increased sperm DNA damage in patients with varicocele: relationship with seminal oxidative stress," *Human Reproduction*, vol. 21, no. 4, pp. 986–993, 2006.

[3] M. Bungum, P. Humaidan, M. Spano, K. Jepson, L. Bungum, and A. Giwercman, "The predictive value of sperm chromatin structure assay (SCSA) parameters for the outcome of intrauterine insemination, IVF and ICSI," *Human Reproduction*, vol. 19, no. 6, pp. 1401–1408, 2004.

[4] D. T. Carrell, L. Liu, C. M. Peterson et al., "Sperm DNA fragmentation is increased in couples with unexplained recurrent pregnancy loss," *Archives of Andrology*, vol. 49, no. 1, pp. 49–55, 2003.

[5] F. F. Pasqualotto, D. P. A. F. Braga, R. C. S. Figueira, A. S. Setti, A. Iaconelli Jr., and E. Borges Jr., "Varicocelectomy does not impact pregnancy outcomes following intracytoplasmic sperm injection procedures," *Journal of Andrology*, vol. 33, no. 2, pp. 239–243, 2012.

[6] D. Sakkas, E. Mariethoz, and J. C. St. John, "Abnormal sperm parameters in humans are indicative of an abortive apoptotic mechanism linked to the Fas-mediated pathway," *Experimental Cell Research*, vol. 251, no. 2, pp. 350–355, 1999.

[7] D. P. Evenson and R. Wixon, "Comparison of the Halosperm test kit with the sperm chromatin structure assay (SCSA) infertility test in relation to patient diagnosis and prognosis," *Fertility and Sterility*, vol. 84, no. 4, pp. 846–849, 2005.

[8] M. B. Shamsi, S. N. Imam, and R. Dada, "Sperm DNA integrity assays: diagnostic and prognostic challenges and implications in management of infertility," *Journal of Assisted Reproduction and Genetics*, vol. 28, no. 11, pp. 1073–1085, 2011.

[9] F. Cornud, X. Belin, E. Amar, D. Delafontaine, O. Hélénon, and J. F. Moreau, "Varicocele: strategies in diagnosis and treatment," *European Radiology*, vol. 9, no. 3, pp. 536–545, 1999.

[10] World Health Organization, *WHO Laboratory Manual for the Examination of Human Semen and Sperm-Cervical Mucus Interaction*, Cambridge University Press, Cambridge, UK, 1999.

[11] K. Hoshi, H. Katayose, K. Yanagida, Y. Kimura, and A. Sato, "The relationship between acridine orange fluorescence of sperm nuclei and the fertilizing ability of human sperm," *Fertility and Sterility*, vol. 66, no. 4, pp. 634–639, 1996.

[12] J. C. Martinez-Soto, J. de Dioshourcade, A. Gutiérrez-Adán, J. L. Landeras, and J. Gadea, "Effect of genistein supplementation of thawing medium on characteristics of frozen human spermatozoa," *Asian Journal of Andrology*, vol. 12, no. 3, pp. 431–441, 2010.

[13] M. H. Schlesinger, I. F. Wilets, and H. M. Nagler, "Treatment outcome after varicocelectomy: a critical analysis," *Urologic Clinics of North America*, vol. 21, no. 3, pp. 517–529, 1994.

[14] I. Madgar, R. Weissenberg, B. Lunenfeld, A. Karasik, and B. Goldwasser, "Controlled trial of high spermatic vein ligation for varicocele in infertile men," *Fertility and Sterility*, vol. 63, no. 1, pp. 120–124, 1995.

[15] A. Agarwal, F. Deepinder, M. Cocuzza et al., "Efficacy of varicocelectomy in improving semen parameters: new meta-analytical approach," *Urology*, vol. 70, no. 3, pp. 532–538, 2007.

[16] P. D. Kantartzi, C. D. Goulis, G. D. Goulis, and I. Papadimas, "Male infertility and varicocele: myths and reality," *Hippokratia*, vol. 11, no. 3, pp. 99–104, 2007.

[17] A. D. Esterhuizen, D. R. Franken, J. G. H. Lourens, E. Prinsloo, and L. H. van Rooyen, "Sperm chromatin packaging as an indicator of in-vitro fertilization rates," *Human Reproduction*, vol. 15, no. 3, pp. 657–661, 2000.

[18] M. Spanò, J. P. Bonde, H. I. Hjøllund et al., "Sperm chromatin damage impairs human fertility," *Fertility and Sterility*, vol. 73, no. 1, pp. 43–50, 2000.

[19] A. Zini, A. Blumenfeld, J. Libman, and J. Willis, "Beneficial effect of microsurgical varicocelectomy on human sperm DNA integrity," *Human Reproduction*, vol. 20, no. 4, pp. 1018–1021, 2005.

[20] R. A. Saleh, A. Agarwal, R. K. Sharma, T. M. Said, S. C. Sikka, and A. J. Thomas Jr., "Evaluation of nuclear DNA damage in spermatozoa from infertile men with varicocele," *Fertility and Sterility*, vol. 80, no. 6, pp. 1431–1436, 2003.

[21] C. G. Blumer, R. M. Fariello, A. E. Restelli, D. M. Spaine, R. P. Bertolla, and A. P. Cedenho, "Sperm nuclear DNA fragmentation and mitochondrial activity in men with varicocele," *Fertility and Sterility*, vol. 90, no. 5, pp. 1716–1722, 2008.

[22] A.-F. Abdel-Maguid and I. Othman, "Microsurgical and non-magnified subinguinal varicocelectomy for infertile men: a comparative study," *Fertility and Sterility*, vol. 94, no. 7, pp. 2600–2603, 2010.

[23] L. Bujan and R. Mieusset, "Male contraception by testicular heating," *Contraception Fertilite Sexualite*, vol. 23, no. 10, pp. 611–614, 1995.

[24] S. H. Benoff, C. Millan, I. R. Hurley, B. Napolitano, and J. L. Marmar, "Bilateral increased apoptosis and bilateral accumulation of cadmium in infertile men with left varicocele," *Human Reproduction*, vol. 19, no. 3, pp. 616–627, 2004.

[25] C.-C. Huang, R.-S. Chen, C.-M. Chen et al., "MELAS syndrome with mitochondrial tRNA(Leu(UUR)) gene mutation in a Chinese family," *Journal of Neurology Neurosurgery and Psychiatry*, vol. 57, no. 5, pp. 586–589, 1994.

[26] World Health Organization, "The influence of varicocele on parameters of fertility in a large group of men presenting to infertility clinics," *Fertility and Sterility*, vol. 57, no. 6, pp. 1289–1293, 1992.

[27] B. N. Hendin, P. N. Kolettis, R. K. Sharma, A. J. Thomas Jr., and A. Agarwal, "Varicocele is associated with elevated spermatozoal reactive oxygen species production and diminished seminal plasma antioxidant capacity," *The Journal of Urology*, vol. 161, no. 6, pp. 1831–1834, 1999.

[28] D. Sakkas, O. Moffatt, G. C. Manicardi, E. Mariethoz, N. Tarozzi, and D. Bizzaro, "Nature of DNA damage in ejaculated human spermatozoa and the possible involvement of apoptosis," *Biology of Reproduction*, vol. 66, no. 4, pp. 1061–1067, 2002.

[29] M. Smit, O. G. Wissenburg, J. C. Romijn, and G. R. Dohle, "Increased sperm DNA fragmentation in patients with vasectomy reversal has no prognostic value for pregnancy rate," *The Journal of Urology*, vol. 183, no. 2, pp. 662–665, 2010.

15

Total Psoas Area Predicts Complications following Radical Cystectomy

Timothy D. Lyon,[1] **Nicholas J. Farber,**[2] **Leo C. Chen,**[3] **Thomas W. Fuller,**[1]
Benjamin J. Davies,[1] **Jeffrey R. Gingrich,**[1] **Ronald L. Hrebinko,**[1] **Jodi K. Maranchie,**[1]
Jennifer M. Taylor,[4] **and Tatum V. Tarin**[1]

[1]*Department of Urology, University of Pittsburgh, Pittsburgh, PA, USA*
[2]*Division of Urology, Rutgers Robert Wood Johnson Medical School, New Brunswick, NJ, USA*
[3]*University of Pittsburgh School of Medicine, Pittsburgh, PA, USA*
[4]*Department of Urology, Baylor College of Medicine, Houston, TX, USA*

Correspondence should be addressed to Timothy D. Lyon; lyontd@upmc.edu

Academic Editor: Fabio Campodonico

Purpose. To determine whether total psoas area (TPA), a simple estimate of muscle mass, is associated with complications after radical cystectomy. *Materials and Methods.* Patients who underwent radical cystectomy at our institution from 2011 to 2012 were retrospectively identified. Total psoas area was measured on preoperative CT scans and normalized for patient height. Multivariable logistic regression was used to determine whether TPA was a predictor of 90-day postoperative complications. Overall survival was compared between TPA quartiles. *Results.* 135 patients were identified for analysis. Median follow-up was 24 months (IQR: 6–37 months). Overall 90-day complication rate was 56% (75/135). TPA was significantly lower for patients who experienced any complication ($7.8 \, \text{cm}^2/\text{m}^2$ versus $8.8 \, \text{cm}^2/\text{m}^2$, $P = 0.023$) and an infectious complication ($7.0 \, \text{cm}^2/\text{m}^2$ versus $8.7 \, \text{cm}^2/\text{m}^2$, $P = 0.032$) than those who did not. On multivariable analysis, TPA (adjusted OR 0.70 (95% CI 0.56–0.89), $P = 0.003$) and Charlson comorbidity index (adjusted OR 1.34 (95% CI 1.01–1.79), $P = 0.045$) were independently associated with 90-day complications. TPA was not a predictor of overall survival. *Conclusions.* Low TPA is associated with infectious complications and is an independent predictor of experiencing a postoperative complication following radical cystectomy.

1. Introduction

Bladder cancer is a common genitourinary malignancy, with an estimated 72,570 new cases reported in the United States in 2013 [1]. Radical cystectomy (RC) with pelvic lymph node dissection remains the standard of care for muscle-invasive bladder cancer. RC is a morbid procedure, with readmission rates approaching 27% and 90-day complication rates as high as 64% [2, 3]. A number of preoperative risk factors portend risk of morbidity and mortality following RC, including age, comorbidities, functional status, and nutritional deficiency [4–6].

Multiple somatometric and serologic markers have been used to quantify nutritional deficiency including body mass index (BMI), weight loss, serum albumin, and skeletal muscle mass [5–7]. Perhaps the least well studied of these is sarcopenia, or loss of total body skeletal muscle mass. Low skeletal muscle index (SMI) is associated with decreased cancer-specific and overall survival following RC [8] but obtaining this measurement requires specialized imaging software and cannot be efficiently determined in a clinical setting. Recent work has investigated whether total psoas area (TPA), which can be more easily determined, provides a reliable estimate of muscle mass and carries the same prognostic value as SMI [9–11]. Smith et al. found an association between low TPA and increased major complication rate following RC in women [12], but this finding requires further validation.

To clarify whether TPA is a useful prognostic marker following RC, we measured TPA on preoperative computed tomography (CT) scans for patients who underwent RC at our institution over a two-year period and compared these to patient outcomes.

2. Materials and Methods

2.1. Patients and Study Design. Following institutional review board approval, we performed a retrospective chart review to identify all patients who underwent RC for bladder cancer at the University of Pittsburgh Medical Center from Jan. 1, 2011, through Dec. 31, 2012. Patients were excluded if a CT scan performed within 30 days prior to RC was not available. RC was performed by one of eight high-volume surgeons in our department. All pathology specimens were reviewed by a dedicated genitourinary pathologist.

Demographic, pathologic, and outcome data were collected for each patient. Complications were categorized according to the Clavien-Dindo classification [13]. The primary outcome was 90-day overall complication rate. Secondary outcomes included major complications (Clavien grades III–V), infectious complications, wound complications, 90-day all-cause mortality, and overall survival. Classification as an infectious complication required a positive culture and treatment with antibiotics, and wound complications referred to fascial dehiscence, enterocutaneous fistula, or incarcerated incisional hernia. Follow-up was determined as of 4/19/2015, with patients censored at the date of their last confirmed visit to our institution or documented death.

2.2. TPA Measurement. TPA was measured at the L3 vertebral level on CT scan by a single investigator blinded to patient outcomes. Measurements were taken on the first image where both transverse processes were visible while traveling in the craniocaudal direction. Images were viewed using iSite PACS radiology software (Phillips, Amsterdam, Netherlands). Cross-sectional area of each psoas muscle was summed. To normalize TPA for body size, each TPA was then divided by the individual's body surface area (BSA), calculated from the height and weight recorded as a routine part of each patient's hospital admission, using the formula BSA = $\sqrt{[(\text{height (cm)} \times \text{weight (kg)})/3600]}$.

2.3. Statistical Analysis. Patients were grouped according to whether or not they experienced a 90-day complication for purposes of comparison. Means with standard deviations (SD) are reported for parametric data and medians with interquartile ranges (IQR) are reported for nonnormal data. TPA was evaluated as a continuous variable. Categorical variables were compared using χ^2 and Fisher's exact tests as appropriate. Means were compared using Student's t-test and medians using the Mann-Whitney U test. A multivariable logistic regression model was used to identify predictors of experiencing a postoperative complication while controlling for patient and disease characteristics known to be associated with adverse outcomes after RC. The Kaplan-Meier method was used to examine overall survival stratified by TPA quartile and compared using the log rank test. Data was analyzed using SPSS software, version 20 (IBM Corp., Armonk, NY). Statistical significance was defined at the $P < 0.05$ level using two-tailed tests.

3. Results

We identified 135 patients for analysis. Mean age was 69 years and 15% of patients (20/135) received neoadjuvant chemotherapy. Other than TPA, there were no significant differences between groups for any measured clinical or pathologic variables (Table 1).

Seventy-five patients experienced 102 postoperative complications (Table 2). Overall 90-day complication rate was 56% (75/135). Forty patients (30%) experienced a Clavien grade I-II complication, and major complications (Clavien grades III–V) occurred in 35 patients (26%). Infectious complications occurred in 22/135 patients (16%) and wound complications in 13/135 (9.4%). On bivariate analysis, infectious complications were not significantly associated with patient age ($P = 0.39$), smoking status ($P = 0.35$), Charlson comorbidity index ($P = 0.45$), EBL ($P = 0.88$), operative time ($P = 0.06$), or diversion type ($P = 0.14$); however, median BMI was higher in patients who had an infectious complication (28.7 kg/m^2 versus 25 kg/m^2, $P = 0.01$) and a wound complication (29.5 kg/m^2 versus 25.7 kg/m^2, $P = 0.046$). Wound complications were not significantly associated with age ($P = 0.6$), smoking status ($P = 0.37$), Charlson comorbidity index ($P = 0.42$), EBL ($P = 0.39$), operative time ($P = 0.09$), or diversion type ($P = 0.06$). Ninety-day mortality was 7.4% (10/135).

Median TPA was significantly lower in patients that experienced a 90-day complication ($7.8 \text{ cm}^2/\text{m}^2$ versus $8.8 \text{ cm}^2/\text{m}^2$, $P = 0.023$) and an infectious complication ($7.0 \text{ cm}^2/\text{m}^2$ versus $8.7 \text{ cm}^2/\text{m}^2$, $P = 0.032$) than in patients who did not. There was no significant difference in TPA between groups for major complications ($8.1 \text{ cm}^2/\text{m}^2$ versus $8.5 \text{ cm}^2/\text{m}^2$, $P = 0.64$), wound complications ($7.3 \text{ cm}^2/\text{m}^2$ versus $8.6 \text{ cm}^2/\text{m}^2$, $P = 0.43$), or 90-day mortality ($7.6 \text{ cm}^2/\text{m}^2$ versus $8.5 \text{ cm}^2/\text{m}^2$, $P = 0.34$).

Multivariable analysis investigating factors associated with experiencing a 90-day complication was performed (Table 3). After adjustment for potential cofounders, independent predictors of postoperative complications included TPA (adjusted OR 0.70 (95% CI 0.56–0.89), $P = 0.003$) and Charlson comorbidity index (adjusted OR 1.34 (95% CI 1.01–1.79), $P = 0.045$).

At a median follow-up of 24 months (IQR: 6–37 months), overall survival was 62% (86/135). When analyzed by quartile, TPA was not a significant predictor of overall survival ($P = 0.65$). Median survival was 34.3 months (95% CI 27.3–41.3), 33.9 months (26.7–41.2), 28.4 months (95% CI 21.6–35.2), and 34.6 months (95% CI 29.2–40.1) for TPA quartiles 1–4, respectively (Figure 1).

4. Discussion

Identifying bladder cancer patients at high risk of postsurgical complications is an important target for improving outcomes after cystectomy. In this study we sought to determine whether TPA, an estimate of skeletal muscle mass, was associated with 90-day outcomes following RC. On multivariable analysis, our data revealed that TPA (adjusted OR 0.70, $P = 0.003$) and Charlson comorbidity index

TABLE 1: Patient characteristics.

	90-day complication n = 75	No complication n = 60	P value
Age, years, mean ± SD	68.5 ± 9.9	69.1 ± 9.4	0.71
Gender (%)			0.99
M	60 (80)	48 (80)	
F	15 (20)	12 (20)	
Race (%)			0.37
White	69 (92)	58 (97)	
Nonwhite	6 (8.0)	2 (3.3)	
Smoker (%)	51 (68)	37 (62)	0.56
BMI, kg/m², median (IQR)	26.2 (22.5–30.4)	25.3 (22.8–29.0)	0.45
Serum albumin*, g/dL, median (IQR)	3.7 (3.0–4.0)	3.8 (3.4–4.0)	0.22
Charlson comorbidity index			0.11
0-1	28 (37)	30 (50)	
2-3	26 (35)	24 (40)	
>3	21 (28)	6 (10)	
Neoadjuvant chemotherapy (%)	13 (17)	7 (12)	0.36
L3 TPA, cm²/m², median (IQR)	7.8 (6.6–9.5)	8.8 (7.5–10.1)	0.023
Diversion type (%)			0.69
Neobladder	21 (28)	18 (30)	
Continent cutaneous	4 (5.3)	1 (1.7)	
Ileal conduit	48 (64)	41 (68)	
No diversion (anephric)	1 (1.3)	0	
Pathologic T Stage (%)			0.23
T0	1 (1.3)	2 (3.3)	
Ta	0	4 (6.7)	
Tis	8 (11)	6 (10)	
T1	5 (6.7)	8 (13)	
T2	14 (19)	9 (15)	
T3	30 (40)	22 (37)	
T4	17 (23)	9 (15)	
Node positive (%)	23 (31)	14 (23)	0.16
Operative time, min, mean ± SD	356 ± 103	334 ± 93	0.20
Estimated blood loss, mL, median (IQR)	850 (550–1075)	850 (675–1525)	0.56

SD: standard deviation, IQR: interquartile range, GFR: glomerular filtration rate, TPA: total psoas area, and mL: milliliter.
*n = 73.

(adjusted OR 1.34, $P = 0.045$) were independent predictors of a postsurgical complication. The odds ratio for TPA corresponds to a 30% decrease in complication risk for each $1 \text{ cm}^2/\text{m}^2$ increase in TPA. TPA was also associated with infectious complications ($P = 0.032$) on bivariate analysis, as was BMI ($P = 0.01$). Unfortunately, due to low event rate a multivariable risk adjustment for infectious complications could not be performed. However, these results are important as they suggest that TPA may be able to identify patients most at risk of complications following RC, potentially improving preoperative risk stratification.

Traditionally associated with aging, sarcopenia, or low skeletal muscle mass, is a prognostic marker of poor overall nutritional status and has been associated with increased mortality in elderly hospitalized patients [7, 14–16] as well as with adverse outcomes in patients undergoing surgery for gastrointestinal malignancies [17–21]. The most well-validated measure of muscle mass is the skeletal muscle index (SMI), obtained by measuring the cross-sectional area of all skeletal muscles including the rectus abdominis; internal, external, and lateral obliques; psoas; quadratus lumborum; and erector spinae muscles at the L3 vertebral level and normalizing for height in m² [22]. Multiple studies have validated the predictive value of skeletal muscle area at the L3 or L4 vertebrae on CT scan as a surrogate measure of whole-body skeletal muscle mass in both healthy and cancer populations [23, 24]. In a cohort of 205 patients who underwent RC, Psutka et al. used validated gender-specific SMI cutoffs to define sarcopenia for each gender and found that SMI was an independent predictor of cancer-specific and overall survival at a median follow-up of 6.7 years [8]. In contrast to these results, we found no difference in overall

TABLE 2: 90-day postoperative complications.

Complication	n (% of patients)
UTI/pyelonephritis	12 (8.9)
Ileus	9 (6.7)
Wound dehiscence	8 (5.9)
DVT/PE	7 (5.2)
Atrial fibrillation	6 (4.4)
Enterocutaneous fistula	5 (3.7)
Renal failure	5 (3.7)
Clostridiumdifficile infection	4 (3.0)
Stroke	4 (3.0)
Pelvic abscess	4 (3.0)
Small bowel obstruction	4 (3.0)
Ureteral obstruction requiring nephrostomy	3 (2.2)
Respiratory failure	3 (2.2)
PEA arrest	2 (1.5)
Ventricular tachycardia	2 (1.5)
Dysphagia	2 (1.5)
Wound infection	2 (1.5)
Hypoxia	2 (1.5)
Hemorrhage requiring transfusion	2 (1.5)
Delirium	2 (1.5)
Intestinal anastomotic leak	1 (0.7)
Pleural effusion	1 (0.7)
AV fistula dissection	1 (0.7)
Critical limb ischemia	1 (0.7)
Malignant hypertension	1 (0.7)
Splenic infarct	1 (0.7)
Ureteroenteric anastomotic stricture	1 (0.7)
Incarcerated incisional hernia	1 (0.7)
Chest pain	1 (0.7)
GI bleed	1 (0.7)
Infected pelvic hematoma	1 (0.7)
Compartment syndrome/rhabdomyolysis	1 (0.7)
Pancreatitis	1 (0.7)
Aspiration pneumonia	1 (0.7)

UTI: urinary tract infection, DVT: deep venous thrombosis, PE: pulmonary embolism, PEA: pulseless electrical activity, AV: arteriovenous, and GI: gastrointestinal.

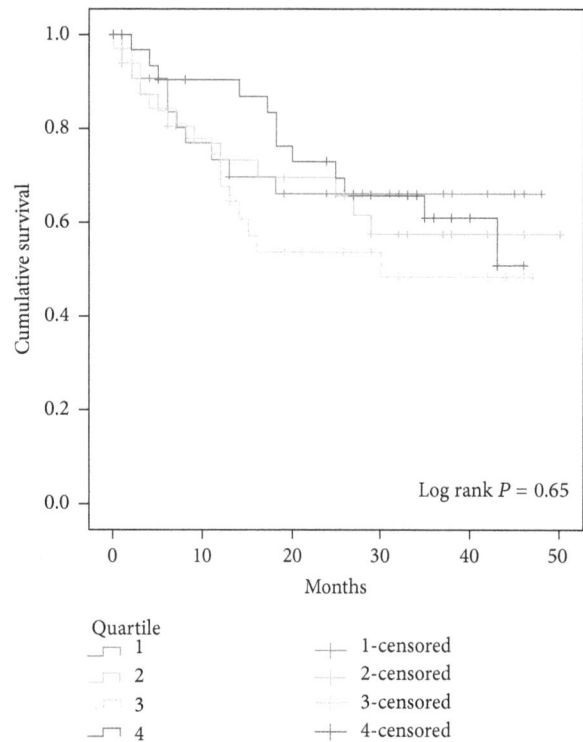

FIGURE 1: Overall survival stratified by TPA quartile.

Number at risk						
Quartile 1	33	22	17	11	4	0
Quartile 2	33	21	18	12	7	0
Quartile 3	33	23	14	10	6	0
Quartile 4	32	26	22	16	9	0

survival in our patients when compared by TPA quartile ($P = 0.65$); however, our median follow-up was only 2 years, and it is possible that with longer follow-up a survival difference would be uncovered.

Total psoas area has also been linked to complications following radical cystectomy; Smith et al. reviewed a series of 200 patients and found that low TPA was a predictor of 30-day major complications in women, but not in men [12]. Similarly, we demonstrated an association between TPA and overall complications ($P = 0.003$) and infectious complications ($P = 0.032$) after RC but did not replicate their finding of an increased risk of major complications. Two protocol differences may account for the differences

in our findings. First, we evaluated 90-day instead of 30-day outcomes. Secondly, Smith et al. normalized TPA using height in m^2, while we opted to normalize it with body surface area to better account for obesity and patient size than height alone [12, 25]. Replication of our findings will be required to determine which of these approaches is optimal.

One potential advantage of using TPA over SMI for the quantification of sarcopenia in surgical patients is the ease with which it can be obtained. Psoas area can be easily and efficiently measured on CT images, a modality very familiar to most surgeons, in an outpatient setting. Further, TPA has been proposed as the surrogate marker best suitable for studying sarcopenia in diseased populations, as the psoas muscle reflects changes of nutritional deficiency in chronically ill patients but not acutely ill ones [14, 26]. Our TPA measurement technique differed slightly from those previously described in that we did not use HU criteria to automatically subtract fatty infiltration from muscle area. Our rationale for doing so was to determine whether a rapidly obtainable clinical measurement could be used in preoperative risk stratification and we did not want to rely on imaging software not available to the average urologist. In centers where SMI is not routinely reported or where radiologists are unfamiliar with the technique, urologists

TABLE 3: Multivariable predictors of 90-day complications.

	Univariate OR (95% CI)	P value	Adjusted OR (95% CI)	P value
Age	0.99 (0.96–1.03)	0.71	0.97 (0.92–1.02)	0.20
Gender (referent female)	1.00 (0.43–2.34)	0.99	2.27 (0.77–6.76)	0.14
Charlson comorbidity index	1.38 (1.07–1.78)	0.014	1.34 (1.01–1.79)	0.045
Neoadjuvant chemotherapy	1.59 (0.59–4.27)	0.36	1.29 (0.40–4.16)	0.67
Total psoas area	0.82 (0.69–0.97)	0.019	0.70 (0.56–0.89)	0.003
Pathologic T Stage				
T0	Referent	0.81	Referent	0.95
Ta	0.0	0.99	0.0	0.99
Tis	2.67 (0.19–36.76)	0.46	3.14 (0.12–83.74)	0.50
T1	1.25 (0.09–17.65)	0.87	1.84 (0.07–46.58)	0.71
T2	3.11 (0.25–39.54)	0.138	3.15 (0.14–73.16)	0.48
T3	2.73 (0.23–32.01)	0.43	3.92 (0.18–84.29)	0.38
T4	3.56 (0.28–44.88)	0.33	2.93 (0.13–64.55)	0.50
Node positive	1.76 (0.80–3.86)	0.16	1.68 (0.65–4.33)	0.29

OR: odds ratio, CI: confidence interval, and TPA: total psoas area.

could more easily calculate TPA than SMI themselves, leading to greater clinical utility.

Nutritional deficiency has been linked to inferior outcomes after RC but has been variably defined, using preoperative albumin levels, body mass index, weight loss, and sarcopenia [4–6, 8, 12]. Confusion exists as to how best to use these markers. Establishing an optimal method of quantifying malnutrition in bladder cancer patients is important, as it may be a factor upon which clinicians can intervene to improve surgical quality. Malnutrition is known to alter the immune response to surgical stress and increase susceptibility to postoperative infections [27, 28]. Specifically, sarcopenia has been shown to predict a greater risk of experiencing serious infections after liver transplantation [9] and of acquiring a nosocomial infection [29]. TPA may be a useful marker in bladder cancer patients as well based on our observed difference in postoperative infection rate. Postcystectomy infectious complications are known to increase perioperative mortality, length of stay, and hospital costs [30]. Preoperative supplementation with immunonutrient high-arginine shakes has been shown to reduce infectious complications and length of stay following gastrointestinal surgery [31–33]. Our results imply that TPA may be able to identify patients at the highest risk of post-RC infectious complications that could potentially benefit from preoperative immunonutrient supplementation or other such targeted interventions, and we are currently enrolling patients at our center in a prospective trial examining whether such supplementation can influence outcomes after RC. Until trial results are available, however, we cannot yet definitively state that preoperative immunonutrient shake supplementation can improve post-RC outcomes in malnourished patients.

Several limitations exist in this study. First, our analysis is retrospective in nature and subject to problems inherent to this approach. The sample size is relatively small, which limits statistical power and the generalizability of our findings. Median follow-up was 2 years, and therefore we were unable to determine whether TPA can predict long-term oncologic outcomes. Subjects are predominantly Caucasian and thus results may not be applicable to persons of other racial backgrounds. Preoperative serum albumin levels were only available for 54% of our cohort, and due to missing data we did not include albumin in our multivariable model despite the fact that low albumin has been previously linked to worse outcomes after cystectomy [5, 6]. For the data that was available, median serum albumin was not significantly different between patients who did and did not experience a postoperative complication, though (Table 1). Future investigations are needed to assess the relationship between TPA, albumin, and other nutritional markers to determine which can best predict patient outcomes. Further work with larger sample sizes and longer follow-up is needed to validate our findings and to better characterize gender-specific normal and abnormal TPA values in a cystectomy population.

Despite these limitations, our data suggest that patients with low TPA have a greater risk of overall and infectious complications after RC, building upon the findings of Smith and colleagues [12] and suggesting that TPA may be able to play a future role in selecting patients at the highest risk of post-RC complications. However, TPA was not associated with long-term survival in our series as has been shown with SMI [8]. On the basis of our findings it would be inappropriate to suggest that TPA be used independently for prognostication prior to RC at this time. Future work is needed to identify whether TPA could be used to predict survival and whether nutritional supplementation in patients with low TPA improves outcomes after RC. For the time being urologists interested in sarcopenia should ask radiologists to report SMI. However, future work may still prove TPA useful to guide targeted interventions to improve the quality of care for patients with bladder cancer.

5. Conclusion

Low total psoas area is associated with overall and infectious complications following radical cystectomy, but not overall survival. TPA may prove useful as a biomarker to identify patients at the highest risk of post-RC complications.

Conflict of Interests

All authors have no relevant financial conflict of interests to report.

References

[1] R. Siegel, D. Naishadham, and A. Jemal, "Cancer statistics, 2013," *CA: A Cancer Journal for Clinicians*, vol. 63, no. 1, pp. 11–30, 2013.

[2] A. Shabsigh, R. Korets, K. C. Vora et al., "Defining early morbidity of radical cystectomy for patients with bladder cancer using a standardized reporting methodology," *European Urology*, vol. 55, no. 1, pp. 164–176, 2009.

[3] C. J. Stimson, S. S. Chang, D. A. Barocas et al., "Early and late perioperative outcomes following radical cystectomy: 90-day readmissions, morbidity and mortality in a contemporary series," *The Journal of Urology*, vol. 184, no. 4, pp. 1296–1300, 2010.

[4] B. K. Hollenbeck, D. C. Miller, D. A. Taub et al., "The effects of adjusting for case mix on mortality and length of stay following radical cystectomy," *The Journal of Urology*, vol. 176, no. 4, pp. 1363–1368, 2006.

[5] J. W. Lambert, M. Ingham, B. B. Gibbs, R. W. Given, R. S. Lance, and S. B. Riggs, "Using preoperative albumin levels as a surrogate marker for outcomes after radical cystectomy for bladder cancer," *Urology*, vol. 81, no. 3, pp. 587–592, 2013.

[6] J. R. Gregg, M. S. Cookson, S. Phillips et al., "Effect of preoperative nutritional deficiency on mortality after radical cystectomy for bladder cancer," *The Journal of Urology*, vol. 185, no. 1, pp. 90–96, 2011.

[7] M. Muscaritoli, S. D. Anker, J. Argilés et al., "Consensus definition of sarcopenia, cachexia and pre-cachexia: joint document elaborated by Special Interest Groups (SIG) 'cachexia-anorexia in chronic wasting diseases' and 'nutrition in geriatrics'," *Clinical Nutrition*, vol. 29, no. 2, pp. 154–159, 2010.

[8] S. P. Psutka, A. Carrasco, G. D. Schmit et al., "Sarcopenia in patients with bladder cancer undergoing radical cystectomy: impact on cancer-specific and all-cause mortality," *Cancer*, vol. 120, no. 18, pp. 2910–2918, 2014.

[9] R. W. Krell, D. R. Kaul, A. R. Martin et al., "Association between sarcopenia and the risk of serious infection among adults undergoing liver transplantation," *Liver Transplantation*, vol. 19, no. 12, pp. 1396–1402, 2013.

[10] P. Peng, O. Hyder, A. Firoozmand et al., "Impact of sarcopenia on outcomes following resection of pancreatic adenocarcinoma," *Journal of Gastrointestinal Surgery*, vol. 16, no. 8, pp. 1478–1486, 2012.

[11] P. D. Peng, M. G. van Vledder, S. Tsai et al., "Sarcopenia negatively impacts short-term outcomes in patients undergoing hepatic resection for colorectal liver metastasis," *HPB*, vol. 13, no. 7, pp. 439–446, 2011.

[12] A. B. Smith, A. M. Deal, H. Yu et al., "Sarcopenia as a predictor of complications and survival following radical cystectomy," *The Journal of Urology*, vol. 191, no. 6, pp. 1714–1720, 2014.

[13] D. Dindo, N. Demartines, and P.-A. Clavien, "Classification of surgical complications: a new proposal with evaluation in a cohort of 6336 patients and results of a survey," *Annals of Surgery*, vol. 240, no. 2, pp. 205–213, 2004.

[14] M. J. Englesbe, S. P. Patel, K. He et al., "Sarcopenia and mortality after liver transplantation," *Journal of the American College of Surgeons*, vol. 211, no. 2, pp. 271–278, 2010.

[15] J. S. W. Lee, T.-W. Auyeung, T. Kwok, E. M. C. Lau, P.-C. Leung, and J. Woo, "Associated factors and health impact of sarcopenia in older Chinese men and women: a cross-sectional study," *Gerontology*, vol. 53, no. 6, pp. 404–410, 2007.

[16] D. L. Vetrano, F. Landi, S. Volpato et al., "Association of sarcopenia with short- and long-term mortality in older adults admitted to acute care wards: Results from the CRIME study," *The Journals of Gerontology—Series A: Biological Sciences and Medical Sciences*, vol. 69, no. 9, pp. 1154–1161, 2014.

[17] N. Harimoto, K. Shirabe, Y.-I. Yamashita et al., "Sarcopenia as a predictor of prognosis in patients following hepatectomy for hepatocellular carcinoma," *The British Journal of Surgery*, vol. 100, no. 11, pp. 1523–1530, 2013.

[18] T. Voron, L. Tselikas, D. Pietrasz et al., "Sarcopenia impacts on short- and long-term results of hepatectomy for hepatocellular carcinoma," *Annals of Surgery*, vol. 261, no. 6, pp. 1173–1183, 2015.

[19] S. Joglekar, A. Asghar, S. L. Mott et al., "Sarcopenia is an independent predictor of complications following pancreatectomy for adenocarcinoma," *Journal of Surgical Oncology*, vol. 111, no. 6, pp. 771–775, 2015.

[20] Y. Miyamoto, Y. Baba, Y. Sakamoto et al., "Sarcopenia is a negative prognostic factor after curative resection of colorectal cancer," *Annals of Surgical Oncology*, vol. 22, no. 8, pp. 2663–2668, 2015.

[21] J. L. A. van Vugt, H. J. Braam, T. R. van Oudheusden et al., "Skeletal muscle depletion is associated with severe postoperative complications in patients undergoing cytoreductive surgery with hyperthermic intraperitoneal chemotherapy for peritoneal carcinomatosis of colorectal cancer," *Annals of Surgical Oncology*, vol. 22, no. 11, pp. 3625–3631, 2015.

[22] K. Fearon, F. Strasser, S. D. Anker et al., "Definition and classification of cancer cachexia: an international consensus," *The Lancet Oncology*, vol. 12, no. 5, pp. 489–495, 2011.

[23] W. Shen, M. Punyanitya, Z. Wang et al., "Total body skeletal muscle and adipose tissue volumes: estimation from a single abdominal cross-sectional image," *Journal of Applied Physiology*, vol. 97, no. 6, pp. 2333–2338, 2004.

[24] M. Mourtzakis, C. M. M. Prado, J. R. Lieffers, T. Reiman, L. J. McCargar, and V. E. Baracos, "A practical and precise approach to quantification of body composition in cancer patients using computed tomography images acquired during routine care," *Applied Physiology, Nutrition and Metabolism*, vol. 33, no. 5, pp. 997–1006, 2008.

[25] J. Verbraecken, P. Van de Heyning, W. De Backer, and L. Van Gaal, "Body surface area in normal-weight, overweight, and obese adults. A comparison study," *Metabolism: Clinical and Experimental*, vol. 55, no. 4, pp. 515–524, 2006.

[26] J. S.-J. Lee, K. He, C. M. Harbaugh et al., "Frailty, core muscle size, and mortality in patients undergoing open abdominal aortic aneurysm repair," *Journal of Vascular Surgery*, vol. 53, no. 4, pp. 912–917, 2011.

[27] J. M. Culebras, "Malnutrition in the twenty-first century: an epidemic affecting surgical outcome," *Surgical Infections*, vol. 14, no. 3, pp. 237–243, 2013.

[28] D. L. Malone, T. Genuit, J. K. Tracy, C. Gannon, and L. M. Napolitano, "Surgical site infections: reanalysis of risk factors," *The Journal of Surgical Research*, vol. 103, no. 1, pp. 89–95, 2002.

[29] G. Cosquëric, A. Sebag, C. Ducolombier, C. Thomas, F. Piette, and S. Weill-Engerer, "Sarcopenia is predictive of nosocomial

infection in care of the elderly," *British Journal of Nutrition*, vol. 96, no. 5, pp. 895–901, 2006.

[30] B. J. Davies, V. Allareddy, and B. R. Konety, "Effect of postcystectomy infectious complications on cost, length of stay, and mortality," *Urology*, vol. 73, no. 3, pp. 598–602, 2009.

[31] B. Jie, Z.-M. Jiang, M. T. Nolan, S.-N. Zhu, K. Yu, and J. Kondrup, "Impact of preoperative nutritional support on clinical outcome in abdominal surgical patients at nutritional risk," *Nutrition*, vol. 28, no. 10, pp. 1022–1027, 2012.

[32] M. Braga, L. Gianotti, A. Vignali, and V. Di Carlo, "Preoperative oral arginine and n-3 fatty acid supplementation improves the immunometabolic host response and outcome after colorectal resection for cancer," *Surgery*, vol. 132, no. 5, pp. 805–814, 2002.

[33] M. Braga, L. Gianotti, G. Radaelli et al., "Perioperative immunonutrition in patients undergoing cancer surgery: results of a randomized double-blind phase 3 trial," *Archives of Surgery*, vol. 134, no. 4, pp. 428–433, 1999.

16

A Prospective Study of Bipolar Transurethral Resection of Prostate Comparing the Efficiency and Safety of the Method in Large and Small Adenomas

Nikolaos Mertziotis,[1] **Diomidis Kozyrakis,**[2] **Christos Kyratsas,**[1] **and Andreas Konandreas**[1]

[1]*Iaso General Hospital, 264 Messogeion Avenue, 15562 Athens, Greece*
[2]*General Hospital of Volos, 134 Polimeri Street, 38222 Volos, Greece*

Correspondence should be addressed to Nikolaos Mertziotis; mertz@hol.gr

Academic Editor: Matthew Rutman

Bipolar technology offers a new perspective in the treatment of BPH. *Purpose.* To present our experience with the TURis system (Olympus, Tokyo, Japan). *Materials and Methods.* From February 2011 till December 2013 in a prospective study, 93 patients were treated for BPH. They were evaluated with IPSS, QoL, uroflow (Q_{max}), and residual urine (RU), preoperatively as well as 6 and 9 months postoperatively. Based on the prostate volume, the patients were divided into two groups: group A ($n = 48$) with prostates $\geq$ 75 cc and group B ($n = 45$) with smaller prostate glands. All patients underwent bipolar TURP or/and plasma vaporization. *Results.* The postoperative improvement for IPSS, QoL, Q_{max}, and RU was statistically significant. The operation time was longer in group A in comparison with group B ($P < 0.001$). The former group also had higher infection and stricture formation rates; however, there was no statistical difference between the two groups. *Conclusions.* Treatment with the TURis constitutes an effective technique and can be offered to large prostates with results equivalent to those in small ones. Regarding safety, large adenomas treated with TURis are not at a higher risk for urethral stricture but their odds to develop urogenital infections are relatively higher compared to the smaller adenomas.

1. Introduction

Benign prostate hyperplasia (BPH) is a high prevalent disease among the middle aged/elderly male population. Even though it is poorly defined, it is encountered at a rate of approximately 50% in ages between 51 and 60 years [1]. Others report a prevalence of 26% in males during their fifth decade of life and up to 46% during their eighth decade [2]. Medical treatment, with a_1 blockers and 5-a reductase inhibitors, offers good results to patients with mild to moderate symptoms, while, for those with more severe lower urinary tract symptoms, an interventional treatment is recommended. For many years, transurethral resection of the prostatic adenoma with monopolar electrocautery (M-TURP) has been the gold standard of surgical treatment due to its effectiveness and its durable results over time but its safety profile is not ideal [3–5]. Postoperative hemorrhage, blood clot retention, and

urethral strictures are a few of the potential complications. The hyponatremia and TUR syndrome are associated with the irrigation of a nonconductive solution (e.g., glycine 1.5%, mannitol 5%) to distend the bladder during the monopolar prostatectomy [6–8]. Prolonged resection time makes patients vulnerable to electrolyte disorders [9] and, for safety reasons, prostates greater than 80–100 mL are excluded from adequate treatment with M-TURP in one single session [10, 11].

Several devices and techniques have been developed to overcome these limitations of M-TURP and the bipolar resection of the prostate (B-TURP) is one of them. This method uses normal saline solution 0.9%, as irrigation fluid, which has the advantage to eliminate the risk of TUR syndrome [12, 13]. This is because the absorption of the irrigation fluid by the vascular system of the prostate is clinically insignificant. The bipolar device is also considered to have an optimal haemostatic effect minimizing the postoperative hemorrhage [14, 15].

We herein present the clinical results of a prospective study, composed of BPH patients treated with the bipolar resectoscope in saline, and we are comparing the surgical results and the complications encountered in large prostates with those in smaller adenomas.

2. Material and Methods

From February 2011 till December 2013, 93 consecutive patients were treated by the same surgeon for BPH with the bipolar 26 F resectoscope OES Pro by Olympus, Tokyo, Japan, in saline. Electric current was delivered by the electrosurgical generator UES-40 SurgMaster. Resection of the prostate was performed using the loop resectoscope combined, in some cases, with vaporization of the adenoma using the plasma button device (TURis).

Before treatment, patient history was taken and clinical examination was performed on each patient, followed by IPSS and quality of life (QoL) questionnaire, transabdominal or transrectal ultrasonography of the urinary tract, and uroflowmetry test with residual urine (RU) echographic assessment. In a prospective follow-up, all these tests were routinely repeated in 6–9 month interval after the operation.

The criteria for surgical treatment were formed based on one or more of the following: high prostate symptom score (IPSS $\geq$ 20), poor BPH related quality of life (score 5 or 6), failure to respond to conservative treatment or recurrence of symptoms after conservative treatment, $Q_{max} \leq 10$ mL/sec, high postvoiding residual urine volume ($\geq$ 200 mL), and urinary retention or patient's preference. Discontinuation of any antiplatelet or anticoagulative treatment was mandatory prior to surgery.

Aiming to perform a comparative analysis, the presurgical prostate volume established the criterion based on which patients were classified into two groups; group A was that of large prostates ($\geq$75 mL) and group B was the one with prostates less than 75 mL and represented the control group of our study.

The two groups were preoperatively examined for statistical significant differences regarding the age, the prostate volume, the IPSS, the QoL, the maximum flow (Q_{max}), and the RU. The surgical outcome was expressed as the postsurgical improvement over the baseline (preoperative) values for each one of the IPSS, QoL, Q_{max}, and RU and a comparison of the results between the two groups was provided. Operation time, hospitalization, postsurgical catheterization, and complication rates were recorded for each group separately and the results were statistically analyzed.

The statistical analysis was performed using the Stata MP 10.1 (StataCorp LP, Texas, USA) software for windows. Normality was examined using the Shapiro-Wilk test. Comparison of the two groups was performed using Wilcoxon rank-sum test and t-test for values in abnormal and normal distribution, respectively. Statistical significance was defined as $P < 0.05$.

TABLE 1: Patients' characteristics at presentation.

Factor	Mean value	Range
Age (years)	71.3	46–92
Prostate volume (mL)	60.98	43–185
IPSS	18.2	7–32
QoL	3.37	2–6
Q_{max} (mL/sec)	8.44	2–14
Residual urine (mL)	167.71	20–700
Urinary retention	6	

3. Results

The patients' characteristics are presented in Table 1. The mean age at presentation was 71.3 years (range: 46–92). The mean prostate volume was 60.98 mL (range: 43–185). The mean IPSS, QoL, Q_{max}, and RU were 18.2, 3.37, 8.44 mL/sec, and 167.71 mL. For both groups, the mean operation time was 63.26 min (range: 36–151), the mean duration of catheterization was 28.06 hours (range: 16–98), and the mean hospital stay was 32.01 hours (range: 22–75). The percentage of improvement for IPSS, QoL, Q_{max}, and RU was 47.41%, −56.67%, 101.07%, and −65.97%, respectively, and statistically significant improvement was noted (Table 2). Two patients were unable to void after surgery. One of them was reoperated on and the other was treated with intermittent catheterization for 6 months. The latter subsequently had a successful voiding without catheterization. Two nonfatal major cardiovascular complications were diagnosed: one myocardial infarction and one pulmonary embolism. Urethral strictures were identified in 8 patients and urogenital infections in 10. Nine patients complained of persistent symptomatology of the lower urinary tract, mainly storage symptoms, for more than 3 months and were treated with anticholinergic regimens. An overview of surgical complications is presented in Table 3.

At the imaging of the lower urinary tract, 48 out of the 93 patients (52%, group A) had prostates greater than 75 mL (mean: 92.13 mL, range: 75–185) while the rest 45 patients (48%, group B) had smaller prostates (mean 51.29 mL, range: 43–66). The preoperative characteristics of both groups are presented in Table 4. When statistically examined, the two groups were comparable in all the preoperative characteristics except for the prostate size and the peak flow in uroflowmetry. The percentage of postsurgical improvement for group A was −52.46%, −47.57%, 157.68%, and −65.03% for IPSS, QoL, Q_{max}, and RU, respectively, and −45.41%, −60.60%, 116.08%, and −65.82% for group B, respectively. The statistical analysis did not reveal any significant difference in the surgical outcome between the two groups. The operation time was longer in large prostates, but the bladder catheterization time and hospital stay were similar (Table 5). The complication rates are presented in Table 6 and although the urogenital infection rate of group A was much higher than that of group B, no statistical significance was revealed.

TABLE 2: Presentation of the operation time, catheterization time, hospital stay, and surgical results for the whole group of patients.

Factor	Mean value (range)	Percentage of change	P value
Operation time (minutes)	63.26 (36–151)		
Catheterization time (hours)	28.06 (16–98)		
Hospital stay (hours)	32.01 (22–75)		
IPSS‡ pre/post	18.2/9.57	−47.41%	0.001
QoL‡ pre/post	3.37/1.46	−56.67%	0.001
Q_{max}† pre/post	8.44/16.97	101.07%	0.001
Residual urine‡ pre/post	167.71/57.08	−65.97%	0.001

‡Abnormal distribution: the comparison was made with the Wilcoxon matched pairs signed ranks test.
†Normal distribution: the comparison was made with the t-test (matched pairs).

TABLE 3: Overview of surgical complications for both groups of patients.

Complication	Number of patients ($n = 93$)	Percentage (%)
Urethral stricture	8	8.6%
Urinary retention	2	2.1%
Blood transfusion	1	1.0%
Urogenital infection	10	10.7%
Prolonged LUTS	9	9.6%
Prolonged hematuria	2	2.1%
Cardiovascular events	2	2.1%

TABLE 4: Comparison of the preoperative characteristics of the two groups of patients.

Variant	Group A ($n = 48$)	Group B ($n = 45$)	P value
Age† (yrs)	72.3 (7.18)	71.0 (10.56)	0.631
V_{prost}‡ (cm^3)	92.1 [75–185]	51.2 [43–66]	<0.001
IPSS†	19.6 (6.26)	17.7 (5.39)	0.221
Qol†	3.7 (0.98)	3.25 (0.93)	0.093
Q_{max}† (mL/sec)	6.6 (2.87)	9.0 (3.12)	0.011
RU‡ (mL)	162.5 [150–240]	150 [100–200]	0.386

‡Abnormal distribution: the median and IQR values are shown and the comparison is based on the Wilcoxon rank-sum test.
†Normal distribution: the mean and SD values are shown and the comparison is based on the t-test.

TABLE 5: Comparison of the surgical outcome, operation time, catheterization time, and hospital stay between the two groups of patients (OK).

Variant	Group A ($n = 48$)	Group B ($n = 45$)	P value
IPSS‡	−52.46%	−45.41%	0.934
QoL†	−47.57%	−60.60%	0.603
Q_{max}† (mL/sec)	157.68%	116.08%	0.384
RU‡ (mL)	−65.03%	−65.82%	0.655
Mean operation time (minutes)‡	88.76	54.23	<0.001
Mean catheterization time (hours)‡	29.41	27.58	0.356
Mean hospital stay (hours)‡	34.06	31.29	0.211

‡Abnormal distribution: the comparison is based on the Wilcoxon rank-sum test.
†Normal distribution: the comparison is based on the t-test.

4. Discussion

Historically, Gyrus (ACMI Southborough, MA, USA) was the first manufacturer that incorporated bipolar technology into the resectoscope device, known as the PlasmaKinetic System (PKS). The prostatectomy was performed using normal saline 0.9% as the irrigant fluid, instead of a nonconductive solution, offering the advantage of minimal absorption by the open vessels and eliminating the risk of electrolytic disorders, particularly the serum sodium level drop [12, 16]. Later on, another bipolar resectoscope, manufactured by Olympus (SurgMaster device, TURis), was released into the market having similar advantages to those of PKS [17]. The use of two interchangeable electrodes, the resection loop and the mushroom shaped plasma button, allows a fast, complete, and precise resection of the adenomas [18].

Nowadays, bipolar technology is a safe and effective method to perform the transurethral prostatectomy. An early meta-analysis published in 2009 showed that the bipolar method had the same efficacy as the monopolar one, but the safety of the former technique was more favorable. In particular, the clot retention rate and the TUR syndrome risk were lower in the bipolar arm. Moreover, the irrigation and catheterization time were significantly shorter [19]. Another meta-analysis published 4 years later, despite the methodological limitations of the RCT incorporated in the study and the short follow-up period, came to similar conclusions, emphasizing once more the better safety profile (non-TUR syndrome, less clot retention, and blood transfusion) encountered in the bipolar arm [13]. Aiming to overcome any methodological flaws, a well-designed multicenter double-blind randomized trial that fulfilled the COCHRANE criteria for high quality trials was performed, comparing the bipolar AutoZone II 400 ESU with the M-TURP. Although the dilutional hyponatremia was diagnosed more frequently in the monopolar group, the TUR syndrome risk was similar in both arms (monopolar: 0.7% versus bipolar: 0%). The authors concluded that the improved safety profile of the B-TURP was only theoretical, bearing minimal clinical significance when the operation was performed by experienced surgeons [20].

Nevertheless, the number of publications that focused on the surgical outcome in large volume prostates is limited.

Table 6: Comparison of surgical complications between the two groups.

Complication	Group A (n = 48): number of patients (%)	Group B (n = 45): number of patients (%)	P value
Urethral stricture	6 (12.5%)	2 (4.4%)	0.163
Urinary retention	1 (2.1%)	1 (2.2%)	0.974
Blood transfusion	1 (2.1%)	0 (0%)	0.328
Urogenital infection	7 (14.6%)	3 (6.6%)	0.219
Prolonged LUTS/incontinence	6 (12.5%)	3 (6.6%)	0.185
Prolonged hematuria	2 (4.2%)	0 (0%)	0.166
Cardiovascular events	2 (4.2%)	0 (0%)	0.166

In a case series of 4 patients with excessive prostate volumes (>160 mL), prostatectomy was performed with the Gyrus PK system. Despite the prolonged operation time, the percentage of complications was favorable regarding the hemoglobin level and serum sodium level drop. The hospitalization time was short (mean: 12 hours) and the catheter was removed after an average of 76 hours [21].

In a prospective randomized study with adenomas greater than 60 gr., the PK system was compared with the conventional M-TURP. The short term surgical outcome (IPSS, Q_{max}, and RU) was similar between the two groups, but the bipolar system had a clear advantage in blood loss, in hyponatremia events, and in catheter stay. The authors stressed the inherent potential of the new technique to become the new gold standard of the minimal invasive prostatectomy [22].

Similar to the PK system, several authors focused on the advantage of the Olympus TURis over the monopolar system in terms of complication rates. In prostates >50 mL, the hemoglobin level drop was minimal, the immediate postoperative complications were fewer, and the hospitalization and catheter stay were shorter [23]. Others underscore the limited postoperative drop in sodium level minimizing the risk of TUR syndrome [24]. All the aforementioned papers have a short follow-up period; therefore, the issue of late complications and durable results over time remains to be answered.

In a study of 136 patients with a follow-up of 3 years, the authors compared the TURis with the M-TURP [25]. In the subgroup of patients with small adenomas, both techniques yield similar results regarding the postoperative complications but in prostates >70 mL the urethral stricture rate was as high as 20% in the TURis arm and only 2.2% in the monopolar one (P = 0.012). Likewise, Rassweiler et al. reported on high stricture formation rates among patients treated either with the PKS or the TURis device [18]. These alarming results were not confirmed in the meta-analysis published by Omar and colleagues, in which the percentage of urethral strictures was not higher than 3.3% [13].

In our series, 8,6% of the patients developed urethral stenosis. The prolonged surgical time and perhaps the large caliber of the resectoscope sheath (26 F) might constitute the explanation for this complication. It could be assumed that, for some urethras, the resectoscope sheath may be large enough as to cause ischemia and urethral trauma.

In addition, the power settings of 310 W and 170 W that we used for resection and coagulation may have produced a thermal damage to the sensitive periurethral tissue and, thus, stricture formation [14, 26]. By adjusting the working settings to a lower power level, we hope that we will be able to reduce the frequency of this complication.

The UTI rate was as high as 14.6% among large prostates and approximately 6,6% in smaller adenomas. It should be stated that we registered not only patients with febrile urogenital infection but those with asymptomatic or minimal bothersome positive urinary culture as well. Except for patients with an indwelling urethral catheter, we performed a preoperative urinary culture and we proceeded to the operation only when the results of the urine culture were negative for bacteria, or sterile. We routinely administered a cephalosporin II or an ampicillin/sulbactam regimen intravenously, 30'–60' before and 5-6 hours after the operation. In some cases with a history of catheterization, or an estimated high risk for infection, particularly in large adenomas, we continued the treatment for 5–7 days orally. Apart from the hypothesis that large prostates may host a plethora of bacterial populations or more aggressive strains that are released into the circulation during prostatectomy and the longer operation time, no clear explanation for the high infection rate could be given.

In our opinion, the disadvantages of the TURis, including the cost of surgical loop and plasma button electrode, are counterbalanced by the short time of postoperative fluid irrigation, catheter stay, and hospitalization. Considering that the majority of patients were discharged after less than 36 hours of hospital stay, it is safe to assume that the benefit for the health care system is major. Although we have not performed an official technoeconomic study, one day less of hospital stay is translated into approximately >400€ of cost savings. The brief postoperative recovery time and the early return to work also have a profound positive effect on the individual's psychological and economic status.

A main drawback of our study is the limited number of patients, and the lack of a control group for a direct comparison of the bipolar technique against the monopolar one. Due to the short follow-up period, the long term effectiveness and the late complications of TURis are impossible to be defined in this series.

5. Conclusions

Treatment of BPH with the bipolar resectoscope is an effective surgical technique and seems to offer patients with large prostates surgical results equivalent to those encountered in smaller prostate volumes. Concerning the safety profile, in our series, large prostates treated with TURis are not at a higher risk for urethral stricture, but their odds to develop urogenital infections are higher compared with the smaller adenomas counterparts. Generally speaking, the percentage of postoperative strictures and infections could be considered suboptimal and should be subjected to investigation in future prospective trials. Candidates for TURis prostatectomy, irrespective of their prostatic volume, should be properly informed about the aforementioned complications before giving their consent for surgery.

Conflict of Interests

The authors declare that there is no conflict of interests regarding the publication of this paper.

References

[1] S. J. Berry, D. S. Coffey, P. C. Walsh, and L. L. Ewing, "The development of human benign prostatic hyperplasia with age," *Journal of Urology*, vol. 132, no. 3, pp. 474–479, 1984.

[2] C. G. Chute, L. A. Panser, C. J. Girman et al., "The prevalence of prostatism: a population-based survey of urinary symptoms," *The Journal of Urology*, vol. 150, no. 1, pp. 85–89, 1993.

[3] W. K. Mebust, H. L. Holtgrewe, A. T. K. Cockett, and P. C. Peters, "Transurethral prostatectomy: immediate and postoperative complications. A cooperative study of 13 participating institutions evaluating 3885 patients," *Journal of Urology*, vol. 141, no. 2, pp. 243–247, 1989.

[4] O. Reich, C. Gratzke, and C. G. Stief, "Techniques and long term results of surgical procedures for BPH," *European Urology*, vol. 49, no. 6, pp. 970–978, 2006.

[5] J. Rassweiler, D. Teber, R. Kuntz, and R. Hofmann, "Complications of transurethral resection of the prostate (TURP)—incidence, management, and prevention," *European Urology*, vol. 50, no. 5, pp. 969–980, 2006.

[6] R. G. Hahn, "Transurethral resection syndrome from extravascular absorption of irrigating fluid," *Scandinavian Journal of Urology and Nephrology*, vol. 27, no. 3, pp. 387–394, 1993.

[7] D. P. Michielsen, T. Debacker, V. De Boe et al., "Bipolar transurethral resection in saline—an alternative surgical treatment for bladder outlet obstruction?" *The Journal of Urology*, vol. 178, no. 5, pp. 2035–2039, 2007.

[8] H. Singh, M. R. Desai, P. Shrivastav, and K. Vani, "Bipolar versus monopolar transurethral resection of prostate: randomized controlled study," *Journal of Endourology*, vol. 19, no. 3, pp. 333–338, 2005.

[9] A. A. Yousef, G. A. Suliman, O. M. Elashry, M. D. Elsharaby, and A. E.-N. K. Elgamasy, "A randomized comparison between three types of irrigating fluids during transurethral resection in benign prostatic hyperplasia," *BMC Anesthesiology*, vol. 10, article 7, 2010.

[10] S. Gravas, A. Bachmann, A. Descazeaud et al., *EAU 2014 Guidelines on the Management of Male Lower Urinary Tract Symptoms (LUTS), incl*, Benign Prostatic Obstruction (BPO), 2014, http://uroweb.org/guideline/treatment-of-non-neurogenic-male-luts/.

[11] O. Reich, C. Gratzke, A. Bachmann et al., "Morbidity, mortality and early outcome of transurethral resection of the prostate: a prospective multicenter evaluation of 10,654 patients," *The Journal of Urology*, vol. 180, no. 1, pp. 246–249, 2008.

[12] H. Botto, T. Lebret, P. Barré, J.-L. Orsoni, J.-M. Hervé, and P.-M. Lugagne, "Electrovaporization of the prostate with the Gyrus device," *Journal of Endourology*, vol. 15, no. 3, pp. 313–316, 2001.

[13] M. I. Omar, T. B. Lam, C. E. Alexander et al., "Systematic review and meta-analysis of the clinical effectiveness of bipolar compared with monopolar transurethral resection of the prostate (TURP)," *BJU International*, vol. 113, no. 1, pp. 24–35, 2014.

[14] L. Qu, X. Wang, X. Huang, Y. Q. Zhang, and X. Zeng, "The hemostatic properties of transurethral plasmakinetic resection of the prostate: comparison with conventional resectoscope in an ex vivo study," *Urologia Internationalis*, vol. 80, no. 3, pp. 292–295, 2008.

[15] X. Huang, L. Wang, X.-H. Wang, H.-B. Shi, X.-J. Zhang, and Z.-Y. Yu, "Bipolar transurethral resection of the prostate causes deeper coagulation depth and less bleeding than monopolar transurethral prostatectomy," *Urology*, vol. 80, no. 5, pp. 1116–1120, 2012.

[16] W. D. Dunsmuir, J. P. McFarlane, A. Tan et al., "Gyrus bipolar electrovaporization vs transurethral resection of the prostate: a randomized prospective single-blind trial with 1 y follow-up," *Prostate Cancer and Prostatic Diseases*, vol. 6, no. 2, pp. 182–186, 2003.

[17] M. Miki, H. Shiozawa, T. Matsumoto, and T. Aizawa, "Transurethral resection in saline (TURis): a newly developed TUR system preventing obturator nerve reflex," *Nihon Hinyokika Gakkai Zasshi*, vol. 94, no. 7, pp. 671–677, 2003 (Japanese).

[18] J. Rassweiler, M. Schulze, C. Stock, D. Teber, and J. De La Rosette, "Bipolar transurethral resection of the prostate—technical modifications and early clinical experience," *Minimally Invasive Therapy and Allied Technologies*, vol. 16, no. 1, pp. 11–21, 2007.

[19] C. Mamoulakis, D. T. Ubbink, and J. J. M. C. H. de la Rosette, "Bipolar versus monopolar transurethral resection of the prostate: a systematic review and metaanalysis of randomized controlled trials," *European Urology*, vol. 56, no. 5, pp. 798–809, 2009.

[20] C. Mamoulakis, A. Skolarikos, M. Schulze et al., "Results from an international multicentre double-blind randomized controlled trial on the perioperative efficacy and safety of bipolar vs monopolar transurethral resection of the prostate," *BJU International*, vol. 109, no. 2, pp. 240–248, 2012.

[21] D. S. Finley, S. Beck, and R. J. Szabo, "Bipolar saline TURP for large prostate glands," *The Scientific World Journal*, vol. 7, pp. 1558–1562, 2007.

[22] M. Bhansali, S. Patankar, S. Dobhada, and S. Khaladkar, "Management of large (>60 g) prostate gland: PlasmaKinetic Superpulse (bipolar) versus conventional (monopolar) transurethral resection of the prostate," *Journal of Endourology*, vol. 23, no. 1, pp. 141–145, 2009.

[23] Q. Chen, L. Zhang, Y. J. Liu, J. D. Lu, and G. M. Wang, "Bipolar transurethral resection in saline system versus traditional monopolar resection system in treating large-volume benign prostatic hyperplasia," *Urologia Internationalis*, vol. 83, no. 1, pp. 55–59, 2009.

[24] D. P. J. Michielsen, D. Coomans, I. Peeters, and J. G. Braeckman, "Conventional monopolar resection or bipolar resection in saline for the management of large (>60 g) benign prostatic hyperplasia: an evaluation of morbidity," *Minimally Invasive Therapy & Allied Technologies*, vol. 19, no. 4, pp. 207–213, 2010.

[25] K. Komura, T. Inamoto, T. Takai et al., "Could transurethral resection of the prostate using the TURis system take over conventional monopolar transurethral resection of the prostate? A randomized controlled trial and midterm results," *Urology*, vol. 84, no. 2, pp. 405–411, 2014.

[26] G. Wendt-Nordahl, A. Häcker, K. Fastenmeer et al., "New bipolar resection device for transurethral resection of the prostate: first ex-vivo and in-vivo evaluation," *Journal of Endourology*, vol. 19, no. 10, pp. 1203–1209, 2005.

17

Lymphoma of the Urinary Bladder

Anthony Kodzo-Grey Venyo

North Manchester General Hospital, Department of Urology, Delaunays Road Crumpsall, Manchester, UK

Correspondence should be addressed to Anthony Kodzo-Grey Venyo; akodzogrey@yahoo.co.uk

Academic Editor: Fabio Campodonico

Background. Lymphoma of the urinary bladder (LUB) is rare. *Aims.* To review the literature on LUB. *Methods.* Various internet databases were used. *Results.* LUB can be either primary or secondary. The tumour has female predominance; most cases occur in middle-age women. Secondary LUB occurs in 10% to 25% of leukemias/lymphomas and in advanced-stage systemic lymphoma. Less than 100 cases have been reported. MALT typically affects adults older than 60 years; 75% are female. Diffuse large B-cell lymphoma is also common and may arise from transformation of MALT. LUB presents with haematuria, dysuria, urinary frequency, nocturia, and abdominal or back pain. Macroscopic examination of LUBs show large discrete tumours centred in the dome or lateral walls of the bladder. Positive staining of LUB varies by the subtype of lymphoma; B-cell lymphomas are CD20 positive. MALT lymphoma is positively stained for CD20, CD19, and FMC7 and negatively stained for CD5, CD10, and CD11c. LUB stains negatively with Pan-keratin, vimentin, CK20, and CK7. MALT lymphoma exhibits t(11; 18)(q21: 21). Radiotherapy is an effective treatment for the MALT type of LUB with no recurrence. *Conclusions.* LUB is diagnosed by its characteristic morphology and immunohistochemical characteristics. Radiotherapy is a useful treatment.

1. Introduction

Lymphoma of the urinary bladder is an uncommon lesion; and its diagnostic features may not be well known by the unaccustomed practitioner. The ensuing document contains a review of the literature on lymphoma of the urinary bladder.

2. Methods

The key words used for the search were Lymphoma of bladder; lymphoma of urinary bladder; vesical lymphoma. Documentations from 46 sources were found which had discussed various aspects relevant to lymphoma of the urinary bladder and information from these 46 sources were used to write the literature review.

3. Literature Review

3.1. Overview

Definition. Lymphoma of the urinary bladder can be either (a) primary lymphoma of the urinary bladder and this is a rare lymphoma originating in the urinary bladder with no known lymphoma elsewhere or (b) secondary lymphoma of the urinary bladder and this is much more common, and this secondary lymphoma is associated with a primary lymphoma originating in an extra vesical site [1].

Epidemiology. Lymphomas of the urinary bladder have a female predominance, and most cases of lymphoma of the urinary bladder occur in middle-age women [1]. Secondary involvement of the urinary bladder occurs in 10% to 25% of leukemias/lymphomas and they occur in advanced-stage systemic lymphoma [1]. Less than 100 cases of lymphoma of the urinary bladder have been reported so far [1]. MALT is the most common subtype of lymphomas in the urinary bladder and this typically affects adults who are more than 60 years old and 75% are female [1]. It has been reported that diffuse large B-cell lymphoma is also common, and it may arise from transformation of MALT [2].

Sites. Lymphoma may involve the urinary bladder and the lower ureteral tract [1].

Clinical Features. Lymphoma comprises 5% of nonurothelial tumours of the urothelial tract [1]. Kempton et al. [3] reported long median survival for either primary lymphoma of bladder or lymphoma with initial presentation in the urinary bladder but other coexisting diseases [3]. Recurrent lymphoma in the urinary bladder is associated with widely disseminated disease and poor prognosis [1]. It has been stated that low-grade MALT lymphoma is the most common lymphoma subtype in the urinary bladder; it is much more common as secondary tumour than primary tumour, and a history of chronic cystitis is commonly associated with this type of tumour [4].

Presentation. Lymphoma of the urinary bladder presents with visible haematuria, dysuria, urinary frequency, nocturia, and abdominal pain or back pain [1].

Radiological Imaging. The radiological investigations of lymphoma of the urinary bladder reveal submucosal masses: 70% of cases are solitary masses; 20% of cases are multiple masses; and 10% of cases show diffuse bladder wall thickening [1].

Macroscopic Description. Macroscopic examination of lymphomas of the urinary bladder shows discrete tumours which are large and centred in the dome or lateral walls of the urinary bladder [1].

Microscopic Description. MALT lymphomas exhibit sheets of low-grade, uniform cells which surround and separate but do not destroy muscle fascicles [1].

Cytology Description. MALT lymphomas of the urinary bladder tend to exhibit monomorphic small- to medium-sized lymphocytes [1].

Immunohistological Staining. Positive staining of lymphomas of the urinary bladder varies by the subtype of lymphoma; B-cell lymphomas are CD20 positive [1].

MALT lymphoma is positively stained for CD20, CD19, and it is negatively stained for CD5, CD10, and CD11c but it is positively stained for FMC7 [1].

Lymphomas of the urinary bladder stain negatively with Pan-keratin, vimentin, CK20, and CK7 [1].

Molecular/Cytogenetics Description. MALT lymphoma exhibits t(11; 18)(q21 : 21) [1].

Prognostic Factors. The prognostic factors of lymphoma of the urinary bladder include histological subtype and the stage of the tumour [1].

Treatment. Radiotherapy is the treatment for the MALT type of lymphoma of the urinary bladder and usually there is no recurrence of tumour following such treatment [1].

Differential Diagnosis. The differential diagnoses of lymphoma of the urinary bladder include

   (i) urothelial carcinoma with prominent lymphoid infiltrate [5];

   (ii) undifferentiated carcinoma [1].

3.2. Narrations from Reported Cases. Cohen et al. [6] stated that the first recorded case of lymphoma of the bladder was reported by Eve and Chaffey in 1885 [6]. They also stated that malignant lymphoma of the urinary bladder can be classified into one of three different clinical groups as follows:

   (i) primary lymphoma localized to the bladder;

   (ii) lymphoma presenting in the bladder as the first sign of disseminated disease (nonlocalized lymphoma);

   (iii) recurrent urinary bladder involvement by lymphoma in patients with a history of malignant lymphoma (secondary lymphoma).

Cohen et al. [6] also stated that primary extranodal marginal zone lymphoma of mucosa-associated lymphoid tissue (MALT type) of the urinary bladder, which was first described by Kempton et al. [3] in 1990, is the most common primary bladder lymphoma and is associated with an excellent prognosis. Cohen et al. [6] also reported a patient with visible haematuria who was found to have a primary lymphoma of the urinary bladder.

Bates et al. [2] reported the clinical and histological features and outcomes of primary and secondary malignant lymphomas of the urinary bladder [2]. They obtained eleven cases of malignant lymphoma of the urinary bladder from the registry of cases of St Bartholomew's and the Royal London Hospitals in the UK. They classified the lymphomas on the basis of their morphology immunophenotype. They also reviewed the clinical records of the patients. Bates et al. [2] reported that there were six primary lymphomas: three extranodal marginal zone lymphomas of mucosa-associated lymphoid tissue (MALT) type and three diffuse large B-cell lymphomas. Of the five secondary cases, four were diffuse large B-cell lymphomas, one secondary to a systemic follicular centre lymphoma, and one nodular sclerosis Hodgkin's disease. Bates et al. [2] also reported the following.

   (i) Four patients with secondary lymphoma, for whom followup was available, had died of disease within 13 months of diagnosis.

   (ii) Primary lymphomas followed a more indolent course.

   (iii) In one case, there was evidence of transformation from low-grade MALT type to diffuse B-cell lymphoma.

   (iv) The most common presenting symptom was haematuria.

   (v) The cystoscopic appearances were of solid, sometimes necrotic, tumours which resembled transitional cell carcinomas, and in one case the tumours were multiple.

Bates et al. [2] stated that these cases represented 0.2% of all neoplasms of the urinary bladder. Bates et al. [2] made the following conclusions.

   (i) Diffuse large B-cell lymphoma and MALT-type lymphoma are the most common primary malignant lymphomas of the bladder.

(ii) Lymphoepithelial lesions in MALT-type lymphoma involve transitional epithelium, and their presence in high-grade lymphoma suggests a primary origin owing to transformation of low-grade MALT-type lymphoma.

(iii) Primary and secondary diffuse large B-cell lymphomas of the bladder are histologically similar, but the prognosis of the former is favourable.

Kempton et al. [3] studied patients with malignant lymphoma of the bladder, and they defined three clinical groups: those with primary lymphoma localized in the bladder, lymphoma presenting in the bladder as the first sign of disseminated disease (nonlocalized lymphoma), and recurrent bladder involvement by lymphoma in patients with a history of malignant lymphoma (secondary lymphoma). They studied differences in these groups regarding lymphoma type, clinical presentation, and clinical outcome. Kempton et al. [3] searched the Mayo Clinic Tissue Registry records from 1940 to 1996 to identify patients with lymphomas involving the bladder. The lymphomas were classified based on review of the histology and immunophenotype performed by immunoperoxidase methods. Kempton et al. [3] also reviewed the clinical records. They reported the following.

(i) The presenting symptoms included urinary frequency, dysuria, haematuria, and lower abdominal and back pain.

(ii) Primary lymphoma was present in six patients. All were B-cell-lineage, low-grade lymphomas of the mucosa-associated lymphoid tissue (MALT) type.

(iii) No patient had recurrent lymphoma or died of lymphoma.

(iv) Nonlocalized bladder lymphoma occurred in 17 patients: one with low-grade lymphoma of the MALT type, four with follicle centre lymphomas, and 12 with large cell lymphomas.

(v) Excluding two patients who died postoperatively, median survival was 9 years. Six patients died of lymphoma in the follow-up period.

(vi) Secondary bladder lymphoma occurred in 13 patients: two with low-grade lymphoma of the MALT type, one with follicle centre lymphoma, one with mantle cell lymphoma, and nine with diffuse large cell lymphomas. Median survival in this group was 0.6 years.

(vii) Low-grade lymphoma of the MALT type was the most frequent type of primary bladder lymphoma and was associated with an excellent prognosis.

They concluded that:

(i) The bladder can be the presenting site of lymphomatous involvement in patients with more widespread disease.

(ii) Survival in this group is quite favourable and is presumably dependent on lymphoma histologic type, stage of disease, and other prognostic factors.

(iii) Bladder involvement by recurrent lymphoma is a sign of widely disseminated disease and is associated with a very poor prognosis.

Al-Maghrabi et al. [4] in 2001 stated that primary lymphoma of the urinary bladder is rare and only 84 cases were reported in the English literature at the time of their publication, but none of these cases had had molecular confirmation of clonal immunoglobulin gene rearrangement. They reviewed all cases with primary urinary bladder lymphoma in their records to classify them using the REAL classification, to confirm their immunophenotype and genotype, and to determine their outcome. They identified 4 cases of primary urinary bladder lymphoma in their medical records from a 30-year period. They performed immunohistochemical detection of immunoglobulin light chains and molecular analysis of immunoglobulin heavy-chain genes using the polymerase chain reaction on paraffin-embedded material. They reported the following.

(i) All patients were older than 60 years.

(ii) The male-female ratio was 1 : 3.

(iii) All patients had a history of chronic cystitis.

(iv) Histologic features of mucosa-associated lymphoid tissue lymphoma with centrocyte-like cells, plasmacytoid occurred.

(v) B cells or both were observed in all cases.

(vi) Monoclonality of B cells was demonstrated by immunohistochemistry, polymerase chain reaction, or both methods in every case.

(vii) All patients presented with stage IAE disease were treated with radiotherapy alone and had been in continuous complete remission for 2 to 13 years.

(viii) On immunophenotyping, light-chain restriction was demonstrated in 3 cases (cases 2, 3, and 4) (results are summarized in Table 2).

(ix) Flow cytometric data were available for case 4 and showed typical marginal zone B-cell immunophenotype (positive for CD45 and CD20; negative for CD5, CD23, and CD10) with k light-chain restriction and an S phase of 1%, which is consistent with a low-grade lymphoma.

(x) PCR for immunoglobulin heavy-chain gene polymerase chain reaction analyses (Figure 3) revealed clonal immunoglobulin heavy-chain (IgH) gene rearrangement in 3 cases (cases 1, 2, and 4); PCR was not informative in case 3. Immunohistochemistry, however, showed k light-chain restriction as well as a heavy-chain restriction in this case.

They concluded the following.

(i) Primary bladder lymphomas are usually of low-grade mucosa-associated lymphoid tissue type.

(ii) They were more common in females and had been associated with a history of chronic cystitis.

TABLE 1: Clinical Summary of the four cases.

Case number	Age, years/sex	Presentation	Stage	Treatment	Follow-up years
1	64, female	Hematuria and frequency	IAE	Radiation	13
2	69, female	Frequency and urgency	IAE	Radiation	5
3	72, female	Hematuria and nocturia	IAE	Radiation	3
4	62, male	Hematuria and urgency	IAE	Radiation	2

Reproduced from [4] with permission of the Editor-in-Chief of Archives of Pathology and Laboratory Medicine on behalf of the editorial team of the journal and the American Association of Pathology.

(iii) Lymphoepithelial lesions were seen only in association with areas of cystitis glandularis.

(iv) B-cell clonality was readily demonstrable by immunohistochemistry and/or polymerase chain reaction analysis.

(v) Local radiotherapy appeared to confer long-term control (see Figures 1, 2, and 3 which show the morphology of 3 of the four tumours and Table 1 which shows the clinical findings of the 4 cases and Table 2 which shows the immunohistochemical and polymerase chain reaction (PCR) findings of the tumours).

Sufrin et al. [7] reported on a study of 599 patients who had died of malignant lymphoma between 1952 and 1972 and this revealed involvement of the bladder in 13 per cent. Bladder involvement was always a secondary event, which occurred in association with disseminated disease and was more common in non-Hodgkin's lymphoma than in Hodgkin's disease. They reported the following.

(i) Direct infiltration from adjacent pelvic foci as well as discrete apparent metastatic foci was noted.

(ii) Involvement was usually microscopic although the presence of gross disease was invariably clinically manifest.

(iii) Cystoscopy and cystography were valuable in the diagnosis of gross lesions.

(iv) In contrast to primary vesical lymphoma, the treatment of secondary vesical lymphoma was symptomatic and an operation was indicated rarely.

(v) Local radiotherapy was effective in treating the symptoms of secondary vesical lymphoma.

Kuhara et al. [8] reported a patient with primary malignant lymphoma of the urinary bladder. They reported that grossly, the bladder showed multiple submucosal masses. Histologically and immunohistochemically, diffuse B-cell lymphoma of the medium-sized cell type was revealed. They stated the following.

(i) On the basis of clinicopathological features, the case resembled previously recorded cases of bladder lymphoma.

(ii) The pathogenesis of the primary bladder lymphoma was presumably associated with follicular or chronic cystitis.

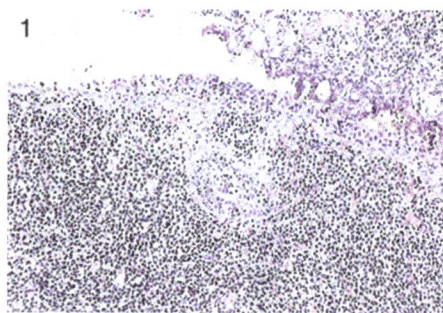

FIGURE 1: The microscopic feature of the second cases (haematoxylin and eosin staining). Case 2: mucosa-associated lymphoid tissue lymphoma involving the lamina propria of the urinary bladder (hematoxylin-eosin, original magnification ×100). Reproduced from [4] with permission of the Editor-in-Chief of Archives of Pathology and Laboratory Medicine on behalf of the editorial team of the journal and the American Association of Pathology.

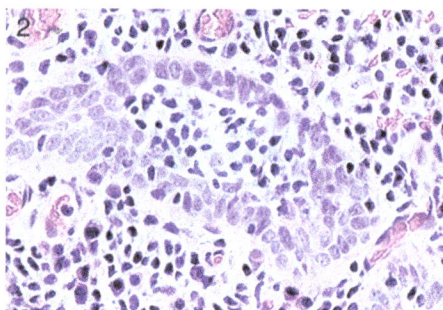

FIGURE 2: The microscopic feature of the second cases (haematoxylin and eosin staining). Case 2: focal lymphoepithelial lesions in area of cystitis glandularis (hematoxylin-eosin, original magnification ×400). Reproduced from [4] with permission of the Editor-in-Chief of Archives of Pathology and Laboratory Medicine on behalf of the editorial team of the journal and the American Association of Pathology.

(iii) Primary lymphoma of the bladder is a condition that is very rarely included in a series of extranodal lymphomas, and there is a curious sex difference in its occurrence rates between Japan and Western countries.

(iv) Primary lymphoma of the bladder may be considered a lymphoma that originates from mucosa-associated lymphoid tissue.

Sönmezer et al. [9] reported a 58-year-old woman who was suffering from chronic pelvic pain, pelvic pressure,

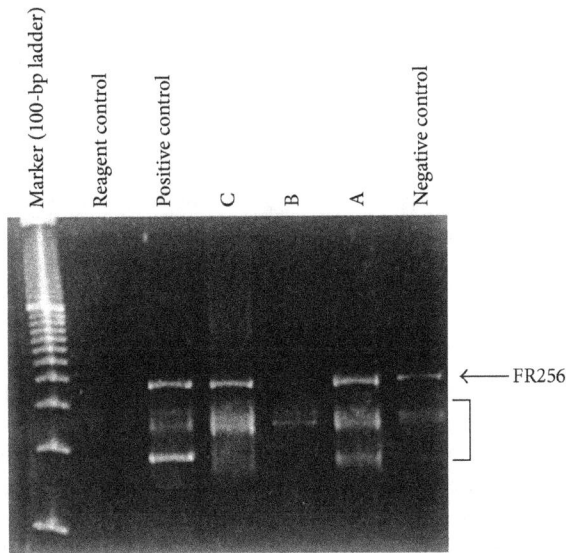

FIGURE 3: Case 4: B-cell-specific polymerase chain reaction using primers directed at the framework 256 (FR256) regions of the immunoglobulin heavy-chain gene (IgH). The top arrow represents the internal control that is used to ensure the presence of amplifiable DNA in each sample. The bracket in the FR256 figure denotes the size range in which IgH gene products can be seen. Although the DNA is degraded and the signal is weak, patient B (case 4) clearly shows the presence of a clonally rearranged IgH gene using the FR256 primers. Clonal rearrangements of IgH genes were also noted in cases 1 and 2 (not shown in figure). Lanes A and C are from cases unrelated to this paper. Reproduced from [4] with permission of the Editor-in-Chief of Archives of Pathology and Laboratory Medicine on behalf of the editorial team of the journal and the American Association of Pathology.

dysuria, and genitourinary bleeding for 2 months. On gynaecological examination, her uterus was found to have a semifixed cervix which was mobile and a solid, irregular mass was also found with a size of 10 cm that was located anterior to her right adnexa. She had ultrasound scan which confirmed a solid mass with indefinite borders. Her CA 125 level was normal. On digital rectal examination, the rectal mucosa was normal. PAP smear and endometrial biopsy were without any pathology. To find out the origin of the bleeding, a cystoscopy evaluation and an intravenous pyelogram were performed which revealed an irregular, necrotic, solid submucosal mass at the dome of the bladder. Histopathological and immunophenotypic evaluation of the biopsy specimen performed thereafter by immunoperoxidase methods using Streptavidin-Biotin peroxidase system revealed a high-grade B-type malignant lymphoma. Following the establishment of the diagnosis as postmenopausal adnexal mass and lymphoma of the urinary bladder, the patient was reevaluated with clinical investigations which included complete blood count, tumour markers, peripheral blood smear and bone marrow biopsy, and radiological investigations which included computed tomography; these revealed no evidence of tumour elsewhere. An exploratory-laparotomy was undertaken which revealed that the urinary bladder was adherent to the anterior abdominal wall, omentum, uterus, and right adnexa forming a conglomerate mass.

The peritoneal surface was free of any metastatic spread. There was no sign of fistula formation. After mobilization of the bladder, a cystotomy was performed and a solid, necrotic mass originating from bladder mucosa at the dome was found which also invaded the bladder wall. The mass was removed completely by partial cystectomy with a 2 cm margin of normal tissue. Total abdominal hysterectomy and bilateral oophorectomy were also performed. The retroperitoneal lymph nodes were found not to be enlarged by palpation. She received four courses of CHOP regimen (cyclophosphamide, vincristine, doxorubicin, and prednisolone). The rebiopsy performed from the dome of the bladder on the 3rd and 6th months postoperatively were normal. During a followup of 6 years, the patient was complaint-free and no local or distant recurrence was found. Sönmezer et al. [9] stated that primary lymphoma of the urinary bladder is a fairly uncommon entity, whereas urinary tract involvement is reported in up to 13% of the cases with advanced systemic disease [7].

Primary malignant lymphoma of the urinary bladder was first described in 1885 and marked female preponderance was reported with a female to male ratio of 6.5 : 1 [10].

The most common types of primary lymphoma of the urinary bladder are

(i) extranodal marginal zone lymphoma of mucosa-associated lymphoid tissue type (MALT-type lymphoma)

(ii) diffuse large B-cell lymphoma.

The development of lymphomas in a site normally not including lymphoid tissue was explained by the MALT concept, which was first described by Isaacson and Wright. They in 1983 [28] reported a 58-year-old woman who had primary high-grade B-type malignant lymphoma and who presented with genitourinary bleeding and a large pelvic mass that appeared as a gynaecological tumour [28].

Ohsawa et al. [10] stated the following.

(i) In mucosa-associated lymphoid tissue, such as neoplasms arising in indigenous lymphoid tissues, primary malignant lymphoma of the urinary bladder is a fairly uncommon disease and this accounts for 0.2% of cases with extranodal lymphoma, mostly appearing in the sixth decade.

(ii) It had been stated that a significant proportion of extranodal non-Hodgkin lymphomas is known to arise from the intestine or lung, or from chronic inflammatory conditions. Since lymphoid tissue is normally not found in the urinary bladder, preexisting chronic inflammation is postulated as the origin. Nevertheless, in most of the cases, as in their case, history of chronic cystitis and histologic evidence of such an inflammation were lacking [2, 10, 27] and therefore uncertainty still exists regarding the role of chronic cystitis in the development of lymphoma.

(iii) A review of the literature revealed that the most apparent symptoms of lymphoma of the urinary bladder are haematuria, dysuria, nocturia, urinary frequency, suprapubic or abdominal pain, weight loss, and anorexia [10, 27].

TABLE 2: Immunohistochemical and polymerase chain reaction (PCR) findings*.

Case number	CD45	CD20	CD45RO	CD5	CD10	CD43	K & L	PCR
1	+	+	I	ND	ND	−	I	Monoclonal
2	+	+	−	−	−	−	LLCR	Monoclonal
3	+	+	−	−	−	−	KLCR	I
4	+	+	−	−	−	F+	K:CR	Monoclonal

*Plus sign indicates positive reaction; I: inconclusive; minus sign: negative reaction; ND: not done; Fl: focally positive; LLCR: l-light chain restriction; and KLCR: k-light chain restriction.
Reproduced from [4] with permission of the Editor-in-Chief of Archives of Pathology and Laboratory Medicine on behalf of the editorial team of the journal and the American Association of Pathology.

Isaacson and Wright [28] stated the following.

(i) In their reported case, the disease (lymphoma of the bladder) presented as a pelvic mass showing strict adhesions with adjacent pelvis organs which resembled a genital cancer. But they initially thought that the patient had both a primary lymphoma of the bladder and an adnexal mass.

(ii) Following an extensive work-up and histopathological evaluation of the biopsy specimen, a high-grade B-type lymphoma was diagnosed.

Lymphoma of the bladder is proposed to have characteristic cystoscopic appearance that can aid in diagnosis and is usually described as a smooth, nonulcerative, friable, or haemorrhagic submucosal tumour [26].

It was stated that treatment of patients with primary lymphoma of the bladder includes many options with favourable prognosis. Ohsawa et al. [10] stated that:

(i) In their review of the literature, they found that multimodality therapy including surgical resection followed by chemotherapy or radiation therapy provided favourable prognosis.

(ii) Only 3 of 27 patients died and 23 of 24 patients had no evidence of disease at the 31-month followup.

(iii) In another review by Kempton et al. [3], none of the 6 patients died as a result of lymphoma.

(iv) The extent of surgery did not seem to affect the prognosis, since a similar proportion died or had recurrence, regardless of total or partial cystectomy/resection performed [27].

(v) The combination therapy including surgery and chemotherapy resulted in a 6-year disease-free survival in their patient.

(vi) Based on the findings in the literature and in their case, they concluded that therapy including surgery along with radiation or chemotherapy for primary lymphoma of the bladder provides a good prognosis, even in case of a large adhesive mass.

Ando et al. [22] reported a 77-year-old woman, who presented with a sensation of urinary retention and symptoms which were suggestive of cystitis and she was treated with antibiotics, but her symptoms did not subside. She had an intravenous pyelogram and cystoscopy which revealed a wide-based submucosal mass which measured 3 cm in the left wall of the urinary bladder. Histological findings of the tissue which was obtained by means of transurethral resection (TUR) revealed a dense, monomorphic atypical lymphoid (centrocyte-like) infiltrate with reactive lymph follicles in the subepithelial tissue. Monocytoid and plasmacytoid features were readily evident in a population of these cells. Lymphoepithelial lesions involving the urothelium were also noticed in some areas. These features were considered to be strongly suggestive of primary low-grade B-cell lymphoma of the MALT type. The diagnosis was confirmed by immunohistochemical and flow cytometric studies, both of which showed a clear immunoglobulin restriction to lambda light chain and also by polymerase chain reaction-based assay using a formalin-fixed paraffin-embedded TUR tissue sample, which showed a clonal Ig heavy-chain gene rearrangement. Clinical staging procedures revealed that the tumour was localized in the urinary bladder. The patient did not receive any chemotherapy and she was alive and well with no evidence of recurrence, 3 years after she had undergone trans-urethral resection (TUR) of her bladder tumour. Ando et al. [22] stated that the case demonstrated that these ancillary tests are worth-performing for the confirmation of B-cell clonality in trans-urethral resected (TUR) tissue samples showing dense B-lymphocytic infiltration.

Tsiriopoulos et al. [25] reported the case of a 76-year-old woman who had a past medical history of low-grade chronic lymphocytic leukaemia. She presented with severe chronic bladder symptoms which were attributed to interstitial cystitis. She underwent cystectomy and ileal conduit formation after the failure of all conventional treatments. Histopathological examination of the bladder revealed primary splenic marginal zone lymphoma. They reviewed the literature which showed the rarity of such nonhematopoietic visceral metastases. They stated that their case may represent the first reported splenic marginal zone lymphoma with bladder involvement and highlighted the clinical and histological similarities with interstitial cystitis.

Rijo et al. [35] reported a 27-year-old female who presented with acute urinary retention. She underwent gynaecological examination which revealed a 30 mm × 40 mm × 30 mm widely pedunculated, firm, smooth, paraurethral mass without discharge, arising close to the external urethral orifice. Her past medical and surgical history was otherwise unremarkable, with no history of previous urinary tract symptoms. She had voiding cystourethrogram (VCUG)

TABLE 3: Some of the reported cases of lymphoma of the urinary bladder mainly primary with other cases of paraurethral lymphoma, their management and outcome.

References of cases	Treatment types	Follow-up duration	Complete remission	Partial remission	No response	Total sex/age histology
Raderer et al. [11]	RCHOP or RCNOP regime	19 months mean Range 10–45	20 (77%)	6 (23%)	0	26 patients with MALT lymphoma of bladder
Terasaki et al. [12]	Radiotherapy Gy 26 and Rituximab chemotherapy after remission	14 months	1 patient			1 female aged 64 years with MALT lymphoma of bladder
Takahara et al. [13]	TURBT and Radiotherapy 40 Gy in 20 fractions	3 monthly intervals to, duration is not available to author	1 patient			1 female aged 85 years with extranodal marginal zone B-cell lymphoma
Kakuta et al. [14]	Rituximab in combination with CHOPP chemotherapy after transurethral biopsy	Duration is not available to author	1 patient			1 female aged 84 years with extranodal marginal zone B-cell lymphoma of bladder
Siegel and Napoli [15]	Extensive resection	Duration is not stated	Alive, but outcome with regard to response is not available to author	Alive, but outcome with regard to response is not available to author		1 elderly female with B-cell lymphoma of dome of bladder with signet ring cell component
Hayashi et al. [16]	3 courses of R CHOPP chemotherapy	Duration is not available to author	1 patient			1 female age not available to author with DCBCL (primary diffuse large B-cell lymphoma of urinary bladder)
Abraham et al. [17]	Resectional biopsy and non-Hodgkin's lymphoma therapy	Duration is not stated	1			1 female aged 72 years with extranodal monocytoid B-cell lymphoma (MBCL) derived from marginal zone lymphocyte
Sundaram and Zhang [18]	Resection but details of further management not available	Details is not available to author				1 female aged 67 years with localized Epstein-Barr virus (EBV) positive B-cell lymphoproliferative disorder (LPD)/polymorphous B-cell lymphoma of the bladder

TABLE 3: Continued.

References of cases	Treatment types	Follow-up duration	Complete remission	Partial remission	No response	Total sex/age histology
Oh and Zang [19]	Transurethral resection biopsy and two cycles of systemic cyclophosphamide, doxorubicin, vincristine, and prednisone (CHOPP) chemotherapy	Duration is not stated	1 patient with simultaneous restoration of urinary function			1 male aged 35 years with diffuse large B-cell lymphoma (non-Hodgkin's lymphoma)
Wang et al. [20]	TURBT and four cycles of CHOPP (cyclophosphamide, doxorubicin, vincristine, and prednisone) chemotherapy	12 months	1 with good response and remained in clinical remission for 12 months after treatment			1 male aged 45 years with T-cell lymphoma of urinary bladder
Mourad et al. [21]	Transurethral resection biopsy of lesion and CHOPP chemotherapy and he received cyclophosphamide, doxorubicin, vincristine, and prednisone	Duration not available to author: appeared case was reported earlier without details of long-term follow-up	Response not available			1 male aged 52 years who had shistosomiasis and found to have T-cell lymphoma of urinary bladder which Mourad et al. [21] felt was induced by shistosomiasis
Ando et al. [22]	Transurethral resection of bladder tumour only	3 years	1			1 female aged 77 years with primary low-grade B-cell lymphoma of the MALT type
Simpson et al. [23]	Details not available to author	Details are not available to author	Details not available to author	—	—	1 female with T-cell primary lymphoma of bladder and urethra
Mearini et al. [24]	Transurethral resection of bladder tumour (Burkitt's lymphoma) plus subsequent antiretroviral treatment with stavudine (40 mg twice daily), lamivudine (150 mg twice daily), and nelfinavir (750 mg 3 times daily), as well as antitumour polychemotherapy (4 cycles of cyclophosphamide, vincristine, doxorubicin, and dexamethasone, alternated with 4 cycles of methotrexate and cytarabine)	8 months of followup	Complete resolution and biopsy of small mucosal lesion at site of previous tumour 8 months later only showed fibrous tissue on immunohisto-chemical and histological examination			27-year-old man with Burkitt's lymphoma

TABLE 3: Continued.

References of cases	Treatment types	Follow-up duration	Complete remission	Partial remission	No response	Total sex/age histology
Tsiriopoulos et al. [25]	Cystectomy and ileal conduit after failure of conservative treatment for presumed interstitial cystitis	Details are not available to author	Details are not available to author	Details are not available to author	Details are not available to author	75-year-old patient with past history of chronic lymphatic leukaemia histology of bladder showed primary splenic marginal zone lymphoma simulating interstitial cystitis
Downs et al. [26]	Details are not available to author	Details are not available to author	Details are not available to author	Details are not available to author	Details are not available to author	They concluded that primary lymphoma of the bladder has a good prognosis and responds to a variety of therapeutic modalities
Simpson et al. [27]	3 cases	7 years. 39 months. Details are not available to author	Alive and free of tumour. Died after 39 months. Details are not available to author			A 70-year-old man with low grade type A 67-year-old woman with intermediate-grade type 76-year-old woman with lymphoma in the urethra
Isaacson and Wright [28]	2 cases, details are not available to author	Details are not available to author	Details are not available to author	Details are not available to author	Details are not available to author	Details are not available to author
Ohsawa et al. [10]	3 cases, details are not available to author	Details are not available to author	Details are not available to author	Details are not available to author	Details are not available to author	Details are not available to author
Sönmezer et al. [9]	Transurethral biopsy, partial cystectomy, total hysterectomy, bilateral oophorectomy, and four courses of CHOP regimen (cyclophosphamide, vincristine, doxorubicin, and prednisolone)	6 years	Alive and well with no local recurrence of distant metastasis			1 female aged 50 years with high-grade B-cell lymphoma

TABLE 3: Continued.

References of cases	Treatment types	Follow-up duration	Complete remission	Partial remission	No response	Total sex/age histology
Kuhara et al. [8]		Details of duration of followup are not available to author	Outcome is not available to author	Outcome is not available to author		Diffuse B-cell lymphoma of medium-sized cell
Sufrin et al. [7]	13% of 599 patients with malignant lymphoma had secondary bladder involvement and were treated with local radiotherapy	1952 to 1972	Good response			13% of 599 patients with secondary bladder lymphoma (details of the various types are not available to author)
Cohen et al. [6]	Details of case are not available to author	Details of case are not available to author	Details of case are not available to author	Details of case are not available to author	Details of case are not available to author	1 case of primary B-cell lymphoma of bladder
Zukerberg et al. [5]	5 cases (diagnosis of malignant lymphoma was excluded in 1 leaving 4 as lymphoma of T-cell type. Of 2 muscle invasive tumours, 2 cases were too recent to have followup	4 Too recent for followup	1 alive with no tumour after 4 years following radiotherapy. and chemotherapy. Details are not available to author			
Al-Maghrabi et al. [4]	Radiotherapy (35 Gy)	13 years, 5 years, 3 years, 2 years, respectively	Alive no recurrence. Alive no recurrence. Alive no recurrence. Alive with no disease			64-year-old female, stage IAE; 69-year-old female, low-grade MALT lymphoma, stage IAE; 72-year-old female, low-grade lymphoma of MALT type-stage IAE; 62-years-old male, B-cell malignant lymphoma of MALT type-stage IAE
Mantzarides et al. [29]	Details of treatment are not available to author	Further details are not available to author	Further details are not available to author	Further details are not available to author	Further details are not available to author	82-year-old female with primary diffuse large B-cell lymphoma of the bladder wall

TABLE 3: Continued.

References of cases	Treatment types	Follow-up duration	Complete remission	Partial remission	No response	Total sex/age histology
Evans and Moore [30]	Transurethral biopsy of bladder tumour and she received a course of R-CHOP (cyclophosphamide, doxorubicin, vincristine, prednisolone, and rituximab) chemotherapy	4 months		CT scan showed regression of lesion and symptomatic improvement		64-year-old female with histologically proven diffuse large B-Cell non-Hodgkin's lymphoma (primary)
Arda et al. [31]	Open biopsy; she refused surgical operation and was referred to oncologist for chemotherapy	Further details are not available to author	Further details are not available to author	Further details are not available to author	Further details are not available to author	54-year-old female had open biopsy proven to be malignant non-Hodgkin's lymphoma
Aceñero, et al. [32]	Details are not available to author	Details are not available to author	Details are not available to author	Details are not available to author	Details are not available to author	3 cases of primary malignant lymphoma of urinary bladder (2 of high grade) of MALT type
Jacobs and Symington [33]	Cystectomy	3 years	Alive and well with no recurrence of locally or distant metastasis			61-year-old woman with primary lymphoma of urinary bladder
Diaz-Peromingo et al. [34]	TUR biopsies and CNOP (cyclophosphamide, mitoxantrone, vincristine, and prednisolone) and monoclonal antibodies anti-CD20	Short period of follow-up case reported shortly after initial treatment	Good initial response			79-year-old man tumour B-cell lymphoma (non-Hodgkin's) which was initially thought to be primary; however, PER scan confirmed that it was a secondary bladder lymphoma

TABLE 3: Continued.

References of cases	Treatment types	Follow-up duration	Complete remission	Partial remission	No response	Total sex/age histology
	Open per vaginal partial excision of paraurerethal lesion. extending to the trigone of the bladder (this was a paraurethal lesion not a bladder lesion). Six cycles of immunochemotherapy: anti-CD20 (Rituximab) combined with chemotherapy (high doses of methotrexate and cytarabine with conventional cystostatics and prophylactic					
Rijo et al. [35]	administration of G-CSF after chemotherapy cycles). After the completion of the third cycle of treatment, the patient achieved near-complete remission as well as a nearly complete regression of the paraurethral tumour and the lesion of the 5th lumbar vertebra. Haematological grade 2 toxicity and gastrointestinal grade 1 toxicity were reported	9 months	1			1 female aged 27 years
Hatano et al. [36]	Transurethral resection of bladder tumour and left total nephroureterectomy; histology adenocarcinoma G2pT2 in renal pelvis and MALT-type lymphoma of bladder; radiotherapy 36 Gy to bladder	14 months	Alive with no evidence of recurrence			84-year-old with MALT-type lymphoma of bladder and adenocarcinoma of left renal pelvis

and computed tomography (CT) scan which revealed a paraurethral mass. Pelvic magnetic resonance imaging (MRI) was performed as a supplementary diagnostic tool and this confirmed the presence of a large, well-circumscribed, paraurethral mass. She underwent cystoscopy which confirmed the urethral protrusions at the bladder neck region. A provisional diagnosis of paraurethral leiomyoma was made on the basis of the cystoscopic examination, as well as radiological and clinical findings. The proposed treatment involved surgical removal of the mass. An open vaginal approach was selected; the paraurethral tissue was diffusely infiltrated and the mass was partially removed. Intraoperative frozen section histological examination showed a small-cell lymphoproliferative tumour, so the surgical procedure was discontinued. The postoperative course was uneventful, and the urethral catheter was left inside the urinary bladder for three weeks. After removal of the urethral catheter, the patient developed mild stress urinary incontinence.

Histology of the haematoxylin-eosin-stained tissue revealed a highly cellularized tumour which displayed a diffuse, infiltrating pattern, a medullary, cohesive proliferation of medium-sized neoplastic cells, monomorphic, medium-sized cells with round nuclei, multiple nucleoli, and a basophilic cytoplasm. A "starry-sky" pattern was observed with frequent mitotic figures.

Immunohistochemical stains were negative for antibodies against CD23, CD3, CD5, bcl2, bcl6, TDT, and p53. Tumour cells were positive for CD79a, CD20, CD43, CD10, MUM1, and Ki67 (100%). Fluorescence in situ hybridization (FISH) for MYC/IGH/CEP8 revealed t(8; 14)(q24; q32). However, Epstein-Barr virus RNA was not detectable. Polymerase chain reaction (PCR) analysis was used to analyse the rearrangement of VH region genes. By amplifying the complementarity-determining region III using PCR, it was discovered that CDRIII, CDRII, and CDRI showed a clonal pattern. All of the phenotypic features mentioned supported the diagnosis of Burkitt's lymphoma.

Based on the presumptive diagnosis of primary paraurethral Burkitt lymphoma (BL), the patient had a full workup that included a bone marrow aspirate/biopsy, viral serologies, MRI evaluation, and PET/CT to rule out metastatic origin of the paraurethral Burkitt's lymphoma (BL). The bone marrow aspirate and biopsy revealed normocellular haematopoiesis, and no tumour cells were detected based on negative immunohistochemical analysis (CD79a, CD20, and CD3). Tumour markers and a screening test for Epstein-Barr virus, human immunodeficiency virus, hepatitis virus, and cytomegalovirus were all negative. She had magnetic resonance imaging (MRI) scan which showed a T2-weighted hypersignal at the fifth lumbar vertebra. The F-2-fluoro-D-deoxyglucose positron emission tomography CT (FDG-PET/CT) revealed increased FDG uptake in pelvic, bilateral iliac internal/external lymph nodes, and significant activity in the fifth lumbar vertebra.

The patient was referred for six cycles of immunochemotherapy: anti-CD20 (Rituximab) combined with chemotherapy (high doses of methotrexate and cytarabine with conventional cystostatics and prophylactic administration of G-CSF after chemotherapy cycles).

After the completion of the third cycle of treatment, the patient achieved near-complete remission as well as a nearly complete regression of the paraurethral tumor and the lesion of the 5th lumbar vertebra. Haematological grade 2 toxicity and gastrointestinal grade 1 toxicity were reported.

Her followup was uneventful, and at the nine-month followup a total body computed tomography (CT) scan revealed no evidence of clinical progression (either local recurrence or other distant metastasis).

The patient was still alive with a good quality of life and without clinical evidence of tumour progression.

Some authors [23, 24] stated that primary genitourinary lymphomas are uncommon, and, in particular, primary Burkitt's lymphoma (BL) of the bladder or genitourinary tissue is extremely rare [23, 37].

Other authors stated that most frequently, genitourinary lymphoma reflects widespread metastasis which was caused by a systemic haematological disease [37].

Burkitt's lymphoma (BL) was first described in 1958 in Uganda by a surgeon who observed children with rapidly enlarging tumours which involved the jaw. Since then, Burkitt's lymphoma (BL) has been categorized by the World Health Organization (WHO) into three types which include the endemic type, the sporadic type, and the immunodeficiency-associated types [38].

It has been stated that the endemic form of Burkitt's lymphoma is found mostly in equatorial Africa and in Papua New Guinea and this form of Burkitt's lymphoma is associated with the Epstein-Barr virus in 95% of cases. The sporadic (or American) form of Burkitt's lymphoma is found in North America, Northern and Eastern Europe, and the Far East and this form of Burkitt's lymphoma is associated with the Epstein-Barr virus in 15% of patients. The immunodeficiency associated form of Burkitt's lymphoma occurs mainly in patients with HIV, but it can also occur in allograft recipients and patients with congenital immunodeficiencies or X-linked lymphoproliferative disease [38, 39].

It was also stated that:

(i) Even though Burkitt's lymphoma can involve the head and neck in children, the gastrointestinal tract, genitourinary tract, gonads, mesentery, peritoneum, and retroperitoneum also represent potentially affected sites.

(ii) Lymphomas arising in the male genitourinary tract are relatively uncommon.

(iii) Malignant lymphoma involving the prostate is rare and accounts for less than 0.1% of newly diagnosed lymphomas.

The most frequent presentation forms are obstructive urinary symptoms. [40–42].

Some authors [43, 44] stated the following.

(i) Bladder outlet obstruction in women is an infrequently diagnosed urological condition.

(ii) A combination of history taking; physical examination; and diagnostic tests provides a consistent way to accurately recognize and diagnose bladder outlet obstruction.

The causes of obstruction are varied and numerous but generally fall within two broad categories: functional and anatomic. In a fertile female, the most likely anatomic causes of bladder outlet obstruction symptoms are bladder and urethral leiomyoma, and an association with female hormone expression has been suggested previously [9, 43, 44].

Other differential diagnoses include urethral caruncle, urethral diverticulum [45, 46], malignant lymphoma, sarcoma, extravesical leiomyoma of the bladder, Gartner's duct cyst, and ectopic urethral orifice [35].

Rijo et al. [35] stated the following.

(i) The diagnosis of Burkitt's lymphoma depends upon morphological findings, immunophenotyping results, and cytogenetic features. Because this lymphoma is one of the most rapidly proliferating neoplasms and is often associated with tumour lysis syndrome, a prompt diagnosis is required.

(ii) Treatment of Burkitt's lymphoma is inclusive of high doses of alkylating agents, frequent administration of chemotherapy, and attention to central nervous system (CNS) prophylaxis with high doses of systemic chemotherapy, intrathecal therapy, or both.

(iii) There is no role for radiation therapy in the modern treatment of Burkitt's lymphoma—even for localized disease or para—spinal presentations, which respond very quickly to chemotherapy.

(iv) To their knowledge, their reported case of female paraurethral Burkitt's lymphoma was the first case of primary paraurethral female Burkitt's lymphoma not related to Epstein-Barr virus which was reported in the literature.

Thomas et al. [46] stated that intensive chemotherapy regimens are required to treat Burkitt's lymphoma. Although several reports utilized initial excision, radiotherapy, chemotherapy, or some combination thereof, their case report suggested that the use of intensive immunochemotherapy should be considered as a possible treatment modality.

Mourad et al. [21] stated that less than 100 cases of primary lymphoma of the urinary bladder had been reported and most of them were B-cell lymphoma. They reported a case of primary T-cell lymphoma of the urinary bladder in a patient with a history of schistosomiasis. They reported a 52-year-old man who presented with suprapubic discomfort and haematuria. On examination, he was found to have a suprapubic mass. He had computed tomography scan of the pelvis which showed a large lobular mass that occupied the urinary bladder. There was no evidence of any pelvic or abdominal lymphadenopathy and the results of metastatic work-up were negative. The patient underwent a trans-urethral biopsy of the bladder mass and histological examination of the biopsy revealed a diffuse large cell lymphoma which was negative for the B-cell marker L-26 (CD20) and positive for the T-cell marker CD-3. Mourad et al. [21] reported that polymerase chain reaction studies of the paraffin-embedded tissue revealed rearrangement of the T-cell receptor gamma gene. The patient was treated by means of CHOPP chemotherapy and he received cyclophosphamide, doxorubicin, vincristine, and prednisone. Mourad et al. [21] stated that their case, represented to their knowledge, a very rare primary lymphoproliferative neoplasm of the urinary bladder that might represent an unusual immune response to schistosomiasis [21].

Wang et al. [20] stated that primary bladder lymphoma, a rare form of non-Hodgkin's lymphoma that is confined to the urinary bladder, is usually of B-cell origin. They reported an extremely rare case of primary T-cell lymphoma of the urinary bladder. Wang et al. [20] reported a 45-year-old man who presented with haematuria, dysuria, and loin pain. He had ultrasound scan and computed tomography scan which showed a thickened left bladder wall and left hydroureteronephrosis. A diagnosis of primary T-cell lymphoma of the urinary bladder was made which was based upon clinical, radiological, and histological findings. The patient underwent trans-urethral resection of his bladder lesion and following this he was treated with four cycles of CHOPP (cyclophosphamide, doxorubicin, vincristine, and prednisone) chemotherapy. He showed good response and remained in clinical remission 12 months after treatment. [20].

Oh and Zang [19] stated that involvement of the lower urinary tract by advanced non-Hodgkin's lymphoma (HL) had been reported in up to 13% of cases; however, primary non-Hodgkin's lymphoma of the urinary bladder is rare. They reported a 35-year-old man who was admitted with a history of visible haematuria and left flank pain. He underwent cystoscopy which revealed an oedematous broad-based mass on the left lateral wall of the bladder. He had trans-urethral biopsy and histological examination of the specimen revealed non-Hodgkin's lymphoma, diffuse large B-cell type. He had computed tomography scan which revealed left-sided hydronephrosis and hydroureter with left proximal ureter infiltration and thickening of the left lateral wall of the bladder with perivesical fat infiltration without lymph node enlargement. He also had full-scale staging work-up which revealed the bone marrow as the solely involved site. The lesions of the urinary bladder and left urinary tract had completely regressed pursuant to two cycles of systemic cyclophosphamide, doxorubicin, vincristine, and prednisone (CHOPP) chemotherapy with simultaneous restoration of urinary function [19].

Sundaram and Zhang [18] reported an unusual case of localized Epstein-Barr virus (EBV) positive B-cell lymphoproliferative disorder (LPD)/polymorphous B-cell lymphoma of the urinary bladder in a 67-year-old female patient. They reported that the patient had no known predisposing immunodeficiencies and she presented with a recent onset of haematuria. She had a computed tomography scan and cystoscopy which revealed a localized 2.5 cm polypoid or plaque-like mucosal mass on the right posterior and lateral wall of the urinary bladder. Histological examination of the biopsy specimen of the mass showed a diffuse and densely polymorphous atypical lymphoid infiltrate admixed with numerous small lymphocytes, histiocytes, and occasional plasma cells and neutrophils. On immunohistochemical staining, the large atypical cells were positively stained for

TABLE 4: List of some of the reported studies on lymphoma of the urinary bladder with outcome.

References	Types and numbers of lymphomas of the urinary bladder	Types of management	Duration of followup	Outcome	Total
Bates et al. [2]	**6 cases of primary lymphoma** 3 extranodal marginal zone lymphoma of MALT type 3 diffuse B-cell lymphomas	Various details are not available 66 years/female, large bladder mass-low-grade MALT-type lymphoma T3	1 year	Indolent course with good prognosis Alive	1
		79 years/female Low-grade MALT-type	No followup	Unknown	1
		59 years female T2-T3 low grade MALT type		Alive with disease	1
		84 years/female, T3 diffuse large B-cell lymphoma	3 years 6 months	Died of disease after 6 months	
		67/years male, Solid tumour diffuse large B-cell lymphoma, had radiotherapy and chemotherapy	16 years	Alive with disease after 16 years	
		80 years/female Diffuse large B-cell lymphoma, had radiotherapy	3 years 8 months	Alive and well after 3 years 8 months	
	5 cases of secondary lymphoma 4 diffuse large B-cell lymphoma 1 nodular sclerosis non-Hodgkin's disease	Various details are not available to author	4 patients had followup up to 13 months	4 patients died within 13 months of followup	
	65-year-old male laparotomy showed mass involving ileum and generalised lymphadenopathy. Diffuse large B-cell lymphoma secondary to systemic follicular lymphoma		13 months	Died of disease after 13 months Died of disease after 10 months	
	41 years/male Diffuse large B-cell lymphoma had caecal mass and abdominal lymph adenopathy biopsy showed malignant lymphoma had radiotherapy and chemotherapy	Radiotherapy and chemotherapy	10 months		
	32 years/male, necropsy showed abdominal mass and lymphadenopathy. Diffuse large B-cell lymphoma		Died of disease. No followup	Died of disease. Died of disease after 1 month	
	76/female, mass in lower abdomen, swollen left leg, lymphadenopathy in left groin, and right axilla. Diffuse large B-cell lymphoma 81-year-old, female known Hodgkin's		1 month No followup	No follow-up	

TABLE 4: Continued.

References	Types and numbers of lymphomas of the urinary bladder	Types of management	Duration of followup	Outcome	Total
	Disease developed to nodular sclerosis Hodgkin's disease of bladder				
Kempton et al. [3]	Primary B-cell MALT-type lymphoma of bladder in 6 patients Nonlocalized lymphoma (17 cases) 1 low-grade lymphoma of MALT type 12 large cell lymphoma 4 follicle centre lymphoma	Various	1940 to 1996	Complete remission. No patient died and no patient developed recurrent disease. Excluding two patients who died postoperatively, median survival was 9 years; 6 patients died of lymphoma in the follow-up group	6 patients
	Secondary lymphoma occurred in 13 patients (2 with low-grade lymphoma of the MALT type; 1 with follicle centre lymphoma; 1 with mantle cell lymphoma; 9 with diffuse large B-cell lymphomas			Median survival was 0.6 years	
Al-Maghrabi et al. [4]	4 cases of primary lymphoma (they had B-cell; centrocyte-like cells plasmacytoid or both)	All patients were treated by radiotherapy	2 to 13 years	Good prognosis (all the four with no recurrence and alive)	4 patients

CD20, CD79a, CD30, and CD43; and they were strongly positive for Epstein-Barr virus (EBV) by in situ hybridization using anti-EBER-1 probe. They also reported that polymerase chain reaction (PCR) for immunoglobulin heavy chain gene rearrangement study showed a clonal gene rearrangement. Sundaram and Zhang [18] made the ensuing statements.

(i) Primary lymphoma of the bladder is rare and primary Epstein-Barr virus (EBV) + lymphoproliferative disorder (LPD) of the bladder had not been previously described.

(ii) Potential misdiagnosis of poorly differentiated urothelial carcinoma can occur and accurate diagnosis depends upon comprehensive immunohistochemical and molecular work-ups [18].

Abraham Jr. et al. [17] stated that monocytoid B-cell lymphoma (MBCL) is a low-grade neoplasm which is considered to be the neoplastic counterpart to monocytoid B-cell lymphocytes, derived from marginal zone lymphocytes. Abraham Jr. et al. [17] reported a 72-year-old woman who presented with urinary symptoms of burning, urgency, and haematuria. Cystoscopic examination revealed an exophytic mass at the base of the urinary bladder. The lesion was suspected based upon the gross examination findings to be a transitional cell carcinoma; however, on initial histological examination of the biopsied specimen, it was found to be lymphoma which was composed of cells with moderately abundant cytoplasm and an overall size reminiscent of a large-cell type. Following detailed histological examination of the specimen, a diagnosis of monocytoid B-cell lymphoma (MBCL) in the submucosal site was made. She underwent clinical staging which did not show any evidence of lymphoma in any other organs. The patient responded to therapy for non-Hodgkin's lymphoma (NHL). Abraham Jr. et al. [17] stated that their case represented an unusual presentation of low-grade non-Hodgkin's lymphoma (NHL) and it may be consistent with previous suggestions of a relationship between monocytoid B-cell lymphoma (MBCL) and lymphomas of mucosa-associated lymphoid tissue.

Hayashi et al. [16] stated that primary lymphoma of the urinary bladder is quite rare and primarily it is extranodal marginal zone B-cell lymphoma-associated lymphoid tissue (MALT-lymphoma). They stated that prior to their publication there was only one case report of primary diffuse large B-cell lymphoma (DLBCL) of the bladder, accompanied by diffuse wall thickening of the urinary bladder. Hayashi et al. [16] reported the second case of primary DLBCL of the urinary bladder in a 75-year-old woman, who initially presented with acute renal failure. She received three courses of R-CHOPP chemotherapy which were effective to treat her acute renal failure caused by postrenal obstruction and to attain clinical remission.

Siegel and Napoli [15] described a malignant lymphoma which involved the dome and the anterior wall of the urinary bladder in an elderly woman. The initial biopsy showed a malignant neoplasm of uncertain cell type. In view of the fact that the clinical presentation was most compatible with urachal adenocarcinoma, an extensive resection was performed. Microscopic examination revealed that the excised tumour was composed of large lymphoid cells with isolated and clustered signet-ring cells. They reported that immunohistochemical analysis of the tumour established the B-cell phenotype of the neoplasm, and electron microscopy of the signet-ring cells revealed endoplasmic reticulum-bound inclusions consistent with immunoglobulin. Siegel and Napoli [15] stated that primary malignant lymphomas of the urinary bladder are rare, and, to their knowledge, their report was the first example with signet-ring cells. They iterated that the histopathological finding would be a cause of potential confusion with urachal adenocarcinoma.

Kakuta et al. [14] stated that primary mucosa-associated lymphoid tissue (MALT) lymphoma of the bladder is a rare disease, and the most effective therapeutic procedure remains unknown. Kakuta et al. [14] reported a case of primary MALT lymphoma of the bladder which regressed after rituximab in combination with CHOPP chemotherapy (R-CHOOP). The patient was an 84-year-old woman who presented with general fatigue and weight loss. She had a computed tomography (CT) scan which showed a solitary mass in the bladder. She had trans-urethral biopsy of the lesion and histological examination of the specimen revealed extranodal marginal zone B-cell lymphoma of MALT. She had one cycle of R-CHOPP chemotherapy which resulted in her complete remission. They stated that their reported case was the fourteenth case of MALT lymphoma of the bladder in Japan.

Takahara et al. [13] reported an 85-year-old woman who presented with macroscopic haematuria and pain on micturition. She had a cystoscopy which revealed a wide-based submucosal mass, and biopsied specimens of the mass were examined histologically which showed a B-cell lymphoma of the MALT type. She had computed tomography scan which showed a 7.5 cm × 3.0 cm solitary mass lesion situated from the anterior wall to the right lateral bladder wall and magnetic resonance imaging (MRI) scan which showed a low intensity in T1W1, high in T2W1 without invasion. She underwent trans-urethral resection of the lesion. Histological examination of the specimen was consistent with extranodal marginal zone B-cell lymphoma of the MALT type. There was no evidence of lymphoma on computed tomography (CT) of the pelvis, chest X-ray, and Gallium scintigraphy. The patient had stages I (AE) lymphoma. She was treated with radiation therapy (radiotherapy) to the urinary bladder and

pelvis (40 Gy in 20 fractions) and she was followed up with computed tomography every 3 months. She had no evidence of recurrence.

Terasaki et al. [12] reported a 64-year-old woman who presented with a history of general malaise. Her haemoglobin level was 9.0 g/dL. She had gastrointestinal endoscopy which revealed a haemorrhagic gastric ulcer, which was considered as aetiology of the anaemia. She had abdominal ultrasound scan which showed bilateral hydronephrosis and hydroureters. Her urine test revealed pyuria and macroscopic haematuria and her urine culture revealed 10(8) colony-forming units of *Escherichia coli* per mL. She had pelvic magnetic resonance imaging which showed thickening of the posterior wall and trigone of the urinary bladder. She underwent trans-urethral resection and biopsy of the mucosa of the urinary bladder which upon histological examination gave a diagnosis of primary mucosa-associated lymphoid tissue (MALT) lymphoma of the urinary bladder. Ann Arbor's clinical stage was IEA. It was planned that she should be administered irradiation at a total dose of 36 Gy to the whole bladder and part of tumour; nevertheless, radiotherapy was discontinued at a dose of 26 Gy because of the fact that she developed pollakisuria. She had pelvic magnetic resonance imaging and pathological examination of the urinary bladder after radiotherapy and these showed that the lymphoma was in complete remission; however, she received rituximab therapy at a dose of 375 mg/m^2/week, 8 times additionally, because of the reduced radiotherapy. The patient had remained in complete remission for 14 months at the time of the report of her case.

Raderer et al. [11] stated that (a) various chemotherapeutic agents as well as the anti-CD20 antibody rituximab (R) had been tested in patients with mucosa-associated lymphoid tissue (MALT) lymphoma; however, no standard chemotherapeutic regimen had emerged so far; (b) judging from the data obtained in various types of lymphoma, the activity of R appears to be enhanced by combination with chemotherapy; (c) as no data on this topic exist for MALT lymphoma, they had retrospectively analysed their experience with R plus cyclophosphamide, doxorubicin/mitoxantrone, vincristine, and prednisone (R-CHOP/R-CNOP) in patients with relapsed MALT lymphoma. Raderer et al. [11] identified a total of 26 patients; 15 of these patients were administered R-CHOP while 11 patients were given R-CNOP due to age greater than 65 years or preexisting cardiac conditions. Cycles were repeated every 21 days, and restaging was performed after 4 cycles of therapy. In cases of complete remission, 2 further cycles were administered for consolidation while the patients who were achieving partial remission or stable disease after restaging were given 4 further courses. Raderer et al. [11] reported the following.

(i) A total of 170 cycles were administered to their patients (median 6, range 2 to 8).

(ii) Twenty of the 26 patients (77%) achieved a complete remission and 6 (23%) a partial remission.

(iii) Toxicities were mainly haematological, with WHO grade III/IV leukocytopenia occurring in 5 patients.

(iv) After a median followup of 19 months (range 10 months to 45 months), all patients were alive: 22 were in ongoing remission, while 4 had relapsed between 12 and 19 months after treatment.

Raderer et al. [11] concluded that their data demonstrated a high activity of R-CHOP/R-CNOP in relapsing MALT lymphoma irrespective of prior therapy.

Finally, Tables 3 and 4 have been provided to summarize the reported experiences of a number of authors regarding the management of various types of lymphomas of the urinary bladder.

4. Conclusions

Lymphoma of the urinary bladder may be either primary or secondary lymphoma.

Diagnosis of lymphoma of the urinary bladder is based upon the characteristic morphology of the bladder lesion which has been resected or biopsied and this must be supported by immunohistochemical analysis.

Lymphoma of the urinary bladder is a rare lesion.

Radiotherapy and chemotherapy are useful and effective in the treatment of lymphoma of the urinary bladder.

Conflict of Interests

The author declares that there is no conflict of interests.

Acknowledgments

Thanks are due to the Editor-in-Chief of Archives of Pathology and Laboratory Medicine for granting the author permission on behalf of the editorial team of the journal and the American Association of Pathology to use figures and tables from [4]: Al-Maghrabi J, Kamel-Reid S, Jewett M, Gospodarowicz M, Wells W, and Banerjee D. Primary low-grade B-cell lymphoma of mucosa-associated lymphoid tissue type arising in the urinary bladder: report of 4 cases with molecular genetic analysis (Arch Pathol Lab Med. 2001 Mar; 125(3): 332–336).

References

[1] G. Levy, "Bladder Other tumors Lymphoma (primary)," PathologyOutlines.com 2011, http://www.pathologyoutlines.com/topic/bladderlymphoma.html.

[2] A. W. Bates, A. J. Norton, and S. I. Baithun, "Malignant lymphoma of the urinary bladder: a clinicopathological study of 11 cases," Journal of Clinical Pathology, vol. 53, no. 6, pp. 458–461, 2000.

[3] C. L. Kempton, P. J. Kurtin, D. J. Inwards, P. Wollan, and D. G. Bostwick, "Malignant lymphoma of the bladder: evidence from 36 cases that low- grade lymphoma of the malt-type is the most common primary bladder lymphoma," American Journal of Surgical Pathology, vol. 21, no. 11, pp. 1324–1333, 1997.

[4] J. Al-Maghrabi, S. Kamel-Reid, M. Jewett, M. Gospodarowicz, W. Wells, and D. Banerjee, "Primary low-grade B-cell lymphoma of mucosa-associated lymphoid tissue type arising in

the urinary bladder: report of 4 cases with molecular genetic analysis," Archives of Pathology and Laboratory Medicine, vol. 125, no. 3, pp. 332–336, 2001.

[5] L. R. Zukerberg, N. L. Harris, and R. H. Young, "Carcinomas of the urinary bladder simulating malignant lymphoma: a report of five cases," American Journal of Surgical Pathology, vol. 15, no. 6, pp. 569–576, 1991.

[6] D. D. Cohen, C. Lamarre, L. Lamarre, and F. S. Fred Saad, "Primary low-grade B-cell lymphoma of the urinary bladder: case report and literature review," The Canadian Journal of Urology, vol. 9, no. 6, pp. 1694–1697, 2002.

[7] G. Sufrin, B. Keogh, R. H. Moore, and G. P. Murphy, "Secondary involvement of the bladder in malignant lymphoma," Journal of Urology, vol. 118, no. 2, pp. 251–253, 1977.

[8] H. Kuhara, Z. Tamura, T. Suchi, R. Hattori, and T. Kinukawa, "Primary malignant lymphoma of the urinary bladder. A case report," Acta Pathologica Japonica, vol. 40, no. 10, pp. 764–769, 1990.

[9] M. Sönmezer, A. Ensari, Y. Üstün, M. Güngör, and F. Ortaç, "Primary lymphoma of the urinary bladder presenting as a large pelvic mass," Journal of the Pakistan Medical Association, vol. 52, no. 5, pp. 228–230, 2002.

[10] M. Ohsawa, K. Aozasa, K. Horiuchi, and A. Kanamaru, "Malignant lymphoma of bladder: report of three cases and review of the literature," Cancer, vol. 72, no. 6, pp. 1969–1974, 1993.

[11] M. Raderer, S. Wöhrer, B. Streubel et al., "Activity of rituximab plus cyclophosphamide, doxorubicin/mitoxantrone, vincristine and prednisone in patients with relapsed MALT lymphoma," Oncology, vol. 70, no. 6, pp. 411–417, 2006.

[12] Y. Terasaki, H. Okumura, Y. Ishiura et al., "Primary mucosa-associated lymphoid tissue lymphoma of the urinary bladder successfully treated by radiotherapy and rituximab," Rinsho Ketsueki, vol. 49, no. 1, pp. 30–34, 2008.

[13] Y. Takahara, H. Kawashima, Y.-S. Han et al., "Primary mucosa-associated lymphoid tissue (MALT) lymphoma of the urinary bladder," Hinyokika Kiyo, vol. 51, no. 1, pp. 45–48, 2005.

[14] Y. Kakuta, T. Katoh, J. Saitoh, K. Yazawa, M. Hosomi, and K. Itoh, "A case of primary mucosa-associated lymphoid tissue lymphoma of the bladder regressed after rituximab in combination with CHOP chemotherapy," Acta Urologica Japonica, vol. 52, no. 12, pp. 951–954, 2006.

[15] R. J. Siegel and V. M. Napoli, "Malignant lymphoma of the urinary bladder: a case with signet-ring cells stimulating urachal adenocarcinoma," Archives of Pathology and Laboratory Medicine, vol. 115, no. 6, pp. 635–637, 1991.

[16] A. Hayashi, Y. Miyakawa, K. Bokuda et al., "Primary diffuse large B-cell lymphoma of the bladder," Internal Medicine, vol. 48, no. 16, pp. 1403–1406, 2009.

[17] N. Z. Abraham Jr., T. J. Maher, and R. E. Hutchison, "Extranodal monocytoid B-cell lymphoma of the urinary bladder," Modern Pathology, vol. 6, no. 2, pp. 145–149, 1993.

[18] S. Sundaram and K. Zhang, "Epstein-Barr virus positive B-cell lymphoproliferative disorder/ polymorphous B-cell lymphoma of the urinary bladder: a case report with review of literature," Indian Journal of Urology, vol. 25, no. 1, pp. 129–131, 2009.

[19] K. C. Oh and D. Y. Zang, "Primary non-Hodgkin's lymphoma of the bladder with bone marrow involvement," The Korean journal of internal medicine, vol. 18, no. 1, pp. 40–44, 2003.

[20] L. Wang, Z. Z. Cao, and L. Qi, "Primary T-cell lymphoma of the urinary bladder presenting with haematuria and hydroureteronephrosis," Journal of International Medical Research, vol. 39, no. 5, pp. 2027–2032, 2011.

[21] W. A. Mourad, S. Khalil, A. Radwi, A. Peracha, and A. Ezzat, "Primary T-cell lymphoma of the urinary bladder," *American Journal of Surgical Pathology*, vol. 22, no. 3, pp. 373–377, 1998.

[22] K. Ando, Y. Matsuno, Y. Kanai et al., "Primary low-grade lymphoma of mucosa-associated lymphoid tissue of the urinary bladder: a case report with special reference to the use of ancillary diagnostic studies," *Japanese Journal of Clinical Oncology*, vol. 29, no. 12, pp. 636–639, 1999.

[23] R. H. W. Simpson, R. S. Amin, and R. D. Pocock, "Malignant lymphoma of the bladder and female urethra," *International Urogynecology Journal*, vol. 5, no. 2, pp. 102–105, 1994.

[24] E. Mearini, A. Zucchi, E. Costantini, P. Fornetti, E. Tiacci, and L. Mearini, "Primary Burkitt's lymphoma of bladder in patient with aids," *Journal of Urology*, vol. 167, no. 3, pp. 1397–1398, 2002.

[25] I. Tsiriopoulos, G. Lee, A. O'Reilly, R. Smith, and M. Pancharatnam, "Primary splenic marginal zone lymphoma with bladder metastases mimicking interstitial cystitis," *International Urology and Nephrology*, vol. 38, no. 3-4, pp. 475–476, 2006.

[26] T. M. Downs, A. S. Kibel, and W. C. DeWolf, "Primary lymphoma of the bladder: a unique cystoscopic appearance," *Urology*, vol. 49, no. 2, pp. 276–278, 1997.

[27] R. H. W. Simpson, J. E. Bridger, P. P. Anthony, K. A. James, and I. Jury, "Malignant lymphoma of the lower urinary tract. A clinicopathological study with review of the literature," *British Journal of Urology*, vol. 65, no. 3, pp. 254–260, 1990.

[28] P. Isaacson and D. H. Wright, "Malignant lymphoma of mucosa-associated lymphoid tissue. A distinctive type of B-cell lymphoma," *Cancer*, vol. 52, no. 8, pp. 1410–1416, 1983.

[29] M. Mantzarides, D. Papathanassiou, G. Bonardel, M. Soret, E. Gontier, and H. Foehrenbach, "High-grade lymphoma of the bladder visualized on PET," *Clinical Nuclear Medicine*, vol. 30, no. 7, pp. 478–480, 2005.

[30] D. A. Evans and A. T. Moore, "The first case of vesico-vaginal fistula in a patient with primary lymphoma of the bladder—a case report," *Journal of Medical Case Reports*, vol. 1, article 105, 2007.

[31] K. Arda, G. Özdemir, Z. Güneş, and H. Özdemir, "Primary malignant lymphoma of the bladder. A case report and review of the literature," *International Urology and Nephrology*, vol. 29, no. 3, pp. 319–322, 1997.

[32] M. J. F. Aceñero, C. M. Rodilla, J. L. García-Asenjo, S. C. Menchero, and J. S. Esponera, "Primary malignant lymphoma of the bladder report of 3 cases," *Pathology, Research and Practice*, vol. 192, 1996.

[33] A. JACOBS and T. SYMINGTON, "Primary lymphosarcoma of urinary bladder," *British journal of urology*, vol. 25, no. 2, pp. 119–126, 1953.

[34] J. A. Diaz-Peromingo, J. T. Tato-Rodriguez, P. M. Pesqueira, S. Molinos-Castro, M. C. Gayol-Fernández, and J. P. Struzik, "Non-Hodgkin's lymphoma presenting as a primary bladder tumour: a case report," *Journal of Medical Case Reports*, vol. 4, pp. 4–114, 2010.

[35] E. Rijo, O. Bielsa, J. A. Lorente, A. Francés, J. Lloreta, and O. Arango, "Female paraurethral primary Burkitt's lymphoma, presenting with symptoms of bladder Outlet obstruction, successfully treated with Chemotherapy," www.bjui.org/ContentFullItem.aspx.

[36] K. Hatano, M. Sato, Y. Tsujimoto et al., "Primary mucosa-associated lymphoid tissue (MALT) lymphoma of the urinary bladder associated with left renal pelvic carcinoma: a case report," *Acta Urologica Japonica*, vol. 53, no. 1, pp. 57–60, 2007.

[37] P. Dahm and J. E. Gschwend, "Malignant non-urothelial neoplasms of the urinary bladder: a review," *European Urology*, vol. 44, no. 6, pp. 672–681, 2003.

[38] J. A. Ferry, "Burkitt's lymphoma: clinicopathologic features and differential diagnosis," *Oncologist*, vol. 11, no. 4, pp. 375–383, 2006.

[39] A. Shad and I. T. Magrath, "Non-Hodgkin's lymphoma in children," in *Principles and Practice of Pediatric Oncology*, P. A. Pizzo and D. G. Poplack, Eds., pp. 545–548, Lippincott-Raven, Philadelphia, Pa, USA, 3rd edition, 1997.

[40] W. W. Choi, R. L. Yap, O. Ozer, M. R. Pins, and A. J. Schaeffer, "Lymphoma of the prostate and bladder presenting as acute urinary obstruction," *Journal of Urology*, vol. 169, no. 3, pp. 1082–1083, 2003.

[41] I. Singh, M. Joshi, S. Agarwal, U. R. Singh, and R. Saran, "Extranodal small cell lymphocytic lymphoma of prostate: an unusual cause of lower urinary tract symptoms," *Urology*, vol. 71, no. 3, pp. 547.e7–549.e7, 2008.

[42] S. D. Schniederjan and A. O. Osunkoya, "Lymphoid neoplasms of the urinary tract and male genital organs: a clinicopathological study of 40 cases," *Modern Pathology*, vol. 22, no. 8, pp. 1057–1065, 2009.

[43] D. E. Shield and R. M. Weiss, "Leiomyoma of the female urethra," *Journal of Urology*, vol. 109, no. 3, pp. 430–431, 1973.

[44] I. E. Yusim, E. Z. Neulander, I. Eidelberg, L. J. Lismer, and J. Kaneti, "Leiomyoma of the genitourinary tract," *Scandinavian Journal of Urology and Nephrology*, vol. 35, no. 4, pp. 295–299, 2001.

[45] A. Gómez Gallo, J. P. Valdevenito Sepúlveda, and M. San Martín Montes, "Giant lithiasis in a female urethral diverticulum," *European Urology*, vol. 51, no. 2, pp. 556–558, 2007.

[46] D. A. Thomas, J. Cortes, S. O'Brien et al., "Hyper-CVAD program in Burkitt's-type adult acute lymphoblastic leukemia," *Journal of Clinical Oncology*, vol. 17, no. 8, pp. 2461–2470, 1999.

18

High Intensity Focused Ultrasound versus Brachytherapy for the Treatment of Localized Prostate Cancer: A Matched-Pair Analysis

Fouad Aoun,[1] Ksenija Limani,[1] Alexandre Peltier,[1]
Quentin Marcelis,[2] Marc Zanaty,[1] Alexandre Chamoun,[2] Marc Vanden Bossche,[2]
Thierry Roumeguère,[2] and Roland van Velthoven[1]

[1]*Department of Urology, Jules Bordet Institute, Université Libre de Bruxelles, 1000 Brussels, Belgium*
[2]*Department of Urology, Erasme Hospital, Université Libre de Bruxelles, 1070 Brussels, Belgium*

Correspondence should be addressed to Fouad Aoun; fouad.aoun@bordet.be

Academic Editor: Nazareno Suardi

Purpose. To evaluate postoperative morbidity and long term oncologic and functional outcomes of high intensity focused ultrasound (HIFU) compared to brachytherapy for the treatment of localized prostate cancer. *Material and Methods.* Patients treated by brachytherapy were matched 1 : 1 with patients who underwent HIFU. Differences in postoperative complications across the two groups were assessed using Wilcoxon's rank-sum or χ^2 test. Kaplan-Meier curves, log-rank tests, and Cox regression models were constructed to assess differences in survival rates between the two groups. *Results.* Brachytherapy was significantly associated with lower voiding LUTS and less frequent acute urinary retention ($p < 0.05$). Median oncologic follow-up was 83 months (13–123 months) in the HIFU cohort and 44 months (13–89 months) in the brachytherapy cohort. Median time to achieve PSA nadir was statistically shorter in the HIFU. Biochemical recurrence-free survival rate was significantly higher in the brachytherapy cohort compared to HIFU cohort (68.5% versus 53%, $p < 0.05$). No statistically significant difference in metastasis-free, cancer specific, and overall survivals was observed between the two groups. *Conclusion.* HIFU and brachytherapy are safe with no significant difference in cancer specific survival on long term oncologic follow-up. Nonetheless, a randomized controlled trial is needed to confirm these results.

1. Introduction

In the last two decades, transperineal low dose rate (LDR) brachytherapy emerged as a therapeutic option for patients with organ confined prostate cancer. This technique was supported by technical advances in transrectal ultrasound (TRUS), advent of template guidance, and improved dosimetry [1]. In 2012, the American Brachytherapy Society (ABS) provided an updated consensus guideline on patient selection, workup, treatment, postimplant dosimetry, and follow-up [2]. The panel recommended prostate brachytherapy as a monotherapy for low risk organ confined prostate cancer patients and some patients with intermediate risk disease [2]. The technique is safe and effective but carries a nonnegligible risk of severe toxicities to the urethra, bladder, neurovascular bundles, and rectum because of their anatomic proximity to the prostate and the high dose intensity close to the radiation source [3]. In addition, the rapid decline in radiation dose can lead to suboptimal control outside the planned area of treatment [4]. Available evidence on oncologic outcomes is based on case series with only one prospective randomized trial comparing brachytherapy to other primary treatment options for organ confined prostate cancer [5]. These facts have contributed to the development and application of new minimally invasive approaches to organ confined prostate cancer. Among these therapies, high intensity focused ultrasound (HIFU) emerged as a valid mini-invasive therapy for organ confined prostate cancer, using focused ultrasound to generate areas of intense heat to induce tissue necrosis. The ability of HIFU to achieve thermoablation of prostatic lesion was proven on MRI imaging and histologically on posttreatment biopsies and on operative specimens [6–9]. Oncologic outcomes were first reported in mid-1990 and subsequently the use of HIFU therapy has expanded [10, 11]. Different case series have been published reporting safety and efficacy of HIFU as well as favorable perioperative and oncologic results. Recently, we published long term results of a cohort of 110 consecutive patients with organ confined prostate cancer primarily treated with whole gland HIFU [12]. At ten years of follow-up, we estimated a biochemical recurrence-free survival (BRFS) rate, an overall survival (OS) rate, and a cancer specific survival (CSS) rate of 40%, 72%, and 90%, respectively. Nonetheless, the European Association of Urology (EAU), the American Urological Association (AUA), and the National Comprehensive Cancer Network (NCCN) do not recommend the routine use of HIFU in the primary treatment of prostate cancer given the absence of prospective randomized controlled trials comparing HIFU with conventional treatment options and the paucity of long term oncologic follow-up data. The aim of this study is to evaluate peri- and postoperative morbidity and long term oncologic and functional outcomes of whole gland HIFU compared with brachytherapy. We thus performed a matched-pair analysis controlling for clinical and pathologic variables comparing patients treated by HIFU and brachytherapy during the same period.

2. Materials and Methods

Patients scheduled to undergo brachytherapy or HIFU for organ confined prostate cancer in our two academic hospitals were prospectively enrolled between September 2001 and December 2012. Pooled prospectively collected data were retrospectively analyzed. Institutional review board approval was obtained from the two centers. Inclusion criteria for the two groups of patients were whole gland primary therapy with curative intent for an organ confined prostate cancer, prostate specific antigen (PSA) < 20 ng/mL, Gleason score ≤ 7 (3 + 4), clinical stage T1N0M0-T2N0M0, and a follow-up longer than 12 months. Baseline physical examination and PSA measurements were obtained for all patients. Extracapsular tumor extension and lymph node status were also assessed for all patients using pelvic CT or MRI. Patients with incomplete oncologic data were excluded from the study.

Our technique of whole gland HIFU had been thoroughly described [12]. All patients were treated by a single experienced surgeon (RVV) with Ablatherm HIFU devices (EDAP-TMS, Vaulx-en-Velin, France). From September 2001 to March 2006, patients were treated with the first commercially available HIFU device from Ablatherm (Maxis-Technomed, Lyon, France) and since April 2006 with Ablatherm Integrated Imaging (Ablatherm, EDAP, Lyon, France). The same team (radiation therapist and physicist) and two experienced surgeons (Alexandre Peltier and Marc Vanden Bossche) performed LDR brachytherapy in the same years. All patients were treated by a permanent transperineal interstitial pre-loaded-free needles implantation of Iode^{125} using a real-time biplanar ultrasound-guided system. The postoperative dosimetric assessment was performed in all patients using computed tomography as recommended by the American Brachytherapy Society guidelines at one month of the implant which is considered essential for maintenance of a satisfactory quality assurance program [2]. In our institution the upper volume limit for HIFU and brachytherapy procedures is set to 40 cc and 50 cc, respectively. Patients with prostates exceeding this threshold are offered neoadjuvant cytoreductive androgen deprivation therapy (ADT). Hormonal treatment is always discontinued at the time of surgery.

2.1. Outcomes. Postoperatively, patients were followed with serial serum PSA determinations and digital rectal examinations at regular intervals. Oncologic outcomes were evaluated using the D'Amico tumor recurrence risk group classification system [13]. Biochemical recurrence rates were defined using the American Society for Therapeutic Radiology and Oncology (ASTRO)/Phoenix criteria (nadir + 2 ng/mL) and the Stuttgart criteria (nadir + 1.2 ng/mL) [14, 15].

Individual PSA nadir was identified in each patient. PSA nadir was defined as the lowest PSA value reached during follow-up. Cause of death was identified from patient file or from physician correspondence and all prostate cancer specific deaths were verified. Overall quality of life and costs were not reported in this study. The follow-up period was defined as the interval between surgery and last available monitoring data or the date of death. Complications were prospectively recorded and retrospectively graded according to the Clavien-Dindo score [16, 17]. Urinary functional outcomes were reported using physician reported rates. De novo or exacerbating postoperative LUTS were noted in the early setting and at long term of follow-up (>1 year). Stress incontinence was graduated according to Stamey into three grades [18]. Grade 1 was defined as loss of urine during heavy exercises, using not more than one pad per day, Grade 2 as loss of urine during light exercises but not at rest or during sleep, and Grade 3 as total loss of urine occurring at rest or during sleep. Patients that were able to penetrate their partner without mechanical or pharmacological support were rated potent.

2.2. Statistics. Patients treated by brachytherapy were matched 1 : 1 with patients undergoing whole gland HIFU in the same years. The matching procedure was blinded to the outcome in order to avoid selection bias. Matching criteria were in the following order: Gleason score, PSA, clinical tumor stage, D'Amico risk, and age. To confirm an appropriate matching, the absence of significant clinical and pathologic differences between the two cohorts of patients was assessed using Wilcoxon's rank-sum or χ^2 test, as appropriate. Similar analyses were conducted to investigate differences in perioperative and pathologic variables.

Univariate logistic regressions were performed to evaluate the impact of the surgical approach on complication occurrence. To evaluate possible amelioration of the technical aspects of the HIFU technique with the new device, we categorized the patients sequentially into two groups and analyzed the changes of the morbidity rate. Kaplan-Meier curves,

TABLE 1: Baseline patient characteristics after matching.

	Brachytherapy (n = 70)	HIFU (n = 70)	p value
Median age (IQR; SD), years	69 (54–79; 6.5)	74 (62–86; 4.47)	<0.01
Clinical stage (T)			0.54
T1a	1	2	
T1b	2	6	
T1c	38	31	
T2a	20	19	
T2b	9	12	
Gleason score			1
≤6	51	51	
7	19	19	
PSA (ng/mL)			0.23
≤10	57	50	
>10 et ≤20	13	20	
D'Amico risk classification			0.33
Low	33	31	
Intermediate	37	39	
Neoadjuvant ADT	14	19	0.43
ASA score			0.68
1	8	10	
2	47	42	
3	15	18	
Median follow-up (IQR), months	44 (21–70)	83 (29–98)	<0.01

TABLE 2: Baseline and tumour characteristics of 110 patients with localized prostate cancer who were treated by a single session of high intensity focused ultrasound.

Mean age, years [range]	76.1 ± 6.2 [61–86]
Mean preoperative PSA, ng/mL [range]	12.1 ± 4.1 [0.55–49.0]
Mean prostate volume, mL [range]	29.3 ± 6.0 [18–39]
Hormone, n (%)	
Yes	37 (33.6)
No	73 (66.4)
Gleason score, n (%)	
≤6	69 (62.7)
7	24 (21.8)
≥8	17 (15.5)
Stage, n (%)	
T1	51 (46.4)
T2	59 (53.6)
D'Amico risk group*, N (%)	
Low	40 (36.4)
Intermediate	49 (44.5)
High	21 (19.1)

*Risk group based on D'Amico definition (according to Stage, Gleason, and PSA).

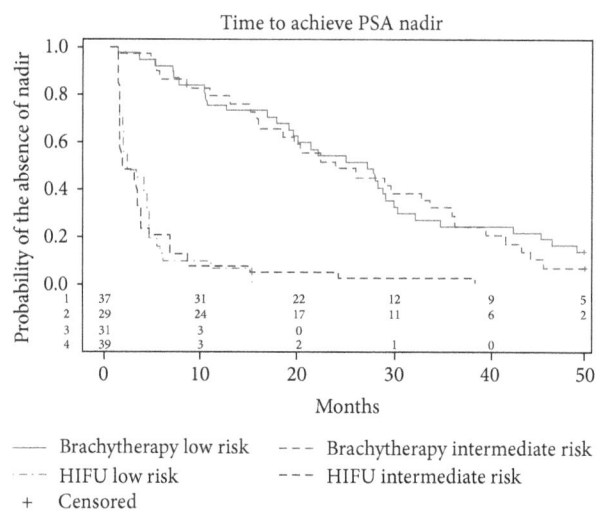

	HIFU	Brachytherapy	p value
Mean PSA nadir (median, SD)	0.55 (0.69 ± 1.32)	0.58 (0.32 ± 1.61)	0.9
Time to achieve PSA nadir (months)	3 (CI 95% 1.3–3.0)	25 (CI 95% 19.3–29.0)	<0.01

FIGURE 1: Time to achieve PSA nadir after HIFU and brachytherapy according to the classification of D'Amico.

log-rank test, and univariate Cox regression were constructed to analyze the influence of the surgical approach on recurrence-free survival, metastasis-free survival, cancer specific survival, and overall survival. A p value < 0.05 was considered to indicate statistical significance. A statistical analysis was performed with SPSS v. 20 (IBM Corp., Armonk, NY, USA).

3. Results

During the period of the study, 106 patients underwent LDR brachytherapy. Patients with incomplete oncologic data (4 patients) or limited follow-up < 12 months (32 patients) were excluded. A total of 70 patients have been included in the final analysis. These patients were matched with an equal number of patients treated by whole gland HIFU during the same years. Matching was successful with no statistically significant difference across the two groups except for the age (Table 1); patients operated by HIFU were older than patients undergoing brachytherapy ($p < 0.01$). The overall clinical and pathologic characteristics of the entire prospective HIFU cohort from which patients were selected for matching can be observed in Table 2. Median oncologic follow-up was statistically higher for the HIFU cohort compared to the brachytherapy cohort (83 months versus 44 months, $p < 0.01$). PSA nadir was noted in 95.7% of patients after HIFU

and in 94.3% of patients after brachytherapy (Figure 1). The median time to achieve the nadir was statistically shorter in the HIFU cohort compared to the brachytherapy cohort (3 months versus 25 months, $p < 0.05$). Oncologic outcomes of the two cohorts are summarized in Table 3. The Phoenix and Stuttgart definitions were used for biochemical recurrence. Hazards ratio was calculated using HIFU cohort as a reference. The 5-year actuarial BRFS rates were significantly higher for the brachytherapy cohort compared to the HIFU cohort

TABLE 3: Oncologic outcomes for the cohort stratified according to the D'Amico risk classification.

	Brachytherapy	HIFU[*]	Hazards ratio (CI[**] 95%)
Biochemical recurrence-free survival rates	Phoenix definition: 68.5%	Phoenix definition: 53.1%	0.41 (0.19–0.81)
	Stuttgart definition: 60.9%	Stuttgart definition: 51.3%	0.39 (0.19–0.74)
Low risk	Phoenix definition: 77.5%	Phoenix definition: 68%	0.31 (0.09–0.94)
	Stuttgart definition: 77.5%	Stuttgart definition: 56.3%	0.31 (0.10–0.84)
Intermediate risk	Phoenix definition: 58.8%	Phoenix definition: 44.9%	0.47 (0.17–1.13)
	Stuttgart definition: 58.8%	Stuttgart definition: 42%	0.41 (0.15–0.97)
Metastasis-free survival rates	79.8%	85%	1.08 (0.36–2.95)
Cancer specific survival rates	92%	89%	0.67 (0.32–1.29)
Overall survival rates	97.5%	88%	0.24 (0.01–1.34)

[*]HIFU: high intensity focused ultrasound; [**]CI: confidence interval.

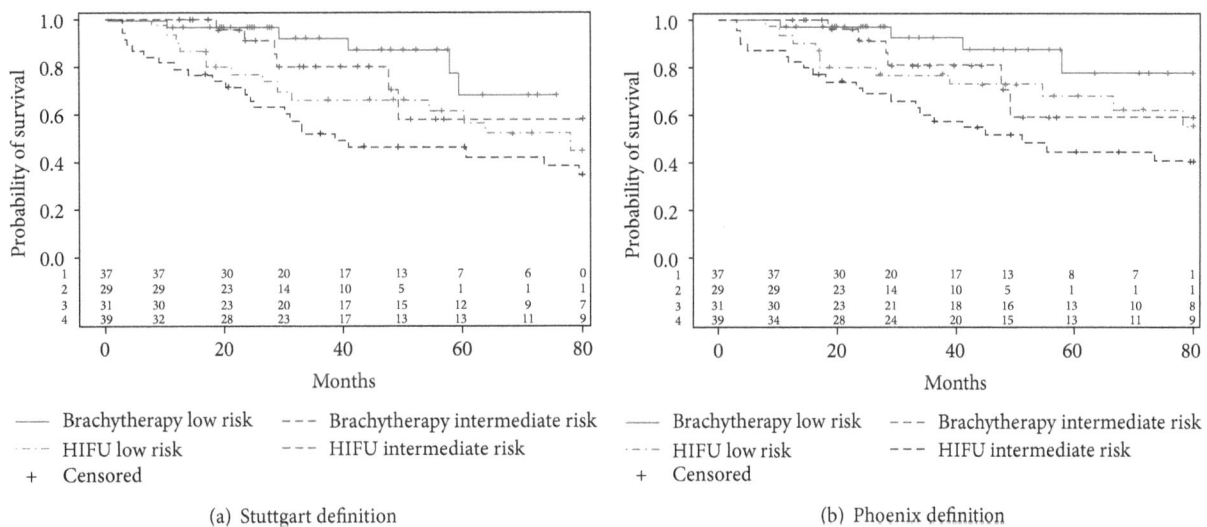

FIGURE 2: Kaplan-Meier curves for biochemical recurrence-free survival using Stuttgart (a) and Phoenix (b) definitions stratified according to D'Amico risk classification.

according to the Phoenix (68.5% versus 53%, HR = 0.41; CI 95%: 0.19–0.81, $p < 0.05$) and Stuttgart definitions (60.9% versus 53%, HR = 0.39; CI 95%: 0.19–0.74, $p < 0.05$), respectively. When stratifying patients according to the D'Amico risk and the technique used, BRFS rates were significantly higher for the low risk group treated by brachytherapy compared to the low risk group treated by HIFU according to Phoenix (77.5% versus 68%, HR = 0.31; CI 95%: 0.09–0.94, $p = 0.05$) and Stuttgart definitions (77.5% versus 56.3%, HR = 0.31; CI 95%: 0.10–0.84, $p = 0.03$), respectively (Figure 2).

For intermediate risk patients, there was no significant difference in BRFS rates between the brachytherapy and HIFU cohorts according to the Phoenix (58.8% versus 44.9%; HR = 0.47; CI 95%: 0.17–1.13, $p = 0.12$) and Stuttgart definitions (58.8% versus 42%; HR = 0.41; CI 95%: 0.15–0.97, $p = 0.05$), respectively. There was no significant difference in the 5-year actuarial metastasis-free survival rates (79.8% versus 85%, HR = 1.08; CI 95%: 0.36–2.95), cancer specific survival rates (92% versus 89%, HR = 0.67; CI 95%: 0.32–1.29), and overall survival (97.5% versus 88%; HR = 0.24; CI 95%: 0.01–1.34), for the brachytherapy and HIFU cohorts,

respectively, even after stratifying according to the D'Amico risk (Figure 3).

The rates of the most common complications associated with these two procedures are reported in Table 4. HIFU cohort was divided into two subgroups according to the technique used. Urinary retention rates and urinary tract infection rates were significantly higher in the subgroup of patients treated with HIFU compared to brachytherapy. Lower urinary tract symptoms (LUTS) were the most frequent early and late postoperative complications with no statistically significant difference across the two cohorts. However, brachytherapy was associated with more storage and less voiding LUTS than HIFU. LUTS and hematuria were self-resolving in the majority of cases and their incidence decreased in the two groups after 1 year of follow-up. Only one patient in the brachytherapy arm had hemorrhagic cystitis in his follow-up managed by an endoscopic fulguration (Grade 3b). Gastrointestinal toxicity was low and comparable across the two cohorts with only one patient in each group developing a rectourethral fistula managed surgically (Grade 3b). Bladder outlet obstructions mainly urethral stricture and chronic pelvic

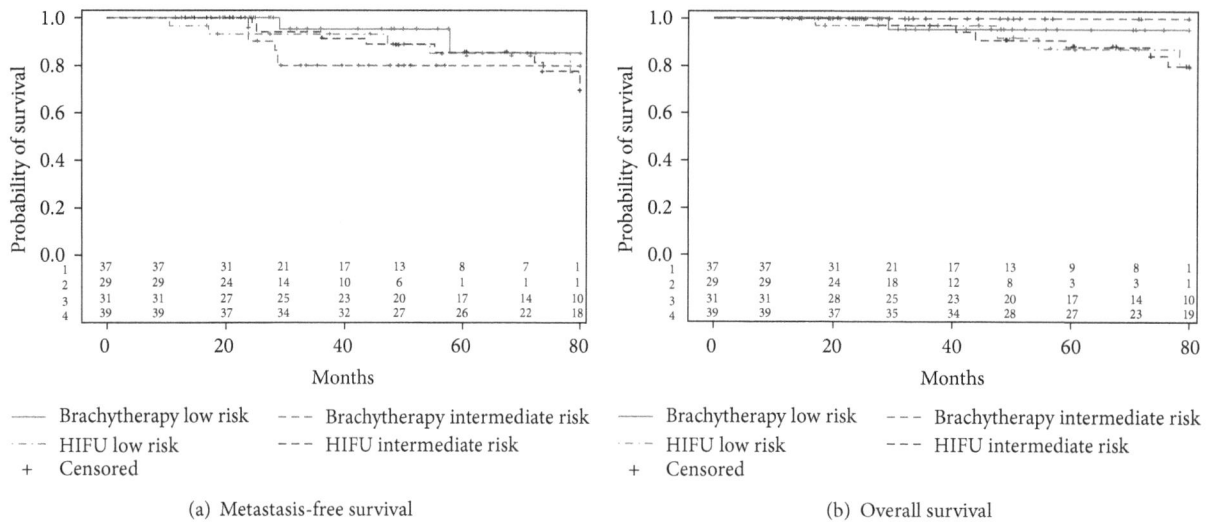

(a) Metastasis-free survival

(b) Overall survival

FIGURE 3: Kaplan-Meier curves for metastasis-free survival (a) and overall survival (b) stratified according to D'Amico risk classification.

TABLE 4: Comparison of early and long term postoperative complications according to the therapeutic approach.

	BT*	HIFU**	Maxis Ablatherm	Ablatherm integrated imaging	p value (BT versus HIFU)	p value (BT versus Maxis)	p value (BT versus integrated imaging)
				(A) Early			
$N =$	59	90	39	31	—	—	—
Acute urinary retention	4 (6.8%)	16 (22.9%)	12 (30.8%)	4 (12.9%)	0.02	<0.01	0.44
Urinary tract infection	5 (8.5%)	15 (21.4%)	12 (30.8%)	3 (9.7%)	0.07	<0.01	0.86
LUTS***	25 (42.4%)	28 (40.0%)	17 (43.6%)	11 (35.5%)	0.93	1	0.68
(i) Storage	19 (32.2%)	5 (7.2%)	3 (7.7%)	2 (6.4%)	<0.01	<0.01	0.01
(ii) Voiding	6 (10.2%)	23 (32.8%)	14 (35.9%)	9 (29.1%)	<0.01	<0.01	0.04
Gastrointestinal toxicity	2 (3.4%)	1 (1.4%)	1 (2.6%)	0 (0.0%)	0.59	1	0.78
				(B) Long term			
$N =$	53	69	39	30	—	—	—
LUTS***	14 (26.4%)	19 (27.5%)	12 (30.8%)	7 (23.3%)	1	0.82	0.96
(i) Storage	10 (18.9%)	7 (10.1%)	4 (10.3%)	3 (10.0%)	0.26	0.30	0.36
(ii) Voiding	4 (7.5%)	12 (17.4%)	8 (20.5%)	4 (13.3%)	0.18	0.18	0.45
Urethral stricture	2 (3.8%)	17 (24.6%)	12 (30.8%)	5 (16.7%)	<0.01	<0.01	0.09
Rectourethral fistula	1 (1.9%)	1 (1.4%)	1 (2.6%)	0 (0.0%)	1	1	1
Chronic pelvic pain	0 (0.0%)	3 (4.3%)	3 (7.7%)	0 (0.0%)	0.34	0.08	1
Urinary incontinence	2 (3.8%)	5 (7.2%)	3 (7.7%)	2 (6.7%)	0.44	0.72	0.62

*Brachytherapy, **high intensity focused ultrasound, and ***lower urinary tract symptoms.

pain were encountered more frequently following HIFU in particular in patients treated early with the first commercially available HIFU device. Finally, no peri- or postoperative deaths were recorded in the two cohorts (Table 5).

Regarding urinary incontinence, no significant difference was found across the two cohorts (7.2% versus 3.8%, $p = 0.44$). Transient urinary incontinence was seen in two patients one in each group. The only patient with persistent incontinence at the last follow-up in the brachytherapy group had a mixed incontinence. This patient had already been treated by optical urethrotomy. In the HIFU cohort, Grade 1 persistent stress urinary incontinence was reported in 2 patients and the 2 other patients had Grade 2 stress urinary incontinence. In preoperatively potent patients in the HIFU cohort ($n = 43$), 5 men (11.6%) had documented post-whole gland ablation erectile dysfunction (ED) and 27 men (62.8%) had erections satisfactory for sexual intercourse with ($n = 9$) or without pharmacotherapy ($n = 20$), and data

TABLE 5: Comparison of overall complications by grade of severity between the two groups.

	Grade 1		Grade 2		Grade 3a		Grade 3b	
	HIFU	BT	HIFU	BT	HIFU	BT	HIFU	BT
LUTS/hematuria (early)	23/70 (32.9%)	18/59 (30.5%)	5/70 (7.1%)	7/59 (11.9%)	0 (0%)	0 (0%)	0 (0%)	0 (0%)
LUTS/hematuria (late)	3/69 (4.3%)	2/53 (3.8%)	16/69 (23.2%)	11/53 (20.7%)	0 (0%)	1/53 (1.9%)	0 (0%)	0 (0%)
Urinary tract infection	0 (0%)	0 (0%)	15/70 (21.4%)	5/59 (8.5%)	0 (0%)	0 (0%)	0 (0%)	0 (0%)
Acute urinary retention	0 (0%)	0 (0%)	0 (0%)	0 (0%)	14/70 (20.0%)	4/59 (6.8%)	2/70 (2.8%)	0 (0%)
Urinary stricture	0 (0%)	0 (0%)	0 (0%)	0 (0%)	2/69 (2.9%)	0 (0%)	15/69 (21.7%)	2/53 (3.8%)
Urinary incontinence	5/69 (7.2%)	1/53 (1.9%)	0 (0%)	1/53 (1.9%)	0 (0%)	0 (0%)	0 (0%)	0 (0%)
Gastrointestinal toxicities	0 (0%)	0 (0%)	0 (0%)	1/59 (1.7%)	0 (0%)	0 (0%)	1/70 (1.4%)	1/59 (1.7%)

were lacking in 9 patients. For the brachytherapy group, data on preoperative erectile function were not available for the majority of patients.

4. Discussion

The aim of this study was to compare retrospectively HIFU and brachytherapy for the curative treatment of organ confined prostate cancer.

The two techniques are effective as demonstrated by the high probability to achieve low PSA nadir following treatment. However, the early achievement of PSA nadir following HIFU compared to brachytherapy provides an immediate feedback on treatment efficacy and identifies quickly patients with residual cancer. This rapid proof of response provides also stringent information about potential cure as demonstrated in most contemporary series [19–21]. In our previous study, only 12.5% of patients achieving PSA nadir < 0.5 ng/mL experienced biochemical failure at 10 years of follow-up [12].

In our clinical practice, assessment of oncologic efficacy is performed by serial PSA testing and random systematic TRUS guided biopsies are offered only for a cause (Phoenix criteria and/or suspicious DRE) in order to minimise burden on the patient. Moreover, systematic post-HIFU biopsy mapping of treated prostates has widely proven the local efficacy of thermoablation. Although PSA testing is accepted as a valid outcome to define biochemical recurrence after brachytherapy, its clinical significance following tissue ablation is not yet determined [22]. To date, studies reporting on HIFU are using the Phoenix definition or the more recent Stuttgart definition to define biochemical recurrence but these two definitions are not validated for the HIFU group. Of note it has to be reminded that HIFU technical procedures leave untreated significant areas of the prostate, that is, up to 7 mm of apical area and anterior sectors of the prostate beyond 26 mm measured from the posterior capsule.

Our results for the two cohorts are in line with the reported rates published in the contemporary literature that had used a combination of biopsy results and PSA threshold values to assess failure [23]. According to these criteria, BRFS was significantly higher for the low risk group following brachytherapy compared to HIFU. This could be explained by the absence of matching for year of treatment across our two groups that resulted in a significantly longer follow-up in the HIFU cohort. The longer follow-up in the HIFU cohort

may lead to the increased number of biochemical recurrences detected in this group. As such, this bias should have also favoured brachytherapy for the intermediate risk. One could argue that the absence of difference is due to an early biochemical recurrence in the intermediate group treated by brachytherapy or even a worse prognosis. In the literature, there has been much discussion on the relative impact of Gleason score 7 on oncologic outcome following treatment by brachytherapy [24–27]. The majority of reports on outcomes after brachytherapy show inferior biochemical control for patients with Gleason 7 [28, 29]. The EAU and ABS exclude patients with a Gleason 7 from the qualification criteria for a brachytherapy alone treatment [2, 30]. For the NCCN, brachytherapy is always combined to external beam radiation therapy (EBRT) for intermediate risk patients [31]. A new study had suggested the need for high quality and high-dose treatment to eradicate Gleason 7 prostate cancer [32]. At present, there is an ongoing phase III prospective randomized controlled open label registered clinical trial (http://www.clinicaltrials.gov/ Identifier: NCT00063882). The trial randomizes patients with intermediate-risk prostate cancer to brachytherapy alone versus combined therapy (brachytherapy and extended beam radiation therapy) in order to define the optimum brachytherapy treatment for patients with intermediate-risk prostate cancer. In the early experience with HIFU, there was much disagreement on treating patients with high risk disease. Some authors have argued that HIFU is a coagulative technology that unlike radiation therapy results in a complete cell destruction independently of Gleason score. However, results have clearly demonstrated that tissue under ablation in high grade tumour may be inadequately ablated (heat sinks phenomenon) and is a high risk site for persistent residual progressive disease and metastatic spread [12, 33]. For patients with intermediate risk of progression, results are contradictory and the debate is ongoing [12]. The main advantage of HIFU over brachytherapy is the possibility to repeat the treatment with a further increase in response rate without substantially increasing side effects [34]. It is also noteworthy to mention that, by using the stricter Stuttgart definition, studies with a short follow-up will experience more failures but possibly achieved a truer picture of outcomes and allow earlier treatment of patients. However, with longer follow-up, the difference between the two criteria will be reduced which is demonstrated in the present study by the small percentages of patients considered as failures according to Stuttgart but not to Phoenix definition. The 5-year actuarial metastasis-free survival, cancer specific survival, and overall survival rates were not significantly different between the two cohorts and are in line with the reported rates in nonrandomized published case series [35]. However, the retrospective design and the insufficient follow-up limit further conclusion.

Early side effects and complications of the two techniques involve primarily the urinary tract. Storage and voiding LUTS develop immediately as a result of implant trauma after brachytherapy or tissue heating following HIFU. Over the first weeks LUTS are due to the effect of radiation and tissue sloughing and necrosis following brachytherapy and HIFU, respectively. At 3 months, HIFU was more associated with voiding LUTS whereas brachytherapy was more associated with storage LUTS. These urinary symptoms are generally mild and self-resolving after several months as evidenced by the lower rate at the last follow-up. Technical improvements with the introduction of the new Ablatherm device (frequency of the ultrasound, length of treatment pulses, and rectal cooling) and the changes in surgical protocol (concomitant TURP and prophylactic antibiotics) had substantially lowered the high rate of urinary tract infection and bladder outlet obstruction encountered at our early experience with HIFU. One patient developed rectourethral fistula in each group.

The incidence of this devastating complication following brachytherapy and HIFU had substantially decreased over the last decade [36]. This is not only due to technical improvements but also to a better understanding of the management of postoperative rectal bleeding. Regarding urinary incontinence, no significant difference was found across the two cohorts. The incidence of urinary incontinence after prostate brachytherapy varies between 0% and 12.9% [37, 38]. The study with the longest follow-up reported a 5.1% risk of urinary incontinence [39]. This result was confirmed by Benoit et al. who estimated the incidence of urinary incontinence to be 6.6% in a study of 2,124 men in a population of Medicare patients with a follow-up from 2 to 3 years [40]. The mechanism is partially elucidated and studies reporting correlation between urinary incontinence and dosimetric or clinical parameters had been published [41]. The incidence of incontinence is also low after HIFU with reported rates varying between 5 and 11% [42]. Safety margins at the level of the apex of the prostate are calculated to avoid temperature diffusion and lesions to the urethra and striated sphincter. The same precautions are taken laterally, to avoid causing lesions to the neurovascular bundles in order to preserve erectile function. These precautions should always be balanced with the risk of oncologic failure [43]. In the HIFU cohort, if we consider patients with lacking data to have ED, the rate after treatment would be 32.5% which is in the range of reported rates in the literature [44]. Recently, we have reported better stress urinary incontinence and erectile function rates with hemiablation HIFU but validated questionnaire and further experience are needed to confirm these findings [45]. Unfortunately, the erectile function data for patients treated by brachytherapy are unavailable. To our knowledge, our study is

the first to compare patients treated by HIFU and brachytherapy. However, we acknowledge the limitations of this retrospective study. Physician reported rates and physician-acquired information have been shown to correlate poorly with data collected from patient self-assessment questionnaires. In addition, the study reported retrospectively on a small cohort of patients. Well-designed, multicenter, prospective, randomized controlled studies are required to assess collateral damage and functional and oncologic outcomes. Another limitation of the present study is the absence of matching for the year of treatment and for the follow-up across the two groups which was already discussed.

5. Conclusion

HIFU and brachytherapy are two minimal invasive safe options for the treatment of organ confined prostate cancer which produce different short term complications but similar long term functional outcomes. Regarding oncologic outcomes, our data reported similar 5-year metastasis-free survival, cancer specific survival, and overall survival in both cohorts of patients. Well-designed, multicenter, prospective, randomized controlled studies with a higher number of patients and a longer follow-up are needed to confirm these results.

Conflict of Interests

There is no conflict of interests.

References

[1] J. Nicholas Lukens, M. Gamez, K. Hu, and L. B. Harrison, "Modern brachytherapy," *Seminars in Oncology*, vol. 41, no. 6, pp. 831–847, 2014.

[2] B. J. Davis, E. M. Horwitz, W. R. Lee et al., "American Brachytherapy Society consensus guidelines for transrectal ultrasound-guided permanent prostate brachytherapy," *Brachytherapy*, vol. 11, no. 1, pp. 6–19, 2012.

[3] N. N. Stone and R. G. Stock, "Complications following permanent prostate brachytherapy," *European Urology*, vol. 41, no. 4, pp. 427–433, 2002.

[4] T. Gupta and C. A. Narayan, "Image-guided radiation therapy: physician's perspectives," *Journal of Medical Physics*, vol. 37, no. 4, pp. 174–182, 2012.

[5] C. Giberti, L. Chiono, F. Gallo, M. Schenone, and E. Gastaldi, "Radical retropubic prostatectomy versus brachytherapy for low-risk prostatic cancer: a prospective study," *World Journal of Urology*, vol. 27, no. 5, pp. 607–612, 2009.

[6] H. P. Beerlage, G. J. L. H. van Leenders, G. O. N. Oosterhof et al., "High-intensity focused ultrasound (HIFU) followed after one to two weeks by radical retropubic prostatectomy: results of a prospective study," *Prostate*, vol. 39, no. 1, pp. 41–46, 1999.

[7] L. Dickinson, Y. Hu, H. U. Ahmed et al., "Image-directed, tissue-preserving focal therapy of prostate cancer: a feasibility study of a novel deformable magnetic resonance-ultrasound (MR-US) registration system," *BJU International*, vol. 112, no. 5, pp. 594–601, 2013.

[8] K. Biermann, R. Montironi, A. Lopez-Beltran, S. Zhang, and L. Cheng, "Histopathological findings after treatment of prostate

cancer using high-intensity focused ultrasound (HIFU)," *Prostate*, vol. 70, no. 11, pp. 1196–1200, 2010.

[9] P. Ryan, A. Finelli, N. Lawrentschuk et al., "Prostatic needle biopsies following primary high intensity focused ultrasound (HIFU) therapy for prostatic adenocarcinoma: histopathological features in tumour and non-tumour tissue," *Journal of Clinical Pathology*, vol. 65, no. 8, pp. 729–734, 2012.

[10] S. Madersbacher, M. Pedevilla, L. Vingers, M. Susani, and M. Marberger, "Effect of high-intensity focused ultrasound on human prostate cancer in vivo," *Cancer Research*, vol. 55, no. 15, pp. 3346–3351, 1995.

[11] A. Gelet, J. Y. Chapelon, R. Bouvier et al., "Treatment of prostate cancer with transrectal focused ultrasound: early clinical experience," *European Urology*, vol. 29, no. 2, pp. 174–183, 1996.

[12] K. Limani, F. Aoun, S. Holz, M. Paesmans, A. Peltier, and R. van Velthoven, "Single high intensity focused ultrasound session as a whole gland primary treatment for clinically localized prostate cancer: 10-year outcomes," *Prostate Cancer*, vol. 2014, Article ID 186782, 7 pages, 2014.

[13] A. V. D'Amico, R. Whittington, S. Bruce Malkowicz et al., "Biochemical outcome after radical prostatectomy, external beam radiation therapy, or interstitial radiation therapy for clinically localized prostate cancer," *Journal of the American Medical Association*, vol. 280, no. 11, pp. 969–974, 1998.

[14] M. Roach III, G. Hanks, H. Thames Jr. et al., "Defining biochemical failure following radiation therapy with or without hormonal therapy in men with clinically localized prostate cancer: recommendation of the RTOG-ASTRO Phoenix Consensus Conference," *International Journal of Radiation Oncology, Biology, Physics*, vol. 65, pp. 965–974, 2006.

[15] A. Blana, S. C. W. Brown, C. Chaussy et al., "High-intensity focused ultrasound for prostate cancer: comparative definitions of biochemical failure," *BJU International*, vol. 104, no. 8, pp. 1058–1062, 2009.

[16] D. Dindo, N. Demartines, and P.-A. Clavien, "Classification of surgical complications: a new proposal with evaluation in a cohort of 6336 patients and results of a survey," *Annals of Surgery*, vol. 240, no. 2, pp. 205–213, 2004.

[17] D. Mitropoulos, W. Artibani, M. Graefen, M. Remzi, M. Rouprêt, and M. Truss, "Reporting and grading of complications after urologic surgical procedures: an ad hoc EAU guidelines panel assessment and recommendations," *European Urology*, vol. 61, no. 2, pp. 341–349, 2012.

[18] T. A. Stamey, "Endoscopic suspension of the vesical neck for urinary incontinence," *Surgery Gynecology and Obstetrics*, vol. 136, no. 4, pp. 547–554, 1973.

[19] R. Ganzer, C. N. Robertson, J. F. Ward et al., "Correlation of prostate-specific antigen nadir and biochemical failure after high-intensity focused ultrasound of localized prostate cancer based on the Stuttgart failure criteria—analysis from the @-Registry," *BJU International*, vol. 108, no. 8, pp. E196–E201, 2011.

[20] J. H. Pinthus, F. Farrokhyar, M. M. Hassouna et al., "Single-session primary high-intensity focused ultrasonography treatment for localized prostate cancer: biochemical outcomes using third generation-based technology," *BJU International*, vol. 110, no. 8, pp. 1142–1148, 2012.

[21] E. R. Cordeiro, X. Cathelineau, S. Thüroff, M. Marberger, S. Crouzet, and J. J. M. C. H. De La Rosette, "High-intensity focused ultrasound (HIFU) for definitive treatment of prostate cancer," *BJU International*, vol. 110, no. 9, pp. 1228–1242, 2012.

[22] T. Uchida, R. O. Illing, P. J. Cathcart, and M. Emberton, "To what extent does the prostate-specific antigen nadir predict subsequent treatment failure after transrectal high-intensity focused ultrasound therapy for presumed localized adenocarcinoma of the prostate?" *BJU International*, vol. 98, no. 3, pp. 537–539, 2006.

[23] H. Lukka, T. Waldron, J. Chin et al., "High-intensity focused ultrasound for prostate cancer: a systematic review," *Clinical Oncology*, vol. 23, no. 2, pp. 117–127, 2011.

[24] S. J. Frank, P. D. Grimm, J. E. Sylvester et al., "Interstitial implant alone or in combination with external beam radiation therapy for intermediate-risk prostate cancer: a survey of practice patterns in the United States," *Brachytherapy*, vol. 6, no. 1, pp. 2–8, 2007.

[25] R. G. Stock, N. N. Stone, J. A. Cesaretti, and B. S. Rosenstein, "Biologically effective dose values for prostate brachytherapy: effects on PSA failure and posttreatment biopsy results," *International Journal of Radiation Oncology Biology Physics*, vol. 64, no. 2, pp. 527–533, 2006.

[26] G. S. Merrick, R. W. Galbreath, W. M. Butler et al., "Primary Gleason pattern does not impact survival after permanent interstitial brachytherapy for gleason score 7 prostate cancer," *Cancer*, vol. 110, no. 2, pp. 289–296, 2007.

[27] R. G. Stock, J. Berkowitz, S. R. Blacksburg, and N. N. Stone, "Gleason 7 prostate cancer treated with low-dose-rate brachytherapy: lack of impact of primary Gleason pattern on biochemical failure," *BJU International*, vol. 110, no. 9, pp. 1257–1261, 2012.

[28] N. N. Stone, M. M. Stone, B. S. Rosenstein, P. Unger, and R. G. Stock, "Influence of pretreatment and treatment factors on intermediate to long-term outcome after prostate brachytherapy," *Journal of Urology*, vol. 185, no. 2, pp. 495–500, 2011.

[29] D. A. Wattson, M.-H. Chen, J. W. Moul et al., "The number of high-risk factors and the risk of prostate cancer-specific mortality after brachytherapy: implications for treatment selection," *International Journal of Radiation Oncology Biology Physics*, vol. 82, no. 5, pp. e773–e779, 2012.

[30] EAU, *Guidelines on Prostate Cancer*, European Association of Urology, 2012.

[31] J. L. Mohler, A. J. Armstrong, R. R. Bahnson et al., "Prostate cancer, version 3.2012: featured updates to the NCCN Guidelines," *Journal of the National Comprehensive Cancer Network*, vol. 10, no. 9, pp. 1081–1087, 2012.

[32] A. Y. Ho, R. J. Burri, J. A. Cesaretti, N. N. Stone, and R. G. Stock, "Radiation dose predicts for biochemical control in intermediate-risk prostate cancer patients treated with low-dose-rate brachytherapy," *International Journal of Radiation Oncology Biology Physics*, vol. 75, no. 1, pp. 16–22, 2009.

[33] D. S. Elterman, J. Barkin, S. B. Radomski et al., "Results of high intensity focused ultrasound treatment of prostate cancer: early Canadian experience at a single center," *Canadian Journal of Urology*, vol. 18, no. 6, pp. 6037–6042, 2011.

[34] A. Blana, S. Rogenhofer, R. Ganzer, P. J. Wild, W. F. Wieland, and B. Walter, "Morbidity associated with repeated transrectal high-intensity focused ultrasound treatment of localized prostate cancer," *World Journal of Urology*, vol. 24, no. 5, pp. 585–590, 2006.

[35] S. Crouzet, X. Rebillard, D. Chevallier et al., "Multicentric oncologic outcomes of high-intensity focused ultrasound for localized prostate cancer in 803 patients," *European Urology*, vol. 58, no. 4, pp. 559–566, 2010.

[36] A. U. Kishan and P. A. Kupelian, "Late rectal toxicity after low-dose-rate brachytherapy: incidence, predictors, and management of side effects," *Brachytherapy*, vol. 14, no. 2, pp. 148–159, 2015.

[37] K. Wallner, L. Henry, S. Wasserman, and M. Dattoli, "Low risk of urinary incontinence following prostate brachytherapy in patients with a prior transurethral prostate resection," *International Journal of Radiation Oncology Biology Physics*, vol. 37, no. 3, pp. 565–569, 1997.

[38] L. Budäus, M. Bolla, A. Bossi et al., "Functional outcomes and complications following radiation therapy for prostate cancer: a critical analysis of the literature," *European Urology*, vol. 61, no. 1, pp. 112–127, 2012.

[39] H. Ragde, J. C. Blasko, P. D. Grimm et al., "Interstitial iodine-125 radiation without adjuvant therapy in the treatment of clinically localized prostate carcinoma," *Cancer*, vol. 80, no. 3, pp. 442–453, 1997.

[40] R. M. Benoit, M. J. Naslund, and J. K. Cohen, "Complications after prostate brachytherapy in the Medicare population," *Urology*, vol. 55, no. 1, pp. 91–96, 2000.

[41] T. L. McElveen, F. M. Waterman, H. Kim, and A. P. Dicker, "Factors predicting for urinary incontinence after prostate brachytherapy," *International Journal of Radiation Oncology Biology Physics*, vol. 59, no. 5, pp. 1395–1404, 2004.

[42] S. Crouzet, J. Y. Chapelon, O. Rouvière et al., "Whole-gland ablation of localized prostate cancer with high-intensity focused ultrasound: oncologic outcomes and morbidity in 1002 patients," *European Urology*, vol. 65, no. 5, pp. 907–914, 2014.

[43] R. Boutier, N. Girouin, A. B. Cheikh et al., "Location of residual cancer after transrectal high-intensity focused ultrasound ablation for clinically localized prostate cancer," *BJU International*, vol. 108, no. 11, pp. 1776–1781, 2011.

[44] X. Rebillard, M. Soulié, E. Chartier-Kastler et al., "High-intensity focused ultrasound in prostate cancer; a systematic literature review of the French Association of Urology," *BJU International*, vol. 101, no. 10, pp. 1205–1213, 2008.

[45] R. Van Velthoven, F. Aoun, K. Limani, K. Narahari, M. Lemort, and A. Peltier, "Primary zonal high intensity focused ultrasound for prostate cancer: results of a prospective phase IIa feasibility study," *Prostate Cancer*, vol. 2014, Article ID 756189, 6 pages, 2014.

19

Treatment of Urethral Strictures from Irradiation and Other Nonsurgical Forms of Pelvic Cancer Treatment

Iyad Khourdaji,[1] **Jacob Parke,**[1] **Avinash Chennamsetty,**[1] **and Frank Burks**[1,2]

[1]*Beaumont Health System, Department of Urology, 3601 W. Thirteen Mile Road, Royal Oak, MI 48073, USA*
[2]*Oakland University William Beaumont School of Medicine, 216 O'Dowd Hall, 2200 N. Squirrel Road, Rochester, MI 48309, USA*

Correspondence should be addressed to Iyad Khourdaji; akhourdaji@gmail.com

Academic Editor: Miroslav L. Djordjevic

Radiation therapy (RT), external beam radiation therapy (EBRT), brachytherapy (BT), photon beam therapy (PBT), high intensity focused ultrasound (HIFU), and cryotherapy are noninvasive treatment options for pelvic malignances and prostate cancer. Though effective in treating cancer, urethral stricture disease is an underrecognized and poorly reported sequela of these treatment modalities. Studies estimate the incidence of stricture from BT to be 1.8%, EBRT 1.7%, combined EBRT and BT 5.2%, and cryotherapy 2.5%. Radiation effects on the genitourinary system can manifest early or months to years after treatment with the onus being on the clinician to investigate and rule-out stricture disease as an underlying etiology for lower urinary tract symptoms. Obliterative endarteritis resulting in ischemia and fibrosis of the irradiated tissue complicates treatment strategies, which include urethral dilation, direct-vision internal urethrotomy (DVIU), urethral stents, and urethroplasty. Failure rates for dilation and DVIU are exceedingly high with several studies indicating that urethroplasty is the most definitive and durable treatment modality for patients with radiation-induced stricture disease. However, a detailed discussion should be offered regarding development or worsening of incontinence after treatment with urethroplasty. Further studies are required to assess the nature and treatment of cryotherapy and HIFU-induced strictures.

1. Introduction

Radiation therapy (RT) is a well-known and effective means of treating pelvic malignancies. External beam radiation therapy (EBRT), brachytherapy (BT), photon beam therapy (PBT), high intensity focused ultrasound (HIFU), and cryotherapy are forms of noninvasive treatments for malignancy. Although an effective form of cancer treatment, radiation therapy is not without complication. Urethral stricture disease is an underrecognized and poorly reported complication that can cause severe morbidity for cancer survivors [1, 2]. Radiated urethral tissue in particular poses a challenge for the reconstructive urologist. It is our goal to provide a comprehensive discussion of etiology, incidence, and available treatment options for urethral stricture disease following pelvic radiation.

2. Epidemiology

The term stricture has previously been the nomenclature applied to any narrowing along the entirety of the urethra. Updated terminology now uses *stenosis* and *stricture* to more appropriately localize the abnormality along the urethra. Narrowed segments of the urethra surrounded by spongiofibrosis have been deemed *stricture*. In contrast, constrictions that occur within the posterior urethra are deemed *stenosis* [3]. It is import to differentiate between the two as treatments can differ depending on location [4].

Radiation effects on the genitourinary system can manifest early after treatment or present months or years after. Acutely, radiation treatment can cause lower urinary tract symptoms (LUTS) such as frequency, urgency, and dysuria requiring symptomatic management [5, 6]. Late urinary toxicity is a prolonged sequelae that can present with hesitancy, retention, stricture, and hematuria [5]. The timing of late toxicity is highly varied and can declare itself decades after initial radiation treatment [7]. Although narrowing can theoretically form at any location along the course of the urethra, bulbomembranous stenosis accounts for 90% of reported strictures after RT [8]. A study investigating the CaPSure registry reported the incidence of stricture from four separate categories of treatment. Their study found the incidence of stricture from BT to be 1.8%, EBRT 1.7%, combined EBRT and BT 5.2%, and cryotherapy as 2.5% [9]. A more recent study documented ranges of bulbomembranous stricture incidence from BT at 1 to 8% versus 2 to 4% for EBRT [2]. Data reporting the incidence of cryotherapy-related stricture disease is also limited; however a recent study comparing 10-year propensity-weighted adverse urinary events after treatment for prostate cancer found incidence of stricture to be 1.05% ($n = 2115$) [10].

3. Etiology

Radiation therapy causes damage on living cells in two main ways: directly, inflicting damage to cellular DNA initiating DNA mutation and apoptosis, and indirectly, interacting with free water within the cell to form hydroxyl free radicals that are highly unstable within the cell. Furthermore, cells that are actively dividing are more sensitive to ionizing radiation than those more stagnant in the cell cycle [11]. Data reviewing the pathophysiology behind urethral stricture in inflammatory, autoimmune, and infectious processes is well-understood and well-described [8]. Unfortunately, studies investigating the underlying mechanism causing stricture after radiation therapy are limited.

Ballek and Gonzalez have studied and described the pathophysiology pertaining to radiation-induced strictures in great detail. Through the aforementioned mechanisms, basement membranes of vascular tissues supplying the urethra become damaged, resulting in occlusion, thrombosis, and impaired neovascularization. Vascular compromise leads to inadequate tissue perfusion and poor wound healing. The result is fibroblasts that are rendered incapable of producing collagen to meet the demands of the healing wound. Collagen maturation is also compromised by poorly functioning fibroblasts leading to contraction and scar formation [12]. Studies have demonstrated this effect to be long lasting and even transmitted to daughter fibroblasts within tissue [13]. Over time, the corpus spongiosum is replaced with fibrotic tissue and subsequent occlusion of the urethral lumen occurs [12].

Healing of these compromised tissues should also be a consideration of the urologist when considering surgical intervention such as reconstructive urethroplasty. Patients receiving radiation therapy weeks to months prior to undergoing surgical intervention experience poor wound healing compared to those who receive similar doses of radiation 6 months or more before surgery [13, 14]. Gorodetsky further found this effect to be dose-dependent; as radiation dose was increased, wound strength decreased. Tissue planes can be distorted making urethroplasty with primary anastomosis or tissue substitution a difficult task [15, 16]. Further

complicating the characteristics of these strictures is their location in the bulbomembranous urethra, higher incidence of postoperative urinary incontinence, erectile dysfunction, and fistula formation [16]. Therefore, these patients should be meticulously informed of the risks and benefits of pursuing surgical intervention.

The overall incidence of urethral stricture disease is also dependent on radiation dosage and the type of radiation used [9, 12]. Merrick et al. found the magnitude and extent of high dose radiation, mean membranous urethral dose, dose 20 mm proximal to the prostatic apex, and the duration of hormonal manipulation to be predictive of stricture formation after radiation therapy [17]. Compared with other side effects of radiation, stricture/stenosis is a relatively uncommon occurrence but is difficult to treat effectively.

4. Diagnosis and Evaluation

Patients presenting with LUTS following pelvic radiotherapy should undergo a thorough history and physical examination with special attention to the patency of the urethral meatus, suprapubic exam, and digital rectal examination. Furthermore, inquiries should be made regarding the dose and type of therapy the patient has received. When indicated, postvoid residual by ultrasound can assess bladder emptying [8, 17].

Cystourethroscopy and retrograde urethrogram provide further detail on the location and length of the urethral stricture [12, 17]. However, exact delineation of the anatomy may be difficult due to distortion from the previously administered therapy. Assessment of external sphincter involvement and the length of the strictured segment are essential [8]. Retrograde urethrography offers the ability to determine the length and location of the obstruction (Figure 1).

If retrograde urethrogram is inconclusive, voiding cystourethrogram allows for full evaluation of the posterior urethra as well as the urethra proximal to the stricture. If a suprapubic tube is present, simultaneous antegrade endoscopy and retrograde urethrography can be performed [12].

Because of the potential deleterious effects of radiation therapy on the bladder, urodynamics can be helpful in evaluating bladder capacity prior to any potential surgery [12, 17]. For patients with bladder volumes less than 200 mL or severe detrusor instability, conservative measures to increase bladder volume may be attempted before reconstruction. However, other options such as bladder augmentation before reconstruction or urinary diversion can be discussed with the patient [12].

5. Treatment

Radiation induces an obliterative endarteritis that results in ischemia and fibrosis of the irradiated tissue. In the perioperative setting, these changes lead to compromised wound healing, altered tissue planes, and impaired blood supply of irradiated tissue [18]. Indeed these pathophysiologic changes induced by radiation are the underlying reasons why treatment can present a challenge.

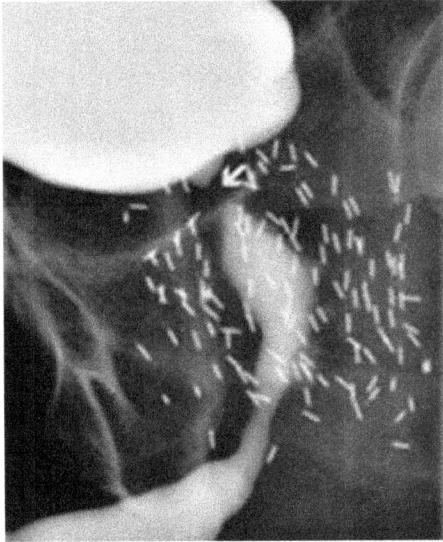

FIGURE 1: Bulbar and bladder neck stricture from combined EBRT and brachytherapy. *Credit to R. Santucci.*

Typical urethral stenosis after single-modality radiation treatment begins at the proximal bulbar urethra and extends through the membranous urethra and prostatic apex [2]. According to the experience of Mundy and Andrich, strictures after EBRT have an average stricture length of approximately 2 cm. Moreover, they report strictures secondary to combination of BT and EBRT are typically longer with nearly half being obliterative [8]. Short strictures are rare and when they happen, anastomotic repairs are rarely successful. Compared with strictures in BT patients, EBRT strictures are not commonly obliterative; they are less complicated to treat and therefore are theoretically amenable to anastomotic urethroplasty. Alternatively, tissue transfer repairs, such as grafts and/or flaps, are more likely to be appropriate and successful in those nonobliterative strictures which are not controlled by interval urethral dilatation [8, 19].

The gold standard for treatment of urethral strictures is urethroplasty with primary anastomosis or substitution urethroplasty being effective techniques depending on the stricture length [19]. Substitution urethroplasty can be accomplished with a graft and/or flap. The difference between the two methods is contingent on the presence (or lack thereof) of the grafted tissue's native blood supply. A graft is tissue that is moved from a donor site to a recipient site without its native blood supply. In contrast, flap tissues maintain their native blood supply on a pedicle that is transferred onto the recipient site [3, 19]. In the previously irradiated patient, several studies have shown urethroplasty to be efficacious. In general, direct-vision internal urethrotomy (DVIU) and dilation carry much higher failure rates than urethroplasty. Urethral stents have been studied in the setting of prostate cancer related urethral stricture disease and their application is discussed below though their use has fallen out of favor.

6. Urethral Dilation and Direct-Vision Internal Urethrotomy

The increased rate of complications associated with reconstruction of the radiated urethra underlies the initial selection of endoscopic therapy for the management of RT induced strictures, regardless of radiation modality. Endoscopic treatment of radiation-induced posterior urethral stenosis [PUS] has been associated with recurrences of approximately 40–60% regardless of the location or etiology [20]. In a study of 76 patients, Santucci and Eisenberg reported a stricture-free rate after first DVIU of 8% with median time to recurrence of 7 months. Subsequent urethrotomies were associated with decreased success rates with 0% stricture-free rate after the fourth and fifth procedures. As such, dilation and DVIU are advocated as temporizing measures, reserved for a select group of patients who have been counseled on the high likelihood of stricture recurrence until definitive curative reconstruction can be planned [1, 21].

Sullivan et al. assessed the nature and outcomes of urethral stricture disease in 38 patients who received high dose rate BT administered either as a boost to EBRT or as monotherapy. 92.1% of these patients experienced a stricture located in the bulbomembranous urethra with a mean time to diagnosis of 22 months. All strictures were initially managed with either dilation ($n = 15$) or DVIU ($n = 20$) with second-line therapy being performed in 17 cases (49%) via repeat dilation, DVIU, or intermittent self-catheterization. Only three cases (9%) required third-line therapy with one patient undergoing urethroplasty. While only one patient underwent invasive surgery with urethroplasty, nearly half of those who initially experienced a urethral stricture subsequently had second-line therapy to treat their stricture disease. However, as the study only provided a median follow-up time after treatment of the initial stricture of 16 months, long-term outcomes of treatment of BT-induced stricture disease cannot truly be reliably assessed based on this data alone [22].

Recently, Hudak et al. investigated the utility and counterproductive effects of repeat DVIU by reviewing 340 consecutive urethroplasties performed by a single surgeon to assess the association of repeat transurethral treatment with stricture complexity. Of 101 urethroplasties meeting inclusion criteria, it was discovered that repeat transurethral manipulation was associated with an eightfold increase in disease duration from stricture diagnosis to curative urethroplasty between patients who had undergone 0 to 1 prior DVIUs versus 2 or more ($p < 0.001$). Moreover, those who had undergone 2 or more previous DVIUs had significantly longer strictures ($p = 0.001$) and were more likely to undergo substitution urethroplasty. Furthermore, though not statistically significant, failure was more common in these patients versus those with 0 or 1 DVIU (12% versus 2%, $p = 0.11$) [23].

Intralesional injection of mitomycin C (MMC) has been assessed as an adjunct to DVIU owing to its ability to mitigate scar formation via inhibition of fibroblast proliferation. Farrell et al. reported a case series prospectively evaluating their experience with DVIU with intralesional MMC and short-term (1 month) clean intermittent catheterization (CIC). 37

patients were enrolled in the study and subsequently underwent DVIU with MMC and once daily CIC for treatment of refractory urethral stricture disease or bladder neck contracture. Radiation-induced urethral strictures were identified in 11 patients with 9 patients (81.8%) having received BT and the other 2 patients receiving EBRT and BT. Though no difference in stricture length was noted between patients with radiation-induced strictures and those without (mean 2.0 cm, $p = 0.651$), patients with prior radiation were noted to have deeper spongiofibrosis. Postoperatively, those with radiation-induced strictures did not experience a significant improvement in flow rate ($p = 0.158$) or PVR ($p = 0.813$) while those with strictures not related to radiation did experience significant improvements in these categories. The overall success rate was found to be 75.7% over the median follow-up period of 23 months. Recurrence-free success was 54.5% in the radiation cohort with a mean time to recurrence of 8 months [24]. The success rate of DVIU with MMC and CIC in patients with radiation-induced strictures is poorer compared to published data assessing urethroplasty [2, 18, 25–30] in this population and is within the estimated overall 40–60% success rate of DVIU/urethral dilation without MMC [20]. Therefore, while conceptually interesting, further large-cohort studies are necessary to the safety and efficacy of intralesional MMC in those with recalcitrant radiation-induced stricture disease.

7. Urethral Stents

The use of urethral stents have been described in the management of urethral stricture disease secondary to prostate cancer therapy. Eisenberg et al. described their experience with urethral stents for treatment of urethral stricture disease in 13 patients, of which 11 had previous history of prostate cancer therapy. The primary indication for urethral stenting versus reconstruction in these patients was to avoid the morbidity of surgery. Of these 11 patients, 3 received EBRT adjuvantly after radical prostatectomy and 4 received combined EBRT and BT with 2 also having undergone concomitant TURP. Overall, 6 of the 13 patients who underwent a urethral stent required additional procedures for stricture recurrence including 5 in previously irradiated patients. Furthermore, 8 of the 13 patients were subsequently rendered incontinent and willing patients underwent AUS placement [31].

In a subsequent study from the same institution, Erickson et al. assessed the efficacy of Urolume stents in 38 men with posterior urethral strictures secondary to prostate cancer treatment. 24 men (63%) received radiation therapy as either the primary treatment (16) or adjuvantly after radical prostatectomy (8). The modalities undertaken to administer radiation treatment were adjuvant EBRT in 8 patients, EBRT with salvage prostatectomy in 2 patients, BT in 8 patients, and BT with EBRT in 6 patients. After a mean follow-up of 2.3 ± 2.5 years, the authors reported an initial success rate of 47% improving to a final success rate of 89% after a total of 33 secondary procedures (including stent placement) in 19 men. Moreover, men who had received radiation therapy experienced recurrence sooner and required more secondary procedures. However, multivariate analysis failed to implicate

radiation therapy as an independent risk factor for failure. The overall postoperative incontinence rate was found to be 82% with a higher rate in men who did versus did not receive previous radiation therapy (96% versus 50%, $p < 0.001$) [32].

Urolume stents are no longer commercially available in the United States and have globally fallen out of favor. However, the aforementioned studies advocate that urethral stenting is a reasonable treatment option for radiation-induced urethral strictures particularly when considering the significant postoperative morbidity patients may experience secondary to open excision. While initial success rates were dismal, secondary procedures led to vast improvements in urethral patency though many required yet further procedures to manage continence. Though incontinence and need for secondary procedures is expected, urethral stenting is a reasonable option for men unwilling or unable to undergo open urethral reconstruction.

8. Urethroplasty

Though urethroplasty is the most invasive approach to the treatment of urethral stricture disease, numerous studies have supported its use given the high rates of success. According to a review by Meeks et al., substitution urethroplasty using a buccal mucosal graft (BMG) has become the primary surgical treatment for long segment bulbar urethral strictures that are not suitable for anastomotic urethroplasty. The success rate for urethroplasty with BMG is between 81% and 96% with an estimated overall 15.6% failure rate for substitution urethroplasty [7]. Furthermore, as previously discussed, repeat DVIUs and/or dilation are destined to fail and may in fact reduce the efficacy of subsequent definitive therapy. In a review of 443 patients who underwent urethroplasty, Erickson et al. determined that a previous history of DVIU ($p = 0.04$) or urethroplasty ($p = 0.03$) was a significant factor predictive of urethroplasty failure [32].Therefore, it stands to reason that further DVIUs and/or dilation should be avoided in favor of more definitive therapy.

Elliott et al. established this notion in 2006 when they prospectively assessed their management of 48 patients presenting with urethral stenosis or rectourinary fistula secondary to prostate cancer therapy. Of the 32 cases of stenosis, 14 occurred secondary to primary radiation therapy while 7 cases involved radical prostatectomy plus EBRT. 23 of 32 patients (73%) experienced successful repair of urethral stenosis, which involved anastomotic urethroplasty (19), flap urethroplasty (2), perineal urethrostomy (2), and urethral stent (9). Regardless of the location of the stricture (i.e., anterior versus posterior), success rates were nearly equal at 70% versus 73%. Moreover, the authors highlight prior EBRT as being a risk factor for urethral reconstruction failure as 9% of RP treated versus 50% of RP plus EBRT treated patients experienced failure after posterior urethroplasty. Of note, the authors excluded patients that had previous treatment with dilation, DVIU, or TUR and also did not subsequently manage any of the patients enrolled in the study with these treatment strategies. However, the study demonstrates that urethroplasty and urethral stenting are viable treatment options with acceptable rates of failure for patients presenting with radiation-induced stricture disease [25].

To further assess the efficacy urethroplasty for treatment of radiation-induced strictures, Meeks et al. performed a review of 30 men undergoing urethroplasty at three separate institutions. EBRT for prostate cancer was etiology of stricture disease in 15 men (50%) with brachytherapy in 7 and a combination of the two in 8. All strictures were noted to be in the proximal bulbar or membranous urethra and on average were 2.9 cm in length. At a mean follow-up of 21 months, 22 men (73%) experienced successful urethral reconstruction with the majority of individuals undergoing excision with primary anastomosis (80%). Incontinence was transient in 10% and persistent in 40%, with 13% subsequently undergoing placement of an artificial urinary sphincter [26].

Glass et al. retrospectively reviewed 29 men with urethral stricture following radiation treatment of prostate cancer of which 11 (38%) were treated with EBRT alone, seven (24%) had radical prostatectomy followed by adjuvant EBRT, seven (24%) had combined EBRT and brachytherapy, and four (14%) were treated with brachytherapy alone. The average stricture length was 2.6 cm. 22 of the cases were reconstructed with excision and primary anastomosis (EPA) (76%), substitution urethroplasty with buccal mucosa in five (17%), and fasciocutaneous flap onlay in two (7%). The overall success rate was 90% at a median follow-up of 40 months (range 12–83 months) with time to stricture recurrence ranging from 6 to 16 months. New onset of urge urinary incontinence was reported in two patients (7%) with one patient opting for an artificial urinary sphincter. Of note, one-third of the patients in this cohort underwent either DVIU or dilation, both of which have been previously shown to contribute to subsequent failure of urethroplasties [18, 33]. Therefore, despite previous treatment, urethroplasty was found to be highly successful in this series.

Further support for the efficacy of excision and primary anastomosis (EPA) for radiation-induced strictures was provided by a 2014 retrospective study conducted by Hofer and colleagues. Of the 72 men identified with radiation-induced urethral strictures, 66 (91.7%) underwent urethral reconstruction with EPA and the remaining 6 (8.3%) were treated with substitution urethroplasty using a graft or flap. Mean stricture length, which was determined intraoperatively, was 2.4 cm. Furthermore, stricture length was 2 cm or less in 37 of 65 men (56.1%) and greater than 2 cm in 28 men (42.4%). Stricture lengths were greater in those who underwent substitution urethroplasty (mean length 4.25 cm, range 3 to 7 cm). 46 (69.7%) men ultimately experienced successful reconstruction. Mean time to recurrence was found to be 10.2 months and was associated with stricture length greater than 2 cm ($p = 0.013$). Moreover, 12 (18.5%) men experienced new onset incontinence while the rate of ED remained stable. Radiotherapy type did not affect stricture length ($p = 0.41$), recurrence risk ($p = 0.91$), postoperative incontinence ($p = 0.88$), or erectile dysfunction ($p = 0.53$). Overall, EPA was found to be a successful treatment strategy for patients with radiation-induced strictures of the bulbomembranous urethra. Furthermore, the study indicates

that men should be counseled on the development of de novo incontinence and the possible need for secondary procedures to provide adequate management [27].

In a 2015 study, Rourke et al. retrospectively reviewed outcomes in 35 patients undergoing urethroplasty for radiation-induced bulbomembranous stenosis. Of the 35 patients, 20 and 15 had stenosis related to EBRT and BT, respectively, with a mean stricture length of 3.5 cm. Nearly half of the patients enrolled in the study presented preoperatively with an indwelling suprapubic catheter indicating baseline. Reconstruction was performed using anastomotic urethroplasty in 23 patients (65.7%) with 12 patients requiring tissue transfer via buccal mucosa graft (20.0%) or penile island flap (14.3%). With 50.5 months of follow-up, thirty patients (85.7%) achieved cystoscopic patency with no significant difference between techniques ($p = 0.32$). 31.4% of patients experienced a reportable 90-day complication all of which were Clavien Grades I-II [2].

The work of Rourke et al. indicates that urethroplasty is efficacious in radiation-induced urethral stenosis. However, even in well-selected patients (i.e., those without extensive prostatic necrosis, cavitation, prostatosymphyseal fistula, osteomyelitis, or small functional bladder capacity) minor complications were fairly common albeit acceptable and manageable. Despite achieving urethral patency many patients continued to experience bothersome LUTS as well as ED and incontinence. This suggests that even though commendable urethral patency rates may be attained, urethroplasty cannot alone mitigate and may even exacerbate, many of the concomitant complaints experienced by this patient population [2].

While the aforementioned studies have largely assessed the efficacy of anastomotic urethroplasties, long-term outcomes reported in men undergoing substitution urethroplasty have demonstrated higher recurrence rates than anastomotic techniques. The failure of substitution urethroplasties is further exacerbated by the use of donor graft or flap tissue that has been irradiated, which can compromise the effects of the previous radiation exposure.

An abstract published by Kuhl et al. specifically assessed the outcomes of buccal mucosa graft (BMG) urethroplasties for the treatment of radiation-induced urethral strictures. Of the 20 patients enrolled in the study with available data, 75% of treated strictures were within the bulbomembranous urethra and less than 6 cm in length. The success rate was found to be 60% after 25 months of follow-up. Postoperatively, patients experienced an improvement in flow rate from 8.4 to 25.6 mL/s, which trended towards significance ($p < 0.07$) in flow rate. Furthermore, 29% and 10% of the patients with preoperative incontinence experienced worsening or de novo incontinence, respectively. However, despite these postoperative changes in continence, BMG substitution urethroplasties were deemed to be successful with high rates of patient satisfaction [28].

Long segment strictures have been found to be challenging to treat. When treated with traditional dorsal or ventral onlay approaches, these strictures carry a high risk of recurrence due to the lack of a well-vascularized graft bed. Moreover, previously irradiated fields are often poorly vascularized thereby impeding wound healing [12, 29, 30]. In order to promote neovascularity and healing of these reconstructions, Palmer et al. assessed the use of a gracilis muscle flap to provide a well-vascularized graft bed for buccal graft substitutions. After performing a ventral buccal graft onlay, the authors describe harvesting and rotating gracilis muscle onto the perineum and buttressing the muscle to the graft. 20 patients with long segment urethral strictures secondary to various etiologies including radiation therapy in 45% (9 of 20) were retrospectively reviewed. Before surgery, 18 patients (90%) had undergone dilatation and/or endoscopic incision. Strictures were located in the posterior urethra with or without bulbar urethral involvement in 50% of cases (10), the bulbomembranous urethra in 35% (7), the bulbar urethra in 10% (2), and the proximal pendulous urethra in 5% (1) with a mean stricture length of 8.2 cm. Urethral reconstruction was found to be successful in 16 cases (80%) at a mean follow-up of 40 months. Mean time to recurrence was observed to be 10 months with 5 patients (25%) experiencing postoperative incontinence requiring an artificial urinary sphincter. Despite significant preoperative risk factors, the authors demonstrate the efficaciousness of substitution urethroplasty with gracilis flap thereby supporting its use in complex patients with a previous history of radiation therapy. However, despite the encouraging results, the study is limited by its retrospective nature and small sample size [30].

Ahyai et al. recently published their experience with ventral onlay buccal mucosa graft urethroplasties in patients with radiation-induced strictures. 35 of the 38 men (92.1%) included in the study underwent radiotherapy for treatment of prostate cancer with 64.9% exclusively undergoing EBRT. BT was performed in 8 patients (21.6%) with EBRT and BT being performed in combination in 6 patients (13.5%). The median length of strictures treated was 3.0 cm. The mean length of implanted buccal graft was 4.9 cm. 27 patients had undergone previous urethral dilation or DVIU. After a median follow-up of 26.5 months, the overall success rate was 71.1% with 4 patients (10.5%) experiencing de novo incontinence and 11 patients (28.9%) experiencing recurrence. Though limited by its retrospective design and small sample size, the study indicates that ventral onlay buccal mucosa urethroplasty is an acceptable treatment strategy with results similar to EPAs particularly for patients with strictures greater than 1 cm [34].

9. Conclusions

Men with urethral strictures secondary to nonsurgical forms of treatment for prostate cancer represent a challenging cohort to treat. Published data suggests that radiation-induced strictures are best treated with urethroplasty via anastomic or substitution techniques. Patients should be counseled on the high likelihood of stricture recurrence after DVIU or dilation. Moreover, a detailed discussion should take place regarding development or worsening of incontinence after treatment with urethroplasty. Further studies are required to assess the nature and treatment of cryotherapy and HIFU-induced strictures.

Conflict of Interests

The authors declare that there is no conflict of interests regarding the publication of this paper.

Acknowledgment

This paper is funded by Ministrelli Program for Urology Research and Education (MPURE).

References

[1] A. C. Chi, J. Han, and C. M. Gonzalez, "Urethral strictures and the cancer survivor," *Current Opinion in Urology*, vol. 24, no. 4, pp. 415–420, 2014.

[2] K. Rourke, A. Kinnaird, and J. Zorn, "Observations and outcomes of urethroplasty for bulbomembranous stenosis after radiation therapy for prostate cancer," *World Journal of Urology*, 2015.

[3] J. M. Latini, J. W. McAninch, S. B. Brandes, J. Y. Chung, and D. Rosenstein, "SIU/ICUD consultation on urethral strictures: epidemiology, etiology, anatomy, and nomenclature of urethral stenoses, strictures, and pelvic fracture urethral disruption injuries," *Urology*, vol. 83, no. 3, supplement, pp. S1–S7, 2014.

[4] L. Zhao, *Contemporary Management of Anterior Urethral Strictures. AUA Update Series*, vol. 33, lesson 18, AUA, 2014.

[5] A. M. McDonald, C. B. Baker, R. A. Popple, R. A. Cardan, and J. B. Fiveash, "Increased radiation dose heterogeneity within the prostate predisposes to urethral strictures in patients receiving moderately hypofractionated prostate radiation therapy," *Practical Radiation Oncology*, vol. 5, no. 5, pp. 338–342, 2015.

[6] A. L. Zietman, M. L. DeSilvio, J. D. Slater et al., "Comparison of conventional-dose vs high-dose conformal radiation therapy in clinically localized adenocarcinoma of the prostate: a randomized controlled trial," *Journal of the American Medical Association*, vol. 294, no. 10, pp. 1233–1239, 2005.

[7] J. J. Meeks, B. A. Erickson, M. A. Granieri, and C. M. Gonzalez, "Stricture recurrence after urethroplasty: a systematic review," *Journal of Urology*, vol. 182, no. 4, pp. 1266–1270, 2009.

[8] A. R. Mundy and D. E. Andrich, "Posterior urethral complications of the treatment of prostate cancer," *British Journal of Urology*, vol. 110, no. 3, pp. 304–325, 2012.

[9] S. P. Elliott, M. V. Meng, E. P. Elkin, J. W. McAninch, J. Duchane, and P. R. Carroll, "Incidence of urethral stricture after primary treatment for prostate cancer: data from CaPSURE," *Journal of Urology*, vol. 178, no. 2, pp. 529–534, 2007.

[10] S. L. Jarosek, B. A. Virnig, H. Chu, and S. P. Elliott, "Propensity-weighted long-term risk of urinary adverse events after prostate cancer surgery, radiation, or both," *European Urology*, vol. 67, no. 2, pp. 273–280, 2014.

[11] N. E. Bolus, "Basic review of radiation biology and terminology," *Journal of Nuclear Medicine Technology*, vol. 29, no. 2, pp. 67–73, 2001.

[12] N. K. Ballek and C. M. Gonzalez, "Reconstruction of radiation-induced injuries of the lower urinary tract," *Urologic Clinics of North America*, vol. 40, no. 3, pp. 407–419, 2013.

[13] D. B. Drake and S. N. Oishi, "Wound healing considerations in chemotherapy and radiation therapy," *Clinics in Plastic Surgery*, vol. 22, no. 1, pp. 31–37, 1995.

[14] D. S. Springfield, "Surgical wound healing," *Cancer Treatment and Research*, vol. 67, pp. 81–98, 1993.

[15] R. Gorodetsky, X. Mou, D. R. Fisher, J. M. G. Taylor, and H. R. Withers, "Radiation effect in mouse skin: dose fractionation and wound healing," *International Journal of Radiation Oncology, Biology, Physics*, vol. 18, no. 5, pp. 1077–1081, 1990.

[16] J. C. Milose and C. M. Gonzalez, "Urethroplasty in radiation-induced strictures," *Current Opinion in Urology*, vol. 25, no. 4, pp. 336–340, 2015.

[17] G. S. Merrick, W. M. Butler, B. G. Tollenaar, R. W. Galbreath, and J. H. Lief, "The dosimetry of prostate brachytherapy-induced urethral stricture," *International Journal of Radiation Oncology Biology Physics*, vol. 52, no. 2, pp. 461–468, 2002.

[18] A. S. Glass, J. W. McAninch, U. B. Zaid, N. M. Cinman, and B. N. Breyer, "Urethroplasty after radiation therapy for prostate cancer," *Urology*, vol. 79, no. 6, pp. 1402–1406, 2012.

[19] D. J. Bryk, Y. Yamaguchi, and L. C. Zhao, "Tissue transfer techniques in reconstructive urology," *Korean Journal of Urology*, vol. 56, no. 7, pp. 478–486, 2015.

[20] S. Herschorn, S. P. Elliott, M. Coburn, H. Wessells, and L. Zinman, "SIU/ICUD consultation on urethral strictures: posterior urethral stenosis after treatment of prostate cancer," *Urology*, vol. 83, no. 3, supplement, pp. S59–S70, 2014.

[21] R. Santucci and L. Eisenberg, "Urethrotomy has a much lower success rate than previously reported," *The Journal of Urology*, vol. 183, no. 5, pp. 1859–1862, 2010.

[22] L. Sullivan, S. G. Williams, K. H. Tai, F. Foroudi, L. Cleeve, and G. M. Duchesne, "Urethral stricture following high dose rate brachytherapy for prostate cancer," *Radiotherapy and Oncology*, vol. 91, no. 2, pp. 232–236, 2009.

[23] S. J. Hudak, T. H. Atkinson, and A. F. Morey, "Repeat transurethral manipulation of bulbar urethral strictures is associated with increased stricture complexity and prolonged disease duration," *Journal of Urology*, vol. 187, no. 5, pp. 1691–1695, 2012.

[24] M. R. Farrell, B. A. Sherer, and L. A. Levine, "Visual internal urethrotomy with intralesional mitomycin C and short-term clean intermittent catheterization for the management of recurrent urethral strictures and bladder neck contractures," *Urology*, vol. 85, no. 6, pp. 1494–1500, 2015.

[25] S. P. Elliott, J. W. McAninch, T. Chi, S. M. Doyle, and V. A. Master, "Management of severe urethral complications of prostate cancer therapy," *Journal of Urology*, vol. 176, no. 6, pp. 2508–2513, 2006.

[26] J. J. Meeks, S. B. Brandes, A. F. Morey et al., "Urethroplasty for radiotherapy induced bulbomembranous strictures: a multi-institutional experience," *Journal of Urology*, vol. 185, no. 5, pp. 1761–1765, 2011.

[27] M. D. Hofer, L. C. Zhao, A. F. Morey et al., "Outcomes after urethroplasty for radiotherapy induced bulbomembranous urethral stricture disease," *Journal of Urology*, vol. 191, no. 5, pp. 1307–1312, 2014.

[28] M. C. Kuhl, R. Dahlem, M. Traumann et al., "935 Outcome of buccal mucosa graft urethroplasty after radiation therapy," *The Journal of Urology*, vol. 187, no. 4, supplement, p. e380, 2012.

[29] L. Zinman, "Muscular, myocutaneous, and fasciocutaneous flaps in complex urethral reconstruction," *Urologic Clinics of North America*, vol. 29, no. 2, pp. 443–466, 2002.

[30] D. A. Palmer, J. C. Buckley, L. N. Zinman, and A. J. Vanni, "Urethroplasty for high risk, long segment urethral strictures with ventral buccal mucosa graft and gracilis muscle flap," *Journal of Urology*, vol. 193, no. 3, pp. 902–905, 2015.

[31] M. L. Eisenberg, S. P. Elliott, and J. W. McAninch, "Preservation of lower urinary tract function in posterior urethral stenosis: selection of appropriate patients for urethral stents," *Journal of Urology*, vol. 178, no. 6, pp. 2456–2461, 2007.

[32] B. A. Erickson, J. W. McAninch, M. L. Eisenberg, S. L. Washington, and B. N. Breyer, "Management for prostate cancer treatment related posterior urethral and bladder neck stenosis with stents," *Journal of Urology*, vol. 185, no. 1, pp. 198–203, 2011.

[33] B. N. Breyer, J. W. McAninch, J. M. Whitson et al., "Multivariate analysis of risk factors for long-term urethroplasty outcome," *The Journal of Urology*, vol. 183, no. 2, pp. 613–617, 2010.

[34] S. A. Ahyai, M. Schmid, M. Kuhl et al., "Outcomes of ventral onlay buccal mucosa graft urethroplasty in patients after radiotherapy," *The Journal of Urology*, vol. 194, no. 2, pp. 441–446, 2015.

20

A Narrative Review on the Pathophysiology and Management for Radiation Cystitis

C. Browne,[1] **N. F. Davis,**[1] **E. Mac Craith,**[1] **G. M. Lennon,**[1] **D. W. Mulvin,**[1] **D. M. Quinlan,**[1] **Gerard P. Mc Vey,**[2] **and D. J. Galvin**[1]

[1]*Department of Urology, St. Vincent's University Hospital, Dublin 4, Ireland*
[2]*Department of Radiation Oncology, St. Vincent's University Hospital, Dublin 4, Ireland*

Correspondence should be addressed to C. Browne; cliodhnabrowne@rcsi.ie

Academic Editor: Fabio Campodonico

Radiation cystitis is a recognised complication of pelvic radiotherapy. Incidence of radiation cystitis ranges from 23 to 80% and the incidence of severe haematuria ranges from 5 to 8%. High quality data on management strategies for radiation cystitis is sparse. Treatment modalities are subclassified into systemic therapies, intravesical therapies, and hyperbaric oxygen and interventional procedures. Short-term cure rates range from 76 to 95% for hyperbaric oxygen therapy and interventional procedures. Adverse effects of these treatment strategies are acceptable. Ultimately, most patients require multimodal treatment for curative purposes. Large randomised trials exploring emergent management strategies are required in order to strengthen evidence-based treatment strategies. Urologists encounter radiation cystitis commonly and should be familiar with diagnostic modalities and treatment strategies.

1. Introduction

Radiotherapy is a common treatment modality for the management of pelvic malignancies. Treatment for prostate, bladder, rectal, and cervical cancers often involves radiotherapy and radiation cystitis is a recognised complication. The response of the urinary bladder to radiation treatment can be classified into acute or subacute reactions that occur within three to six months of radiation treatment and late reactions that occur after six months. Urinary symptoms include dysuria, frequency, urgency, and haematuria [1]. Haemorrhagic cystitis is a recognised late complication of pelvic radiation and is commonly encountered by urologists. Modern technologies in radiotherapy aim to reduce the dose administered to organs at risk, including the bladder. Differences in toxicities between radiotherapy modalities are explained by total radiation dose to the genitourinary tract [2]. The bladder is sensitive to small increments of radiation dose [3]. The introduction of intensity modulated radiotherapy (IMRT) has allowed reduction in planning target volume (PTV) margins, resulting in significantly less genitourinary toxicity compared to 3D conformal radiotherapy [4–7]. Stereotactic radiotherapy has acceptable and comparable toxicity rates to external beam radiotherapy [8]. In this narrative review, we discuss the pathophysiology, epidemiology, and management options for radiation cystitis. Our aim is to objectively assess the systemic, intravesical, and surgical management options for this problematic condition.

2. Materials and Methods

A literature search was performed using PubMed database and the Cochrane Central Register of Controlled Trials, aiming to identify peer-reviewed articles that outlined epidemiology, pathophysiology, diagnosis, and management of radiation cystitis. The following terms were entered into the search function for each database: "radiation" AND "cystitis" OR "radiation cystitis". One hundred and fifty-four studies published between 1953 and 2015 were identified. The bibliographies of these studies were interrogated to identify other studies for possible inclusion.

The latest search was conducted on 24 September 2015. One author (CB) examined the title and abstract of all retrieved studies and obtained full texts of all papers for

TABLE 1: The proposed pathophysiology of radiation cystitis [1, 9, 10].

Anatomical location in bladder	The proposed mechanism of radiation damage
Urothelium	Nuclear irregularity
	Cellular oedema
	Increased cytoplasmic elements
	Disruption of tight junctions & polysaccharide layer
Vasculature	Vascular endothelial cell oedema
	Endothelial cell proliferation
	Perivascular fibrosis
Muscle	Smooth muscle oedema
	Replacement of smooth muscle with fibroblasts
	Increased collagen deposition
	Vascular ischaemia of bladder wall

potential inclusion. These full texts were analysed for suitability for reporting. American Urological Association and European Association of Urology guidelines were also included. Case reports were excluded. A total of fifty-five papers were included for review.

3. Epidemiology

The reported incidence of radiation cystitis varies from 23% to 80% and this wide range is due to variable types and doses of radiotherapy among different medical subspecialties [1]. The mean duration for developing radiation cystitis is 31.8 months after treatment [10]. Males are more likely to develop radiation cystitis than females (2.8 : 1) due to frequent use of radiotherapy in the treatment of prostate cancer [10]. The reported incidence of severe haematuria ranges from 5% to 8% and haematuria can develop up to fourteen years following radiotherapy treatment [9, 28–30]. The actuarial risk of developing haematuria is 5.8% at five years and 9.6% at twenty years [31].

4. Pathophysiology

The pathophysiology of radiation cystitis is poorly understood. Multiple mechanisms of radiation damage to the bladder have been described (Table 1). The proposed mechanisms of pathology include inflammatory effects of ionising radiation traumatising the urothelium, vasculature, and detrusor muscle [10] with radiation effects on the urothelium most evident after four months [1].

Postradiation intermediate and basal urothelium displays nuclear irregularity and cellular oedema. The tight junctions and polysaccharide layer are disrupted, allowing hypertonic urine and isotonic tissue in contact with one another which results in tissue inflammation and early symptomatic acute radiation cystitis [1]. Vascular endothelial cells are thought to be the main target cell for bladder damage after radiation with late bladder fibrosis occurring secondary to vascular

ischaemia of the bladder wall [1]. Vascular endothelial cell oedema is evident at three months and endothelial cell proliferation is evident after six months. Vascular ischaemia, oedema, and cellular destruction cause replacement of bladder smooth muscle fibres with fibroblasts and lead to increased collagen deposition and subsequent decreases in bladder compliance and capacity [9].

5. Diagnosis

The diagnosis of radiation cystitis is mainly based on exclusion of other causes of the patient's symptoms. An initial assessment involves a full patient history, physical examination, urinalysis, urine culture, urine cytology, and cystoscopy. Computed tomography (CT) may exclude an upper tract lesion as the cause of haematuria and magnetic resonance imaging (MRI) should be considered in the presence of a previous pelvic malignancy [32]. The Radiation Therapy Oncology Group guidelines on late radiation morbidity outline a grading system for radiation cystitis [11] (Table 2).

6. Treatment

A number of treatment options are described for radiation cystitis. However, a multitude of these are anecdotal and presented in case reports or very small case series and the paucity of high quality evidence in the form of randomised control trials makes development of meaningful evidence-based treatment algorithms difficult (Table 5). Management options can be divided into systemic treatments, intravesical treatments, and interventional procedures.

6.1. Systemic Treatments. As outlined above, one of the proposed mechanisms for the pathophysiology of radiation cystitis is disruption of the urothelium which affects the integrity of the bladder-urine interface and propagates inflammation that causes bladder damage. The rationale behind systemic treatments is to replace or enhance the polysaccharide layer of the bladder and reduce vascular fragility. Glucosamine and pentosan polysulfate have been postulated as possible systemic treatment options, but there is no evidence in the literature to support this [31]. Outlined below are some of the more commonly used agents and their relevant evidence (Table 3).

6.1.1. TCDO/WF10. TCDO/WF10 is a chemically stabilised chlorite matrix that has previously been shown to have a positive effect in chronic inflammatory conditions [31]. It induces natural immunity and stimulates cellular defence mechanisms through its actions on natural killer cells, cytotoxic T lymphocytes, and modification of the monocyte-macrophage system. It reduces inflammation quickly so that healing can begin [13]. A prospective case series from 2006 reports on a cohort of patients with cystoscopically confirmed late grade 2/3 radiation cystitis following treatment of gynaecologic cancers. 88% of patients showed improvement of haematuria to grade 0/1 after two to four cycles of therapy with WF10 [13].

Another prospective case series of twenty patients with grade three radiation cystitis showed an 80% response rate

TABLE 2: Radiation Therapy Oncology Group Late Radiation Morbidity Scoring Schema [11].

Grade	Presentation
Grade 0	Normal
Grade 1	Slight epithelial atrophy
	Minor telangiectasia
	Microscopic haematuria
Grade 2	Moderate frequency
	Generalised telangiectasia
	Intermittent macroscopic haematuria
Grade 3	Severe frequency and dysuria
	Severe generalised telangiectasia with petechiae
	Frequent haematuria
	Reduction in bladder capacity (<150 cc)
Grade 4	Necrosis
	Contracted bladder (<100 cc)
	Severe haemorrhagic cystitis

TABLE 3: The proposed systemic treatments for radiation cystitis and their levels of evidence.

Systemic agent	Level of evidence	Data
TCDO/WF10	1b	Reduction in use of antibiotics and antispasmodics
		Reduction in recurrence of haematuria at one year [12]
		Side effects include nausea, headache, and anaemia [13]
Flavoxate hydrochloride	2b	Higher doses of 1200 mg improve urodynamic measures [14]
Cranberry products	1b	Reduction in cystitis symptoms with cranberry capsules [15]
		No evidence for use of cranberry juice [16, 17]
Conjugated oestrogen	3	Resolution of haematuria in severe haemorrhagic cystitis [18]

to TCDO with 30% showing complete response after one cycle [33]. A multicentre randomised control trial showed significantly lower use of antibiotics and antispasmodics in the group treated with WF10. This study also showed a significant reduction in recurrence of haematuria one year following WF10 treatment; however, cystoscopy at one year showed objective improvement in both groups, with no significant difference [12]. Side effects include nausea, headache, and transient anaemia [12, 13]. TCDO/WF10 is not currently licensed for the treatment of radiation cystitis.

6.1.2. Flavoxate Hydrochloride.
Flavoxate hydrochloride is an antimuscarinic medication used to treat lower urinary tract symptoms. A nonrandomised, uncontrolled, unblinded study of 34 patients with urgency following pelvic radiotherapy compared two doses of this medication. Patients receiving 1200 mg per day demonstrated improvement on urodynamics in first desire volume, bladder capacity, and pressure at

capacity, compared to patients who received 600 mg per day [14]. Flavoxate hydrochloride is licensed for use in cystitis.

6.1.3. Cranberry Capsules/Juice.
Cranberry capsules were initially investigated for prevention of UTIs, but a recent Cochrane review does not support the use of cranberry products for UTI prevention. Cranberries are high in antioxidants including flavonoids, anthocyanins, and proanthocyanidins, but bioavailability is very poor. It should also be noted that standardisation of cranberry products is difficult. A randomised, double blinded, placebo-controlled trial from New Zealand examined the use of cranberry capsules in prevention of development of radiation cystitis in men receiving radiotherapy for prostate cancer. All measures of cystitis on a self-reported quality of life index, with the exception of visible haematuria, were lower in the cranberry capsule arm of the study compared to the placebo group. It should be noted however that the hydration regime for patients was changed during the study [15].

Another randomised, double blinded, placebo-controlled trial from Scotland assessed the use of cranberry juice in prevention of radiation cystitis in patients undergoing pelvic radiotherapy for bladder or cervical cancer. They found no significant difference in rates of cystitis between the groups, but the power of the study was significantly undermined by poor compliance, underrecruitment, and high baseline levels of urinary toxicity in the study population [16]. A Canadian randomised control trial compared cranberry juice to apple juice for preventing radiation cystitis in men undergoing radiotherapy for prostate cancer and found no significant difference between the two arms [17].

6.1.4. Conjugated Oestrogen.
Conjugated oestrogen is thought to have an effect on the vascular wall, resulting in decreased vascular fragility [31]. Studies in this area are lacking with only one small uncontrolled prospective study from 1990 finding that systemic conjugated oestrogen therapy resolved haematuria in a group of patients with severe radiation and/or cyclophosphamide-induced haemorrhagic cystitis [18]. Conjugated oestrogen is not licenced for use in radiation cystitis.

6.2. Intravesical Treatments.
Several different intravesical agents have been used in the treatment of radiation cystitis. High quality evidence in support of many of these agents is lacking. Aluminium has appeared historically in the literature in a number of case reports outlining severe refractory haemorrhagic cystitis. It was thought to act as an astringent and cause contraction, wrinkling, and blanching of the surface of the bladder. No studies exist to support its use. Prostaglandins have been used in the gastrointestinal tract to prevent mucosal ulceration and are postulated to work similarly in the bladder, but there are no studies to support this [31]. Outlined below are some of the more commonly used agents and their relevant evidence (Table 4).

6.2.1. Botulinum Toxin A.
A retrospective review of six patients with radiation cystitis following pelvic radiotherapy

TABLE 4: The proposed intravesical treatments for radiation cystitis and their levels of evidence.

Intravesical agent	Level of evidence	Data
Botulinum toxin A	4	Increase in bladder capacity
		Reduction in urinary frequency from 14 to 11 episodes
		No side effects reported [19]
Hyaluronic acid	1b	Significant reduction in voiding frequency
		Significant reduction in pelvic pain
		Reduction of haematuria equal to that of hyperbaric oxygen
		Side effects: increased rate of UTIs at 6 months [20]
Chondroitin sulfate	2b	Reduction in self-reported bladder symptoms
		No side effects reported [21]
Formalin	4	Significant reduction in haematuria
		High complication rate including mortality [22–24]
Polydeoxyribonucleotides	3	Improvement in reported cystitis symptoms [25]
Early placental extract	3B	Symptomatic improvement in radiation cystitis
		Cystoscopic improvement in radiation cystitis [26]

TABLE 5: Levels of evidence [27].

Level of evidence	Type of evidence
1a	Systematic review (with homogeneity) of randomised control trials
1b	Individual randomised control trials (with narrow confidence intervals)
1c	All or none randomised control trials
2a	Systematic review (with homogeneity) of cohort studies
2b	Individual cohort study or low quality randomised control trials
2c	Outcomes research
3a	Systematic review (with homogeneity) of case-control studies
3b	Individual case-control study
4	Case series (and poor quality cohort and case-control studies)
5	Expert opinion

for prostate and cervical cancer suggested some benefit from intravesical botulinum toxin A injection. In five of the six patients, there was an increase in mean bladder capacity and a moderate reduction in urinary frequency from fourteen to eleven episodes per day. No side effects were reported [19]. Botulinum toxin A is currently licenced for the treatment of overactive bladder.

6.2.2. Hyaluronic Acid and Chondroitin Sulfate. Hyaluronic acid is a major mucopolysaccharide that contributes to the protective function of the urothelium. It is also thought to have immunomodulatory properties and to enhance connective tissue healing. Chondroitin sulfate and hyaluronic acid are components of the glycosaminoglycan layer of the bladder. A randomised control trial compared intravesical treatment with hyaluronic acid to hyperbaric oxygen therapy

and found that hyaluronic acid provided a significant reduction in pelvic pain and voiding frequency up to eighteen months of follow-up. Hyaluronic acid was equivalent to hyperbaric oxygen therapy for ameliorating haematuria [20].

A nonrandomised prospective cohort study of a mixed group of patients with both chemical and radiation-induced cystitis reported a significant increase in bladder capacity, relief of pelvic pain, and dysuria in 97% of patients with intravesical treatment with hyaluronic acid [34]. A small, nonrandomised case-control study looked at self-reported symptom scores in a group of patients who received intravesical chondroitin sulfate while undergoing pelvic radiotherapy for cervical cancer. Over an eight-week study period, patients who received intravesical chondroitin sulfate scored lower than control patients in the areas of overactive bladder, incontinence, obstructive voiding, and pelvic pain [21]. A small prospective pilot study looked at intravesical treatment with hyaluronic acid and chondroitin sulfate in patients with radiation cystitis following radiotherapy for prostate cancer. A significant reduction in nocturia following treatment was noted; however, the absence of a control group in this trial makes definitive conclusions about treatment efficacy difficult [35]. Hyaluronic acid is licenced for use in interstitial cystitis/painful bladder syndrome.

6.2.3. Formalin. Formalin precipitates cellular proteins in the mucosa of the bladder which occludes telangiectatic tissue and small capillaries. It is extremely caustic to skin and precautions apply when handling this substance [31]. Reports of use of intravesical formalin are relatively small retrospective reviews and rates of resolution of haematuria with intravesical therapy range from 70 to 89%. However, rates of serious complication are as high as 30% [22–24]. Serious complications included bilateral hydronephrosis with anuria, vesicovaginal fistula, and death ($n = 2/41$, due to sepsis) [24]. Five patients in a series of 35 required subsequent urinary diversion due to complications from intravesical formalin therapy [22]. 1% formalin is as effective as higher concentrations and has less associated morbidity [22].

6.2.4. Polydeoxyribonucleotides (PDRN). Polydeoxyribonucleotides reduce inflammation and improve tissue perfusion and angiogenesis. Evidence for their use in radiation cystitis is sparse. One small prospective observational cohort study of eight patients with late radiation cystitis suggested an improvement in reported cystitis symptoms following biweekly PDRN bladder instillations for two months [25].

6.2.5. Early Placental Extract. Growth factors and angiogenic factors have been identified in early placenta and this has been reported for the healing of venous ulcers [31]. One nonrandomised case-control study reports that patients receiving intravesical placental extract have symptomatic and cystoscopic improvements in radiation cystitis compared to a saline control group over a study period of twelve months [26].

6.3. Hyperbaric Oxygen. Hyperbaric oxygen therapy causes hyperoxygenation of tissues, capillary growth into scarred submucosal tissues, and neovascularisation of the bladder. Studies reporting on outcomes of hyperbaric oxygen therapy are mostly retrospective reviews of reasonably large numbers of patients who have failed conservative management of radiation-induced haemorrhagic cystitis. The usual course of treatment involves thirty-five to forty sessions of ninety to one hundred minutes each, five days per week, breathing 100% oxygen at 2-atmosphere absolute pressure per session. Success rates range from 76 to 95% for short-term results and from 72 to 83% for long-term results where success is defined as a symptomatic and/or cystoscopic improvement in radiation cystitis [29, 36–40]. Rates of cure range from 57 to 92%, where cure is defined as complete resolution of visible haematuria [38, 39, 41–44]. Earlier studies with smaller numbers report poor long-term outcomes, with one group reporting 45% of patients who initially responded to hyperbaric oxygen therapy requiring eventual urinary diversion for recurrent haemorrhagic cystitis [45]. However, more recent retrospective studies with larger patient numbers report recurrence rates of 0.12 per year [46]. The longest follow-up was eleven years and this group reported that 74% of patients had no recurrence of symptoms [37]. Outcome also depends on the severity of haematuria prior to treatment and the type of radiotherapy used [36, 37]. Retrospective reviews of large numbers of patients suggest that longer time from onset of haematuria to commencement of hyperbaric oxygen therapy results in significantly poorer clinical response, with optimal results obtained when therapy is commenced within six months of onset of haematuria [36, 37, 47]. The main reported side effect of hyperbaric oxygen therapy is otalgia in 33% of patients [29].

6.4. Interventional Procedures. Options for interventional radiological or surgical management of radiation cystitis are limited to case reports or very small case series.

6.4.1. Surgery. Surgical options include cystoscopic management of bleeding, long-term percutaneous nephrostomies, and urinary diversion with or without cystectomy; however, small and large bowel can often be compromised by radiation. A retrospective review of cystoscopic management of radiation cystitis reported that the majority of patients required more than one cystoscopy to attain resolution of haematuria [48]. Cutaneous ureterostomies are reported in the literature as a last resort in intractable radiation-induced haemorrhagic cystitis [49]. A retrospective review of twenty-eight patients with intractable radiation cystitis after radiotherapy for cervical cancer who underwent ileal conduit diversion with or without concomitant vesicovaginostomy suggested that early diversion is prudent in severe disease [50].

6.4.2. Interventional Radiology. Selective radiological embolization of vesical arteries is a minimally invasive option, but no long-term follow-up with large numbers is described.

6.4.3. Argon Beam Coagulator (ABC). A case series of seven patients with refractory radiation cystitis, who had failed various treatments including intravesical agents and radiological embolization, reports good outcomes with cystoscopic use of an argon beam coagulator. The bladder is distended with carbon dioxide and the ABC is used to treat telangiectatic regions of the bladder. No patients required further catheterisation or blood transfusions. One patient required a hospital readmission for haematuria but this settled spontaneously [51].

6.4.4. Laser. Two small case series of patients with radiation-induced haemorrhagic cystitis report clearance of haematuria after one treatment with the GreenLight Xcelerated Performance System (XPS) or GreenLight potassium-titanyl-phosphate (KTP) laser [52, 53]. A second case series of twenty patients undergoing endoscopic treatment with the GreenLight KTP laser reported a 92.3% rate of resolution of haematuria, although 25% of patients required multiple treatments. The average haematuria-free interval was 11.8 months (1–37 months) [54]. A larger series of forty-two patients reported that thirty-nine patients achieved resolution of haematuria after one session of endoscopic neodymium: YAG laser coagulation under local anaesthesia [55].

7. Conclusions

High quality evidence describing the management of radiation cystitis is sparse. Reports of evolving interventional techniques such as laser coagulation of haemorrhagic cystitis continue to emerge; however, radiation cystitis remains a difficult condition to treat. The strongest evidence exists for systemic therapy with TCDO/WF10, cranberry capsules, hyperbaric oxygen therapy, and intravesical hyaluronic acid, but even evidence for these modalities is not of high quality. In the absence of robust evidence for any one treatment modality, most patients are managed supportively in the first instance. Ultimately, most patients require multimodal treatment for curative purposes. In future, large randomised trials exploring emergent management strategies are required in order to strengthen evidence-based treatment strategies.

Conflict of Interests

The authors declare there is no conflict of interests regarding the publication of this paper.

References

[1] L. B. Marks, P. R. Carroll, T. C. Dugan, and M. S. Anscher, "The response of the urinary bladder, urethra, and ureter to radiation and chemotherapy," *International Journal of Radiation Oncology, Biology, Physics*, vol. 31, no. 5, pp. 1257–1280, 1995.

[2] S. Sutani, T. Ohashi, M. Sakayori et al., "Comparison of genitourinary and gastrointestinal toxicity among four radiotherapy modalities for prostate cancer: conventional radiotherapy, intensity-modulated radiotherapy, and permanent iodine-125 implantation with or without external beam radiotherapy," *Radiotherapy and Oncology*, vol. 117, no. 2, pp. 270–276, 2015.

[3] T. P. Kole, M. Tong, B. Wu et al., "Late urinary toxicity modeling after stereotactic body radiotherapy (SBRT) in the definitive treatment of localized prostate cancer," *Acta Oncologica*, pp. 1–7, 2015.

[4] J. Sveistrup, P. M. af Rosenschöld, J. O. Deasy et al., "Improvement in toxicity in high risk prostate cancer patients treated with image-guided intensity-modulated radiotherapy compared to 3D conformal radiotherapy without daily image guidance," *Radiation Oncology*, vol. 9, no. 1, article 44, 2014.

[5] V. Fonteyne, G. Villeirs, N. Lumen, and G. De Meerleer, "Urinary toxicity after high dose intensity modulated radiotherapy as primary therapy for prostate cancer," *Radiotherapy and Oncology*, vol. 92, no. 1, pp. 42–47, 2009.

[6] G. O. De Meerleer, L. A. M. L. Vakaet, W. R. T. De Gersem, C. De Wagter, B. De Naeyer, and W. De Neve, "Radiotherapy of prostate cancer with or without intensity modulated beams: a planning comparison," *International Journal of Radiation Oncology Biology Physics*, vol. 47, no. 3, pp. 639–648, 2000.

[7] S. Jain, D. A. Loblaw, G. C. Morton et al., "The effect of radiation technique and bladder filling on the acute toxicity of pelvic radiotherapy for localized high risk prostate cancer," *Radiotherapy and Oncology*, vol. 105, no. 2, pp. 193–197, 2012.

[8] A. Katz and J. Kang, "Stereotactic body radiotherapy as treatment for organ confined low and intermediate risk prostate carcinoma, a 7-year study," *Frontiers in Oncology*, vol. 4, article 240, 2014.

[9] P. G. Pavlidakey and G. T. MacLennan, "Radiation cystitis," *Journal of Urology*, vol. 182, no. 3, pp. 1172–1173, 2009.

[10] M. Rapariz-González, D. Castro-Díaz, and D. Mejía-Rendón, "Evaluation of the impact of the urinary symptoms on quality of life of patients with painful bladder syndrome/chronic pelvic pain and radiation cystitis: EURCIS study," *Actas Urologicas Espanolas*, vol. 38, no. 4, pp. 224–231, 2014.

[11] RTOG/EORTC Late Radiation Morbidity Scoring Schema, September 2015, https://www.rtog.org/researchassociates/adverseeventreporting/rtogeortclateradiationmorbidityscoring-schema.aspx.

[12] V. Veerasarn, C. Khorprasert, V. Lorvidhaya et al., "Reduced recurrence of late hemorrhagic radiation cystitis by WF10 therapy in cervical cancer patients: a multicenter, randomized, two-arm, open-label trial," *Radiotherapy and Oncology*, vol. 73, no. 2, pp. 179–185, 2004.

[13] V. Veerasarn, W. Boonnuch, and C. Kakanaporn, "A phase II study to evaluate WF10 in patients with late hemorrhagic radiation cystitis and proctitis," *Gynecologic Oncology*, vol. 100, no. 1, pp. 179–184, 2006.

[14] R. Milani, S. Scalambrino, S. Carrera, P. Pezzoli, and R. Ruffmann, "Flavoxate hydrochloride for urinary urgency after pelvic radiotherapy: comparison of 600 mg versus 1200 mg daily dosages," *Journal of International Medical Research*, vol. 16, no. 1, pp. 71–74, 1988.

[15] K. Hamilton, N. C. Bennett, G. Purdie, and P. M. Herst, "Standardized cranberry capsules for radiation cystitis in prostate cancer patients in New Zealand: a randomized double blinded, placebo controlled pilot study," *Supportive Care in Cancer*, vol. 23, no. 1, pp. 95–102, 2015.

[16] C. C. Cowan, C. Hutchison, T. Cole et al., "A randomised double-blind placebo-controlled trial to determine the effect of cranberry juice on decreasing the incidence of urinary symptoms and urinary tract infections in patients undergoing radiotherapy for cancer of the bladder or cervix," *Clinical Oncology*, vol. 24, no. 2, pp. e31–e38, 2012.

[17] G. Campbell, T. Pickles, and Y. D'yachkova, "A randomised trial of cranberry versus apple juice in the management of urinary symptoms during external beam radiation therapy for prostate cancer," *Clinical Oncology*, vol. 15, no. 6, pp. 322–328, 2003.

[18] Y. K. Liu, J. I. Harty, G. S. Steinbock, H. A. Holt Jr., D. H. Goldstein, and M. Amin, "Treatment of radiation or cyclophosphamide induced hemorrhagic cystitis using conjugated estrogen," *Journal of Urology*, vol. 144, no. 1, pp. 41–43, 1990.

[19] Y.-C. Chuang, D. K. Kim, P.-H. Chiang, and M. B. Chancellor, "Bladder botulinum toxin A injection can benefit patients with radiation and chemical cystitis," *BJU International*, vol. 102, no. 6, pp. 704–706, 2008.

[20] Y. Shao, G.-L. Lu, and Z.-J. Shen, "Comparison of intravesical hyaluronic acid instillation and hyperbaric oxygen in the treatment of radiation-induced hemorrhagic cystitis," *BJU International*, vol. 109, no. 5, pp. 691–694, 2012.

[21] M. H. Hazewinkel, L. J. A. Stalpers, M. G. Dijkgraaf, and J.-P. W. R. Roovers, "Prophylactic vesical instillations with 0.2% chondroitin sulfate may reduce symptoms of acute radiation cystitis in patients undergoing radiotherapy for gynecological malignancies," *International Urogynecology Journal*, vol. 22, no. 6, pp. 725–730, 2011.

[22] A. K. Dewan, G. Madan Mohan, and R. Ravi, "Intravesical formalin for hemorrhagic cystitis following irradiation of cancer of the cervix," *International Journal of Gynecology and Obstetrics*, vol. 42, no. 2, pp. 131–135, 1993.

[23] M. Likourinas, A. Cranides, B. Jiannopoulos, A. Kostakopoulos, and C. Dimopoulos, "Intravesical formalin for the control of intractable bladder haemorrhage secondary to radiation cystitis or bladder cancer," *Urological Research*, vol. 7, no. 2, pp. 125–126, 1979.

[24] B. Lojanapiwat, S. Sripralakrit, S. Soonthornphan, and S. Wudhikarn, "Intravesicle formalin instillation with a modified technique for controlling haemorrhage secondary to radiation cystitis," *Asian Journal of Surgery*, vol. 25, no. 3, pp. 232–235, 2002.

[25] P. Bonfili, P. Franzese, F. Marampon et al., "Intravesical instillations with polydeoxyribonucleotides reduce symptoms of radiation-induced cystitis in patients treated with radiotherapy for pelvic cancer: a pilot study," *Supportive Care in Cancer*, vol. 22, no. 5, pp. 1155–1159, 2014.

[26] S. Micic and O. Genbacev, "Post-irradiation cystitis improved by instillation of early placental extract in saline," *European Urology*, vol. 14, no. 4, pp. 291–293, 1988.

[27] Oxford Centre for Evidence-Based Medicine—Levels of Evidence, CEBM, March 2009, http://www.cebm.net/oxford-centre-evidence-based-medicine-levels-evidence-march-2009/.

[28] J. P. Crew, C. R. Jephcott, and J. M. Reynard, "Radiation-induced haemorrhagic cystitis," *European Urology*, vol. 40, pp. 111–123, 2001.

[29] C. Oliai, B. Fisher, A. Jani et al., "Hyperbaric oxygen therapy for radiation-induced cystitis and proctitis," *International Journal of Radiation Oncology, Biology, Physics*, vol. 84, no. 3, pp. 733–740, 2012.

[30] C. Levenback, P. J. Eifel, T. W. Burke, M. Morris, and D. M. Gershenson, "Hemorrhagic cystitis following radiotherapy for stage Ib cancer of the cervix," *Gynecologic Oncology*, vol. 55, no. 2, pp. 206–210, 1994.

[31] A. S. Denton, N. W. Clarke, and E. J. Maher, "Non-surgical interventions for late radiation cystitis in patients who have received radical radiotherapy to the pelvis," *Cochrane Database of Systematic Reviews*, vol. 3, Article ID CD001773, 2002.

[32] A. Thompson, A. Adamson, A. Bahl et al., "Guidelines for the diagnosis, prevention and management of chemical- and radiation-induced cystitis," *Journal of Clinical Urology*, vol. 7, no. 1, pp. 25–35, 2015.

[33] S. Srisupundit, P. Kraiphibul, S. Sangruchi, V. Linasmita, K. Chingskol, and V. Veerasarn, "The efficacy of chemically-stabilized chlorite-matrix (TCDO) in the management of late postradiation cystitis," *Journal of the Medical Association of Thailand*, vol. 82, pp. 798–802, 1999.

[34] M. L. Sommariva, S. D. Sandri, and V. Ceriani, "Efficacy of sodium hyaluronate in the management of chemical and radiation cystitis," *Minerva Urologica e Nefrologica*, vol. 62, no. 2, pp. 145–150, 2010.

[35] M. Gacci, O. Saleh, C. Giannessi et al., "Sodium hyaluronate and chondroitin sulfate replenishment therapy can improve nocturia in men with post-radiation cystitis: results of a prospective pilot study," *BMC Urology*, vol. 15, article 65, 2015.

[36] K. T. Chong, N. B. Hampson, and J. M. Corman, "Early hyperbaric oxygen therapy improves outcome for radiation-induced hemorrhagic cystitis," *Urology*, vol. 65, no. 4, pp. 649–653, 2005.

[37] T. Nakada, H. Nakada, Y. Yoshida et al., "Hyperbaric oxygen therapy for radiation cystitis in patients with prostate cancer: a long-term follow-up study," *Urologia Internationalis*, vol. 89, no. 2, pp. 208–214, 2012.

[38] D. M. Norkool, N. B. Hampson, R. P. Gibbons, and R. M. Weissman, "Hyperbaric oxygen therapy for radiation-induced hemorrhagic cystitis," *Journal of Urology*, vol. 150, no. 2, pp. 332–334, 1993.

[39] T. Yoshida, A. Kawashima, T. Ujike, M. Uemura, K. Nishimura, and S. Miyoshi, "Hyperbaric oxygen therapy for radiation-induced hemorrhagic cystitis," *International Journal of Urology*, vol. 15, no. 7, pp. 639–641, 2008.

[40] N. Oscarsson, P. Arnell, P. Lodding, S.-E. Ricksten, and H. Seeman-Lodding, "Hyperbaric oxygen treatment in radiation-induced cystitis and proctitis: a prospective cohort study on patient-perceived quality of recovery," *International Journal of Radiation Oncology Biology Physics*, vol. 87, no. 4, pp. 670–675, 2013.

[41] H. C. Lee, C. S. Liu, C. Chiao, and S. N. Lin, "Hyperbaric oxygen therapy in hemorrhagic radiation cystitis: a report of 20 cases," *Undersea & Hyperbaric Medicine*, vol. 21, no. 3, pp. 321–327, 1994.

[42] J. P. Weiss, D. M. Mattei, E. C. Neville, and P. M. Hanno, "Primary treatment of radiation-induced hemorrhagic cystitis with hyperbaric oxygen: 10-year experience," *Journal of Urology*, vol. 151, no. 6, pp. 1514–1517, 1994.

[43] B. G. Rijkmans, D. J. Bakker, N. F. Dabhoiwala, and K. H. Kurth, "Successful treatment of radiation cystitis with hyperbaric oxygen," *European Urology*, vol. 16, no. 5, pp. 354–356, 1989.

[44] J. M. Corman, D. McClure, R. Pritchett, P. Kozlowski, and N. B. Hampson, "Treatment of radiation induced hemorrhagic cystitis with hyperbaric oxygen," *The Journal of Urology*, vol. 169, no. 6, pp. 2200–2202, 2003.

[45] J. J. Del Pizzo, B. H. Chew, S. C. Jacobs, and G. N. Sklar, "Treatment of radiation induced hemorrhagic cystitis with hyperbaric oxygen: long-term follow up," *The Journal of Urology*, vol. 160, no. 3, pp. 731–733, 1998.

[46] R. F. M. Bevers, D. J. Bakker, and K. H. Kurth, "Hyperbaric oxygen treatment for haemorrhagic radiation cystitis," *The Lancet*, vol. 346, no. 8978, pp. 803–805, 1995.

[47] A. Dellis, C. Deliveliotis, V. Kalentzos, P. Vavasis, and A. Skolarikos, "Is there a role for hyberbaric oxygen as primary treatment for grade IV radiation-induced haemorrhagic cystitis? A prospective pilot-feasibility study and review of literature," *International Braz J Urol*, vol. 40, no. 3, pp. 296–305, 2014.

[48] J. R. Kaplan and J. S. Wolf, "Efficacy and survival associated with cystoscopy and clot evacuation for radiation or cyclophosphamide induced hemorrhagic cystitis," *The Journal of Urology*, vol. 181, no. 2, pp. 641–646, 2009.

[49] S. Pomer, G. Karcher, and W. Simon, "Cutaneous ureterostomy as last resort treatment of intractable haemorrhagic cystitis following radiation," *British Journal of Urology*, vol. 55, no. 4, pp. 392–394, 1983.

[50] J. S. Banerji, A. Devasia, N. S. Kekre, and N. Chacko, "Early urinary diversion with ileal conduit and vesicovaginostomy in the treatment of radiation cystitis due to carcinoma cervix: a study from a tertiary care hospital in South India," *ANZ Journal of Surgery*, vol. 85, no. 10, pp. 770–773, 2015.

[51] M. P. Wines and W. D. Lynch, "A new minimally invasive technique for treating radiation cystitis: the argon-beam coagulator," *BJU International*, vol. 98, no. 3, pp. 610–612, 2006.

[52] D. R. Martinez, C. E. Ercole, J. G. Lopez, J. Parker, and M. K. Hall, "A novel approach for the treatment of radiation-induced hemorrhagic cystitis with the GreenLight XPS laser," *International Brazilian Journal of Urology*, vol. 41, no. 3, pp. 584–587, 2015.

[53] J. Zhu, B. Xue, Y. Shan, D. Yang, and Y. Zang, "Transurethral coagulation for radiation-induced hemorrhagic cystitis using greenlight potassium-titanyl-phosphate laser," *Photomedicine and Laser Surgery*, vol. 31, no. 2, pp. 78–81, 2013.

[54] S. S. Talab, W. S. McDougal, C.-L. Wu, and S. Tabatabaei, "Mucosa-sparing, KTP laser coagulation of submucosal telangiectatic vessels in patients with radiation-induced cystitis: a novel approach," *Urology*, vol. 84, no. 2, pp. 478–483, 2014.

[55] R. Ravi, "Endoscopic neodymium:YAG laser treatment of radiation-induced hemorrhagic cystitis," *Lasers in Surgery and Medicine*, vol. 14, no. 1, pp. 83–87, 1994.

21

Bipolar Transurethral Incision of Bladder Neck Stenoses with Mitomycin C Injection

Timothy D. Lyon, Omar M. Ayyash, Matthew C. Ferroni, Kevin J. Rycyna, and Mang L. Chen

Department of Urology, University of Pittsburgh School of Medicine, Pittsburgh, PA 15213, USA

Correspondence should be addressed to Timothy D. Lyon; lyontd@upmc.edu

Academic Editor: Francisco E. Martins

Introduction. To determine the efficacy of bipolar transurethral incision with mitomycin C (MMC) injection for the treatment of refractory bladder neck stenosis (BNS). *Materials and Methods.* Patients who underwent bipolar transurethral incision of BNS (TUIBNS) with MMC injection at our institution from 2013 to 2014 were retrospectively reviewed. A total of 2 mg of 40% mitomycin C solution was injected in four quadrants of the treated BNS. Treatment failure was defined as the need for subsequent intervention. *Results.* Thirteen patients underwent 17 bipolar TUIBNS with MMC injection. Twelve (92%) patients had failed a mean of 2.2 ± 1.1 prior endoscopic procedures. Median follow-up was 16.5 months (IQR: 14–18.4 months). Initial success was 62%; five (38%) patients had a recurrence with a median time to recurrence of 7.3 months. Four patients underwent a repeat procedure, 2 (50%) of which failed. Overall success was achieved in 77% (10/13) of patients after a mean of 1.3 ± 0.5 procedures. BNS recurrence was not significantly associated with history of pelvic radiation (33% versus 43%, $p = 0.9$). There were no serious adverse events. *Conclusions.* Bipolar TUIBNS with MMC injection was comparable in efficacy to previously reported techniques and did not result in any serious adverse events.

1. Introduction

Bladder neck stenosis (BNS) is a known complication of prostatectomy, prostate radiotherapy, and transurethral resection of the prostate (TURP) [1]. Although the majority of patients can be treated successfully with one to two endoscopic procedures, approximately 27% develop refractory bladder neck stenoses requiring multiple and increasingly complex treatments, potentially culminating in open reconstruction [2–6]. Many go on to require intermittent self-dilation to avoid major reconstruction, which has been shown to decrease quality of life [7]. More effective endoscopic treatments for refractory BNS are therefore needed.

There has been recent enthusiasm for the use of scar modulators such as mitomycin C to help increase success rates of transurethral incision of bladder neck stenoses (TUIBNS). Mitomycin C is a DNA cross-linker that decreases collagen deposition and leads to fibroblast apoptosis [8]. Patency rates for TUIBNS alone in the setting of recurrent stenoses are around 17% per procedure [2]. In contrast, TUIBNS with MMC injection has urethral patency rates ranging from 58 to 72% per procedure [9, 10]; however, MMC injection has also been associated with severe complications including rectourethral fistula, osteitis pubis, and bladder neck necrosis in a minority of patients [9]. Deep cuts into the fat with high dose MMC injection may be the culprit for these complications.

Monopolar electrocautery has greater depth of tissue penetration than bipolar technology [11, 12]. We hypothesize that bipolar cutting current could be associated with increased success following TUIBNS with MMC since less adjacent tissue damage could decrease scar reformation. We also hypothesize that avoiding deep incisions with bipolar electrocautery with MMC could minimize adverse events. To examine these hypotheses, we reviewed our institutional series of bipolar TUIBNS with intralesional MMC injection.

2. Materials and Methods

2.1. Data Collection. Following institutional review board approval, a retrospective review of all patients who underwent bipolar TUIBNS by a single surgeon (Mang L. Chen) at our institution from January 1, 2013, to December 31, 2014, was completed. Demographic information was collected including age, race, BNS etiology, number and type of prior interventions, and whether or not the patient had previously received pelvic radiation. Operative time and total dose of mitomycin C used were recorded. Postoperative complications were categorized according to the Clavien-Dindo classification [13]. Data were censored as of March 6, 2015.

Postoperatively, patients were monitored every 3 months for stricture recurrence using a combination of serial postvoid residuals, uroflowmetry, and self-reported obstructive voiding symptoms. Flexible cystoscopy was performed as indicated. Recurrence was defined as the need for any subsequent BNS procedure.

2.2. Operative Technique. Rigid cystoscopy was performed and guidewire passed through the stenotic lumen into the bladder. Scar resection was accomplished utilizing either a bipolar PK button electrode or PK Plasma-CISE (Gyrus ACMI, Southborough, MA). The PK Plasma-CISE was placed through a traditional 22-French cystoscope; the PK button electrode required use of a 26-French continuous flow resectoscope. The decision as to which instrument to use was made intraoperatively by the attending surgeon on a case-by-case basis. Severe stenosis required cannulation first with the smaller Plasma-CISE. Less severe but symptomatic stenoses were treated first with the Plasma-CISE, and if scar tissue ablation was unsatisfactory for cystoscopic passage into the bladder, the button was used. Scar incision and sometimes resection were accomplished using a cutting current at the 3, 9, and 12 o'clock positions and were continued until the lumen easily permitted the passage of the operating instrument into the bladder. We avoided 6 o'clock incisions to minimize risk of rectal injury. No fat was identified after the incision and/or resection was complete.

Mitomycin C was injected into four quadrants of the treated BNS following incision and/or resection. The needle was advanced approximately 5 mm into the tissue at the 1, 4, 8, and 11 o'clock positions for injection. A total dose of 2 mg of 40% mitomycin C in saline solution was used in all patients. Foley catheter was left in place for 3 days postoperatively.

2.3. Data Analysis. Demographic information is reported as frequencies and percentages. Means and standard deviations (SD) are reported for normally distributed data and medians with interquartile ranges (IQR) for nonnormal data. Fisher's exact test was used to compare the likelihood of recurrence between patients who did and did not receive pelvic radiation. Time to recurrence following the initial procedure was modeled with the Kaplan-Meier method. Success rates for initial and repeat procedures were analyzed separately so as not to compare MMC-naïve patients with those who had previously received MMC. Statistical significance was defined at the $p < 0.05$ level using two-tailed tests. Data was analyzed using SPSS software, version 20 (IBM Corp., Armonk, NY).

TABLE 1: Patient demographics.

	$n = 13$
Age, years, mean ± SD	67 ± 8.0
BMI, kg/m^2, mean ± SD	31 ± 6.0
Charlson comorbidity index (%)	
0-1	4 (31)
2	5 (38)
3	4 (31)
Etiology (%)	
RRP	5 (33)
RALP	3 (20)
TURP	3 (20)
Brachytherapy	2 (13)
Prior BNS treatment (%)	12 (92)
Number of prior interventions, mean ± SD	2.2 ± 1.1
Prior radiation (%)	6 (46)

SD: standard deviation, RRP: radical retropubic prostatectomy, RALP: robot-assisted laparoscopic prostatectomy, TURP: transurethral resection of prostate, and TUIBN: transurethral incision bladder neck.

3. Results

Thirteen consecutive patients underwent seventeen bipolar TUIBNS with MMC procedures over the study period. Median follow-up was 16.5 months (IQR: 14–18.4 months). Patient characteristics are summarized in Table 1. Stenosis etiology included radical prostatectomy in 8, prostate brachytherapy in 2, and TURP in 3. Four radical prostatectomy patients received postoperative radiation. Ninety-two percent of patients had failed a mean of 2.2 ± 1.1 prior endoscopic BNS procedures, but all were MMC-naïve.

Success following a single bipolar TUIBNS with MMC injection was 62% (8/13), as shown in Figure 1. Five patients (38%) had a recurrence with a median time to recurrence of 7.3 months (IQR: 3.7–10.9 months). Of the five patients who had a recurrence, one was retreated with TUIBNS alone due to a pharmacy shortage and 4 underwent a repeat TUIBNS with MMC procedure. Retreated patients were given the same MMC dosage of 2 mg. Two of the four (50%) repeat MMC procedures failed, one at four months and one at eight months, and these patients did not receive any further MMC with subsequent treatment. Both patients who failed a repeat procedure had a history of pelvic radiation whereas the two patients with successful repeat procedures did not; further the patients who failed repeat procedures had higher Charlson comorbidity index scores (2 and 3 versus 1) than the patients who responded to a second round. Overall, 77% (10/13) of patients had a patent bladder neck after a mean of 1.3 ± 0.5 procedures. Success rate per procedure was 59% (10/17).

Five of thirteen patients (38%) had some degree of stress urinary incontinence prior to undergoing TUIBNS. Incontinence was significantly worsened in two patients (15%) with preexisting incontinence; one subsequently underwent artificial urinary sphincter placement after BNS resolution and the other was managed with a Cunningham clamp per patient preference. Both of these patients had a history

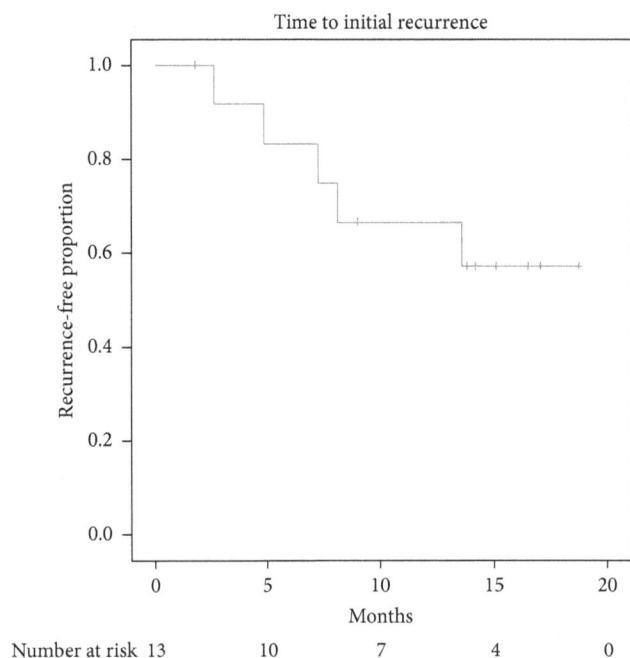

FIGURE 1: Time to stenosis recurrence following first transurethral incision of bladder neck stenosis with intralesional mitomycin C (MMC) injection in MMC-naïve patients. Censored cases marked by vertical line.

of pelvic radiation. De novo incontinence occurred in one patient (8%), which was mild and required one pad/day.

BNS recurrence was not significantly associated with a history of pelvic radiation (33% versus 43%, $p = 0.9$). One postoperative complication occurred, namely, urinary retention after catheter removal necessitating clean intermittent catheterization, classified as Clavien 1.

4. Discussion

Management of refractory BNS is a vexing problem for urologists and patients given its high recurrence rates following endoscopic treatments. Approximately 27% of patients with BNS develop refractory stenoses highly resistant to traditional therapy, with success rates of 0–20% following dilation or urethrotomy alone [2, 4]. Injection of mitomycin C as an inhibitor of scar formation has gained some traction for use in this subset of patients. Also, previous work has shown that use of electrocautery over cold knife incision may increase success rates [9]. In this paper we reviewed our institutional series of bipolar TUIBNS with MMC injection to determine whether the addition of bipolar electrocautery could maintain or improve upon previously reported patency rates. Using this approach, we report an initial success rate of 62% (8/13) and an overall patency rate of 77% (10/13) at a median follow-up of 16.5 months, which is consistent with recently reported results [9, 10].

Two previous studies have examined the efficacy of intralesional MMC injection in the treatment of refractory

BNS. Vanni and colleagues report a series of 18 patients— all of whom had failed prior endoscopic therapy for BNS— treated with cold knife TUIBNS followed by injection of 0.3–0.4 mg/mL MMC [10]. At a median follow-up of 12 months, they report patency rates of 72% after a single procedure and 89% after two procedures. These are confounding results as other reports have suggested superiority of monopolar TUIBNS over cold knife incision [9, 14]. MMC injection may explain the higher than expected patency rates. Building upon this study, Redshaw et al. (TURNS study) reported a multi-institutional series of 55 patients treated with TUIBNS plus MMC [9]. Eighty percent of included patients had failed prior endoscopic treatment, and mean MMC dose was 3.5 mg. Initial and overall success rates in their series were 58% and 75%, respectively. Patients in the TURNS study had TUIBNS by either cold knife or monopolar incision depending on individual surgeon preference. Interestingly, use of electrocautery was associated with success on univariate analysis (OR 10.7 [95% CI 1.2–197], $p = 0.03$), although the confidence interval was wide and no multivariable risk adjustment was possible due to sample size. Our initial and overall success rates of 62% and 77% compare favorably with these two series. It should be noted, however, that our definition of treatment failure as based on clinical symptoms may be causing us to overestimate success relative to the TURNS experience, which defined recurrence based on urethral caliber noted on cystoscopy regardless of whether obstructive voiding symptoms were present.

Two of four patients in our series who failed an initial TUIBNS with MMC responded to a second round of treatment. Subsequent procedures were performed in an identical manner with the same MMC dosage as initial treatments. Both patients who responded to a second procedure had no history of pelvic radiation and a Charlson comorbidity index of 1; conversely the two patients who failed had both received pelvic radiation and had higher Charlson scores of 2 and 3. Unfortunately comparative statistics were not possible in this subset of patients due to the small overall numbers; however our data suggest that a history of pelvic radiation and greater number of comorbidities may be associated with decreased success rates for subsequent TUIBNS with MMC procedures. This finding needs to be validated in a larger sample size before this statement can be definitively made, however.

It is not clear from the literature that concomitant MMC injection is necessary to achieve high success rates following TUIBNS. In contrast to the above, Ramirez and colleagues were able to demonstrate an overall patency rate of 86% after 2 procedures at a mean follow-up of 13 months in 50 patients who underwent TUIBNS with electrocautery alone [14]. It is also not clear whether our ability to achieve similar success to this is due principally to the use of electrocautery, MMC injection, or a combination of the two. Unfortunately the present study is not designed or powered to delineate these differences.

Data from TURP procedures has shown that bipolar current is associated with a more superficial depth of tissue penetration than monopolar electrocautery, ranging from 0.5–1 mm in bipolar procedures to 3–5 mm in monopolar cases [11, 12]. As such, we hypothesized that bipolar cutting current would be associated with increased success following TUIBNS with MMC as there would theoretically be less adjacent tissue damage and therefore less of an impetus for scar reformation. However, with initial success in 62% of our patients compared to 58% in a series of mixed cold and hot knife procedures [9], we are unable to conclude that bipolar electrocautery meaningfully improved success. Due to our small sample size, the power to detect a true difference between techniques is low, and it is possible that with a larger sample a significant difference between the two techniques could emerge.

No patients in our study required diversion, and the only postoperative complication was one case of retention following catheter removal, requiring clean intermittent catheterization. The TURNS group noted 4 adverse events with 3 patients needing cystectomy [9]. There are two key protocol differences that may account for this discrepancy. First, our study exclusively used a 2 mg dose of mitomycin C, lower than the doses ranging from 0.4 to 10 mg in their series. Second, no perivesicular fat was visualized after incision in our series. This is in stark contrast to nearly every other research protocol where, as a prerequisite to injection, incisions were routinely made until the fat was visualized [9, 10, 14, 15]. These deeper incisions may account for the prevalence of serious complications observed in prior studies by allowing extravasation of MMC into the perivesicular fat, resulting in instances of rectourethral fistula, osteitis pubis, and bladder neck necrosis. It should be noted that our series achieved equivalent urethral patency rates to the TURNS study without requiring deep bladder neck incision into the perivesicular fat.

This study has several significant limitations. As with all retrospective studies, the potential for a selection bias exists. The small number of patients included limits statistical power to find differences in outcome. Follow-up was relatively short with a median of 16.5 months and long-term outcomes in these patients are not known. All patients included in this study were Caucasian, which limits generalizability to those of other racial backgrounds. The makeup of our cohort was heterogeneous, including patients who did and did not receive pelvic radiation as well as those with stenosis developing after varying treatments for both benign and malignant prostatic diseases. Unfortunately, the uncommon nature of this problem is a barrier to reaching a large enough sample size to compare these discrete groups directly, and this is reflected in the sample sizes of 18 and 55 seen in the Vanni and Redshaw papers, respectively [9, 10].

Despite these limitations, our results are meaningful for several reasons. We report the first series to our knowledge using bipolar TUIBNS with concomitant MMC injection for the treatment of refractory BNS. We achieved initial success in 62% and overall success in 77% of patients after a mean of 1.3 procedures, which is comparable to prior studies. Importantly, none of the serious adverse events that have previously been reported with the use of MMC were found in our series, possibly due to the previously described alterations in dosage and technique. Although the sample size is small, our results indicate that TUIBNS with MMC can achieve reasonable success without major morbidity. Further

study with larger sample size, less patient heterogeneity, and longer follow-up is needed both to determine whether the use of bipolar electrocautery can confer an advantage over other techniques and to confirm that serious morbidity can effectively be avoided without compromising treatment success.

5. Conclusions

Bipolar TUIBNS with MMC done without deep incisions into the perivesicular fat can achieve comparable success to previously published techniques while also avoiding serious adverse events. A prospective, randomized study is needed to determine which factors (dilation, cold knife DVIU, monopolar/bipolar electrocautery, and scar modulator injection) are the most important in decreasing BNS recurrence.

Conflict of Interests

The authors declare that there is no conflict of interests regarding the publication of this paper.

References

[1] J. M. Latini, J. W. McAninch, S. B. Brandes, J. Y. Chung, and D. Rosenstein, "SIU/ICUD consultation on urethral strictures: epidemiology, etiology, anatomy, and nomenclature of urethral stenoses, strictures, and pelvic fracture urethral disruption injuries," *Urology*, vol. 83, no. 3, pp. S1–S7, 2014.

[2] P. G. Borboroglu, J. P. Sands, J. L. Roberts, and C. L. Amling, "Risk factors for vesicourethral anastomotic stricture after radical prostatectomy," *Urology*, vol. 56, no. 1, pp. 96–100, 2000.

[3] D. Ramirez, J. Simhan, S. J. Hudak, and A. F. Morey, "Standardized approach for the treatment of refractory bladder neck contractures," *The Urologic Clinics of North America*, vol. 40, no. 3, pp. 371–380, 2013.

[4] G. Giannarini, F. Manassero, A. Mogorovich et al., "Cold-knife incision of anastomotic strictures after radical retropubic prostatectomy with bladder neck preservation: efficacy and impact on urinary continence status," *European Urology*, vol. 54, no. 3, pp. 647–656, 2008.

[5] R. Park, S. Martin, J. D. Goldberg, and H. Lepor, "Anastomotic strictures following radical prostatectomy: insights into incidence, effectiveness of intervention, effect on continence, and factors predisposing to occurrence," *Urology*, vol. 57, no. 4, pp. 742–746, 2001.

[6] A. R. Mundy and D. E. Andrich, "Posterior urethral complications of the treatment of prostate cancer," *BJU International*, vol. 110, no. 3, pp. 304–325, 2012.

[7] J. D. Lubahn, L. C. Zhao, J. F. Scott et al., "Poor quality of life in patients with urethral stricture treated with intermittent self-dilation," *The Journal of Urology*, vol. 191, no. 1, pp. 143–147, 2014.

[8] B. Ferguson, S. D. Gray, and S. Thibeault, "Time and dose effects of mitomycin C on extracellular matrix fibroblasts and proteins," *The Laryngoscope*, vol. 115, no. 1 I, pp. 110–115, 2005.

[9] J. D. Redshaw, J. A. Broghammer, T. G. Smith et al., "Intralesional injection of mitomycin C at transurethral incision of bladder neck contracture may offer limited benefit: TURNS Study Group," *Journal of Urology*, vol. 193, no. 2, pp. 587–592, 2015.

[10] A. J. Vanni, L. N. Zinman, and J. C. Buckley, "Radial urethrotomy and intralesional mitomycin C for the management of recurrent bladder neck contractures," *Journal of Urology*, vol. 186, no. 1, pp. 156–160, 2011.

[11] O. Sinanoglu, S. Ekici, M. N. Tatar, G. Turan, A. Keles, and Z. Erdem, "Postoperative outcomes of plasmakinetic transurethral resection of the prostate compared to monopolar transurethral resection of the prostate in patients with comorbidities," *Urology*, vol. 80, no. 2, pp. 402–406, 2012.

[12] C. Dincel, M. M. Samli, C. Guler, M. Demirbas, and M. Karalar, "Plasma kinetic vaporization of the prostate: clinical evaluation of a new technique," *Journal of Endourology*, vol. 18, no. 3, pp. 293–298, 2004.

[13] D. Dindo, N. Demartines, and P.-A. Clavien, "Classification of surgical complications: a new proposal with evaluation in a cohort of 6336 patients and results of a survey," *Annals of Surgery*, vol. 240, no. 2, pp. 205–213, 2004.

[14] D. Ramirez, L. C. Zhao, A. Bagrodia, J. F. Scott, S. J. Hudak, and A. F. Morey, "Deep lateral transurethral incisions for recurrent bladder neck contracture: promising 5-year experience using a standardized approach," *Urology*, vol. 82, no. 6, pp. 1430–1435, 2013.

[15] S. Kumar, N. Garg, S. K. Singh, and A. K. Mandal, "Efficacy of optical internal urethrotomy and intralesional injection of Vatsala-Santosh PGI tri-inject (triamcinolone, mitomycin C, and hyaluronidase) in the treatment of anterior urethral stricture," *Advances in Urology*, vol. 2014, Article ID 192710, 4 pages, 2014.

22

Ureteral Dilatation with No Apparent Cause on Intravenous Urography: Normal or Abnormal? A Pilot Study

Vinita Rathi, Sachin Agrawal, Shuchi Bhatt, and Naveen Sharma

University College of Medical Sciences and Guru Teg Bahadur Hospital, Dilshad Garden, Delhi 110095, India

Correspondence should be addressed to Vinita Rathi; vineetarathi@yahoo.com

Academic Editor: Hiep T. Nguyen

A pilot study was done in 18 adults to assess the significance of ureteral dilatation having no apparent cause seen on Intravenous Urography (IVU). A clinicoradiological evaluation was undertaken to evaluate the cause of ureteral dilatation, including laboratory investigations and sonography of the genitourinary tract. This was followed, if required, by CT Urography (using a modified technique). In 9 out of 18 cases, the cause of ureteral dilatation on laboratory investigations was urinary tract infection (6) and tuberculosis (3). In the remaining 9 cases, CTU identified the cause as extrinsic compression by a vessel (3), extrinsic vascular compression of the ureter along with ureteritis (2), extrinsic vascular impression on the right ureter and ureteritis in the left ureter (1), ureteral stricture (2), and ureteral calculus (1). Extrinsic vascular compression and strictures did not appear to be clinically significant in our study. Hence, ureteral dilatation without any apparent cause on intravenous urogram was found to be clinically significant in 12 out of 18 (66.6%) cases. We conclude that ureteral dilatation with no apparent cause on IVU may indicate urinary tract tuberculosis, urinary tract infection (*E. coli*), or a missed calculus. Thus, cases with a dilated ureter on IVU, having no obvious cause, should undergo a detailed clinicoradiological evaluation and CTU should be used judiciously.

1. Introduction

Ureteral dilatation, showing no apparent cause, is frequently observed in Intravenous Urography (IVU) done using ionic contrast, with or without the use of an abdominal binder, especially involving the right ureter. Spiro and Fry had reported that minor dilatation of the ureter is considered to be the residue of past pregnancy changes and of no significance [1].

Experimental studies have demonstrated that inflammatory changes in the wall of the ureter, as well as bacterial toxins, are associated with marked loss of ureteral muscle tone which is at least partly responsible for the dilatation [1]. According to Flower, the radiologist's inability to demonstrate reflux up a dilated ureter should not mislead him into suggesting that it is obstructed, as this unfortunate misinterpretation may lead to a needless or incorrect operation [2]. The concept of the "nonobstructed, nonrefluxing wide ureter" implies that the primary defect, either congenital or acquired, lies in the wall of the ureter [2].

Assessing the cause of ureteral dilatation may play an important role in influencing patient management. Ultrasonography (US) and MR imaging have been used to compensate for the limitations of IVU in the evaluation of ureters, as they do not involve ionizing radiation. However, while large portions of the ureters may not be visualized at US due to bowel gases, obesity, and so forth, MR imaging may not demonstrate ureteral calculi.

CT Urography (CTU) can clearly delineate obscure causes of ureteral dilatation, for example, presence of minute stones, radiolucent stones, or even a recently passed out stone that can be confirmed on CTU [3]. It can be used to depict unsuspected extraurinary disease [4]. Inflammatory processes adjacent to the ureter, such as appendicitis or diverticulitis, which may impair ureteral peristalsis and result in ureteral dilatation, can be identified on CTU [3]. CTU can even detect subtle benign abnormalities (e.g., ureteritis cystica) and urothelial carcinoma causing ureteral dilatation [5].

The aim of this pilot study was to assess the significance, if any, of ureteral dilatation (without any obvious cause) seen on IVU in a developing country. A clinicoradiological evaluation was done, including modified CT Urography in selected cases.

2. Materials and Methods

2.1. Patient Selection. Between November 2011 and January 2013, 18 adults showing no obvious cause of ureteral dilatation on IVU underwent a clinicoradiological evaluation. This pilot study was approved by the Institutional Ethics Committee and a written informed consent was taken from all cases. 14 cases had presented for IVU with renal calculus disease and 4 with unilateral flank pain of unknown cause.

IVU had been conducted using 40 mL ionic contrast meglumine/sodium diatrizoate (Urografin 76%, Schering AG, Germany) and abdominal binder was not applied in any of the cases.

Intravenous urograms with any obvious cause of ureteral dilatation, for example, calculus, stricture, ureterocele, megaureter, pelvic tumors, lower urinary tract obstruction, and vesicoureteral reflux, were excluded. Cases with a known cause of ureteral dilatation, for example, history of recent passage of calculus; pregnancy in the last three months, surgery involving the ureter, history of diabetes mellitus, diabetes insipidus, estrogen therapy, analgesic abuse (which causes papillary necrosis), and intake of diuretic, were also excluded.

2.2. IVU Evaluation. On IVU, the ureter was considered dilated if the transverse ureteral diameter was >7.0 mm at the site of maximum dilatation [1, 6], involving at least a 10 cm long segment of the ureter on supine IVU films, and the dilatation persisted in two or more radiographic exposures taken at an interval of at least 5 minutes [1]. The ureter was measured at three points, at least 1.0 cm apart (using electronic calipers on the workstation), at the widest part of the ureter; and a mean of the three measurements was recorded as the ureteral diameter in mm by Sachin Agrawal and Vinita Rathi (VR).

2.3. Investigations. All the patients underwent a number of investigations to exclude known causes of ureteral dilatation, for example, stone formation due to hypercalcemia and hyperuricemia, urinary tract infection, tuberculosis, diabetes insipidus, diabetes mellitus, and papillary necrosis, due to sickle cell anaemia. The investigations included assessment of urinary pH, urine specific gravity, routine and microscopic examination of urine, urine culture, microscopic examination of urine for acid-fast bacilli (AFB), urine culture for *M. tuberculosis*, haemogram with ESR, peripheral smear examination to exclude sickle cell anaemia, serum uric acid, serum calcium, fasting blood sugar, Mantoux test, and chest radiograph and sonography of the genitourinary tract (to exclude ureteral calculi and tumors involving pelvic organs).

2.4. Study Design. Those cases, in which the cause of ureteral dilatation on IVU was apparent on laboratory investigations and sonography, were excluded from further examination to avoid undue exposure to radiation. The remaining cases underwent CT Urography, within one week of IVU, to identify any other obscure cause of ureteral dilatation.

Voiding cystourethrography or cystourethroscopy was done, if clinically indicated. All cases were followed up clinically by the surgeon (Naveen Sharma) and on sonography till the end of the study period (i.e., 3 months to 1 year).

2.5. CT Scan Protocol. CT Urography was carried out by a modified technique on a 64-slice scanner (Somatom Definition AS, Siemens, Forchheim, Germany). Axial sections of 3.0 mm slice thickness were acquired and reconstructed at 1.0 mm interval. Scans were started one vertebral level above the region of maximum dilatation of the ureter on IVU and continued till the level of the ischial spines.

A noncontrast CT scan was performed at 120 kVp and 165 mAs to identify any small radiopaque calculus in the ureter. If the cause of ureteral dilatation was identified on noncontrast scans, the subsequent phases of CT Urography with contrast were abandoned, to avoid unnecessary irradiation.

100 mL nonionic contrast iohexol 300 mg I/mL (Omnipaque 300 GE Healthcare) was injected intravenously, and nephrogenic phase scans were acquired after a delay of 80–100 seconds at 120 kVp and 165 mAs, to evaluate the ureteral walls and periureteral disease.

Excretory phase of CT Urography was performed at low dose, that is, 120 kVp and 100 mAs, to reduce the radiation exposure.

The cause of ureteral dilatation was evaluated on CT Urography by two radiologists, VR and Shuchi Bhatt, independently. Ureteritis was diagnosed in the presence of diffuse, mild to moderate, circumferential ureteral wall thickening and enhancement associated with periureteric stranding [7]. Vascular compression was defined as extrinsic pressure effect on the ureter at the level where it crosses the iliac vessels [8], resulting in an abrupt change in the caliber of the ureter.

3. Results

The study comprised 18 cases (12 females and 6 males) with age ranging between 18 and 60 years and the mean age being 32.2 years. 50% of the cases were less than 30 years of age.

Out of the 12 females, 10 were in the reproductive age group, while 2 were postmenopausal. In the former group, 8 were multiparous (having 2 to 7 issues) and 2 were nulliparous.

On IVU, 35 out of 37 ureters were measured (1 case had a duplicated left ureter, and in two cases, one of the ureters was not opacified due to complete obstruction by a renal calculus). The maximum ureteral diameter on IVU ranged from 3.0 to 20.0 mm. 22 out of 35 ureters were dilated: 15 on the right and 7 on the left. Ureteral diameter was normal (<7.0 mm) in 13 of the 35 ureters: 2 on the right and 11 on the left. In both sexes, ureteral dilatation was more frequent on the right side: in 10 out of 15 (66.66%) females and 5 out of 7 (71.43%) males. 12 ureters were dilated on the symptomatic side and 8 ureters were found dilated on the urinary pH and specific gravity and routine examination for albumin and sugar were normal in all cases. Details of the urine analysis done for assessing infection are shown in Table 1. Total leucocyte count, differential leucocyte count, serum uric acid, and fasting blood sugar levels were also normal in all cases. Seven cases had anemia, of which 4 had iron-deficiency anaemia. ESR was elevated in 6 cases. Four cases had a positive Mantoux test and three cases had hypocalcemia. Chest radiographs were normal in all cases except Case 14, in which left-sided pleural thickening was seen.

Sonography of the genitourinary tract revealed renal calculus disease causing hydronephrosis in 13 out of 18 cases. Hydroureter was found in 5 of the 18 cases, which had shown a dilated ureter on IVU. The cause of hydroureter could not be identified on sonography. Vesicoureteral reflux was absent on colour Doppler in all cases. Urinary tract infection/tuberculosis was diagnosed in 8 out of the mentioned 13 cases on laboratory investigations, while the remaining 7 cases underwent CT Urography.

Based on the laboratory investigations and sonography, the cause of ureteral dilatation was identified in 9 out of 18 (50%) cases. Ureteral dilatation was attributed to urinary tract infection in 6 cases (pus cells on urine microscopy: 3 cases; positive urine culture: 3 cases) and urinary tract tuberculosis in 3 cases. Thus, excluding these (6 + 3 = 9 cases), the remaining 9 cases underwent a modified CT Urography to evaluate the cause of ureteral dilatation. The causes of ureteral dilatation revealed on CT Urography are listed in Table 2. In Case 1, noncontrast CT detected a ureteral calculus as a cause of ureteral dilatation; hence, contrast phase and excretory phase of CTU were not performed.

Voiding cystourethrography was done in Case 12 to evaluate the cause of the left-sided ureteritis and chronic pyelonephritis of the left kidney; but no vesicoureteral reflux was demonstrated. Ureteroscopy was not done to evaluate ureteral stricture in Cases 7 and 8, as it was not indicated clinically.

Ureteral dilatation caused by extrinsic compression by iliac arteries (seen on CTU) in four ureters (Cases 5, 6, 12, and 18) and the strictures reported in Cases 7 and 8 (on CTU) showed no clinical significance, since after undergoing pyelolithotomy these patients were asymptomatic during the follow-up period. Thus, excluding these six cases, a dilated ureter on IVU was found to be clinically significant in 12 out of 18, that is, 66.6% cases.

4. Discussion

The causes of ureteral dilatation are divided into obstructive and nonobstructive. Dilatation of the right ureter with associated urinary tract infection in previously gravid women is often ascribed to pressure upon this structure by an incompletely involuted, aberrant, dilated, right ovarian vein [8].

TABLE 1: Urine analysis ($n = 18$).

Investigation	Abnormal	Normal
Microscopic urine examination		
Pus cells*	8	10
RBCs	3	15
Urine culture	3 (*E. coli* > 100000 CFU/mL)	15
Microscopic examination for acid-fast bacilli (AFB)	3	15
Culture for *Mycobacterium tuberculosis*	3	15

*1 case showed microscopic field full of pus cells; 7 cases showed 4–10 pus cells/HPF.
Urinary tract infection was found in 8 patients with a dilated ureter, out of which 3 showed growth of *E. coli* on urine culture, while in 2 cases *Mycobacterium tuberculosis* was isolated on culture (1 patient with genitourinary tuberculosis had no pus cells in urine).

With the advent of multislice CT (MSCT) scan in developing countries and its inherent advantages in detecting urinary and extraurinary causes of ureteral dilatation, we performed a pilot study to assess the reason for ureteral dilatation on Intravenous Urography in those cases where this was not apparent. However, considering the lack of easy availability and high cost of MSCT in developing nations, we used a detailed clinicoradiological evaluation including laboratory investigations and CT Urography (using a modified technique), if necessary.

The present study had been conducted in patients with renal calculi (14) or undiagnosed flank pain (4), who presented for IVU to the department of radiodiagnosis. Only 18 out of 200 IVU cases presenting during the study period had dilated ureters with no apparent cause.

The right ureter was dilated in 90% (9 out of 10) parous women in our study. Our findings were similar to Flower who had stated that dilated ureters on the right, particularly, are sometimes seen in adult parous females. A combination of hormonal effect and past or present urinary tract infection had been postulated and evidence of obstruction and reflux could not be demonstrated [2]. On IVU of 26 parous women, Dure-Smith also found the width of the right ureter was greater than the left one in 76% of cases [9]. In our study in male patients too, dilatation was more commonly seen in the right ureter.

Ureteral dilatation with no obvious cause on Intravenous Urography was found to be clinically significant in 12 out of 18 (66.6%) cases. In 8 out of these 12 cases, it was associated with urinary tract infection (pus cells on urine microscopic examination: two; *E. coli* infection on urine culture: three; ureteritis on CTU: three). Identification of urinary tract infection (UTI) is important in patients with renal calculi to prevent postoperative complications and also in patients with flank pain in the absence of calculus. Thus in patients with ureteral dilatation with no obvious cause on IVU, if urinary tract infection is detected, it should be adequately

TABLE 2: Causes of ureteral dilatation on CT Urography ($n = 9$).

Number	Right ureter	Left ureter
Case 1	Ureteral calculus	Normal ureter
Case 2	Extrinsic vascular impression (internal iliac artery); ureteritis	Normal ureter
Case 4	Not assessed*	Extrinsic vascular impression (common iliac artery); ureteritis
Case 5	Extrinsic vascular impression (common iliac artery)	Normal ureter
Case 6	Extrinsic vascular impression (bifurcation of common iliac artery)	Normal ureter
Case 7	Ureteral stricture at external iliac artery origin level	Normal ureter
Case 8	Ureteral stricture at lumbosacral junction level	Normal ureter
Case 12	Extrinsic vascular impression (common iliac artery)	Ureteritis
Case 18	Extrinsic vascular impression (common iliac artery)	Normal ureter

*Case 4: right ureter was not assessed on CT Urography as it was not visible on Intravenous Urography and hence not dilated.

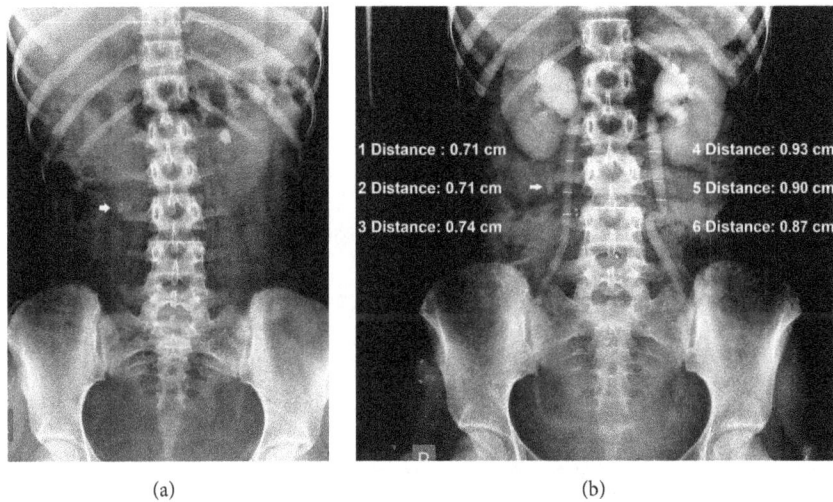

FIGURE 1: (a) Scout film shows a left renal calculus. An oval calcified node (arrow) lies outside the line of the ureter in (b). (b) Intravenous urogram shows dilated ureters with no apparent cause. Acid-fast bacilli on microscopic examination and culture of urine confirmed tuberculosis.

treated. Zelenko et al. had stated that *E. coli*, *Pseudomonas*, and *Citrobacter* infections can impair ureteral peristalsis and cause ureteral dilatation [3]. Findings of Spiro and Fry had also suggested that ureteral dilatation is associated with infection, that is, pelvi-ureteritis, past or present [1].

In 3 out of the 12 cases, dilated ureters on IVU were likely to be a manifestation of tuberculosis (confirmed on urine examination) in our study, as no other signs suggestive of tuberculosis had been seen on either IVU or sonography. In 2 out of these 3 cases (having dilated ureters with no apparent cause on IVU), patients had presented with renal calculi and IVU had been requested preoperatively (Figure 1). Hence, urinary tract tuberculosis would have remained undiagnosed and untreated in these 3 cases, if they had not undergone a detailed clinicoradiological evaluation for the cause of ureteral dilatation (Figure 2).

In one case, ureteral dilatation on IVU was due to a ureteral calculus (identified on CTU), which had been missed on a plain radiograph and not detected by sonography.

CTU played a very important role in the management of this case, as ureteroscopic removal of stone was done.

CT Urography was performed in 9 out of the 18 (50%) cases and identified the cause of ureteral dilatation in all the 10 dilated ureters (100%) (Table 2). But the cause of dilatation was clinically significant in only 4 of the dilated ureters (calculus: 1, ureteritis: 1, and ureteritis along with extrinsic compression by a vessel: 2) (Figure 3).

In another 4 ureters, CTU showed no significant cause of ureteral dilatation other than extrinsic vascular compression. According to Chait et al., minor degrees of obstruction of the ureter caused by iliac vessels do not appear to be clinically significant [8].

In two cases, stricture was the possible cause of ureteral dilatation on CTU, but these patients developed no fresh clinical complaints till one year, after undergoing surgery for renal calculus. Thus, these strictures were not considered clinically significant. Ureteroscopy was not warranted clinically and hence was not performed. However, a prolonged

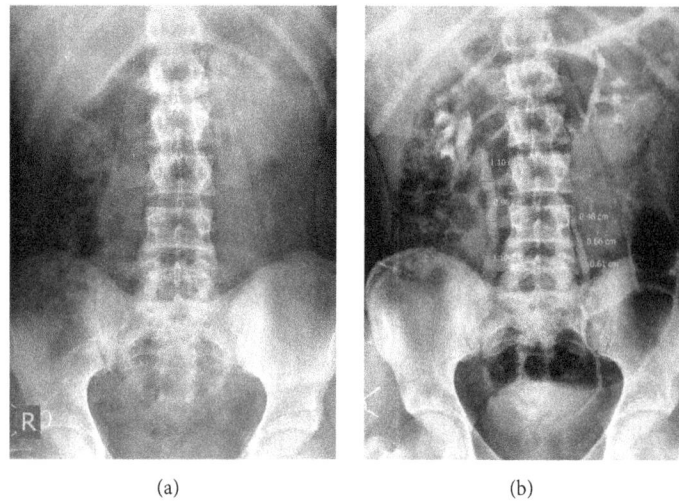

FIGURE 2: (a) Scout film: male patient with right-sided flank pain. No radiopaque calculus seen. (b) IVU: right ureter was dilated, but the cause was not obvious. No vesicoureteral reflux seen on color Doppler. Urine examination revealed tuberculosis.

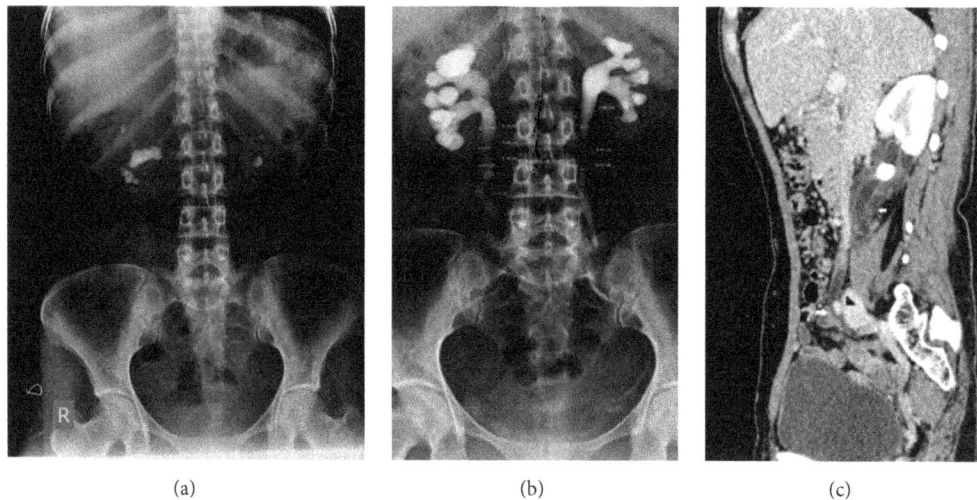

FIGURE 3: (a) Scout film: bilateral renal calculi. (b) IVU: a dilated right ureter, but the cause was not apparent. No ureteral calculus on noncontrast CT. (c) Contrast-enhanced CT scan: marked wall thickening in the region of ureteral dilatation (arrow) indicating ureteritis and also an extrinsic vascular compression of the right ureter (between arrowhead and lower white arrow).

follow-up is required to assess the significance of the ureteral strictures seen on CTU in these two cases.

5. Conclusions

In developing countries, availability and cost of MSCT are major limitations. Hence cases having a dilated ureter with no apparent cause on IVU should undergo a detailed clinicoradiological evaluation that includes laboratory investigations to identify the cause. CT Urography should be used judiciously and the technique should be modified (e.g., restricting scan length to identify cause of ureteral dilatation and using low dose technique) to limit the radiation dose.

Conflict of Interests

The authors declare that there is no conflict of interests regarding the publication of this paper.

References

[1] F. I. Spiro and I. K. Fry, "Ureteric dilatation in non-pregnant women," *Proceedings of the Royal Society of Medicine*, vol. 63, no. 5, pp. 462–466, 1970.

[2] C. D. R. Flower, "Radiology now. Wide ureters, a dilemma in diagnosis," *British Journal of Radiology*, vol. 50, no. 596, pp. 539–540, 1977.

[3] N. Zelenko, D. Coll, A. T. Rosenfeld, and R. C. Smith, "Normal ureter size on unenhanced helical CT," *American Journal of Roentgenology*, vol. 182, no. 4, pp. 1039–1041, 2004.

[4] S. G. Silverman, J. R. Leyendecker, and E. S. Amis Jr., "What is the current role of CT urography and MR urography in the evaluation of the urinary tract?" *Radiology*, vol. 250, no. 2, pp. 309–323, 2009.

[5] M. Noroozian, R. H. Cohan, E. M. Caoili, N. C. Cowan, and J. H. Ellis, "Multislice CT urography: state of the art," *British Journal of Radiology*, vol. 77, pp. S74–S86, 2004.

[6] R. B. Dyer, M. Y. M. Chen, and R. J. Zagoria, "Intravenous urography: technique and interpretation," *Radiographics*, vol. 21, no. 4, pp. 799–824, 2001.

[7] A. P. Wasnik, K. M. Elsayes, R. K. Kaza, M. M. Al-Hawary, R. H. Cohan, and I. R. Francis, "Multimodality imaging in ureteric and periureteric pathologic abnormalities," *American Journal of Roentgenology*, vol. 197, no. 6, pp. W1083–W1092, 2011.

[8] A. Chait, K. W. Matasar, C. E. Fabian, and H. Z. Mellins, "Vascular impressions on the ureters," *The American Journal of Roentgenology, Radium Therapy, and Nuclear Medicine*, vol. 111, no. 4, pp. 729–749, 1971.

[9] P. Dure-Smith, "The female ureter and pyelonephritis," *British Journal of Urology*, vol. 40, no. 4, pp. 415–417, 1968.

23

Measurement of the Physical Properties during Laparoscopic Surgery Performed on Pigs by Using Forceps with Pressure Sensors

Hiroyuki Yamanaka,[1] **Kazuhide Makiyama,**[1] **Kimito Osaka,**[1] **Manabu Nagasaka,**[2] **Masato Ogata,**[2] **Takahiro Yamada,**[3] **and Yoshinobu Kubota**[1]

[1]*Department of Urology, Yokohama City University, Yokohama 236-0004, Japan*
[2]*Mitsubishi Precision Co., Ltd., Kamakura 247-8505, Japan*
[3]*Graduate School of Environment and Information Sciences, Yokohama National University, Yokohama 240-8501, Japan*

Correspondence should be addressed to Hiroyuki Yamanaka; hymnk@yokohama-cu.ac.jp

Academic Editor: Walid A. Farhat

Objectives. Here we developed a unique training system, a patient specific virtual reality simulator, for laparoscopic renal surgery. To develop the simulator, it was important to first identify the physical properties of the organ. *Methods.* We recorded the force measured during laparoscopic surgery performed on pigs by using forceps with pressure sensors. Several sensors, including strain gauges, accelerometers, and a potentiometer, are attached to the forceps. *Results.* Throughout the experiment, we measured the reaction force in response to the forceps movement in real time. *Conclusions.* The experiment showed the possibility of digitizing these physical properties in humans as well.

1. Background

Laparoscopic surgery has become an increasingly common practice in recent years because it is less invasive than traditional methods [1]. However, surgeons must be highly skilled to perform laparoscopic surgery since it is one of the most difficult surgical techniques to learn and involves a steep learning curve [1]. Surgeons must acquire laparoscopic skills before performing laparoscopy in the operating room [2–6].

Like flight and driving simulators, laparoscopy simulators must provide a virtual yet accurate simulation of the task at hand. For example, in a flight simulator, the view and sounds in the cockpit are very real. Some flight simulators also demonstrate acceleration.

The latest laparoscopy simulators can reproduce an entire laparoscopic surgery [7–9]. Some training systems that simulate surgical processes are commercially available. Such systems are useful for basic training. They demonstrated initial construct validity regarding force and position sensing and capable of detecting differences between novices and

experts in a laparoscopic suturing task with respect to force and position [10, 11]. However, they do not provide surgeons with the necessary experience to respond to specific conditions in individual patients. Therefore, we have developed a unique training system, called a PSVR type simulator, for laparoscopic surgery [12–15]. Using data specific to each individual patient, this system facilitates "rehearsal" operations for surgeons. We use multislice CT imaging technology in laparoscopic surgery, and CT images of individual patients who are scheduled to undergo surgery are transferred into the simulation system (Figure 1). Each patient's specific organ volume data are extracted by our simulator to allow surgeons to perform a preoperative "rehearsal." Some PSVR simulators are reportedly in commercial use, but no PSVR simulator is currently available in the field of urology [16, 17].

In an effort to make our simulator performance more "real," we considered the importance of the subjective sensation that surgeons feel while using it. Other commercial surgical simulators are validated by the adjustment of the

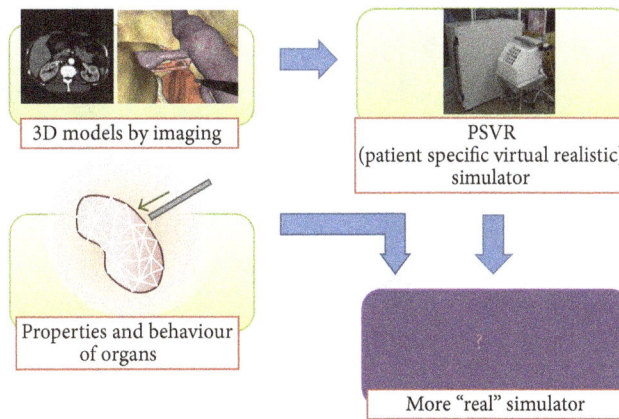

FIGURE 1: To make our simulator performance more "real," we considered the importance of the subjective sensation that surgeons feel while using it.

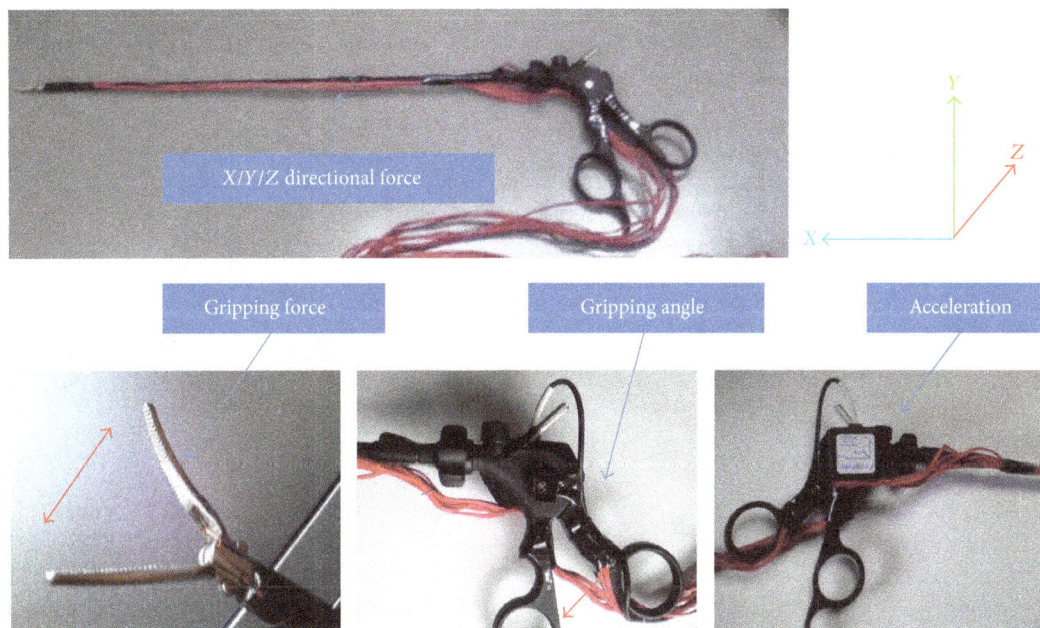

FIGURE 2: The forceps we developed.

physical parameters of the deformable model and reliance on the surgeon's subjective sensation [11, 16, 17]. Those simulators might present a reaction force to the surgeon that is similar to a certain degree to that of a real operation. However, an evaluation that relies only on the surgeon's sensation is subjective and lacks objectivity. Our mechanical model, based on the corotated finite element method [15, 18], has not been numerically verified with real soft tissue during surgery.

To resolve these issues, the collection of numerical data such as the forceps reaction force, grabbing angle, and moving speed is necessary. Unfortunately, no such measurement data currently exist. Therefore, as a first step, we recorded the force measured during laparoscopic surgery performed on pigs by using forceps with pressure sensors. During the experiment, we measured the reaction force and gripping force of the membrane, kidney, liver, and vessels.

2. Materials and Methods

We developed a multimodal measuring device that interferes very little with the surgeon's movements. The system was developed through collaboration among Yokohama City University, Mitsubishi Precision, and Yokohama National University (our homepage: http://www-user.yokohama-cu .ac.jp/~urology/kenkyu/surgicalsimulatorindex.html). The measuring device is illustrated in Figure 2 and Table 1.

Figure 2 shows the forceps and the sensor wires. The running sensor wires are packed inside of the instrument and we use special guide when we insert the forceps to the trocar. So the forceps is free from contact or damage and we can observe the accurate measurements.

The block diagram is presented in Figure 3. Several sensors (e.g., strain gauges, accelerometers, and a potentiometer)

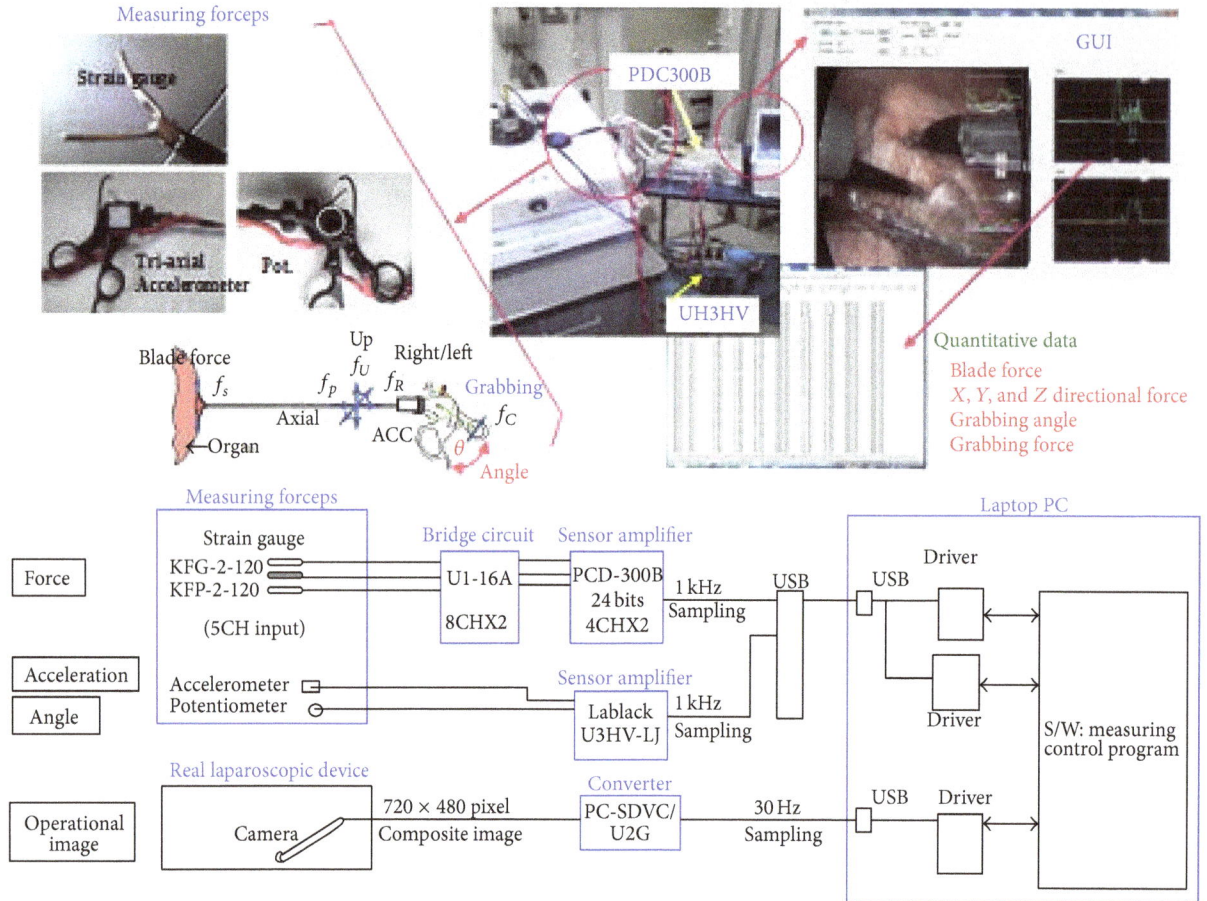

FIGURE 3: The system we developed to detect the sensation of the forceps.

TABLE 1: The equipment we used.

	Name	Type
1	Forceps	K3331OMD, KARL STORZ
2	Controller & amplifier	PDC300B, Kyowa
3	Controller & amplifier	U3HV, Lab Jack
4	Bridge	U1-16A, Kyowa
5	Laptop PC	CF-S10, Panasonic, Windows 7 64 bits
6	Acc.	CXL17LF3, Crossbow
7	Converter	PC-SDVC/U2G, BUFFALO

are attached to the forceps to measure the $X/Y/Z$ directional forces, blade force, grabbing force, grabbing angle, and acceleration. All of these parameters are measured over 0.1 ms and stored on a hard disk drive for later analysis. To synchronize the acquired physical quantities, such as the reaction force, with the corresponding surgical operations, we adopted a method to overlap a plotted graphical image of quantitative data.

We calibrated the system and then checked the control. Under this condition, we performed a laparoscopic nephrectomy on a pig by using multimodal measuring forceps.

We performed the laparoscopic nephrectomy as follows: (1) we made an incision in the peritoneum and displaced the colon; (2) we exposed the ureter and renal artery and vein; (3) we exposed the renal capsule; (4(A)) we ruptured the kidney by using forceps; (5) we sutured the ruptured kidney by using a surgical needle; and (6) we dissected the renal artery and vein after ligation.

During and after the nephrectomy, we measured the reaction force of the organs as follows: (B) we gripped the gonadal vein; (C) we pulled on the renal artery; (D) we pulled on the renal vein; (E) we pulled on the ureter; (F) we gripped the liver softly; (G) we gripped the liver strongly; (H) we gripped and pulled the liver; (I) we gripped the kidney softly; (J) we gripped the kidney strongly; and (K) we gripped and pulled the kidney.

The forceps used for the measurements are fragile, so we used normal forceps or energy devices when not taking the measurements. We collected these measurements three or four times to obtain an appropriate average reaction force as well as the max reaction force. This experiment was examined by ethical committee of Yokohama City University and accepted (Research number B100902033: the measurement

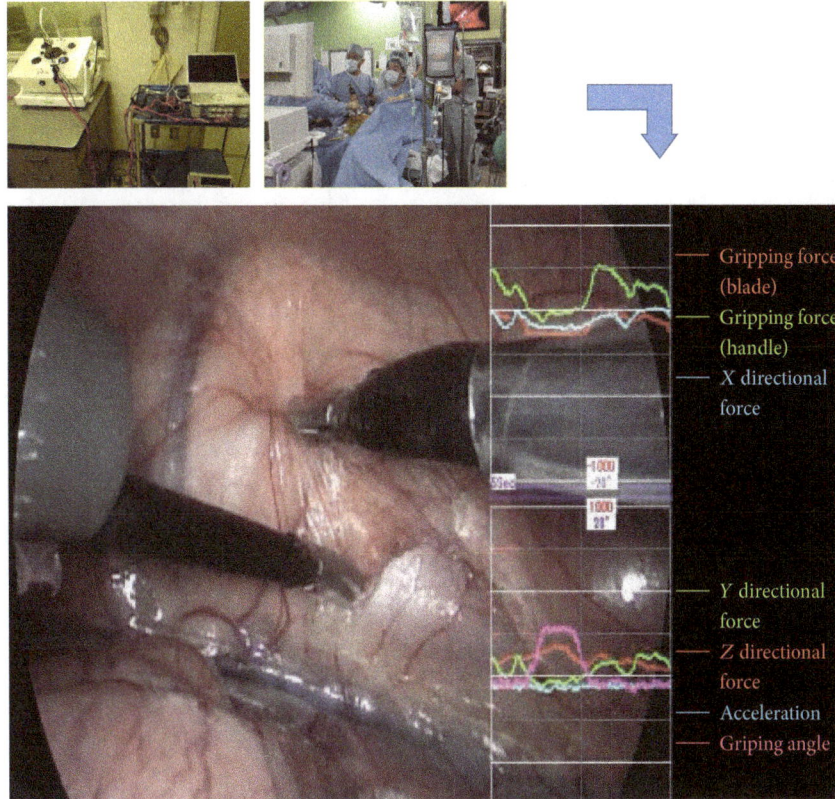

FIGURE 4: To synchronize the acquired physical quantities, such as the reaction force, with the corresponding surgical operations, we adopted a method to overlap a plotted graphical image of quantitative data.

of transformation and physical properties of organ by the external force). The experiment was performed under the ethical consideration.

3. Results

The results are shown in Table 2. The force (N) is determined as the maximum force during the experiment.

The sample results presented in Figures 4 and 5 show the reaction force on the blade and the corresponding grabbing force. The green line represents the X directional force, the red line represents the grabbing force, and the blue line represents the sum of the Y and Z directional forces. The angles of the blade are shown as a purple line, and the measurements are synchronized with the blade opening and closing, suggesting that the experimental data interference is small.

(A) Rupture the Kidney. The surgeon tried to rupture the kidney by using the tip of the closed forceps. When the tip of the blade pushed on the kidney, the forceps received a reaction force (green line). When we pushed kidney with 4.5 N, it ruptured. As such, we assume that the reaction force required to rupture the kidney was 4.5 N from the X directional force with the tip of the closed forceps (Figure 6).

(B) Grip the Gonadal Vein. When the surgeon gripped the gonadal vein softly and strongly, the gripping force reached

TABLE 2: The results of the experiments.

	Pulling/X directional force (N)	Gripping force (N)
(A) Rupture the kidney	5	4
(B) Grip the gonadal vein	—	2 (soft)–17 (strong)
(B) Pull on the gonadal vein	3	8–15
(C) Pull on the renal artery	3	15–20
(D) Pull on the renal vein	2	15–20
(E) Pull on the ureter	2	10–16
(F) Grip the liver softly	—	2–4
(G) Grip the liver strongly	—	18–42
(H) Grip and pull on the liver	9	26
(I) Grip the kidney softly	—	10–13
(J) Grip the kidney strongly	—	11–18
(K) Grip and pull on the kidney	4	12

2 and 17 N, respectively. A total of 8–15 N of gripping force and 3 N of pulling force were required (Figure 7).

(C) Grip and Pull on the Renal Artery. When we gripped the renal artery softly and strongly to stop the blood flow, the

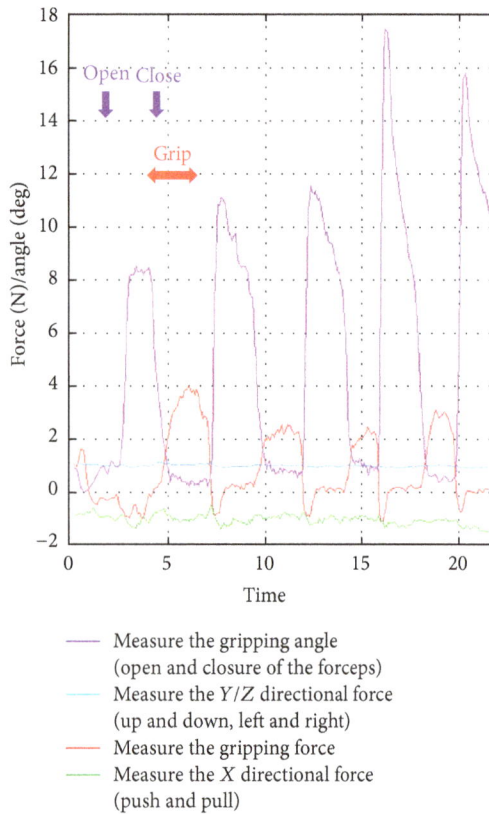

FIGURE 5: The green line represents the X directional force, the red line represents the grabbing force, and the blue line represents the sum of the Y and Z directional forces. The angles of the blade are shown as a purple line, and the measurements are synchronized with the blade opening and closing.

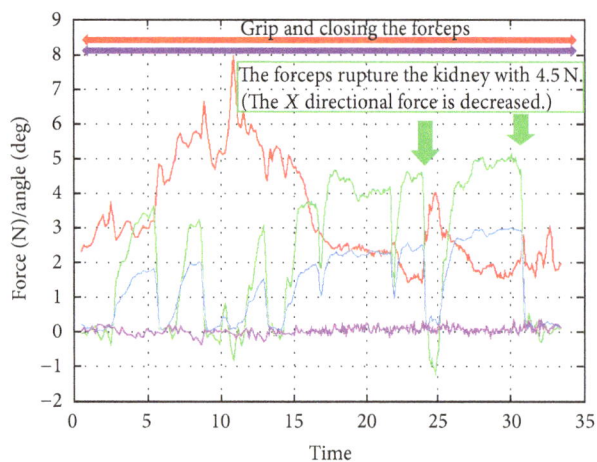

FIGURE 6: Experiment (A), rupture the kidney.

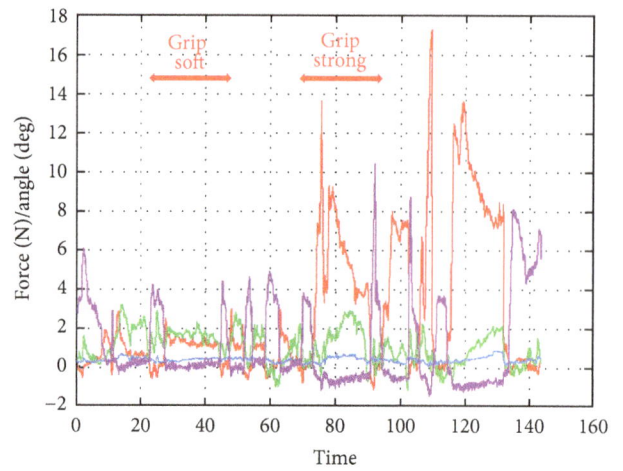

(a)

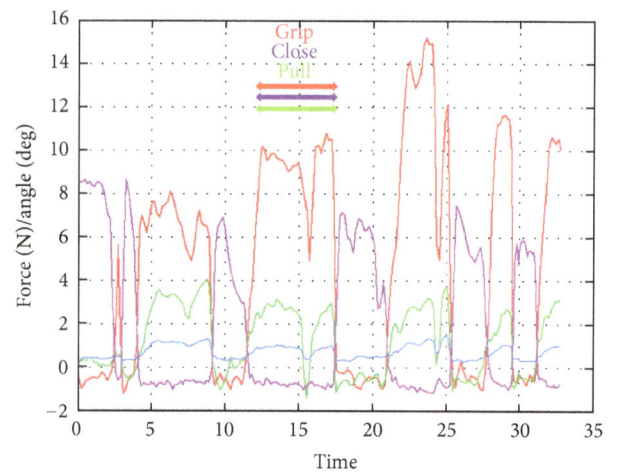

(b)

FIGURE 7: Experiment (B), grip the gonadal vein.

gripping force reached 6 and 16 N, respectively. When the surgeon pulled and gripped the renal artery to stretch it, 8–10 N of gripping force and 3 N of pulling force were needed (Figure 8).

(D) Grip and Pull on the Renal Vein. When we gripped the renal vein softly and strongly to stop the blood flow, the

gripping forces reached 10 and 16 N, respectively. We gripped and pulled the renal vein, and just before it tore off, it needed 15–20 N of gripping force and 2 N of pulling force (Figure 9).

(E) Grip and Pull the Ureter. The ureter required 10–16 N of gripping force and 2 N of pulling force to be torn off (Figure 10).

(F) Grip of Liver Softly; (G) Grip the Liver Strongly; (H) Grip and Pull on the Liver. When the surgeon gripped the liver softly, the forceps received 2–4 N of force. On the other hand, when the surgeon gripped the liver strongly, the forceps received 18–42 N of force. Moreover, he could tear off the liver by gripping the forceps with 26 N of force and pulling with 9 N of force (Figure 11).

(I) Grip the Kidney Softly; (J) Grip the Kidney Strongly; (K) Grip and Pull on the Kidney. When the surgeon gripped the liver softly, the forceps received 10–13 N of force. On the other hand, when the surgeon gripped the liver strongly, the forceps received 11–18 N of force. Moreover, the liver was torn off with 12 N of gripping force and 4 N of pulling force (Figure 12).

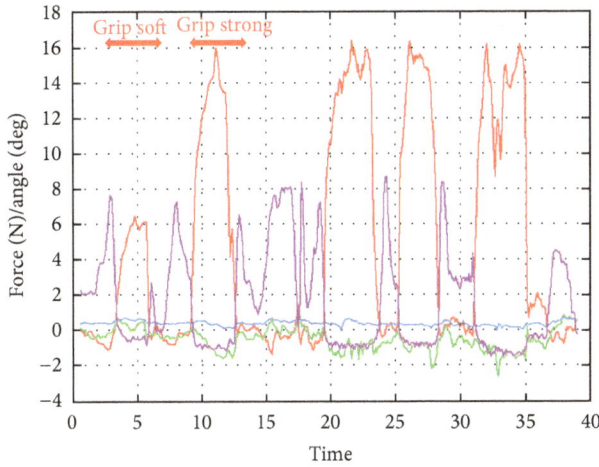

(a)

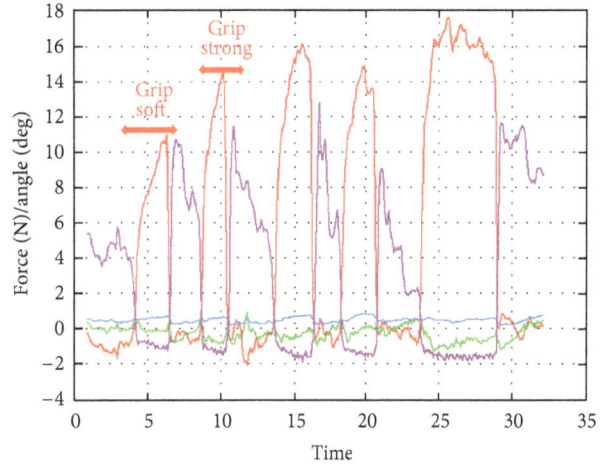

(b)

FIGURE 8: Experiment (C), grip and pull on the renal artery.

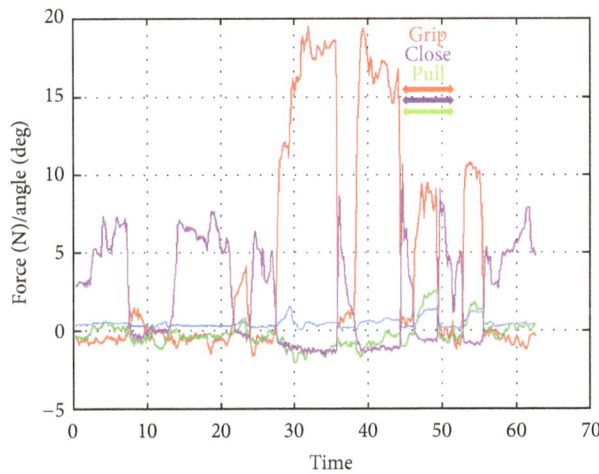

(a)

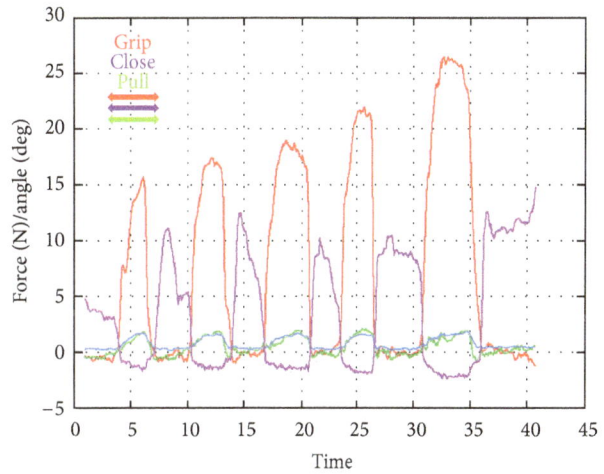

(b)

FIGURE 9: Experiment (D), grip and pull on the renal vein.

4. Discussion

When the surgeon pulled on the renal artery, renal vein, gonadal vein, and ureter just before tearing them off, the forceps received large gripping forces. As such, we believe the following: the renal artery bears 10 N of gripping force and 3 N of pulling force; the renal vein bears 20 N of gripping force and 2 N of pulling force; the gonadal vain bears 15 N of gripping force and 3 N of pulling force; and the ureter bears 16 N of gripping force and 2 N of pulling force. These findings show that if a surgeon grips and pulls the renal artery, renal vein, gonadal vein, or ureter rather roughly, each can resist the surgical force to some extent. To stop the blood flow during an operation, we must know blood pressure and vessel properties. These properties may be changed by patient age or history [19], so we need to perform more experiments.

We gripped and pulled the liver and kidney, to measure their properties and determine the force at which they tear off. The edge of the liver is flat, while that of the kidney is round, so the surgeon can easily grip the liver with less gripping force.

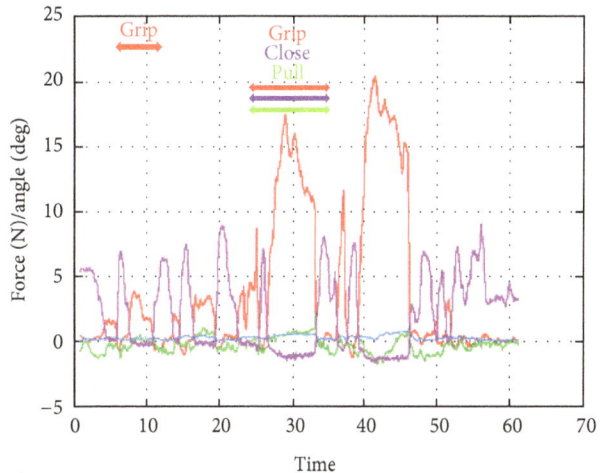

FIGURE 10: Experiment (E), grip and pull the ureter.

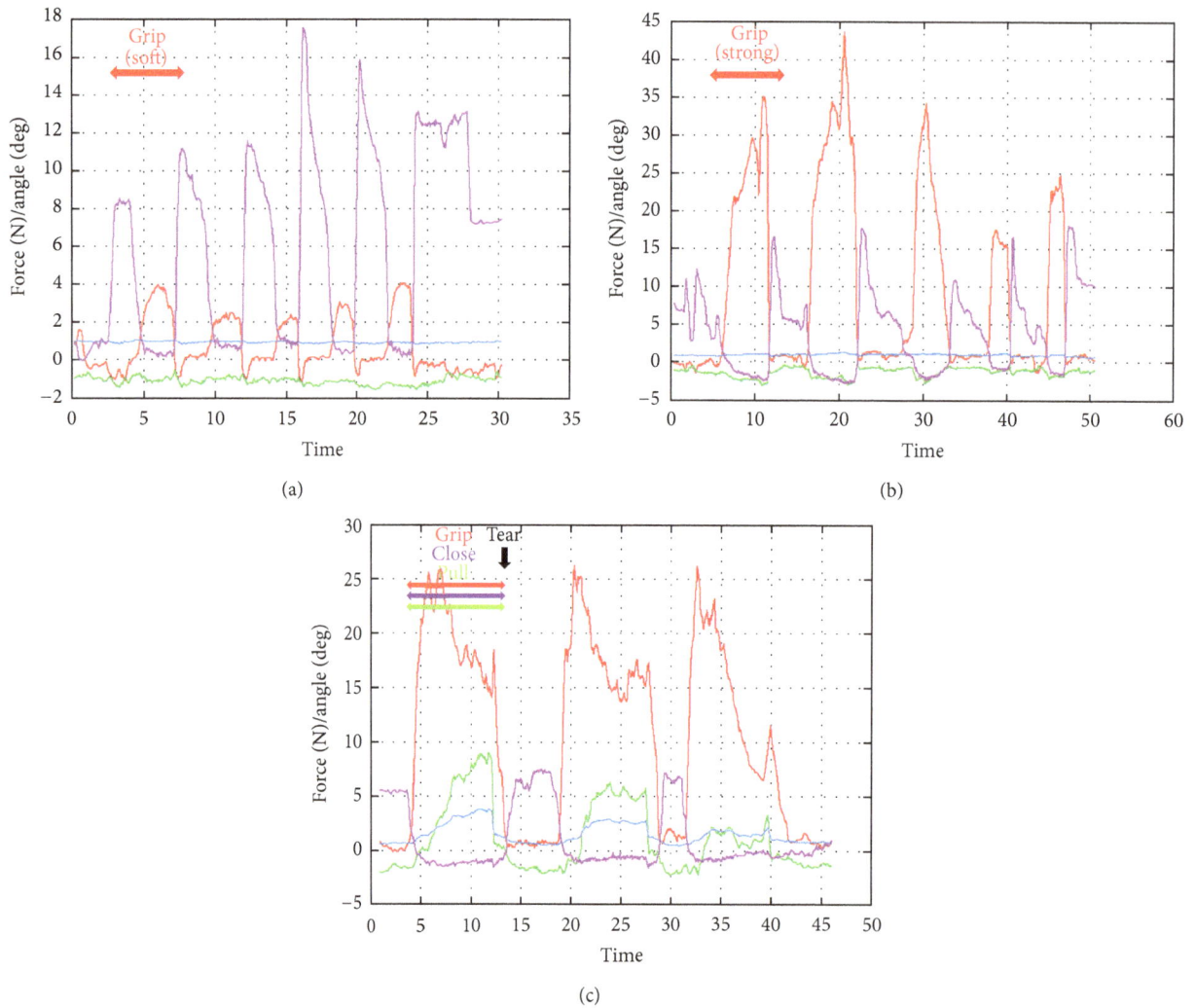

(a)

(b)

(c)

FIGURE 11: Experiment (F), grip liver softly; (G) grip the liver strongly; (H) grip and pull on the liver.

However, more force is needed to tear it off. This shows that the liver is solid compared with the kidney.

Figure 6 shows that, to rupture the kidney, for example, the surgeon gripped the forceps strongly to push the forceps into the kidney. He initially gripped the forceps too strongly. The red line demonstrated 8 N of force. After he got used to handling the forceps and was familiar with the moderate amount of power needed to grip and push the kidney, the gripping force tended to decrease (red line demonstrated 2 N of force). The gripping force increased to 4 N the moment of rupture, as the surgeon gripped the forceps strongly because he noticed the sudden shock when the kidney was ruptured.

These findings demonstrated that the operator tends to grip the forceps strongly when he notices the sudden shock of the forceps. As such, it may be possible to use gripping force to detect an operator's skill level since beginners tend to grip the forceps strongly. The gripping force as well as the moving speed or acceleration may be signs of operator proficiency. Thus, surgical techniques between operators can be evaluated and scored. Indeed, Yoshida et al. examined forceps forces and application time, and their results suggest that experts

should try to keep the instrument tip within the operative field [20]. Trejos et al. also show that force-based metrics were able to provide stronger correlations with experience than those found with task completion time or position based metrics [11].

Many experiments have tried to detect the properties of the organs or materials using operative devices or other kinds of equipment [10, 11, 19–24]. While many other experiments have been performed in a Dry-Box with a metal cylinder, our experiment was performed in a real operative environment and with real forceps that can measure gripping force, directional force, and the blade's angle. Here we used Maryland-type dissecting forceps. If the shape of the blade is changed, the X directional force or gripping force may be changed. In fact, it has been shown that 15 N of force is needed to destroy liver tissue by using a rubber plate [21], whereas our experimental data showed that 30–42 N is required to destroy liver tissue and 26 N is required to tear it off.

Some experiments have been performed with real forceps and dead pig organs [20, 23]. These gripping or directional forces are assumed by the gripping of the handle's angle and

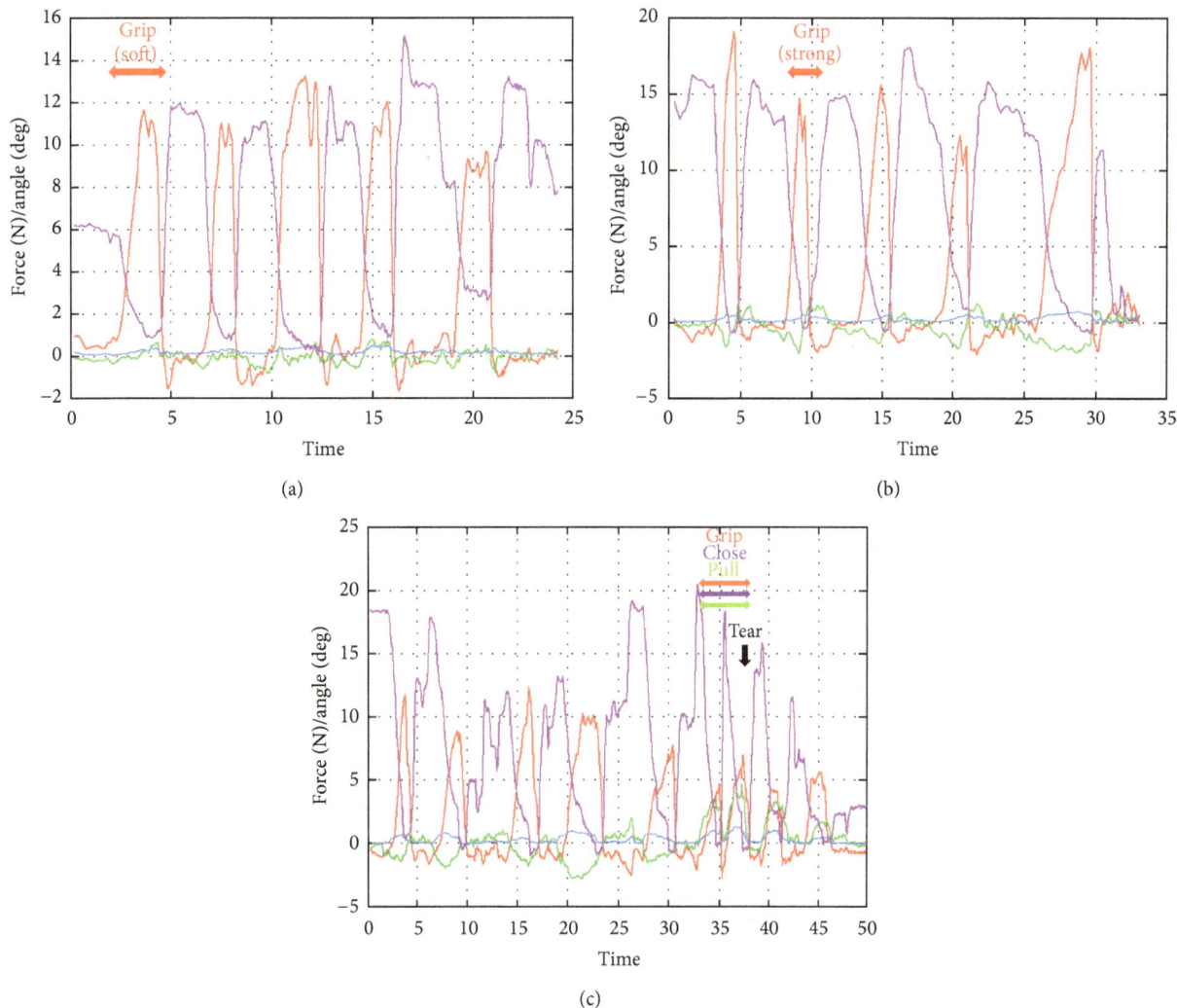

FIGURE 12: Experiment (I), grip the kidney softly; (J) grip the kidney strongly; (K) grip and pull on the kidney.

the force or sensor attached to the forceps shaft or handle. On the other hand, our dynamic sensors are attached to not only the shaft and handle but also the tip of the blade. Since our forceps directly detect the gripping force from the shaft and the directional force from the blade, our results are free of functional noise. Moreover, our forceps can be used in a real operative environment and can be inserted with the trocar in laparoscopic surgery, making it technically possible to perform such experiments in humans. However, there are associated ethical problems. Of course, we should also perform this kind of experiment in a Dry-Box to fine-tune our simulator and complement the shortage of actual experiments. We never have an intention to perform our experiment on living human body but we may perform this kind of experiment in a Dry-Box with use of extracted organs by carcinoma with patient's agreement. In that case, we will compare measurement data of pig with human and improve the simulator's sensors. Certainly, this experiment does not improve our "patient specific" simulation. However, this acquired data improves general sensation or action of our simulator and is efficacious for good compulsory training programs. As such we believe that our result is realistic and will lead to a more "real" simulation experience.

5. Conclusions

Here we recorded the force measured during laparoscopic surgery performed on pigs by using forceps with pressure sensors and performed a laparoscopic nephrectomy on a pig by using multimodal measuring forceps. The forceps measured the $X/Y/Z$ directional forces, blade force, grabbing force, and grabbing angle in real operative situations within a pig. The experiment showed the possibility of digitizing the physical properties in humans as well.

Abbreviations and Acronyms

CT: Computed tomography
PSVR: Patient specific virtual reality.

Ethical Approval

This experiment was examined by ethical committee of Yokohama City University and accepted (Research number B100902033: the measurement of transformation and physical properties of organ by the external force).

Disclosure

The authors have no intention to perform their experiment on living human body.

Conflict of Interests

Yamanaka, Makiyama, Osaka, Nagasaka, Ogata, Yamada, and Kubota have no conflict of interests or financial ties to disclose.

Authors' Contribution

Hiroyuki Yamanaka made conception and designing and drafted the paper. Kazuhide Makiyama participated in the design of the study and revised the paper. Hiroyuki Yamanaka, Kazuhide Makiyama, Kimito Osaka, Manabu Nagasaka, and Masato Ogata collected and assembled the data. Manabu Nagasaka, Masato Ogata, and Takahiro Yamada developed the equipment used in this study. Yoshinobu Kubota conceived of the study and helped to draft the paper. All authors read and approved the final paper. Kazuhide Makiyama, Kimito Osaka, Manabu Nagasaka, Masato Ogata, Takahiro Yamada, and Yoshinobu Kubota contributed equally to this work.

Acknowledgment

This work was supported by Grant-in-Aid for Scientists (no. 30550347) from Japan Society for the Promotion of Science.

References

[1] R. P. W. F. Wijn, M. C. Persoon, B. M. A. Schout, E. J. Martens, A. J. J. A. Scherpbier, and A. J. M. Hendrikx, "Virtual reality laparoscopic nephrectomy simulator is lacking in construct validity," *Journal of Endourology*, vol. 24, no. 1, pp. 117–122, 2010.

[2] Japan Society for Endoscopic Surgery, "Guideline for performing endoscopy surgery," *Japan Society for Endoscopic Surgery*, vol. 2, p. 7, 1997.

[3] A. Miyajima, M. Hasegawa, T. Takeda et al., "How do young residents practice laparoscopic surgical skills?" *Urology*, vol. 76, no. 2, pp. 352–356, 2010.

[4] P. D. Vlaovic, E. R. Sargent, J. R. Boker et al., "Immediate impact of an intensive one-week laparoscopy training program on laparoscopic skills among postgraduate urologists," *Journal of the Society of Laparoendoscopic Surgeons*, vol. 12, no. 1, pp. 1–8, 2008.

[5] C. Q. Le, D. J. Lightner, L. VanderLei, J. W. Segura, and M. T. Gettman, "The current role of medical simulation in American urological residency training programs: an assessment by program directors," *The Journal of Urology*, vol. 177, no. 1, pp. 288–291, 2007.

[6] J. R. Korndorffer Jr., D. Stefanidis, and D. J. Scott, "Laparoscopic skills laboratories: current assessment and a call for resident training standards," *American Journal of Surgery*, vol. 191, no. 1, pp. 17–22, 2006.

[7] K. Maschuw, I. Hassan, and D. K. Bartsch, "Surgical training using simulator: virtual reality," *Chirurg*, vol. 81, no. 1, pp. 19–24, 2010.

[8] L. Beyer, J. D. Troyer, J. Mancini, F. Bladou, S. V. Berdah, and G. Karsenty, "Impact of laparoscopy simulator training on the technical skills of future surgeons in the operating room: a prospective study," *The American Journal of Surgery*, vol. 202, no. 3, pp. 265–272, 2011.

[9] D. L. Diesen, L. Erhunmwunsee, K. M. Bennett et al., "Effectiveness of laparoscopic computer simulator versus usage of box trainer for endoscopic surgery training of novices," *Journal of Surgical Education*, vol. 68, no. 4, pp. 282–289, 2011.

[10] S. Jayaraman, A. L. Trejos, M. D. Naish, A. Lyle, R. V. Patel, and C. M. Schlachta, "Toward construct validity for a novel sensorized instrument-based minimally invasive surgery simulation system," *Surgical Endoscopy and Other Interventional Techniques*, vol. 25, no. 5, pp. 1439–1445, 2011.

[11] A. L. Trejos, R. V. Patel, R. A. Malthaner, and C. M. Schlachta, "Development of force-based metrics for skills assessment in minimally invasive surgery," *Surgical Endoscopy*, vol. 8, no. 7, pp. 2106–2019, 2014.

[12] H. Yamanaka, K. Makiyama, T. Tatenuma, R. Sakata, F. Sano, and Y. Kubota, "Preparation for pyeloplasty for ureteropelvic junction obstruction using a patient-specific laparoscopic simulator: a case report," *Journal of Medical Case Reports*, vol. 6, article 338, 2012.

[13] K. Makiyama, M. Nagasaka, T. Inuiya, K. Takanami, M. Ogata, and Y. Kubota, "Development of a patient-specific simulator for laparoscopic renal surgery," *International Journal of Urology*, vol. 19, no. 9, pp. 829–835, 2012.

[14] K. Makiyama, R. Sakata, H. Yamanaka, T. Tatenuma, F. Sano, and Y. Kubota, "Laparoscopic nephroureterectomy in renal pelvic urothelial carcinoma with situs inversus totalis: preoperative training using a patient-specific simulator," *Urology*, vol. 80, no. 6, pp. 1375–1378, 2012.

[15] M. Ogata, M. Nagasaka, T. Inuiya, K. Makiyama, and Y. Kubota, "A development of surgical simulator for training of operative skills using patient-specific data," in *Medicine Meets Virtual Reality 19*, pp. 361–373, IOS Press, 2010.

[16] J. Brewin, T. Nedas, B. Challacombe, O. Elhage, J. Keisu, and P. Dasgupta, "Face, content and construct validation of the first virtual reality laparoscopic nephrectomy simulator," *BJU International*, vol. 106, no. 6, pp. 850–854, 2010.

[17] R. P. W. F. Wijn, M. C. Persoon, B. M. A. Schout, E. J. Martens, A. J. J. A. Scherpbier, and A. J. M. Hendrikx, "Virtual reality laparoscopic nephrectomy simulator is lacking in construct validity," *Journal of Endourology*, vol. 24, no. 1, pp. 117–122, 2010.

[18] M. Ogata, K. Makiyama, T. Yamada, M. Nagasaka, H. Yamanaka, and Y. Kubota, "Dynamic measuring of physical properties for developing a sophisticated preoperative surgical simulator: how much reaction force should a surgical simulator represent to the surgeon?" *Studies in Health Technology and Informatics*, vol. 184, pp. 312–318, 2013.

[19] I. S. Mackenzie, I. B. Wilkinson, and J. R. Cockcroft, "Assessment of arterial stiffness in clinical practice," *QJM—Monthly Journal of the Association of Physicians*, vol. 95, no. 2, pp. 67–74, 2002.

[20] K. Yoshida, Y. Kuroda, Y. Kagiyama et al., "Pressure measurement in three axial directions on the tip of the laparoscopic forceps and skill analysis in a dissection procedure," *Transactions of Japanese Society for Medical and Biological Engineering*, vol. 48, no. 1, pp. 25–32, 2010.

[21] I. Sakuma, T. Hisada, C. K. Chui et al., "In vitro measurement of mechanical propertiesof liver tissue under compression and elongation using a new test piece holding method with surgical glue," in *Surgery Simulation and Soft Tissue Modeling: International Symposium, IS4TM 2003 Juan-Les-Pins, France, June 12-13, 2003, Proceedings*, vol. 2673 of *Lecture Notes in Computer Science*, pp. 284–292, 2003.

[22] Y. Hayashi, K. Kiguchi, K. Konishi, H. Nakashima, and M. Hashizume, "Estimation of forceps nonlinear haptic parameters for laparoscopic surgery simulator," in *Proceedings of the 1st International Conference of Applied Bionics and Biomechanics*, 2010.

[23] K. Kiguchi, M. Yamamoto, K. Konishi et al., "1A1-A11 Development of Laparoscopic Surgery Simulators-Dynamic Properties of Operated Forceps during the Laparoscopic Surgery," Nippon Kikai Gakkai Robotikusu, Mekatoronikusu Koenkai Koen Ronbunshu (CD-ROM), 2006.

[24] C. Sarkissian, G. S. Marchini, and M. Monga, "Endoscopic forceps for ureteroscopy: a comparative in vitro analysis," *Urology*, vol. 81, no. 3, pp. 690–695, 2013.

24

A Review of the Literature on Primary Leiomyosarcoma of the Prostate Gland

Anthony Kodzo-Grey Venyo

Department of Urology, North Manchester General Hospital, Delaunays Road, Manchester, UK

Correspondence should be addressed to Anthony Kodzo-Grey Venyo; akodzogrey@yahoo.co.uk

Academic Editor: In Ho Chang

Primary leiomyosarcoma of the prostate (PLSOP) is rare, with less than 200 cases reported so far. PLSOPs present with lower urinary tract symptoms, haematuria, and perineal pain; may or may not be associated with a history of previous treatment for adenocarcinoma of prostate by means of radiotherapy and or hormonal treatment; may afflict children and adult male. Examination may reveal benign enlarged prostate and hard enlarged mass. PLSOPs may be diagnosed by histological examination findings of spindle-shaped carcinoma cells in prostate specimens. Immunohistochemical staining tends to be positive for vimentin, CD44, smooth muscle actin, and calponin, focally positive for desmin, and at times positive for keratin. They stain negatively for PSA, S-100, CD34, CD117, and cytokeratin. Cytogenetic study on primary leiomyosarcoma of the prostate gland may show clonal chromosomal rearrangement involving Chromosomes 2, 3, 9, 11, and 19. On the whole the prognosis is poor. Surgery with or without chemotherapy would appear to be the mainstay of treatment for PLSOPs that are operable, but generally there is no consensus opinion on the best therapeutic approach. Most cases of PLSOPs are diagnosed in an advanced stage of the disease. A global multicenter trial is required to find therapies that would improve the prognosis.

1. Introduction

Sarcoma of the prostate gland is rare and this accounts for only 0.1% of all malignant tumours of the prostate gland [1]. Leiomyosarcoma of the prostate gland is rare and globally less than 200 cases have been reported in the literature and less than 100 PLSOPs have been reported in the English literature [2]. Leiomyosarcoma accounts for approximately 25% of all sarcomas of the prostate gland. [3] Leiomyosarcoma of the prostate was first described in 1853 by Sambert as stated by Riba et al. [4] in 1950. Leiomyosarcoma of the prostate gland is an aggressive tumour which most clinicians globally have not encountered; in view of this most clinicians would not be familiar with its biological behaviour. The ensuing literature review on primary leiomyosarcoma of the prostate gland is divided into two parts: (A) an overview and (B) miscellaneous narrations and discussions from some reported cases of leiomyosarcoma of the prostate gland.

2. Methods

Various internet data bases were searched, including Google, Google Scholar, PubMed, and Educus, for information on primary leiomyosarcoma of the prostate gland. The search terms used included primary leiomyosarcoma of the prostate gland; leiomyosarcoma of the prostate gland; leiomyosarcoma of prostate; prostatic leiomyosarcoma; primary prostatic leiomyosarcoma. Fifty-five references related to case reports, case series, and other types of the literature related to primary leiomyosarcoma of the prostate gland were identified suitable for writing the literature review.

3. Literature Review

(A) Overview

General Comments

> Primary leiomyosarcoma of the prostate gland (PLSOP) is the commonest sarcoma affecting the prostate gland, even though on the whole it is a rare tumour [5].

> PLSOPs cause obstruction and tend to involve adjacent organs [5].

> PLSOPs tend to recur [5].

PLSOP metastasizes to the liver and lung [5].

PLSOP tends to be associated with a mean survival of 3 to 4 years [5].

Definition. Sarcoma of the prostate is a rare type of malignancy of mesenchymal origin that can rarely afflict the prostate gland. Various types of sarcoma of the prostate gland can occur including leiomyosarcoma, which is a smooth muscle sarcoma, and rhabdomyosarcoma, a skeletal muscle-type sarcoma.

Aetiology of Sarcoma of the Prostate Gland. On the whole the aetiology of PLSOP is unknown or not well understood.

Sarcomatous Dedifferentiation [6]. A number of cases of leiomyosarcoma of the prostate gland develop a number of years after patients had undergone treatment by means of radiotherapy and/or hormonal treatment for adenocarcinoma of the prostate gland. Even though there may be absence of any residual adenocarcinoma of the prostate, evidence of a new malignancy in the form of leiomyosarcoma of the prostate could be conjectured to be a sequel of dedifferentiation of totipotential cells in the prostate gland as an emanation from previous effect of the radiotherapy or hormonal therapy on the totipotential cells.

Li-Fraumeni Syndrome [6–8]. Li-Fraumeni syndrome has been postulated to be associated with mutation of p53 tumour suppressor gene and this leads in some children to the development of sarcomas and their mothers tend to have an increased risk of carcinoma of the breast with siblings having an increased risk for the development of malignancy [7, 8].

Age Distribution. Leiomyosarcoma of the prostate gland has been reported in children and adults whose ages have ranged from 2.5 years to 80 years (see the case of the 2.5-year-old boy in [9]).

Presentation. Patients with PLSOPs tend to present with the following (see [2, 10, 11] for some of the presentations):

(1) "Lower urinary tract symptoms" including urinary frequency, poor flow, hesitancy, urinary urgency, and inability to void. The presentation of lower urinary tract symptoms may mimic benign prostatic hypertrophy clinically in that rectal examination findings may indicate benign prostatic hypertrophy and the diagnosis is established after the patient has undergone transurethral resection of prostate and the histology result would indicate leiomyosarcoma of the prostate.

(2) Haematuria: sometimes a history of previous treatment for adenocarcinoma of prostate by means of hormonal therapy and/or radiotherapy in the form of external beam radiotherapy or brachytherapy may be obtained

(3) Retention of urine may occur.

(4) They may present with an exophytic mass of prostate projecting towards or infiltrating the rectum or a perineal mass.

(5) Leiomyosarcomas of the prostate may manifest with metastases to the liver and lung [12].

Clinical Findings. Digital rectal examination may reveal the following:

(1) An enlarged prostate which may feel benign.

(2) An enlarged/firm prostate gland.

(3) A hard prostate which has extended to the capsule or distorted the capsule.

(4) An enlarged hard mass arising from the prostate and extending to the rectum, pelvic side wall, perineum, and seminal vesicle or involving the base of the urinary bladder.

(5) An enlarged mass arising in the prostate gland in a child with voiding symptoms.

Laboratory Investigations. The following investigations tend to be undertaken in cases of PLSOP:

(1) Urine: urinalysis may be normal or may show evidence of visible or nonvisible haematuria and these are not specific for a diagnosis of leiomyosarcoma of the prostate but form part of the general assessment of the patient. Urine microscopy and culture may or may not show evidence of infection and this examination is used as part of the general assessment of the patient.

(2) Blood tests: routine blood tests are undertaken in the assessment of the patient including full blood count, serum urea and electrolytes, liver function tests, serum glucose, and coagulation screen. If the patient is anaemic, then the appropriate management is undertaken to correct the anaemia. Furthermore attempts tend to be made to correct any impairment noticed in the blood test results to improve upon the general management of the patient. Serum PSA may be normal or raised, but this would not be diagnostic of leiomyosarcoma of the prostate and the level of serum PSA would not be helpful to determine the progress of leiomyosarcoma of the prostate following treatment (see [13], e.g., when serum PSA was normal).

Radiological Investigations. Radiological investigations which may be undertaken in PLSOP include the following:

(1) Ultrasound scan (see [14] when ultrasound scan of abdomen and pelvis was done): ultrasound scan of the abdomen and pelvis would assess whether or not the patient has hydronephrosis; it can also indicate whether or not there is thickening of the bladder wall or trabeculation or sacculation or if there is a blood clot in the urinary bladder. Infiltration of

the base of the bladder or any part of the bladder can be illustrated by ultrasound scan. Enlargement of the prostate as well as the characteristic features of the prostate gland and its relationship to nearby structures can be illustrated by ultrasound scan.

(2) Transrectal ultrasound scan of prostate (TRUSP) and biopsies (see [10, 15] in which transrectal ultrasound scan of prostate and biopsies were undertaken): transrectal ultrasound scan of prostate is a useful technique for the assessment of the characteristics of the prostate gland which may show enlargement of the whole or part of the prostate gland involved. It may show heterogeneous hypoechoic lesions in the prostate, invasion of the capsule or extension into the rectum, pelvic side wall, seminal vesicle, ejaculatory duct, or protrusion into the urinary bladder or infiltration of the wall of the urinary bladder. Transrectal ultrasound-guided biopsy tends to be the usual approach for obtaining specimens of the prostatic lesion for histological examination which would establish the diagnosis of leiomyosarcoma of the prostate. A patient who had previously undergone radiotherapy by means of external beam method or brachytherapy or who has been having hormonal treatment for adenocarcinoma of prostate gland upon subsequent development of relapse and further enlargement of prostate may undergo a further ultrasound-guided biopsy of the prostate gland and its histological examination on the second occasion may reveal leiomyosarcoma of the prostate.

(3) Computed tomography (CT) scan (see [10, 11, 13] in which CT scan was used): CT scan of abdomen, pelvis, and thorax can be used to assess the features of the prostatic lesion, the relation of the lesion to nearby structures, and the extent of the disease locally. It can also show whether or not there is lymphadenopathy or metastases in the abdomen or within the thorax. CT scan can also be used in the follow-up assessment of the patient following treatment.

(4) Magnetic resonance imaging (MRI scan) (see [15] in which MRI scan was used): MRI scan of abdomen, pelvis, and thorax can be used to assess the features of the prostatic lesion, the relation of the lesion to nearby structures, and the extent of the disease locally. It can also show whether or not there is lymphadenopathy or metastases in the abdomen or within the thorax. MRI scan can also be used in the follow-up assessment of the patient following treatment.

(5) Isotope bone scan (see [10] in which isotope bone scan was used): isotope bone scan can be used in the initial as well as follow-up assessment of the patient to ascertain whether or not there is bone metastasis.

Cystoscopy Findings

(i) Cystoscopy may be undertaken in the assessment of the patient and this may show an enlarged prostate gland. Cystoscopy may at times show enlarged necrotic or bleeding median lobe of the prostate; it may also show protrusion or invasion of the prostatic lesion into the urinary bladder as well as trabeculation of the urinary bladder or blood clot in the urinary bladder. Nevertheless, these findings are not specific to leiomyosarcoma of the prostate gland.

(ii) Transurethral resection biopsy of a bleeding or necrotic median lobe can be undertaken after cystoscopy for histological examination which may lead to a diagnosis of leiomyosarcoma of the prostate.

(iii) At the end of cystoscopy transurethral resection of the prostate gland may be done for a presumed benign prostatic hypertrophy requiring resection to improve urinary flow or to relieve urinary retention and the histological examination may incidentally reveal leiomyosarcoma of the prostate gland.

Macroscopic Features

(i) Leiomyosarcomas of the prostate tend to be large tumours arising from the prostate and breaching the capsule of the prostate, extending into the perineum, towards the side wall of the pelvis or projecting into or invading the urinary bladder. When the median lobe is involved necrotic areas and bleeding areas may be seen of the median lobe of the prostate. The macroscopic features of leiomyosarcoma of the prostate gland are not specific features.

(ii) The size of PLSOPs tends to vary from 3 cm to 21 cm and infiltrative [2].

(iii) Macroscopic examination of PLSOPs tends to reveal a non-well-defined mass which may be fleshy with areas of necrosis and bleeding.

Microscopic Features

(i) Microscopic examination of leiomyosarcoma of the prostate tends to reveal spindle cells with enlarged hyperchromatic nuclei with evidence of increased mitotic activity [10].

(ii) Most cases of PLSOP tend to have high-grade features on microscopic examination associated with areas of viable tumour which comprise hypercellular, intersecting bundles of eosinophilic, spindle-shaped cells that have variable degrees of nuclear mitotic activity as well as nuclear atypia. Some cases may have low-grade features [13].

Immunohistochemistry

Positive Immunohistochemistry. Leiomyosarcomas of the prostate tend to stain positively for the following:

(i) Vimentin [2, 13].

(ii) CD44 [13].

(iii) Smooth muscle actin—about 63% may stain positive for actin [2].

(iv) Calponin—focally positive [11].

(v) Desmin—20% of cases may stain weakly for desmin [2].

(vi) Keratin—27% of cases may stain positive for keratin [2].

Negative Immunohistochemistry. Leiomyosarcomas of the prostate gland tend to stain negatively for the following:

(i) S-100 [13].

(ii) Cytokeratin [13].

(iii) CD117 (c-kit) [13].

(iv) PSA [11].

(v) CD34 [11].

Cytogenetics/Molecular Genetic Tests. Cytogenetic study on primary leiomyosarcoma of the prostate gland may show clonal chromosomal rearrangement involving Chromosomes 2, 3, 9, 11, and 19 [16].

Electron Microscopic Features. Electron microscopic examination of specimens of leiomyosarcoma of the prostate gland may show the bulk of the cytoplasm to be filled with microfilaments which are arranged on a long axis [15].

Differential Diagnoses. The differential diagnoses of PLSOP include the following:

(i) Nodular hyperplasia of prostate with atypical changes: in this case microscopic examination would reveal no evidence of invasion and no evidence of mitotic figures [2]. In nodular hyperplasia of the prostate gland microscopic examination of the specimen of the prostate tends to show hyperplasia of stroma and glandular tissue with evidence of papillary buds; in-folding and cysts, associated with squamous metaplasia and necrosis; the microscopic features which tend to begin around the urethra where the ejaculatory ducts enter the prostate gland (in the transitional and periurethral zone); the basal layer which tends to be continuous, evidence of stromal changes including increased smooth muscle, lymphocytes, and ducts which in the majority of cases are not associated with infectious process of prostatitis, reduced elastic tissue; various other features including sclerosing adenosis, fibroadenoma-like and phyllodes-like hyperplasia, leiomyoma-like nodules, and fibromyxoid nodules associated with infarct [17]. Nodular hyperplasia of prostate gland on immunohistochemistry tends to be positive for CD10 [18]. It has been stated that in nodular hyperplasia of the prostate gland no well-organized fascicles are seen on microscopic examination of the prostatic lesion and also there is

hyalinization, no necrosis, and no calcification on microscopic examination [12].

(ii) Postoperative spindle cell nodules: diagnosis of this condition could be based upon history of previous prostatic operation and microscopic examination tends to reveal no evidence of invasion and no evidence of mitotic figures [2]. Microscopic examination of the prostate specimen involved with postoperative spindle cell nodule tends to show evidence of cellular tissue with high mitotic activity, interlacing fascicles of spindle cells with extravasation of red blood cells which resemble Kaposi's sarcoma, minimal nuclear pleomorphism, and no atypical mitosis, and the size of the lesion tends to be relatively small [19].

(iii) Gastrointestinal stromal tumour of rectum (Rectal GIST): it has been stated that there may be difficulties differentiating between PLSOP and Rectal GIST [20]. In Rectal GIST microscopic examination tends to show transmural, usually plump, spindle cells with eosinophilic cytoplasm within stroma that tend to be variably hyalinised or oedematous, skeinoid fibres which are extracellular globules tend to be commonly seen, muscle infiltration may also be seen, there may be evidence of epithelioid morphology, and one to two mitotic figures may be seen per ten high-power fields [21]; on rare occasions there may be evidence of osteoclast-like giant cells [21, 22]. In Rectal GIST immunohistochemistry tends to reveal positive staining with CD117, CD34, and vimentin; immunohistochemistry also tends to show positive staining in 30% to 40% of cases for alpha smooth muscle actin and in 5% of cases for S100. Variable weak positive staining for keratin may also be seen in Rectal GIST [21]. In Rectal GIST electron microscopic examination of the specimen tends to show predominantly features of smooth muscle differentiation including long interdigitating cytoplasmic processes, intercellular junctions, and dense core granules [21]. In Rectal GIST electron microscopic examination also tends to show features of predominant neural differentiation including neuron-like cells which have axonal cytoplasmic processes, synapse-like structures, and dense core neurosecretory granules [21].

(iv) Some PLSOPs mimic stromal sarcoma of the prostate and sarcomatoid carcinoma of the prostate. Macroscopic examination of stromal sarcoma of the prostate specimen may reveal a whitish-yellow multinodular appearance with focal necrosis; microscopic examination of the specimen may show sarcomatoid oval to spindle cells; immunohistochemical staining of the specimen tends to show the membrane of the tumour cells to be positive with CD56, focal positivity in the cytoplasm of the tumour cells for synaptophysin, and positive staining on the cell membrane of the tumour cells for CD99 [23]. Microscopic examination of sarcomatoid carcinoma of the prostate gland (carcinosarcoma of the prostate) tends to reveal a biphasic tumour with adenocarcinoma and recognizable sarcoma components including chondrosarcoma, rhabdomyosarcoma, angiosarcoma, osteosarcoma, and leiomyosarcoma [24]. Immunohistochemistry of sarcomatoid carcinomas of the prostate tends to exhibit positive staining for the epithelial component for cytokeratin and PAP but negative staining for PSA [25]. Immunohistochemistry of the sarcoma component of sarcomatoid carcinoma of the prostate tends to reveal negative staining for PSA, EMA, and keratin [24].

(v) Other PLSOPs may mimic leiomyomas. In leiomyomas of the prostate gland microscopic examination of the prostate tends to show well-organized fascicles of spindle cells [12]. In leiomyoma of the prostate the lesion tends to be normocellular with no or rare mitotic activity and no or rare nuclear atypia, but there may be evidence of atypical bizarre stromal cells [26, 27]. Leiomyomas of the prostate gland tend to stain positively with desmin, actin, and androgen receptor on immunohistochemical staining [12]. On the other hand, leiomyosarcomas of the prostate gland microscopic examination of the prostatic lesion tend to show hypercellularity, evidence of infiltration, variable atypia, definite mitotic activity, and necrosis [12].

Treatment. Treatment options that can be undertaken in cases of leiomyosarcoma of the prostate gland include the following:

(1) Radical surgery in the form of radical prostatectomy or exenteration alone or plus or minus chemotherapy alone or plus radiotherapy (see, e.g., [15, 28]).

(2) Chemotherapy and radiotherapy (see, e.g., [29]).

(3) Chemotherapy alone (see, e.g., [10]).

(4) Radiotherapy alone (see, e.g., [13]).

(5) Palliative care including pain control and overall supportive care by a multidisciplinary team approach.

(6) Patients who have stomas in the form of ileal conduit or colostomies in cases where the rectum is involved and colostomy performed would require support from the stoma nurse.

Outcome. The outcome of the disease may be summarized as follows:

(1) On the whole the prognosis of leiomyosarcoma of the prostate is poor, but variable survival rates have been reported (see [2]), but it has been stated that the best survival occurs following curative surgery without evidence of residual or metastatic disease. It would appear that curative surgery together with multimodal therapy with chemotherapy would be the best form of treatment if the patient is fit to undergo multimodal treatment, but this approach may be hampered by the advanced stage of the disease at presentation and the general condition of the patients who may not be fit for multimodal treatment.

(2) There is no consensus opinion on the best therapeutic approach in view of the rarity of leiomyosarcoma of the prostate; therefore there is need for a global multicentre trial on management of leiomyosarcoma of the prostate in order to form an opinion on the best treatment option that would improve the prognosis.

(3) Perhaps if leiomyosarcoma of the prostate is diagnosed at an early stage, then the prognosis may improve following treatment. It may be that if patients who had previously undergone radiotherapy and/or hormonal therapy for adenocarcinoma of prostate are made to undergo prostate biopsies early when there is evidence of relapse or recurrence of their prostate carcinomas those whose tumours may have dedifferentiated into leiomyosarcoma of the prostate would be detected early, but this is conjectural.

(4) Leiomyosarcomas of the prostate gland are aggressive tumours with a median survival of 3 to 4 years and they tend to recur as well as metastasize to the liver and the lungs [5].

(B) Miscellaneous Narrations and Discussions from Some Reported Cases (See Table 1 for a List of Some of the Reported Cases and Case Series). Cheville et al. [2] undertook a clinicopathological study of all of the cases of leiomyosarcoma of prostate that had been managed in their institution from 1929 to 1994. They had retrieved twenty-three cases from their files and out of these clinical follow-up data were available for 14 patients. Immunohistochemical studies had been undertaken including actin, desmin, S-100 protein, keratin, and vimentin. With regard to the results, Cheville et al. [2] reported the following:

(i) The ages of the patient had ranged between 41 years and 78 years and their mean age was 61 years.

(ii) All of the patients (100%) presented with urinary obstruction. Twenty-five percent of the patients presented with perineal pain. Seven percent of the patients had presented with burning on ejaculation and seven percent of the patients had presented with weight loss.

(iii) The dimensions of the prostatic tumours had ranged from 3.3 cm to 21 cm in the greatest dimension with a mean dimension of 9 cm.

(iv) The tumours quite often were associated with necrosis.

(v) With regard to the histological grading of the tumours 7 tumours were assigned grade 2; 10 tumours were assigned grade 3 and 6 tumours were assigned grade 4. The grading of the tumours was based upon Broder's grading system (scale, 1–4).

(vi) The mitotic figure counts had varied between 2 and 24 per 10 high-power fields.

TABLE 1: List of some of the reported cases of primary leiomyosarcoma of the prostate gland.

Authors and reference	Year of publication	Number of cases
Dotan et al. [30]	2006	8
Talapatra et al. [31]	2006	1
Sexton et al. [32]	2001	12
Cheville et al. [2]	1995	23
Dundore et al. [33]	1995	5
Russo et al. [34]	1993	1
Ahlering et al. [35]	1988	4
Vandoros et al. [13]	2008	1
Singh et al. [10]	2013	1
Dubey et al. [11]	2010	1
Chen et al. [15]	2000	1
Vakilha et al. [29]	2004	1
Horiguchi et al. [28]	2014	1
Sastri et al. [14]	2002	1
Germiyanoglu et al. [9]	1994	1
Barone and Joelson [36]	1950	1
Yee et al. [37]	2009	1
Lida et al. [38]	1998	2 cases, but they also reviewed 57 cases in the Japanese literature previously published
Palma et al. [39]	1983	1
Stallwoodand Davidson [40]	1977	1
Moreira et al. [41]	2004	1
Limon et al. [16]	1986	1
Cambronero et al. [42]	1999	1
Cuesta Alcaca et al. [43]	2000	1
Chen et al. [44]	2005	1
Camuzzi et al. [45]	1981	1
Kuroda et al. [46]	1994	1
Tazi et al. [47]	2001	2
Mansouri et al. [48]	2001	1 (14-year-old boy)
Mondaini et al. [49]	2005	3

(vii) With regard to immunohistochemistry, fifteen of 15 (100%) of the tumours were immunohistochemically positively stained for vimentin, 10 out of 16 (63%) were positively stained for actin, and 3 out of 15 (20%) were weakly reactive for desmin. Immunohistochemical expression was observed for keratin in 15 (27%) of the cases and, furthermore, all of the tumours (100%) were negatively stained for S-100.

(viii) With regard to treatment, the patients underwent various types of treatment which usually included a combination of radiotherapy, chemotherapy, and radical prostatectomy or cystoprostatectomy.

(ix) The follow-up of the patients had ranged from 2 months to 72 months and the mean follow-up was 19 months.

(x) With regard to the outcome of the patients, 10 patients had died 3 months to 72 months (mean, 22 months) pursuant to their diagnosis and 4 patients were alive at the time of publication of the paper which included three patients who had residual tumour and one patient who did not have any evidence of tumour at 1 month, 4 months, 30 months, and 4.5 months, respectively. Ten out of 11 patients had developed local recurrence which included 5 patients who had gross residual tumour present after their surgery. Metastases had developed up to 40 months pursuant to their surgery (with a mean time of 10.3 months after their surgeries) and most of the metastases had involved the lungs.

Cheville et al. [2] made the ensuing conclusions:

(i) Their findings indicated that leiomyosarcoma of the prostate gland has a variable histological appearance which ranges from spindle cell tumours reminiscent of smooth muscle to pleomorphic sarcoma.

(ii) Epithelioid characteristics may be present in the tumours.

(iii) The majority of the tumours on immunohistochemical staining were positively stained with vimentin and actin and immunoreactivity with antikeratin antibodies would not exclude the diagnosis of leiomyosarcoma.

(iv) Leiomyosarcoma of the prostate gland has a poor prognosis, even though the duration of survival has been variable.

(v) Radical surgery had been the treatment modality of choice in their series, but it was difficult to achieve complete excision of tumour in the majority of cases and the surgical operations did not result in cure.

Vandoros et al. [13] reported an 80-year-old man who had presented with urinary frequency, dysuria, poor urinary stream, and nocturia. His rectal examination showed a firm nodular mass of 3 cm to 4 cm diameter which had involved the left lobe of the prostate gland and which had extended to the edge of the gland. The right lobe of the prostate gland was noted to be diffusely firm. His serum prostate specific antigen (PSA) level at presentation was 2.7 ng/mL and this had not changed over 3 years. He underwent transurethral resection of prostate (TURP) and histological examination of the specimen showed a dominant population neoplastic spindle cells which were intermingled with giant neoplastic cells and multifocal necrosis which had involved almost the entire tumour (see Figures 1(a) and 1(b)). Immunohistochemical staining of the tumour was reported to have confirmed the diagnosis of leiomyosarcoma of the prostate gland in that the tumour cells on immunohistochemistry expressed

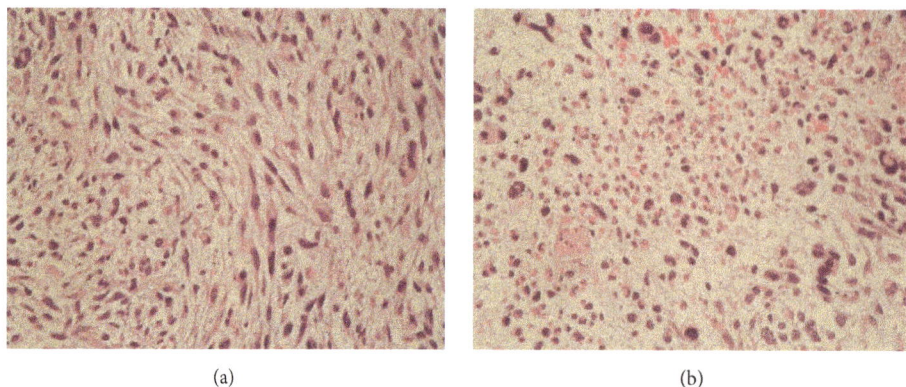

(a)

(b)

FIGURE 1: (a) Leiomyosarcoma composed of a dominant population of neoplastic spindle cells: (a) intermingled with giant neoplastic cells and multifocal and multifocal necrosis (b). Reproduced from [13].

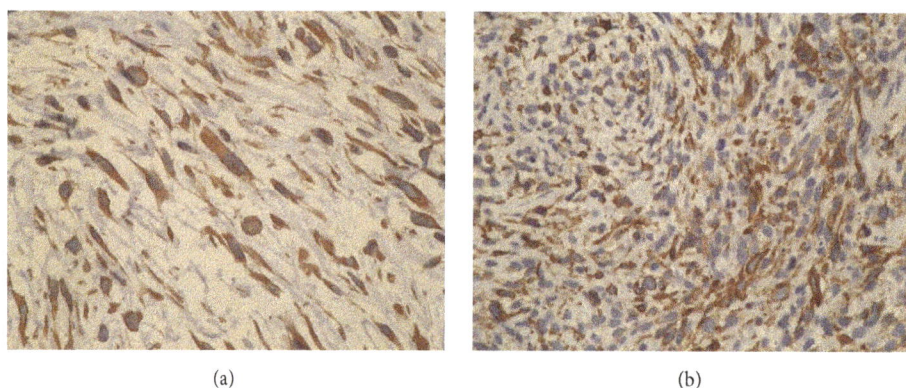

(a)

(b)

FIGURE 2: (a) and (b) Immunohistochemistry demonstrates that tumour cells express smooth muscle actin (a) and vimentin (b). Reproduced from [13].

positive staining with smooth muscle actin (see Figure 2(a)), vimentin (see Figure 2(b)), and CD44, and the tumours on immunohistochemistry exhibited negative staining for S-100, cytokeratins, and CD117 (c-KIT). He had computed tomography (CT) scan of the abdomen and thorax which had revealed two hypodense liver lesions, multiple pulmonary nodules, and mediastinal and left hilar lymphadenopathy, which were all considered to be suspicious of metastases. He also had CT scan of the brain which did not show any metastasis. He did not want any intervention; therefore, he was treated symptomatically. Three months subsequently, he presented with retention of urine and acute renal failure for which a long-term urinary catheter was inserted and for which palliative external beam radiotherapy was recommended, but he refused to undergo radiotherapy, so he was discharged home with hospice care. He died 2 months later. Vandoros et al. [13] stated that they had reviewed 54 cases of leiomyosarcoma which had been reported prior to the publication of their case and their review had revealed the following:

(i) The mean survival of leiomyosarcoma of the prostate gland was estimated at 17 months (95% CI, 20.7–43.7 months).

(ii) The 1-, 3-, and 5-year actuarial survival rates were 68%, 34%, and 26%, respectively.

(iii) The only factors predictive of long-term survival were negative surgical margins and absence of metastatic disease at the time of initial presentation.

Vandoros et al. [13] concluded that a multidisciplinary approach to the management of leiomyosarcoma of the prostate gland is necessary for the appropriate management of this dire (aggressive) disease.

Singh et al. [10] reported a 35-year-old man who had presented with lower urinary tract symptoms and progressive perineal pain. He was found on examination to have a palpable urinary bladder and a nontender, lobulated asymmetrically enlarged, prostate gland of variegated consistency. His serum PSA level was slightly raised at 5.31 ng/mL. His urine analysis and the rest of his serum biochemical analyses were normal. He had transrectal ultrasound scan of prostate which revealed an enlarged prostate gland with a heterogeneous mass on the left posterolateral aspect of the prostate gland. He had transrectal ultrasound-guided biopsies of the prostate gland and histological examination of the specimens had revealed the tumour to be composed of spindle-shaped cells, with elongated, plump nuclei, nuclear pleomorphism, and brisk bizarre multipolar mitotic activity. A diagnosis of leiomyosarcoma of the prostate gland was made. He had a CT scan of abdomen, pelvis, and thorax which had shown a heterogeneous mass arising from the left posterolateral aspect of the prostate gland with an area of infiltration in the base of the urinary bladder, anterior wall of the rectum, and left posterolateral wall of the pelvis. The CT scan also showed multiple enlarged presacral lymph nodes and small nodules on the base of the lung on the left side. He had isotope bone scan which was normal with no evidence of bone metastasis. The patient received two cycles of combination chemotherapy which consisted of ifosfamide (1600 mg/m^2) and epirubicin at 40 mg/m^2 for three days at three-weekly intervals. However, he died one month after receiving his second cycle of chemotherapy.

Dubey et al. [11] reported a 73-year-old man who presented with memory loss. His wife reported that he had been having problems with his bowel movements and at times he had had episodes of severe rectal burning. He had also been having lower urinary tract symptoms. He had colonoscopy which was on the whole normal but which showed a benign polyp at 35 cm. His serum biochemistry tests were normal except for evidence of hyponatraemia which was considered to be the reason for his confusion. His serum PSA at initial manifestation was 2.7 ng/mL and this had not changed over 3 years. He had a CT scan of brain, thorax abdomen, and pelvis which had shown a very large nodular prostate gland of about 6 cm in size and which had projected into the left posterior inferior aspect of the urinary bladder and had indented into the lumen of the rectum and this was adjudged to have almost obstructed the lumen of the rectum at the level of the dentate line. There was no evidence of lymphadenopathy or metastasis. He had a digital rectal examination which had revealed a very large, hard, nodular prostate gland projecting into the lumen of the rectum and almost causing obstruction of the lower gastrointestinal tract. He could not tolerate transrectal ultrasound-guided biopsy of the prostate under local anaesthesia because it was too painful. He underwent trocar needle biopsy of prostate under sedation in the operating theatre. During assessment at the time of the prostate biopsy upon assessment of the prostate gland it was felt that the tumour was far more advanced than was previously envisaged. The histopathological findings of the biopsy specimens showed malignant spindle cell tumour which was adjudged to favour leiomyosarcoma of the prostate gland. Immunohistochemichal staining had shown that the spindle cell proliferation was negatively stained for PSA, S100, pancytokeratin, CD117, and CD34. Immunohistochemical staining had shown that the tumour was strongly positively stained for smooth muscle actin, calponin, and CD44 and focally positive for desmin. His perineal pain deteriorated subsequently and he developed urinary retention which required insertion of suprapubic cystostomy. The case was discussed at a multidisciplinary team meeting which concluded that the lesion was leiomyosarcoma of prostate and the treatment would require surgery which should involve total pelvic exenteration or if the tumour was bulky then

neoadjuvant chemotherapy with or without radiotherapy, followed by surgery. His hyponatraemia resolved and his mentation had improved; however, with his low performance status, he was adjudged unsuitable to undergo surgical operation as well as not fit to receive chemotherapy. He developed persistent haematuria for which he was able to tolerate a single high dose 8-gray radiotherapy out of the 30 Gy/10 fractions which was planned. His bleeding had stopped in a few weeks, but he had severe pelvic pain which was not controlled by regular narcotics and he required palliative care and he received methadone but died of his disease after two weeks.

Chen et al. [15] reported a 27-year-old man who had had difficulty with voiding. He developed acute retention of urine and was catheterized and one week later was referred to a different institution. He had rectal examination which revealed a solid mass of approximately 11 cm × 8 cm × 7 cm with a smooth surface and elastic consistency. His serum PSA level was 4.8 ng/mL. But his urine analysis and his blood biochemistry were on the whole normal otherwise. He had transrectal ultrasound scan-guided biopsy of prostate and histological examination of the specimen revealed features consistent with spindle cell sarcoma. He had a chest X-ray which was normal. He also had intravenous urography which had shown an atonic urinary bladder with marked residual urine volume after voiding. He had magnetic resonance imaging (MRI) scan of pelvis which showed a large lesion in the pelvis arising from the prostate gland and which had invaded the urinary bladder. He underwent radical cystoprostatectomy and during the operation it was noted that there was involvement of the rectum by the tumour; therefore low anterior resection was undertaken with segmental resection of the rectum and construction of an ileal conduit. Microscopic examination of the tumour had revealed that the tumour had consisted of spindle cells with enlarged hyperchromatic nuclei as well as increased mitotic activity. Immunohistochemical staining of the tumour had shown positive staining for vimentin and weakly positive staining for actin as well as negative staining for desmin. The tumour was therefore adjudged to have illustrated leiomyosarcoma of the prostate gland with invasion of the urinary bladder and rectum. Furthermore, electron microscopic examination of the tumour revealed features of spindle cell sarcoma which established a definite pathological diagnosis of leiomyosarcoma of the prostate gland. He had remained alive for 48 months at the time of publication of the paper with no evidence of recurrence of his tumour. Lessons learnt from this case would indicate the following: leiomyosarcoma of the prostate gland could be locally advanced, but if radical surgery is undertaken and there is complete clearance of tumour without any evidence of residual disease even without adjuvant chemotherapy or radiotherapy some of the patients would tend to have a medium/long-term survival.

Vakilha et al. [29] reported a 72-year-old man who presented with urinary dribbling, hesitancy, and perineal pain. He had rectal examination which revealed a firm and immobile prostatic mass. He had CT scan which showed a nonhomogeneous prostatic mass which was confined to the prostate gland and not invading other organs and it also showed no evidence of lymph node involvement. He had CT scan of thorax and chest X-ray which were normal. His serum PSA level at presentation was 4.2 ng/mL. He had transrectal ultrasound-guided biopsy of prostate and histological examination of the specimen revealed features which were considered to be suspicious of malignancy and the patient underwent radical surgery (prostatectomy). Histological examination of the specimen showed a high-grade spindle cell sarcoma which was diagnosed as leiomyosarcoma of prostate with clear surgical margin. Immunohistological examination of the tumour showed that the tumour cells were weakly stained with desmin, but EMA staining was negative. This result was adjudged to be consistent with a diagnosis of leiomyosarcoma of prostate gland. He initially received one course of chemotherapy with three drug regimens which consisted of ifosfamide, dacarbazine, and farmorubicin. He did not want to continue having chemotherapy. He, therefore, received 4500 cGy of radiotherapy to the pelvis and 1500 cGy to the prostatic bed. He was initially well for 10 months; nevertheless, he represented with shortness of breath and he had CT scan of thorax which showed multiple lung metastases. He had a rectal examination which revealed a nontender firm nodule. He was started on chemotherapy with the MAID regimen (mesna, Adriamycin, ifosfamide, and dacarbazine). After he had received four courses of chemotherapy, a partial response was observed both in his radiological image findings and with regard to his symptoms. He was still receiving chemotherapy at the time of publication of the paper.

Horiguchi et al. [28] reported a 69-year-old man who had been diagnosed as having adenocarcinoma of prostate gland and who had been treated by means of brachytherapy. Six years after he had undergone brachytherapy, he developed dysuria and visible haematuria. He underwent urethroscopy which had shown a stenosis caused by a tumour at the level of the prostate. He underwent transurethral resection of the prostate and histological examination of the tumour showed features consistent with a diagnosis of leiomyosarcoma of the prostate gland. He was treated by means of three cycles of neoadjuvant chemotherapy which consisted of doxorubicin and ifosfamide. And this was followed by radical cystoprostatectomy and pelvic lymphadenectomy. It was found that the tumour originated from the prostate gland and had infiltrated the wall of the urinary bladder and serosa with lymphatic and venous invasion. The surgical margin was clear of tumour and there was no evidence of residual adenocarcinoma of the prostate gland on histological examination. Histological examination had also revealed that the proportion of necrotic tumour cells which had been induced by the chemotherapy was 50%. He was offered adjuvant chemotherapy later on, but he opted to be followed up without receiving any further chemotherapy. At three months pursuant to his surgical operation, he had a CT scan of abdomen, pelvis, and thorax which showed local recurrence and lung metastasis. He was then treated with ifosfamide; nevertheless, he did not respond to chemotherapy and he died six months after the operation. Horiguchi et al. [28] concluded that effective treatment strategy for sarcoma of the prostate gland should be developed in the near future,

although the clinical features of sarcoma of the prostate gland remain unclear due to its rare incidence. The development of dedifferentiation of totipotential cells in the prostate gland following radiotherapy to the prostate gland or hormonal therapy for adenocarcinoma has been known.

Sastri et al. [14] reported a 60-year-old man who presented with dysuria, lower abdominal pain, and pain in his left lower limb. He had undergone open prostatectomy in another hospital from where he was referred. On examination he was found to have on palpation underneath his hypogastric surgical scar a 5 cm diameter, almost globular nontender, immobile mass. He had a rectal examination which revealed a large, hard growth anterior to his rectum with obliteration of the median sulcus of the prostate gland and the upper border of the prostate gland could not be reached. He had ultrasound scan of the abdomen and pelvis and this revealed a mass which measured 104 mm × 94 mm in the region of the prostate gland. He had transrectal ultrasound scan of the prostate which showed the mass to be predominantly echogenic in the central part of the prostate with compression of the peripheral zone. A provisional diagnosis of benign prostatic hyperplasia was made. His serum PSA was 3 ng/mL. He later on had open biopsy of the prostate gland and histological examination of the specimen showed diffusely infiltrating spindle cell tumour which was arranged in interlacing fascicles. There was also evidence of moderate to marked nuclear pleomorphism and high mitotic activity. But there was no evidence of epithelial elements. Immunohistochemical staining of the tumours showed positive staining for desmin and smooth muscle actin; however, immunohistochemistry was negative for cytokeratin and PSA. A diagnosis of primary leiomyosarcoma of the prostate gland was made. He received 30 Gy of palliative external beam radiotherapy in 10 fractions over two weeks. The patient was doing well at his six-month follow-up. This case had illustrated the use of external beam radiotherapy in the palliative treatment of primary leiomyosarcoma of prostate, but considering the fact that the case was reported after 6-month follow-up one cannot predict the medium-term and long-term outcome of the patient with regard to the effect of the radiotherapy alone as treatment.

Germiyanoglu et al. [9] reported a 2.5-year-old boy who had presented with difficulty in voiding. He had had urinary frequency for 7 days prior to the onset of his voiding difficulty. He had a rectal examination which revealed a mass which measured 6 cm × 4 cm × 2 cm in the prostatic fossa. His urine examination and blood biochemistry results were normal except for his serum urea nitrogen which was raised at 40 mg/dL. He had an X-ray of the chest which was normal. He also had a cystogram which had shown that the urinary bladder had been displaced superiorly. He had computed tomography (CT) scan which had shown a 51 mm diameter hypodense homogeneous mass within the location of the prostate gland. He had transrectal ultrasound-guided biopsy of the prostate gland and histological examination of the specimen had shown leiomyosarcoma of the prostate gland. The family of the patient did not accept the offer of radical surgical operation and in view of this a suprapubic cystostomy was carried out and chemotherapy and radiotherapy were planned. After the initial days of receiving chemotherapy, the patient was not brought back to complete the planned treatment. He died 4 months later. Germiyanoglu et al. [9] stated the following: Mottola et al. [50] had postulated that chronic inflammatory processes are responsible for causing leiomyosarcoma of the prostate gland in view of the fact that it had been known that hyperplasia had been observed in the smooth muscles of the prostate gland in chronic prostatitis; nevertheless, the reason behind the aetiology of leiomyosarcoma of the prostate has not been clarified; Palma et al. [39] had stated that leiomyosarcoma reaches a peak in childhood; however, leiomyosarcoma of the prostate gland is most often encountered in the 6th decade; the commonest manifestations tend to be symptoms associated with urinary obstruction and these include dysuria, nocturia, urinary frequency, or retention of urine; Barone and Joelson [36] had stated that leiomyosarcoma of the prostate gland should be differentiated from benign prostatic hyperplasia, carcinoma of the prostate gland, prostatic abscess, mullerian duct cysts, and retrovesical tumours [36].

Yee et al. [37] reported a 75-year-old man who presented with haematuria. He had rectal examination which had revealed a mass in the prostate. He had a history of having been diagnosed 8 years earlier with a stage T2b adenocarcinoma of the prostate gland which was treated by means of external beam radiotherapy and brachytherapy. Both his treatments had failed in that his serum prostate specific antigen (PSA) had been increasing. Four years subsequently he had undergone cryosurgical ablation for a poorly differentiated Gleason 4 + 5 = 9, adenocarcinoma of the prostate gland which was clinically staged as T2b. He had isotope bone scan and CT scan of abdomen and pelvis which showed absence of metastasis. His serum PSA prior to his cryosurgical ablation treatment was 11.4 μg/L and his prostate volume was 26 cc and his rectal examination had revealed a small irregular prostate with induration over both lobes of the prostate. Pursuant to his cryotherapy his serum PSA had decreased to 0.2. After the cryotherapy his serum PSA had increased to 1.5 after one year and 2.7 after two years and he was found to have a questionable induration at the base of the prostate. He had a CT scan which had shown a 2.3 cm mass anterior to the rectum behind the seminal vesicles. He was commenced on hormonal therapy and he received bicalutamide 50 mg orally daily and 30 mg leuprolide depot injections every 4 months and after 8 months his serum PSA had dropped to 0.1. Rectal examination then had revealed a small benign feeling prostate gland. The serum PSA had remained at 0.1 whilst he remained on hormonal therapy, but 2 years later he developed visible haematuria at which time his serum PSA had remained at 0.1 and his rectal examination had shown his prostate gland to be indurated and of about 30 grams. He underwent cystoscopy which had revealed an enlarged necrotic and bleeding median lobe of his prostate gland. He had CT scan which had shown an increase in the size of the prostatic neoplasm which had invaded the rectum, but it had not invaded the pelvic side wall and there was no lymph adenopathy. He had prostate biopsies and histological examination of the specimens showed infiltrative, interlacing fascicles of spindle cells which had

eosinophilic cytoplasm and had exhibited high cellularity, marked nuclear atypia, and many atypical mitotic figures which were suggestive of sarcoma of the prostate gland. Immunohistochemical staining of the specimen revealed negative staining for PAS, PCA3, CK A1/A3, CK 903, PSA, and hormone receptor ER/PR which had ruled out any residual adenocarcinoma of the prostate gland. Immunohistochemichal stains for leiomyosarcoma were positive in that desmin and smooth muscle actin were weakly positive, and vimentin was strongly positive. He underwent radical cystoprostatectomy and bilateral pelvic lymph adenectomy, resection of sigmoid colon, and rectum, colostomy, and ileal conduit construction. Histopathological examination of the specimen had revealed features consistent with high-grade leiomyosarcoma of the prostate gland. Pathological examination had shown that the tumour had replaced the prostate gland completely and had extended into the periprostatic fat and the urinary bladder. There was evidence of perineural invasion but no evidence of angiolymphatic involvement. The tumour had also extended and involved the full thickness of the rectum. The tumour additionally had involved the posterior margin of the prostate gland and the deep margin of the rectum; therefore additional deep margins were excised which were free of the designated ink margin. The apex of the prostate was also positive for tumour. Pathological examination of the resected rectum had shown infiltration by high-grade leiomyosarcoma which had involved the full thickness of the bowel wall and numerous ulcerations of the bowel mucosa. There was no tumour in the sigmoid colon and the pelvic lymph nodes. Immunohistochemical staining was positive for desmin and smooth muscle actin which supported a diagnosis of leiomyosarcoma. With regard to the differential diagnosis of mesenchymal neoplasms and sarcomatoid carcinoma, these were ruled out by means of immunohistochemical staining which were negative for myogenin, S100, CD34, high molecular weight cytokeratin, and pancytokeratin. His tumour continued to progress and three months later there was evidence of a nodule in the middle lobe of the right lung and a lesion in the area of the prostatic bed as well as rectal stump which was adjudged to represent tumour recurrence and in view of this he received chemotherapy. Several months later he had CT scan which had shown that the tumour near the prostatic bed had increased in size and extended to involve the perineum and abdominal wall and this had resulted in a cutaneous fistula. It had also shown many new pulmonary metastases. Twenty-five months after the surgical operation and chemotherapy he had remained alive with adjudged poor prognosis. Yee et al. [37] stated the following:

(i) Leiomyosarcoma of the prostate gland is associated with poor prognosis in view of the aggressive biological behaviour of the tumour, lack of early symptoms, and late presentation; the rate of survival varies between 0% and 60% and the survival rates vary from months to years.

(ii) Miedler and MacLennan [51] had stated that 50% to 75% of patients die as a sequel of leiomyosarcoma of the prostate gland after 2.5 years.

(iii) Mondaini et al. [49] had recommended surgical treatment in the form of cystoprostatectomy followed by chemotherapy or radiotherapy for leiomyosarcoma of the prostate gland.

(iv) Surgical operation may give symptomatic relief and may be an option of palliation for patients rather than cure in view of the fact that development of local recurrence and metastasis tends to be common.

(v) There is no treatment option that has been regarded as optimum; nevertheless, Mansouri et al. [48] had iterated that radical surgery with complete resection of tumour is the therapeutic option which offers the chance of prolonged survival when the tumour has low mitotic activity.

(vi) Dotan et al. [30] had shown that complete surgical resection of tumour can lead to decreased local recurrence and decreased metastasis which prolongs survival. Nevertheless, leiomyosarcomas of the prostate are often diagnosed late in the process of the disease; in view of this the size of the tumour at the time of resection tends to be extensive.

(vii) Sexton et al. [32] did not find any association between survival and negative surgical margins, the tumour size, or stage of the tumour.

(viii) With regard to adjuvant treatment, Sexton et al. [32] and Janet et al. [52] had shown that survival advantage may exist for a combined multimodality therapeutic strategies to improve the outcome of leiomyosarcoma of the prostate gland. However, studies had revealed that uncommon carcinomas which develop pursuant to radiotherapy tend to be aggressive tumours which manifest with metastatic deposits, for which the prognosis tends to be poor irrespective of treatment.

(ix) In view of the fact that sarcomas tend to be associated with a high recurrence rate, it had been recommended that patients with leiomyosarcoma of the prostate gland should be monitored closely with imaging of the chest, abdomen, and pelvis. The reported sites of metastasis in leiomyosarcoma of the prostate gland in order of frequency include the lung, bone, lymph nodes, and brain [53].

(x) The exact aetiology of leiomyosarcoma of the prostate gland has not been ascertained and there has been an ongoing debate regarding whether radiotherapy to the prostate gland can induce a secondary cancer.

(xi) Moreira et al. [41] had postulated a causal effect of leiomyosarcoma of prostate pursuant to brachytherapy to the prostate gland. Moreira et al. [41] had discussed the complications of brachytherapy, in which 3 patients had developed carcinoma of the prostate gland after they had received brachytherapy. One of the patients had subsequently developed recurrence of adenocarcinoma of the prostate gland, another patient had developed subsequently neuroendocrine

tumour of the rectum, and the third patient had subsequently developed leiomyosarcoma of the prostate gland.

(xii) McKenzie et al. [54] had reported three cases of postradiotherapy sarcoma which had developed in the pelvis, 8 years, 15 years, and 16 years, ensuing localized adenocarcinoma of the prostate gland.

(xiii) Mazzucchelli et al. [53] had undertaken a study on histological variants of carcinoma of the prostate gland and reported that half of the sarcomatous components (SC) and carcinosarcomas of the prostate gland had developed following hormonal treatment or radiotherapy treatment ensuing an initial diagnosis of acinar adenocarcinoma of the prostate gland. Nevertheless, Mazzucchelli et al. [53] stated that sarcomatous component of carcinosarcoma status of the prostate gland after radiotherapy is not necessarily the only cause of malignancy and that de novo carcinosarcoma of the prostate gland can also develop.

(xiv) Prevost et al. [55] had also reported a case of postradiotherapy sarcoma which did develop 8 years after the patient had received extended beam radiotherapy for adenocarcinoma of the prostate gland.

Talapatra et al. [31] reported a 67-year-old man who had presented with a history of recurrent episodes of haematuria and poor urinary stream. He had previously been diagnosed as having had a benign prostatic hypertrophy for which he had undergone transurethral resection of prostate (TURP) tumour elsewhere two years earlier. The histology slides had not been available for review. He had rectal examination which revealed an enlarged, hard prostate gland with obliteration of the median sulcus and the right lobe of the prostate gland was noted to be enlarged and abutting the rectum but not fixed to it. The examination also revealed a mass which had infiltrated the periprostatic tissue and extended to the pelvic side wall. His serum PSA level at presentation was normal. He had ultrasound scan of abdomen and pelvis which revealed a hypoechoic heterogeneous mass within the prostate gland and infiltrating the base of the urinary bladder and invading the lumen of the urinary bladder. The urinary bladder was noted to have a thick wall and it also contained blood clots. He had magnetic resonance imaging (MRI) scan of the pelvis which had revealed a 7.5 cm × 4.3 cm tumour mass in the right lobe of the prostate and which had distorted the capsule and had extended into the periprostatic fat, neurovascular bundle, and the base of the urinary bladder. He underwent cystoscopy which revealed a large fleshy growth in his prostatic urethra and within the lumen of the urinary bladder in association with blood clot in the urinary bladder. The right lobe of the prostate was enlarged especially at the apex. He had biopsy of the tumour mass and histological examination of the specimen had revealed spindle cell sarcoma which had destroyed the prostate gland with only the occasional benign prostatic gland entrapped within the tumour. With regard to the details of the microscopic features of the tumour, the tumour was laid out in intergrating fascicles. The spindle-shaped cells had elongated blunt ended cigar-shaped hyperchromatic nuclei and eosinophilic fibrillary cytoplasm which had the characteristics of leiomyosarcoma. Other characteristics of the tumour which confirmed the diagnosis include nuclear pleomorphism, raised mitotic activity, and areas of necrosis. He had metastatic work-up which showed no evidence of metastatic disease. He was adjudged to be unsuitable for curative surgery in view of the extent of the disease and the associated expected morbidity. He was treated by means of adjuvant chemotherapy which included ifosfamide and this was followed by external beam radiotherapy. Upon completion of the chemotherapy and radiotherapy treatments the patient's symptoms had resolved. At his six-month follow-up, he was asymptomatic in that he did not have any haematuria and his lower urinary tract symptoms had resolved. He had a CT scan which showed significant reduction in the size of the prostatic mass and minimal periprostatic stranding as well as normal looking urinary bladder. His serum PSA was normal. Talapatra et al. [31] stated the following: Limon et al. [16] had studied the cytogenetic analysis of primary leiomyosarcoma of the prostate and reported that their study had revealed clonal chromosomal rearrangement involving Chromosomes 2, 3, 9, 11, and 19; Cambronero et al. [42] reported a case of leiomyosarcoma of prostate which presented as an exophytic tumour mass in the rectum as a rare presentation of leiomyosarcoma of the prostate gland; Cuesta Alcaca et al. [43] reported leiomyosarcoma of the prostate gland which was detected in a patient who underwent TURP for lower urinary tract symptoms diagnosed as benign prostatic hypertrophy, but histological examination of the specimen had revealed leiomyosarcoma of the prostate gland; Chen et al. [44] had stated that rectal examination in leiomyosarcoma of the prostate gland generally tends to reveal a prostatic mass; however, biopsy of the prostatic mass is required for histological examination to confirm the diagnosis; Ahlering et al. [35] reported 11 patients who had leiomyosarcoma; of these 11 patients, 7 had leiomyosarcoma of the urinary bladder, and 4 patients had leiomyosarcoma of the prostate gland. They reported that the patients who did not have bulky tumours underwent surgical resection and they were observed as to if their operative surgical margins and lymph nodes were negative for tumour. The patients who were found to have surgical margins or lymph node positive for tumour received adjuvant external beam radiotherapy and chemotherapy. With regard to the patients who had bulky tumours, they received preoperative chemotherapy with or without radiotherapy which was followed by exenteration. With regard to the outcome, Ahlering et al. [35] reported that, out of the 11 patients, 9 patients did not have any evidence of disease after a mean follow-up of 61 months and the follow-up had ranged between 35 months and 96 months; Camuzzi et al. [45] had reported a patient with leiomyosarcoma of the prostate gland who was successfully treated by means of transperineal radon seed implantation and external beam radiotherapy; Kuroda et al. [46] had reported a case of leiomyosarcoma of the prostate gland which was accompanied by multiple hepatocellular carcinomas who had received combination chemotherapy that consisted of cyclophosphamide, vincristine, Adriamycin, and

DTIC (CYDAVIC). He died one year and two months after his initial diagnosis as a result of liver failure. During postmortem examination it was revealed that the histology of the liver tumours was hepatocellular carcinoma and even though the leiomyosarcoma of the prostate gland had invaded the wall of the urinary bladder and the rectum, there was no obvious distant metastasis from the leiomyosarcoma of the prostate gland; Tazi et al. [47] stated the following: a number of treatment modalities had been adopted including radical surgery, radiotherapy, and chemotherapy for the treatment of primary leiomyosarcoma of the prostate gland, but in their opinion a successful outcome had not been achieved in any instance. Leiomyosarcoma of the prostate gland has a poor prognosis, even though the survival time is variable. In view of the aforementioned reasons, it is very important that leiomyosarcoma of the prostate gland is correctly identified and that occurrence of each case of the disease, type of treatment given, and response to treatment should be reported in order to enable the understanding of the natural history of the disease.

Russo et al. [34] reported a 57-year-old man who had a high-grade leiomyosarcoma of the prostate. MRI scan was used to define the extent of the tumour. He was treated by means of chemotherapy and he had a further MRI scan which had shown that the size of the tumour had reduced by 60% and based upon the MRI scan findings the tumour was adjudged to be clinically resectable. He underwent radical cystoprostatectomy but subsequently died of metastatic disease.

Dundore et al. [33] reviewed the notes and pathological findings of 21 cases of carcinosarcoma of the prostate in the Mayo Clinic and reported the results as follows: the mean age of the patients was 68 years and the ages had ranged between 50 years and 89 years; ten of the patients (48%) were previously diagnosed as having acinar adenocarcinoma of the prostate gland two to seventy-three months prior to the diagnosis of carcinosarcoma and the mean time of the diagnosis of acinar adenocarcinoma prior to the diagnosis of carcinosarcoma was 33 months. Eight of the patients, meanwhile, had received androgen deprivation treatment and/or radiotherapy; the Gleason scores of the adenocarcinomas had ranged from Gleason 7 to Gleason 10 and the mean Gleason score was 9 and, furthermore, the median Gleason score was also 9; the various types of sarcomas which were diagnosed were as follows: 13 cases of osteosarcoma, 5 cases of leiomyosarcoma, 1 case of fibrosarcoma, 1 case of malignant fibrous histiocytoma, and 1 case of rhabdomyosarcoma. The grades of the sarcoma components of the tumours had ranged from 2 to 4 and the mean grade was 4. The median grade of the sarcomatous components of the tumour was 4; with regard to the dominant component of the tumours, adenocarcinoma was the dominant histological pattern in 7 cases and sarcoma was the dominant component in 14 cases; with regard to the immunohistochemistry of the tumours, positive immunohistochemical staining cytoplasmic reactivity was revealed for prostate specific antigen or keratin in 16 of 16 cases in the adenocarcinoma component. The sarcoma component exhibited positive staining: in 16 out of 16 cases for vimentin, in 8 out of 16 cases of which 2 were focally positive, in 2 out of 16 cases for S-100 protein, and in 1 out of 16 for desmin; at the time of the initial diagnosis of carcinosarcoma, 11 of the patients were found to have had metastases and of these patients 4 had had metastatic adenocarcinoma prior to the diagnosis of adenocarcinoma; the patients had undergone various types of treatment and they had found that nonsurgical treatment was ineffective; the sites of the metastatic lesions included the lung in 10 cases, bone in 7 cases, brain in 4 cases, liver in 1 case, and the peritoneum in 1 case; with regard to the follow-up of patients, this had ranged between 1 month and 107 months pursuant to the diagnosis of carcinosarcoma and the mean follow-up was 34 months, but the median follow-up was 10 months; with regard to outcome, the mean time to progression of tumour was 23 months, but this had ranged between 1 month and 96 months and the median time to progression was 18 months. Eighteen of the patients had died of carcinosarcoma from 2 months to 107 months following their diagnosis, but the mean and median times of their deaths pursuant to their diagnosis were 34 months and 9.5 months, respectively. The 5-year survival was 41% and the 7-year survival was 14%. The progression and survival of the patients were observed not to be affected by the histological pattern of the carcinosarcomas. Dundore et al. [33] concluded that carcinosarcoma of the prostate gland is an aggressive malignancy, irrespective of the histological type of the carcinosarcoma of the prostate gland.

Globally, a large number of patients undergo treatment for adenocarcinoma of the prostate gland with curative intent in the form of radiotherapy (external beam radiotherapy or brachytherapy) plus or minus adjuvant hormonal therapy and out of these patients a number of patients subsequently develop relapse or progress of their tumours. What is not known globally is the percentage of patients who were initially diagnosed as having adenocarcinoma of prostate who subsequently develop either de novo carcinosarcoma including leiomyosarcoma of the prostate or dedifferentiated carcinoma of the prostate gland including leiomyosarcoma of the prostate. Perhaps the reason behind the lack of information regarding the percentage of patients globally who develop carcinosarcoma alone or in association with adenocarcinoma may be due to the fact that globally routine rebiopsies are not generally undertaken in the majority of patients who are treated globally for adenocarcinoma of prostate gland in the form of radiotherapy plus or minus hormonal therapy. It would be argued perhaps if all patients who develop relapse after radiotherapy/hormonal treatment for adenocarcinoma of the prostate gland undergo rebiopsies of the prostate a number of cases of dedifferentiated carcinomas would be found alone or in association with adenocarcinoma. In view of the finding that carcinosarcomas have been found to be aggressive tumours that would require aggressive treatment with curative intent in the form multimodal treatment including radical surgery, chemotherapy, and radiotherapy in cases of patients who are fit to undergo aggressive treatment, it would be argued that a global multicentre study should be undertaken in which patients whose adenocarcinomas have relapsed given the chance to undergo rebiopsies of their prostates to see if their carcinomas remain the same or they have subsequently developed different types of prostate

cancers. If a pilot study shows a high percentage of patients developing other types of prostate cancers, then perhaps new guidelines could be formulated globally for the follow-up of patients with adenocarcinoma of the prostate. Finally, it is conjectural, but it may be that the percentage of other types of carcinomas of the prostate that are reported globally is higher than is believed and this would hopefully be known in the future if lots of patients undergo rebiopsies of their prostatic lesions for histological examination.

Lida et al. [38] in 1998 reported two patients with PLSOPs. The first patient was a 45-year-old man who presented with lower urinary tract symptoms. He had ultrasound scan and CT scan which revealed a tumour in his prostate gland. He had ultrasound-guided biopsy of the prostatic lesion and histological examination of the specimen revealed leiomyosarcoma of the prostate gland. He underwent radical cystoprostatectomy. He was alive at the time of publication of the paper 12 months after his operation. The second patient was a 63-year-old man who was admitted for the treatment of lung and colon cancers. He had CT scan which had shown multiple tumours in the lung, in the liver, and bilaterally in the kidney as well as prostate gland. Histological examination of biopsies from the prostate gland had confirmed the presence of leiomyosarcoma of the prostate. Lida et al. [38] also reviewed 57 cases of primary leiomyosarcoma of the prostate gland which had been reported in the Japanese literature.

Palma et al. [39] reported a case of leiomyosarcoma of the prostate gland in association with an incidental adenocarcinoma of the prostate gland in 1983 and in 1997 Stallwood and Davidson [40] reported leiomyosarcoma of the rectum and prostate gland.

Mansouri et al. [48] reported a 14-year-old boy who presented with perineal pain on voiding and during defecation as well as dysuria and haematuria. His rectal examination revealed an indurated left lobe of the prostate gland. He had intravenous urography and CT scan of abdomen and pelvis which showed the urinary bladder displaced anteriorly compressed by a large pelvic mass, 15 cm × 11 cm, multiseptated pelvic mass with thickened irregular walls which had displaced the urinary bladder and rectum. He had surgical biopsy of the mass elsewhere and histological examination of the specimen had shown a smooth muscle neoplasm which did not have any features that would exclude leiomyosarcoma. He underwent radical cystoprostatectomy and pelvic lymph node dissection. The radical prostatectomy specimen contained a tumour on the left side which was not circumscribed and the tumour had extended from the apex to the base. Histological examination of the tumour had shown an infiltrative tumour that had invaded and displaced the normal prostate stroma of glands and these tumours had abnormal mitotic figures and giant cells. Necrosis was observed and a high mitotic count of 14 per 10 high-power fields was also observed. Immunohistochemical staining of the tumour revealed strong cytoplasmic positive staining for actin, desmin, and vimentin, but there was negative staining for keratin and S-100 protein. The surgical margin at the resection site was involved by tumour as well as extraprostatic extension. Three left iliac nodes contained metastatic tumour. He was treated by means of adjuvant radiotherapy and received 46 Gy of therapy, but he died as a result of metastases in the lung, liver, and bone as well as gross local recurrence 4 months following his initial diagnosis.

All the aforementioned information could be confusing to a clinician who is faced with a patient who is diagnosed with PLSOP. One of the questions that would be on the mind of the clinician is what is the best treatment option for the disease (PLSOP) Sexton et al. [32] had recommended that multimodality treatment include surgery, radiotherapy, and chemotherapy. Some authors [2, 11, 26, 32] had iterated that the overall outcome for PLSOPs is not good, and 50% to 75% of patients tend to die of their leiomyosarcoma between 3 months and 72 months. Sexton et al. [32] stated that the outcome of PLSOPs tends to improve in patients who do not have evidence of distant metastasis at initial manifestation and in those patients who have localized disease in whom complete resection of the tumour can be undertaken with histological evidence of negative surgical margins.

4. Conclusions

Leiomyosarcoma of the prostate gland is a rare tumour which can afflict children and adults. On the whole the prognosis is poor. Surgery with or without chemotherapy/radiotherapy would appear to be the mainstay of treatment for leiomyosarcoma of the prostate for operable cases, but generally there is no consensus opinion on the best therapeutic approach. Most cases of PLSOP at the time of initial presentation tend to be diagnosed in an advanced stage of the disease. There is the need for all cases of PLSOP diagnosed to be entered into a global multicentre trial in order to find therapeutic modalities that would improve the prognosis of this aggressive disease. Perhaps if all patients who have developed progressive disease or relapse of local disease in cases of adenocarcinoma prostate undergo repeat prostate biopsies early, some cases of dedifferentiated leiomyosarcomas of the prostate may be diagnosed early.

Conflict of Interests

The author declares that there is no conflict of interests regarding the publication of this paper.

Acknowledgment

Sarcoma is acknowledged for granting copyright permission for contents of the articles to be reproduced under the Creative Commons Attribution License: Copyright © 2008 Gerasimos P. Vandoros et al.

References

[1] S. C. Quay and K. H. Proppe, "Carcinosarcoma of the prostate: case report and review of the literature," *Journal of Urology*, vol. 125, no. 3, pp. 436–438, 1981.

[2] J. C. Cheville, P. A. Dundore, A. G. Nascimento et al., "Leiomyosarcoma of the prostate. Report of 23 cases," *Cancer*, vol. 76, no. 8, pp. 1422–1427, 1995.

[3] B. H. Smith and L. P. Dehner, "Sarcoma of the prostate gland," *American Journal of Clinical Pathology*, vol. 58, no. 1, pp. 43–50, 1972.

[4] L. W. Riba and M. C. Wheelock, "Leiomyosarcoma of the prostate," *The Journal of Urology*, vol. 63, no. 1, pp. 162–164, 1950.

[5] K. Arora, "Prostate Leiomyosarcoma Pathology Outlines," Pathology Outlines, http://www.Pathologyoutlines.com/topic/prostatelms.html.

[6] Prostate sarcoma Oral B Official Website, http://www.urology-textbook.com/.

[7] Li-Fraumeni Syndrome—Genetics Home Reference, http://ghr.nlm.nih.gov/condition/li-fraumeni-syndrome .

[8] Prostate Sarcoma Oral B, http://www.urology-textbook.com/.

[9] C. Germiyanoglu, H. Özkardes, Ü. Kurt, A. Öztokatli, and D. Erol, "Leiomyosarcoma of the prostate. A case report," *International Urology and Nephrology*, vol. 26, no. 2, pp. 189–191, 1994.

[10] J. P. Singh, D. Chakraborty, M. K. Bera, and D. Pal, "Leiomyosarcoma of prostate: a rare aggressive tumor," *Journal of Cancer Research and Therapeutics*, vol. 9, no. 4, pp. 743–745, 2013.

[11] A. Dubey, G. Sivananthan, T. Bradel, and R. Koul, "Prostatic leiomyosarcoma—a rare case report with review of literature," *The Internet Journal of Oncology*, vol. 8, no. 1, 2010, http://ispub.com/IJO/8/1/9519.

[12] K. Arora, "Prostate Benign lesions/conditions Leiomyoma," Pathology Outlines, 2014, http://www.pathologyoutlines.com/topicprostatelms.html.

[13] G. P. Vandoros, T. Manglidis, M. V. Karamouzis et al., "Leiomyosarcoma of the prostate: case report and review of 54 previously published cases," *Sarcoma*, vol. 2008, Article ID 458709, 5 pages, 2008.

[14] G. J. Sastri, S. K. Mohanty, A. Munshi, S. Ghosal, S. C. Sharma, and F. D. Patel, "Leiomyosarcoma of the prostate—a case report," *Indian Journal of Urology*, vol. 18, no. 2, pp. 171–172, 2002.

[15] K. C. Chen, C. M. Lin, T. S. Hsieh et al., "Leiomyosarcoma of the prostate," *The Journal of Urology*, vol. 11, pp. 39–42, 2000.

[16] J. Limon, P. Dal Cin, and A. A. Sandberg, "Cytogenetic findings in a primary leiomyosarcoma of the prostate," *Cancer Genetics and Cytogenetics*, vol. 22, no. 2, pp. 159–167, 1986.

[17] A. Amin, "Prostate Benign lesions/conditions. Nodularhyperplasia," PathologyOutlines.com, January 2012, http://www.pathologyoutlines.com/topicprostatelms.html.

[18] S. Tawfic, G. A. Niehans, and J. C. Manivel, "The pattern of CD10 expression in selected pathologic entities of the prostate gland," *Human Pathology*, vol. 34, no. 5, pp. 450–456, 2003.

[19] M. Roychowdhury, "Prostate Benign lesions/conditions Postoperative spindle cell nodules," Pathology Outlines, 2012, http://www.pathologyoutlines.com/topic/prostatepostop.html.

[20] H. Koruma, T. Ao, K. Suyama et al., "A case of gastrointestinal stromal tumor of rectum, difficult to differentiate from leiomyosarcoma of rectum," *Nihon Hinyokika Gakkai Zasshi*, vol. 92, no. 6, pp. 624–627, 2001.

[21] C. Singh, "Colon tumor Mesenchymal tumors Gastrointestinal stromal tumors (GIST) of colon Pathology," Pathology Outlines, 2014, http://pathologyoutlines.com/topic/colontumorgist.html.

[22] L. Insanato, D. Di Vizio, G. Ciancia, G. Pettinato, L. Tormillio, and L. Terracciano, "Malignant gastrointestinal leiomyosarcoma and gastrointestinal stromal tumor with prominent osteoclast-like giant cells," *Archives of Pathology & Laboratory Medicine*, vol. 128, no. 4, pp. 444–443, 2004.

[23] H. Yamazaki, T. Ohyama, T. Tsuboi et al., "Prostatic stromal sarcoma with neuroectodermal differentiation," *Diagnostic Pathology*, vol. 7, article 173, 2012.

[24] K. Arora, "Prostate Other carcinomas. Carcinosara," PathologyOutlines.com, March 2012, http://www.pathologyoutlines.com/topic/prostatecarcinosarcoma.html.

[25] M. R. Wick, R. H. Young, R. Malvesta, D. S. Beebe, J. J. Hansen, and L. P. Dehner, "Prostatic carcinosarcomas. Clinical, histologic, and immunohistochemical data on two cases, with a review of the literature," *American Journal of Clinical Pathology*, vol. 92, no. 2, pp. 131–139, 1989.

[26] D. E. Hansel, M. Herawi, E. Montgomery, and J. I. Epstein, "Spindle cell lesions of the adult prostate," *Modern Pathology*, vol. 20, no. 1, pp. 148–158, 2007.

[27] D. Hossain, I. Meiers, J. Qian, G. T. MacLennan, and D. G. Bostwick, "Prostatic leiomyoma with atypia: follow-up study of 10 cases," *Annals of Diagnostic Pathology*, vol. 12, no. 5, pp. 328–332, 2008.

[28] H. Horiguchi, K. Tukada, R. Takimoto et al., "Radiation-induced leiomyosarcoma of the prostate after brachytherapy for prostatic adenocarcinoma," *Case Reports in Oncology*, vol. 7, no. 2, pp. 565–570, 2014.

[29] M. Vakilha, F. N. Dadgar, and T. Tuirgani, "Leiomyosarcoma of prostate: report of a case," *Iranian Journal of Radiation Research*, vol. 1, no. 4, pp. 229–231, 2004.

[30] Z. A. Dotan, R. Tal, D. Golijanin et al., "Adult genitourinary sarcoma: the 25-year Memorial Sloan-Kettering experience," *Journal of Urology*, vol. 176, no. 5, pp. 2033–2038, 2006.

[31] K. Talapatra, B. Nemade, R. Bhutani et al., "Recurrent episodes of hematuria: a rare presentation of leiomyosarcoma of prostate," *Journal of Cancer Research and Therapeutics*, vol. 2, no. 4, pp. 212–214, 2006.

[32] W. J. Sexton, R. E. Lance, A. O. Reyes, P. W. T. Pisters, S.-M. Tu, and L. L. Pisters, "Adult prostate sarcoma: the M. D. Anderson cancer center experience," *The Journal of Urology*, vol. 166, no. 2, pp. 521–525, 2001.

[33] P. A. Dundore, J. C. Cheville, A. G. Nascimento, G. M. Farrow, and D. G. Bostwick, "Carcinosarcoma of the prostate. Report of 21 cases," *Cancer*, vol. 76, no. 6, pp. 1035–1042, 1995.

[34] P. Russo, B. Demas, and V. Reuter, "Adult prostatic sarcoma," *Abdominal Imaging*, vol. 18, no. 4, pp. 399–401, 1993.

[35] T. E. Ahlering, P. Weintraub, and D. G. Skinner, "Management of adult sarcomas of the bladder and prostate," *The Journal of Urology*, vol. 140, no. 6, pp. 1397–1399, 1988.

[36] J. M. Barone and J. J. Joelson, "Leiomyosarcoma of the prostate: report of a case," *The Journal of Urology*, vol. 63, pp. 533–538, 1950.

[37] S. Yee, M. J. Goldfischer, R. J. Rosenbluth, D. A. McCain, I. Jackson, and I. S. Sawczuk, "Post radiotherapy leiomyosarcoma of the prostate: can radiation therapy induce a secondary cancer? A case report," *UroToday International Journal*, vol. 2, no. 3, 2009.

[38] K. Lida, M. Tanaka, S. Matsumoto et al., "Leiomyosarcoma of the prostate: report of two cases," *Hinyokika Kiyo*, vol. 44, no. 10, pp. 739–742, 1998.

[39] P. C. R. Palma, N. R. Netto Jr., O. Ikari, C. A. D'Ancona, and A. Billis, "Leiomyosarcoma in association with incidental adenocarcinoma of the prostate," *The Journal of Urology*, vol. 129, no. 1, pp. 156–157, 1983.

[40] G. Stallwood and J. W. Davidson, "Leiomyosarcoma of the rectum and prostate," *Canadian Journal of Surgery*, vol. 20, no. 5, pp. 446–449, 1977.

[41] S. G. Moreira Jr., J. D. Seigne, R. C. Ordorica, J. Marcet, J. M. Pow-Sang, and J. L. Lockhart, "Devastating complications after brachytherapy in the treatment of prostate adenocarcinoma," *BJU International*, vol. 93, no. 1, pp. 31–35, 2004.

[42] S. J. Cambronero, M. M. Martín, A. F. Villacampa, A. C. Hörndler, O. R. Espuela, and G. O. Leiva, "Prostate leiomyosarcoma with perineal exophytic mass," *Actas Urologicas Espanolas*, vol. 23, no. 9, pp. 797–800, 1999.

[43] J. A. Cuesta Alcaca, P. I. Pascual, J. L. Arrondo et al., "Stromal tumor of the rectum and leiomyosarcoma of the prostate as a cause of urinary syndrome attributable to BPH," *Archivos Españoles de Urología*, vol. 53, no. 9, pp. 763–768, 2000.

[44] H.-J. Chen, M. Xu, L. Zhang, Y.-K. Zhang, and G.-M. Wang, "Prostate sarcoma: a report of 14 cases," *Zhonghua Nan Ke Xue*, vol. 11, no. 9, pp. 683–685, 2005.

[45] F. A. Camuzzi, N. L. Block, K. Charyulu, S. Thomsen, and V. A. Politano, "Leiomyosarcoma of prostate gland," *Urology*, vol. 18, no. 3, pp. 295–297, 1981.

[46] H. Kuroda, Y. Yasunaga, H. Takatera, H. Fujioka, and M. Tsujimoto, "Leiomyosarcoma of the prostate accompanied by multiple hepatocellular carcinoma: report of a case," *Acta Urologica Japonica*, vol. 40, no. 2, pp. 147–149, 1994.

[47] K. Tazi, S. M. Moudouni, J. Elfassi et al., "Leiomyosarcoma of prostate: a study of two cases," *Annales d'Urologie. EMC-Urologie*, vol. 35, no. 1, pp. 56–59, 2001.

[48] H. Mansouri, L. Kanouni, T. Kebdani, K. Hassouni, H. Sifat, and B. El Gueddari, "Primary prostatic leiomyosarcoma," *Journal of Urology*, vol. 165, no. 5, p. 1676, 2001.

[49] N. Mondaini, D. Palli, C. Saieva et al., "Clinical characteristics and overall survival in genitourinary sarcomas treated with curative intent: a multicenter study," *European Urology*, vol. 47, no. 4, pp. 468–473, 2005.

[50] A. Mottola, C. Selli, M. Carini, A. Natali, and G. Gambacorta, "Leiomyosarcoma of the prostate," *European Urology*, vol. 11, no. 2, pp. 131–133, 1985.

[51] J. D. Miedler and G. T. MacLennan, "Leiomyosarcoma of the prostate," *Journal of Urology*, vol. 178, no. 2, p. 668, 2007.

[52] N. L. Janet, A.-W. May, and R. S. Akins, "Sarcoma of the prostate: a single institutional review," *American Journal of Clinical Oncology*, vol. 32, no. 1, pp. 27–29, 2009.

[53] R. Mazzucchelli, A. Lopez-Beltran, L. Cheng, M. Scarpelli, Z. Kirkali, and R. Montironi, "Rare and unusual histological variants of prostatic carcinoma: clinical significance," *BJU International*, vol. 102, no. 10, pp. 1369–1374, 2008.

[54] M. McKenzie, I. MacLennan, E. Kostashuk, and T. Bainbridge, "Postirradiation sarcoma after external beam radiation therapy for localized adenocarcinoma of the prostate: report of three cases," *Urology*, vol. 53, no. 6, p. 1228, 1999.

[55] J.-B. Prevost, A. Bossi, R. Sciot, and M. Debiec-Rychter, "Postirradiation sarcoma after external beam radiation therapy for localized adenocarcinoma of the prostate," *Tumori*, vol. 90, no. 6, pp. 618–621, 2004.

25

Impact of Short-Stay Urethroplasty on Health-Related Quality of Life and Patient's Perception of Timing of Discharge

Henry Okafor and Dmitriy Nikolavsky

Department of Urology, Upstate Medical University, 750 East Adams Street, Syracuse, NY 13210, USA

Correspondence should be addressed to Dmitriy Nikolavsky; nikolavd@upstate.edu

Academic Editor: Francisco E. Martins

Objective. To evaluate health-related quality of life in patients after a short-stay or outpatient urethroplasty. *Methods.* Over a 2-year period a validated health-related quality-of-life questionnaire, EuroQol (EQ-5D), was administered to all patients after urethroplasty. Postoperatively patients were offered to be sent home immediately or to stay overnight. Within 24 hours after discharge they were assessed for mobility, self-care, usual activities, pain or discomfort, and anxiety and depression. An additional question assessing timing of discharge was added to the survey. Clinical and operative characteristics were examined. *Results.* Forty-eight patients after anterior urethroplasty completed the survey. Mean age and mean stricture length were 51.6 years (21–78) and 60 mm (5–200 mm), respectively. Most etiologies were idiopathic (50% *n* = 24), trauma (19%, *n* = 9), and iatrogenic (19%, *n* = 9). Forty-one patients (85%) stayed overnight, while 7 patients (15%) chose to be discharged the same day. Overall, ninety-six percent were discharged within 23 hours of surgery. In the short stay and the outpatient cohorts, 90% and 86%, respectively, felt they were discharged on time. No patient reported a severe problem with postoperative pain or mobility. *Conclusions.* The majority of patients discharged soon after their procedure felt that discharge timing was appropriate and their health-related quality of life was only minimally affected.

1. Introduction

Urethroplasty is recognized as the gold standard treatment of anterior urethral stricture disease, given the reasonably high long-term success rates and acceptable morbidity [1–3]. While, traditionally, urethroplasty was followed by inpatient hospital stay, there has been an increasing trend for urological procedures to be performed on an outpatient basis [4], a pattern reflected in urologic reconstruction as well [5, 6]. While numerous studies have been published reporting the clinical outcomes of urethroplasty, patient perception, satisfaction, and subjective outcomes are not well studied. There is also a paucity of data examining patient perception of early return home from the hospital. The purpose of this study was to examine the patient's perception of appropriateness of timing of discharge and to evaluate immediate health-related quality of life immediately after discharge.

2. Methods

With institutional board review approval, electronic charts of 80 consecutive patients who underwent anterior urethral reconstruction at our institution from August 2012 to May 2014 were analyzed. Patients under 18 years of age, those with documented intellectual disability, incarcerated patients, and transgender patients were excluded, as were patients with planned multistage procedures.

All patients underwent preoperative evaluation with retrograde urethrogram and/or voiding cystourethrogram, uroflowmetry, and AUA symptom scores. All patients were counseled at the time of the preoperative evaluation of possible immediate postoperative discharge or overnight stay based on their postoperative condition and desire. Patients were assured that from our previous experience most prior patients safely returned home either immediately following urethroplasty or after an overnight stay providing pain is controlled and there are no other health concerns. Patients were educated on proper use of all postoperative medications and care for Foley catheter. Each patient was given contact information for the clinic and additionally a mobile phone number of the surgeon and were encouraged to call with additional questions or concerns before or after the surgery. The same points were reiterated immediately before the surgery in the Preoperative Unit.

The type of urethroplasty performed was dependent on stricture length, location, and etiology as well as surgeon preference. For substitution or augmentation urethroplasties, only buccal mucosal grafts (BMG) were used. The BMG was harvested as described by Morey and McAninch [7]; however, the harvest site was left open after harvest. The midline perineal incisions were closed in layers and no wound drains were used. A urethral catheter was left in place in all patients. When present, a suprapubic catheter remained capped on discharge.

In the postanesthesia recovery area all patients were assessed and given a choice of immediate discharge or an overnight hospital stay. Patients who elected to return home on the day of surgery were placed in the "outpatient cohort" while those who stayed overnight were a "short-stay" group. Discharge criteria in both groups included hemodynamic stability, adequate pain control with oral analgesics, and sufficient mobility to ambulate without difficulty. Patients were routinely sent home with prescriptions for nonsteroidal anti-inflammatory agents, oral narcotic medications for breakthrough pain, anticholinergics, stool softeners, and anesthetic/antiseptic mouthwash.

Within 24 hours of discharge, a routine postoperative check was conducted over the phone by a nurse or non-medical administrative assistant. The assessment included questions from the EuroQol (EQ-5D), a validated health-related quality of life (QOL) questionnaire [8, 9]. The questions are designed to assess mobility, self-care, usual activities, pain or discomfort, and anxiety/depression. The choices were scored from 1 to 3 as having "no problems," "moderate," or "severe problems," respectively. An additional question assessing perception of the timing of discharge as "right on time," "too soon," or "too late" was added to the interview.

We also reviewed the charts for hospital readmissions, emergency room visits, and unplanned clinic visits to capture any additional potential burden on patients or the healthcare system due to early postoperative discharge.

3. Results and Discussion

A total of 48 patients who underwent anterior urethroplasty between August 2012 and May 2014 were included. Mean age of the group was 51.6 years (21–78). Mean stricture length was 59.7 mm (5–200 mm). Preoperative patient characteristics and stricture etiology are shown in Table 1. The most common type of repair was a single stage, one sided dissection, dorsal onlay buccal urethroplasty in 13 (27%) patients as described by Kulkarni [10], followed by excision and primary anastomosis in 11 (23%) and augmented anastomotic urethroplasty in 10 (21%) patients (Table 2). Overall, 37 of the 48 patients (77%)

TABLE 1: Patient characteristics.

	Mean (Std. Dev.)	Range
Age (years)	51.6 (±15.65)	21–78
BMI (kg/m^2)	30.6 (±6.2)	18.6–44.7
Stricture length (mm)	60 (±51)	5–200
Stricture etiology	Number	%
Idiopathic	24	50
Trauma	9	19
Iatrogenic	9	19
Infectious	2	4
Radiation	2	4
Lichen sclerosis	2	4
Stricture location	Number	%
Bulbar	20	42
Bulbomembranous	12	25
Panurethral	9	18
Pendulous	5	10.4
Fossa navicularis	2	4

TABLE 2: Type of urethroplasty.

Repair type	Number (%)
One sided dissection, dorsal onlay (Kulkarni)	13 (27%)
Excision and primary anastomosis (EPA)	11 (23%)
Augmented anastomotic urethroplasty (AAU)	10 (21%)
Dorsal onlay	9 (19%)
Ventral onlay	4 (8%)
Others	1 (2%)

had buccal mucosa harvest for augmentation or substitution urethroplasty of which 8 required bilateral buccal mucosa harvest.

Forty-one patients made a postoperative decision to stay overnight, while seven elected to return home the same day. All except two patients (96%) were discharged within 23 hours of surgery.

Forty-six out of 48 patients (96%) responded to the EuroQuol-5 questionnaire as well as the question on timing of discharge within 24 hours of discharge. Overall, 89.1 % of all patients felt they were discharged on time (Figure 1).

With regard to the 5 dimensions on the EuroQuol-5, severe problems with "mobility" were not reported by any patient: 26 (56%) patients reported moderate problems with mobility compared to 20 (44%) that reported no problems (Figure 2). Only 2 patients (4%) reported severe problems in the "self-care" domain; a majority of patients, 31 (67%), reported no problems with self-care. Eleven patients (24%) reported severe problems with "usual activities," while 23 (50%) reported moderate problems. When asked about "pain or discomfort," no patients reported severe problems, but the majority 38 (83%) did indicate having moderate problems with pain or discomfort. On the question of "anxiety/depression," only one patient (2%) reported severe problems with anxiety or depression, while the majority of

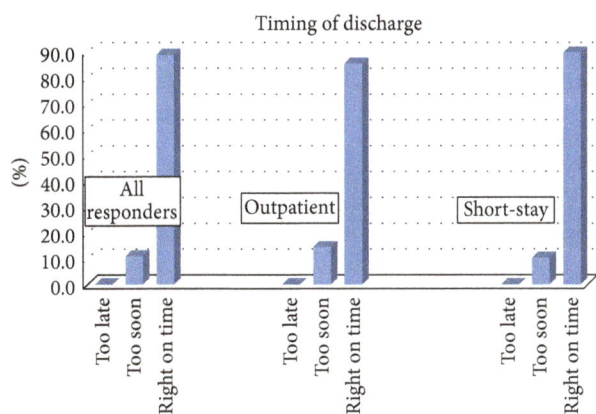

FIGURE 1: Timing of discharge.

TABLE 3: EQ-5 patient responses by group.

EQ-5D dimension	All responders (%)	Outpatient (%)	Short-stay (%)
Mobility			
1 = no problem	20 (44%)	3 (43%)	17 (56%)
2 = moderate	26 (56%)	4 (57%)	22 (44%)
3 = severe	0	0	0
Self-care			
1 = no problem	31 (68%)	6 (86%)	25 (64%)
2 = moderate	13 (28%)	1 (14%)	12 (31%)
3 = severe	2 (4%)	0	2 (5%)
Usual activity			
1 = no problem	12 (26%)	3 (43%)	9 (23%)
2 = moderate	23 (50%)	3 (43%)	20 (51%)
3 = severe	11 (24%)	1 (14%)	10 (26%)
Pain/discomfort			
1 = no problem	8 (17%)	1 (14%)	7 (18%)
2 = moderate	38 (83%)	6 (86%)	32 (82%)
3 = severe	0	0	0
Anxiety/depression			
1 = no problem	35 (76%)	7 (100%)	28 (72%)
2 = moderate	10 (22%)	0	10 (26%)
3 = severe	1 (2%)	0	1 (2%)

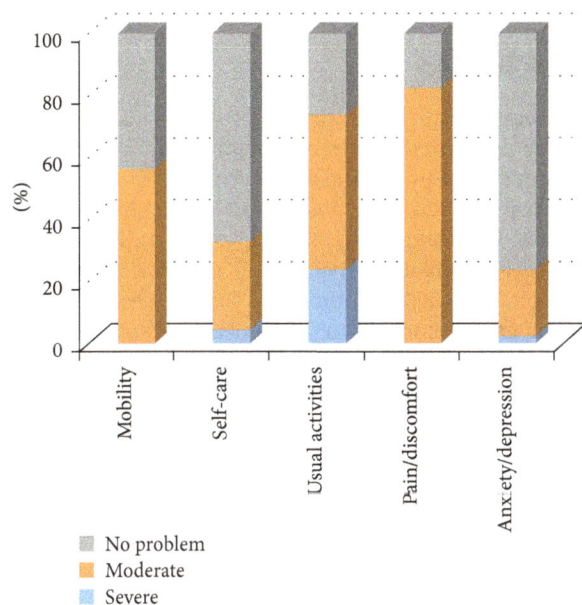

FIGURE 2: EQ-5 patient responses (all patients).

patients, 35 (76%), reported no problems. Table 3 summarizes the EQ-5 data collected from each group.

There were two Emergency Room visits recorded, one of which was readmitted to the hospital for incision and drainage of a perineal hematoma. No unscheduled clinic visits were identified.

In light of increasing emphasis on patient reported outcome measures (PROMs), a concerted effort has been made to have a questionnaire specific to urethral stricture disease. This has culminated in Jackson et al. developing the validated urethral stricture PROM, part of which assesses health-related quality of life [11]. Prior to that, various tools developed for other disease states were utilized for the urethral stricture patient [12]. We utilized the EuroQuol-5 validated questionnaire as it seeks to identify general health-related difficulties these patients may face, particularly in the context of an elective procedure (urethroplasty) intended to improve quality of life. Most patients, 82.6%, did report

moderate problems with pain and discomfort. However, despite the added morbidity of buccal harvest in most of the patients, none reported severe pain within 24 hours after discharge. In this population the donor site was left open; however, there are several studies with contradicting conclusions on effect of donor site closure on postoperative pain [13–16].

In this cohort, the majority of patients reported moderate and severe problems in performing usual activities (74%). This was expected as the patients were sent home with an indwelling catheter for 3 weeks and strict instructions to avoid strenuous physical activity and abstain from any sexual activity. Given the varying types of urethroplasty performed in this small population it is difficult to ascertain whether the type of procedure correlates with the increased perception of pain postoperatively. One patient reported severe problems with anxiety or depression, which was unexpected considering that the procedure was performed with a goal of improving the patient's quality of life. This finding highlighted an important limitation of this study, a lack of preoperative data on patients' baseline health-related quality of life. We have since changed our practice and administer all PROM questionnaires pre- and postoperatively.

To our knowledge, there are no published studies on patient-reported perception of appropriateness of timing of discharge after anterior urethroplasty. The only studies on short-stay or outpatient urethroplasty published by Lewis et al. and MacDonald et al. have concentrated on clinical outcomes [5, 6].

Results of anterior urethroplasty performed in the outpatient setting were first described in 2002 by Lewis et al. [5]. The authors described a cohort of patients who underwent bulbar urethroplasty and were then discharged home within 23 hours of surgery. In 2006, MacDonald et al. published outcomes of the "same day urethroplasty," which he defined as being discharged home within 4 hours after surgery [6]. In both series the outcomes of the surgery were excellent but the cohorts were small.

In detail, the first study described 78 bulbar urethroplasties of which 54 (69%) were performed on a short-stay basis (patients discharged <24 hours after surgery) [5]. Overall success in the short-stay cohort was 93% compared with 88% of the admitted inpatient cohort. The authors noted that the short-stay status depended on the type of urethroplasty (90% after EPA, 64% after penile skin flaps, and 45% after buccal mucosal grafts), younger patient's age (36 versus 46 years), and shorter stricture length (3.1 versus 6.6 cm.). The study did not comment on readmissions, ER visits, or unscheduled clinic visits.

In the second study, MacDonald et al. retrospectively describes 54 patients after anterior urethroplasty performed over 4 consecutive years [6]. Over the study period, the rate of the outpatient (same day) urethroplasty increased from 27% to 85%. In this study the outpatient and the admitted inpatient cohorts had similar stricture length, but the outpatient cohort was slightly younger age (42 versus 49 years of age). Over the 27 months of follow-up the success rate was similar in both groups (94% versus 97% in the inpatient group) as were the long-term complications (19% versus 18%, resp.). The authors reported that no readmissions or emergency room visits occurred in this study.

For both studies, overall clinical outcomes were similar between the outpatient or short-stay group and admitted patients. These two studies represent the only studies published on "minimal-impact urethroplasty" and further evaluation of outpatient urethroplasty, as far as patient reported outcome measures have been lacking.

In our series, the majority of patients were comfortable with the timing of discharge in both the outpatient and short-stay cohorts. Given the relative small size of the outpatient cohort, we did not attempt further statistical comparison of the two groups. Additionally, the decision to leave or stay was made by the patient and as might be expected the majority of patients later agreed with their own choices. We surmised that the few "too soon" responses represented a later regret of their original decision. Overall, majority of patients were satisfied with leaving the hospital within 23 hours after urethral reconstruction, even for long or panurethral strictures requiring extensive dissection and bilateral BMG harvest. This data is reassuring as it shows that majority of patients did not feel rushed out of the hospital. This study can serve for a future counseling of patients considering a short-stay urethroplasty showing it as a reasonable option from patients' perspective.

With prompt postoperative discharge, there is a concern about increased readmission rates; this failed to materialize in this series [17]. In our cohort there were two ER visits, one of which was related to patient's concern of scrotal bruising and another for perineal hematoma. The latter resulted in the only readmission to the hospital and subsequent incision and drainage. There were no unscheduled visits to the outpatient clinic in this group showing that early discharge from the hospital did not shift the burden of care from the inpatient to outpatient setting.

Some limitations of the study include its retrospective nature and the nonrandomization of the two groups, which led to an uneven distribution of the outpatient versus short-stay groups. This limited the ability to perform a multivariate or comparative analysis for each group. No preoperative EuroQuol-5 questionnaires were administered making it difficult to identify patients with preexisting problems in any of the 5 dimensions. This study is limited by the assumption that every patient was in sufficiently good health prior to surgery. However, even with this assumption, the majority of patients did not report severe changes in the health-related quality of life shortly after urethroplasty.

4. Conclusion

Early return home after urethroplasty seems to be well tolerated by patients as reported on their health-related quality of life questionnaire. When using EQ-5 as a quality of life indicator in the early postoperative period, the patient's QOL was only minimally affected, except when otherwise expected in domains of "pain" and "usual activities." Most patients are satisfied with timing of their discharge from the hospital after a short-stay or outpatient urethroplasty. Early discharge did not result in numerous catastrophes leading to ER visits, readmissions, or unscheduled office visits.

Conflict of Interests

The authors declare that there is no conflict of interests regarding the publication of this paper.

References

[1] G. Barbagli, S. B. Kulkarni, N. Fossati et al., "Long-term followup and deterioration rate of anterior substitution urethroplasty," *Journal of Urology*, vol. 192, no. 3, pp. 808–813, 2014.

[2] A. S. Kinnaird, M. A. Levine, D. Ambati, J. D. Zorn, and K. F. Rourke, "Stricture length and etiology as preoperative independent predictors of recurrence after urethroplasty: a multivariate analysis of 604 urethroplasties," *Journal of the Canadian Urological Association*, vol. 8, no. 5-6, pp. 296–300, 2014.

[3] H. S. Al-Quadah and R. A. Santucci, "Extended complications of urethroplasty," *International Brazilian Journal of Urology*, vol. 31, no. 4, pp. 315–325, 2005.

[4] K. W. Kaye, "Changing trends in urology practice: increasing outpatient surgery," *Australian and New Zealand Journal of Surgery*, vol. 65, no. 1, pp. 31–34, 1995.

[5] J. B. Lewis, K. A. Wolgast, J. A. Ward, and A. F. Morey, "Outpatient anterior urethroplasty: outcome analysis and patient selection criteria," *The Journal of Urology*, vol. 168, no. 3, pp. 1024–1026, 2002.

[6] M. F. MacDonald, H. S. Al-Qudah, and R. A. Santucci, "Minimal impact urethroplasty allows same-day surgery in most patients," *Urology*, vol. 66, no. 4, pp. 850–853, 2005.

[7] A. F. Morey and J. W. McAninch, "When and how to use buccal mucosal grafts in adult bulbar urethroplasty," *Urology*, vol. 48, no. 2, pp. 194–198, 1996.

[8] EuroQol Group, "EuroQol—a new facility for the measurement of health-related quality of life," *Health Policy*, vol. 16, no. 3, pp. 199–208, 1990.

[9] R. Brooks, "EuroQol: the current state of play," *Health Policy*, vol. 37, no. 1, pp. 53–72, 1996.

[10] S. Kulkarni, G. Barbagli, S. Sansalone, and M. Lazzeri, "One-sided anterior urethroplasty: a new dorsal onlay graft technique," *BJU International*, vol. 104, no. 8, pp. 1150–1155, 2009.

[11] M. J. Jackson, J. Sciberras, A. Mangera et al., "Defining a patient-reported outcome measure for urethral stricture surgery," *European Urology*, vol. 60, no. 1, pp. 60–68, 2011.

[12] B. B. Voelzke, "Critical review of existing patient reported outcome measures after male anterior urethroplasty," *Journal of Urology*, vol. 189, no. 1, pp. 182–188, 2013.

[13] D. N. Wood, S. E. Allen, D. E. Andrich, T. J. Greenwell, and A. R. Mundy, "The morbidity of buccal mucosal graft harvest for urethroplasty and the effect of nonclosure of the graft harvest site on postoperative pain," *The Journal of Urology*, vol. 172, no. 2, pp. 580–583, 2004.

[14] K. Rourke, S. McKinny, and B. St. Martin, "Effect of wound closure on buccal mucosal graft harvest site morbidity: results of a randomized prospective trial," *Urology*, vol. 79, no. 2, pp. 443–447, 2012.

[15] K. Muruganandam, D. Dubey, A. Gulia et al., "Closure versus nonclosure of buccal mucosal graft harvest site: a prospective randomized study on post operative morbidity," *Indian Journal of Urology*, vol. 25, no. 1, pp. 72–75, 2009.

[16] E. Wong, A. Fernando, A. Alhasso, and L. Stewart, "Does closure of the buccal mucosal graft bed matter? Results from a randomized controlled trial," *Urology*, vol. 84, no. 5, pp. 1223–1227, 2014.

[17] J. P. Crew, K. J. Turner, J. Millar, and D. W. Cranston, "Is day case surgery in urology associated with high admission rates?" *Annals of The Royal College of Surgeons of England*, vol. 79, no. 6, pp. 416–419, 1997.

26

The Natural History and Predictors for Intervention in Patients with Small Renal Mass Undergoing Active Surveillance

Zaher Bahouth,[1,2] **Sarel Halachmi,**[1,2] **Gil Meyer,**[1,2] **Ofir Avitan,**[1,2] **Boaz Moskovitz,**[1,2] **and Ofer Nativ**[1,2]

[1]*Department of Urology, Bnai Zion Medical Center, 3339414 Haifa, Israel*
[2]*Faculty of Medicine, Technion-Israel Institute of Technology, 3200003 Haifa, Israel*

Correspondence should be addressed to Zaher Bahouth; zaher.bahouth@b-zion.org.il

Academic Editor: Maxwell V. Meng

Aim. To describe the natural history of small renal mass on active surveillance and identify parameters that could help in predicting the need for intervention in patients with small renal masses undergoing active surveillance. We also discuss the need for renal biopsy in the management of these patients. *Methods.* A retrospective analysis of 78 renal masses ≤4 cm diagnosed at our Urology Department at Bnai Zion Medical Center between September 2003 and March 2012. *Results.* Seventy patients with 78 small renal masses were analyzed. The mean age at diagnosis was 68 years (47–89). The mean follow-up period was 34 months (12–112). In 54 of 78 masses there was a growth of at least 2 mm between imaging on last available follow-up and diagnosis. Eight of the 54 (15%) masses which grew in size underwent a nephron-sparing surgery, of which two were oncocytomas and six were renal cell carcinoma. Growth rate and mass diameter on diagnosis were significantly greater in the group of patients who underwent a surgery. *Conclusions.* Small renal masses might eventually be managed by active surveillance without compromising survival or surgical approach. All masses that were eventually excised underwent a nephron-sparing surgery. None of the patients developed metastases.

1. Introduction

Renal cell carcinoma (RCC) represents 2-3% of all cancers, with an age-adjusted incidence of 5.8 per 100,000 in developed countries [1]. During the last two decades, there has been an annual increase of about 2% in the incidence of RCC worldwide [2]. RCC is the most common solid lesion in the kidney and accounts for 90% of all kidney malignancies. Small renal mass (SRM) is defined as solid enhancing tumors up to 4 cm in maximal diameter and accounts for up to 66% of all renal tumors [3], most of them being diagnosed incidentally.

At least 20% of SRMs presumed to be RCC are in fact benign masses when biopsied or excised [4]. In a retrospective study of 2770 patients with renal masses, Frank et al. showed a direct correlation between tumor size and probability of malignancy, with an increase of 17% for each growth of 1 cm in size of mass [5]. Most SRMs show a slow growth rate and rarely progress to metastatic disease

[6]. Because of the slow growth rate and the low risk of metastases, active surveillance with delayed treatment for patients showing progression can be considered in patients with a newly diagnosed SRM [7], especially those with significant comorbidities, but it could also be acceptable regardless of the patient age in very small renal masses (<1 cm) as suggested by Gill et al. [8]. However, indications for active treatment and predictors for progression are not well defined.

In addition, other treatment options exist for small masses especially for patients who do not fit for surgery or prefer a less radical treatment. Such treatment options include renal cryoablation and radiofrequency ablation.

Even though NSS is considered the gold-standard in managing small renal masses, it has been shown that surgery could adversely affect the renal function, adversely affecting survival [9], although far less than radical nephrectomy.

The aim of the current study was to assess the results of active surveillance for SRMs and to define parameters that could differentiate those who need surgery from those that can be managed by surveillance only. We also discuss the need for biopsy in these patients.

2. Materials and Methods

We retrospectively analyzed the radiological and clinical data collected from a total of 101 contrast-enhancing SRMs diagnosed between September 2003 and January 2013 at our Urology Department at Bnai Zion Medical Center. The inclusion criteria for surveillance were contrast-enhancing renal mass of 4 cm or less in maximal diameter, risk factors for end-stage renal disease, multiple major comorbidities, and patient preference. Risk factors for end-stage renal failure (e.g., impaired baseline renal function, poorly controlled hypertension, and long-standing or poorly controlled diabetes) were included because of the risk of subsequent decrease in renal function and the need for renal replacement therapy following renal surgery. Exclusion criteria included patients who did not have a follow-up of at least 12 months (n = 23). We ended up with a total of 70 patients with 78 masses clinically staged as T1aN0M0. The following data was obtained from the medical records: age, gender, comorbidities, history of renal and nonrenal malignancies, laterality, number and size of the lesions, date and modality of follow-up imaging, and all relevant information concerning surgery when it was done. Follow-up protocol included reimaging every six months in the first year by CT-Urography or MR-Urography in order to determine any change in the lesion size and assess disease progression. Starting in the second year, follow-up protocol included an alternating CT-Urography or MR-Urography (in patients with impaired renal function) and sonography every six months. Masses measurement was done by one radiologist who was not aware of patients' outcome and was based on the measurement of the maximal tumor diameter. Indications for intervention were high growth rate, a lesion that grew beyond 40 mm, and patient or doctor preference.

Statistical Analysis. The mean tumor growth rate was calculated by the absolute change in maximal diameter in imaging at last available follow-up and at diagnosis and stated as cm/year. Categorical data were analyzed using Fisher's exact test and Chi-square test. Continuous variables were analyzed using t-test. Significance level was set as P value < 0.05. A multivariate analysis was done using a stepwise logistic regression and included the following parameters: sex, age, laterality, size of mass on diagnosis, previous NSS, history of cancer, and growth rate. For statistical analysis, MedCalc version 12.5 was used.

3. Results

Among the 70 patients, 39 were males and 31 were females. Mean patients age was 68 years (range 47–89 years). Mean Charlson Comorbidity Index was 4.5, with minority of patients having a score of less than 2. Fifty-six percent of the masses were in men. Six of 70 patients had multiple SRMs; of them three had bilateral synchronous lesions. One

TABLE 1: Patients and masses characteristics with statistical significance.

Feature	Active surveillance	NSS	P value
Age			0.88
Mean (range)	68.6 (49–89)	69 (47–87)	
Sex			0.63
Men	34	5	
Women	29	2	
Side			0.19
Right	30	6	
Left	40	2	
Follow-up, months	34.9 (12–112)	25.9 (13–46)	0.28
Size at Dx, mm	18 (5–40)	24.9 (8–40)	**0.04**
Growth rate, cm/year	0.12 (−0.29–0.65)	0.53 (0.18–0.88)	**<0.0001**

patient had SRM in a single kidney (first kidney removed of RCC) and 6 patients had previously undergone renal surgery, one for oncocytoma and five for RCC. Mean follow-up time was 34 months (range 12–112 months). Patients and masses characteristics are summarized in Table 1.

Seven patients (10%) with 8 SRMs underwent treatment, all of them by NSS. All patients were referred to NSS as it is considered the gold-standard treatment and because of limited data and experience in other treatment options (e.g., ablative therapies). On histopathology, six of the excised masses were RCC and two oncocytomas (Table 2). None of the surgically treated patients had recurrence during the study follow-up.

The mean growth rate of all SRMs in our study was 0.17 cm/year (range −0.29 to 0.88 cm/year). Fifty-four of the 78 masses (69%) showed growth in size of at least 2 mm between diagnosis and last available imaging study. All other 24 masses (31%) did not show any growth during follow-up period. Among the 54 masses that increased in size, the mean growth rate was 0.25 cm/year. Table 3 shows the growth rate of SRMs as seen in our study compared to previous studies.

Three patients from the surveillance group had indications for intervention as detailed before, but none of them underwent such a surgery, one because of benign histology on biopsy and two because of very advanced age.

We did a univariate and multivariate analysis to check for differences in patients' parameters in both groups. Univariate analysis showed size at diagnosis and tumor growth rate as the only parameters with significant difference. The mean growth rate of the lesions that were actively treated was 0.53 cm/year (95% CI 0.33, 0.71) as opposed to 0.12 cm/year (95% CI 0.08, 0.17) for masses managed expectantly (P < 0.0001) (Figure 1).

Mean tumor diameter at diagnosis for the entire group was 18.7 mm (range 5–40 mm). Patients who remained on active surveillance had significantly smaller masses at diagnosis as compared to patients who underwent surgery, 18 mm (95% CI 15.9, 20.2) and 24.9 mm (95% CI 16.7,33), respectively,

TABLE 2: Characteristics of patients who underwent NSS.

Number	Age	Sex	Size at Dx (mm)	Size on Sx (mm)	Growth rate (cm/year)	Time to surgery (months)	Histopathology	Mass
1	77	M	30	45	0.47	38	Oncocytoma	Exophytic
2	57	F	40	59	0.88	26	Oncocytoma	Exophytic
3	54	M	31	37	0.31	23	Pap RCC	Exophytic
4	47	F	8	20	0.46	32	CC RCC, G2	Hilar
5	82	M	28	37	0.67	16	CC RCC, G3	Exophytic
6	87	M	25	43	0.47	46	CC RCC, G3	Exophytic
7a	75	M	20	28	0.74	13	CC RCC, G2	Endophytic
7b	75	M	17	19	0.18	13	Pap RCC	Exophytic
Average	69		24.8	36	0.53	25.9		

Pap RCC: papillary renal cell carcinoma; CC RCC: clear-cell type renal cell carcinoma; G = Fuhrman grade; 7a and 7b represent two lesions in the same patient; lesion 7b was excised because the patient was undergoing an excision for lesion 7a; otherwise it could still be on active surveillance. Mean growth rate without lesion 7b is 0.57 cm/year compared to 0.53 cm/year with lesion 7b.

TABLE 3: Growth rate of SRMs as seen in several studies.

Study	Year	Number of lesions	Number of patients	Mean mass size (cm)	Mean growth rate (cm/year)	Mean follow-up (months)
Chawla et al. [10][‡]	2006	234	NA	2.6	0.28	34
Kunkle et al. [11]	2007	106	89	2.0[*]	0.19[*]	29[*]
Jewett et al. [12]	2011	151	82	2.1	0.13	28
Mason et al. [13]	2011	84	82	2.3[*]	0.25[*]	36[*]
Smaldone et al. [14][‡]	2012	284	259	2.3	0.31	33.5
Current study	2015	78	70	1.9	0.17	34

NA: not available. [*]Median. [‡]Review article.

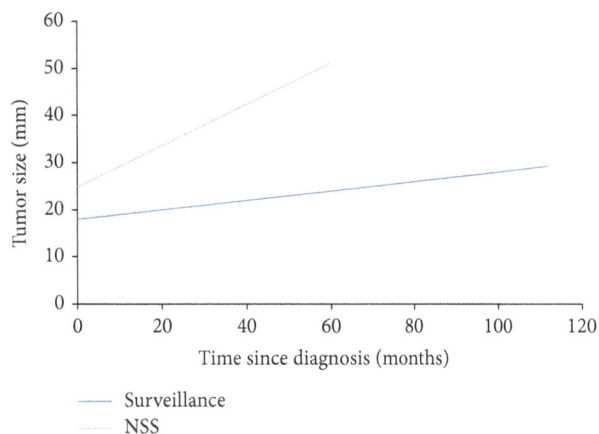

FIGURE 1: Growth rate of small renal masses. Growth rate of masses that underwent active treatment was 0.53 cm/year (light line) which was significantly higher than that observed for masses which were managed expectantly, 0.12 cm/year (dark line). $P < 0.0001$.

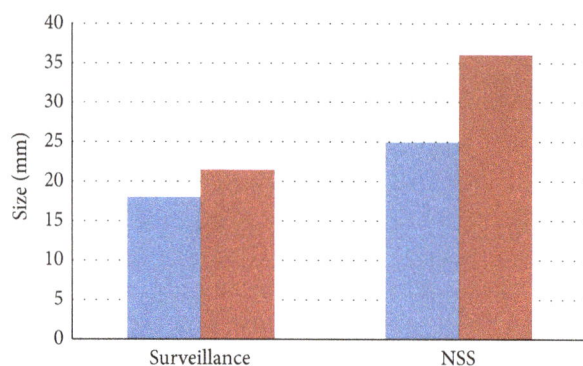

FIGURE 2: Masses size in both groups as observed at diagnosis and on last follow-up. Blue demonstrates size at diagnosis and red demonstrates size at last available follow-up. Masses diameter at diagnosis was significantly ($P = 0.04$) smaller in the group of patients who were managed conservatively (18 mm versus 24.9 mm).

$P = 0.04$. The mean tumor diameter on last available follow-up was 21.4 mm (range 7–40) in the group of patients who remained on active surveillance and 36 mm (range 19–59) in patients who underwent a NSS (Figure 2).

In multivariate analysis the only parameter with significant difference between the intervention group and the follow-up was tumor growth rate.

4. Discussion

Our data demonstrated that a significant number (31%) of SRMs did not grow at all, while many (59%) demonstrated a slow growth rate (0.25 cm/year). Only 8 masses in 7 patients (10%) underwent an intervention, in which the growth rate was significantly higher (4.5-fold increase, $P < 0.0001$).

Similar data was reported by Jewett et al. showing that 37% of SRMs did not grow [12]. Mason et al. reported 15% of masses not growing in size [13], in a cohort of 84 masses with a mean size of 2.3 cm at diagnosis. The mean growth rate of the 54 masses that increased in size was 0.25 cm/year in our study. This rate is similar to other previous studies [12, 13].

Follow-up revealed stage progression in only 3 patients (4%) who increased from clinical stage T1a to T1b. None of the patients showed progression to clinical stage T $\geq$ 2 nor to metastatic disease. No functional deterioration among the study participants was observed, and no patient required a renal replacement therapy. Such limited stage progression was also reported in previous studies [13].

Our initial conservative treatment approach, that is, active surveillance, did not compromise our ability to carry out a nephron-sparing surgery in patients mandated to active treatment, which is the gold-standard surgery. Moreover, postoperative follow-up of the 7 patients who were operated on did not demonstrate locoregional or metastatic progression. Several studies reported favorable outcomes for patients with SRMs who were managed conservatively, with only sporadic cases of stage progression [13, 15].

Tumor size at diagnosis was significantly higher (24.9 mm versus 18 mm, $P = 0.04$) in masses that were eventually subjected to surgical intervention. Similarly, Mason et al. demonstrated that larger tumors ($\geq$24.5 mm) have a higher growth rate leading to higher rate of intervention [13]. We saw a similar trend in the current study, with a growth rate of 0.23 cm/year for masses $\geq$24.5 mm and 0.14 cm/year for masses <24.5 mm, but without statistical significance ($P = 0.17$). This fact shows that the size of tumor at diagnosis could be helpful in selecting the optimal management, as larger masses tend to grow faster than smaller ones.

In our study, we did not require a pretreatment biopsy for enrollment. Among our patients, only three underwent a renal biopsy, all of them because of personal preference. One patient was an 80-year-old patient, with a mass of 18 mm at diagnosis, who remained under follow-up for additional 46 months without progression, and his biopsy showed G1 clear-cell RCC. The second patient was diagnosed with a 25 mm mass, whose biopsy showed G2 clear-cell RCC and underwent a surgery when the mass was 43 mm, 4 years after initial diagnosis. The last patient was from the surveillance group who had a mass of 40 mm who underwent a biopsy that showed a benign lesion.

It should be mentioned that two of the eight SRMs that were excised were oncocytoma. One could argue that a biopsy could have changed the management by omitting surgical treatment. However, even in the presence of oncocytic cells in the biopsy specimen, the possibility of hybrid tumor cannot be ruled out. The issue of a pretreatment biopsy is still under debate and requires further studies. Other reasons to omit biopsy include nondiagnostic results in as high as 20% in some studies, the need for a repeat biopsy in 3%, and grade 1 and grade 3 complications in 10.1% and 0.3%, respectively [16]. However, more recent studies suggest better results and less nondiagnostic biopsies [17].

Taken together, the results of the current study and of previously published studies indicate that most SRMs possess a favorable biology. Conservative treatment approach is safe and effective, and if a surgery is needed during the follow-up, a NSS could still be performed.

In our experience, the most significant predictors for intervention were tumor growth rate and tumor size at diagnosis. Larger tumors and high growth rate should mandate an early intervention rather than active surveillance because of the higher tendency of being operated on.

Eventually, the major limitation of our study was the fact that it was retrospective. Another limitation is the relatively small number of patients. One more limitation is the relatively short mean follow-up. A prospective study with a larger number should be done in order to validate our results and to better define thresholds for initiating treatment.

5. Conclusions

Active surveillance with serial imaging studies is a reasonable and safe management option for newly diagnosed SRMs. A small percentage of these masses require intervention and delayed treatment with NSS can still be carried out although the masses grew in size. Moreover, delayed treatment does not compromise overall long-term outcomes.

Conflict of Interests

The authors have no conflict of interests to disclose.

References

[1] A. Jemal, F. Bray, M. M. Center, J. Ferlay, E. Ward, and D. Forman, "Global cancer statistics," *CA: Cancer Journal for Clinicians*, vol. 61, no. 2, pp. 69–90, 2011.

[2] P. Lindblad, "Epidemiology of renal cell carcinoma," *Scandinavian Journal of Surgery*, vol. 93, no. 2, pp. 88–96, 2004.

[3] M. M. Nguyen, I. S. Gill, and L. M. Ellison, "The evolving presentation of renal carcinoma in the united states: trends from the surveillance, epidemiology, and end results program," *The Journal of Urology*, vol. 176, no. 6, pp. 2397–2400, 2006.

[4] S. C. Campbell, A. C. Novick, A. Belldegrun et al., "Guideline for management of the clinical T1 renal mass," *The Journal of Urology*, vol. 182, no. 4, pp. 1271–1279, 2009.

[5] I. Frank, M. L. Blute, J. C. Cheville, C. M. Lohse, A. L. Weaver, and H. Zincke, "Solid renal tumors: an analysis of pathological features related to tumor size," *The Journal of Urology*, vol. 170, no. 6, part 1, pp. 2217–2220, 2003.

[6] G. Lughezzani, C. Jeldres, H. Isbarn et al., "Tumor size is a determinant of the rate of stage T1 renal cell cancer synchronous metastasis," *The Journal of Urology*, vol. 182, no. 4, pp. 1287–1293, 2009.

[7] M. J. Wehle, D. D. Thiel, S. P. Petrou, P. R. Young, I. Frank, and N. Karstead, "Conservative management of incidental contrast-enhancing renal masses as safe alternative to invasive therapy," *Urology*, vol. 64, no. 1, pp. 49–52, 2004.

[8] I. S. Gill, M. Aron, D. A. Gervais, and M. A. S. Jewett, "Small renal mass," *The New England Journal of Medicine*, vol. 362, no. 7, pp. 624–634, 2010.

[9] A. F. Fergany, K. S. Hafez, and A. C. Novick, "Long-term results of nephron sparing surgery for localized renal cell carcinoma:

10-year followup," *The Journal of Urology*, vol. 163, no. 2, pp. 442–445, 2000.

[10] S. N. Chawla, P. L. Crispen, A. L. Hanlon, R. E. Greenberg, D. Y. T. Chen, and R. G. Uzzo, "The natural history of observed enhancing renal masses: meta-analysis and review of the world literature," *Journal of Urology*, vol. 175, no. 2, pp. 425–431, 2006.

[11] D. A. Kunkle, P. L. Crispen, D. Y. T. Chen, R. E. Greenberg, and R. G. Uzzo, "Enhancing renal masses with zero net growth during active surveillance," *The Journal of Urology*, vol. 177, no. 3, pp. 849–854, 2007.

[12] M. A. S. Jewett, K. Mattar, J. Basiuk et al., "Active surveillance of small renal masses: progression patterns of early stage kidney cancer," *European Urology*, vol. 60, no. 1, pp. 39–44, 2011.

[13] R. J. Mason, M. Abdolell, G. Trottier et al., "Growth kinetics of renal masses: analysis of a prospective cohort of patients undergoing active surveillance," *European Urology*, vol. 59, no. 5, pp. 863–867, 2011.

[14] M. C. Smaldone, A. Kutikov, B. L. Egleston et al., "Small renal masses progressing to metastases under active surveillance," *Cancer*, vol. 118, no. 4, pp. 997–1006, 2012.

[15] P. L. Crispen, R. Viterbo, S. A. Boorjian, R. E. Greenberg, D. Y. T. Chen, and R. G. Uzzo, "Natural history, growth kinetics, and outcomes of untreated clinically localized renal tumors under active surveillance," *Cancer*, vol. 115, no. 13, pp. 2844–2852, 2009.

[16] M. J. Leveridge, A. Finelli, J. R. Kachura et al., "Outcomes of small renal mass needle core biopsy, nondiagnostic percutaneous biopsy, and the role of repeat biopsy," *European Urology*, vol. 60, no. 3, pp. 578–584, 2011.

[17] S. M. Korbet, K. C. Volpini, and W. L. Whittier, "Percutaneous renal biopsy of native kidneys: a single-center experience of 1,055 biopsies," *American Journal of Nephrology*, vol. 39, no. 2, pp. 153–162, 2014.

27

Predictors of Incisional Hernia after Robotic Assisted Radical Prostatectomy

Avinash Chennamsetty,[1] Jason Hafron,[1,2] Luke Edwards,[1] Scott Pew,[2] Behdod Poushanchi,[2] Jay Hollander,[1,2] Kim A. Killinger,[1] Mary P. Coffey,[3] and Kenneth M. Peters[1,2]

[1]Beaumont Health System, Department of Urology, Royal Oak, MI 48073, USA
[2]Oakland University William Beaumont School of Medicine, Rochester, MI 48309, USA
[3]Beaumont Health System, Department of Biostatistics, Research Institute, Royal Oak, MI 48073, USA

Correspondence should be addressed to Avinash Chennamsetty; avinash.chennamsetty@beaumont.edu

Academic Editor: Maxwell V. Meng

Introduction. To explore the long term incidence and predictors of incisional hernia in patients that had RARP. *Methods.* All patients who underwent RARP between 2003 and 2012 were mailed a survey reviewing hernia type, location, and repair. *Results.* Of 577 patients, 48 (8.3%) had a hernia at an incisional site (35 men had umbilical), diagnosed at (median) 1.2 years after RARP (mean follow-up of 5.05 years). No statistically significant differences were found in preoperative diabetes, smoking, pathological stage, age, intraoperative/postoperative complications, operative time, blood loss, BMI, and drain type between patients with and without incisional hernias. Incisional hernia patients had larger median prostate weight (45 versus 38 grams; $P = 0.001$) and a higher proportion had prior laparoscopic cholecystectomy (12.5% (6/48) versus 4.6% (22/480); $P = 0.033$). Overall, 4% (23/577) of patients underwent surgical repair of 24 incisional hernias, 22 umbilical and 2 other port site hernias. *Conclusion.* Incisional hernia is a known complication of RARP and may be associated with a larger prostate weight and history of prior laparoscopic cholecystectomy. There is concern about the underreporting of incisional hernia after RARP, as it is a complication often requiring surgical revision and is of significance for patient counseling before surgery.

1. Introduction

Robot assisted radical prostatectomy (RARP) has emerged as the leading operation for patients with localized prostate cancer. In 2010, almost 80% of all prostatectomies in the USA were performed with robotic assistance [1]. The procedure provides patients with excellent clinical, functional, aesthetic, and oncologic results with decreased postoperative pain and quicker recovery [2]. However, in patients who develop incisional hernias, the benefits may be negated as incisional hernias can lead not only to bothersome symptoms but also to severe complications, such as bowel obstruction, strangulation, and perforation. Another reason the incidence of incisional hernias remains a concern is its reoperation rate (Grade III Clavien Classifcation); secondary repair failures as great as 45% have been reported [3, 4].

For patients who had a RARP, the incidence of incisional hernia in several large series is estimated at 0.2%–4.8% [5–13]. However, some of these studies have inadequate follow-up. Without longer follow-up, it is commonly accepted that a large number of incisional hernias are undiagnosed. In some series, 35% of all incisional hernias occurred 3 years after the operation [14]. Additionally, many asymptomatic patients may not seek medical care or present to a general surgeon directly for repair leading to a lower reported incidence. A recent review of the SEER (surveillance, epidemiology, and end results) database reported an incisional hernia repair rate after minimally invasive prostatectomy of 5.3% within 3.1 years, notably higher than previously reported in the literature [15].

Factors predisposing patients to incisional hernias include technical factors, such as trocar type and size, lack of fascial defect closure, and location of trocar placement [16]. Furthermore, the development of incisional hernias can also be affected by many predisposing host factors that decrease wound healing. When factors such as diabetes, morbid obesity, smoking, surgical site infection, malnutrition, and immunosuppression are present, optimal wound healing is impeded. The objective of our study was to explore the incidence and potential predictors of incisional hernia in patients who underwent RARP at our single teaching institution.

2. Materials and Methods

After receiving institutional review board approval, we identified all men who underwent RARP for prostate cancer between January 1, 2003, and December 31, 2012, by multiple surgeons at our institution. Patients of eight surgeons with varied levels of experience were included in the analysis. All patients underwent a transperitoneal approach through 6 ports using bladeless sharp or blunt obturators. Trocar placement included a 12 mm supraumbilical camera port, two 8 mm ports in the left and right lower quadrant just lateral to the rectus muscle, a 8 mm port two finger breaths above the left anterior iliac spine, a 12 mm lateral port two finger breaths above the right anterior iliac spine, and 5 mm port in the right upper quadrant. The 12 mm supraumbilical camera port site was vertically incised by all surgeons, except for one surgeon who utilized a horizontal incision. At the end of the procedure, the specimen was extracted by extending the supraumbilical site camera port site as needed. The extraction incision site was closed in an interrupted fashion with figure of eights. However suture type varied based on each individual surgeon's preference and included #0 Vicryl, #0 Prolene, #0 PDS, and #0 Ethibond. The 12 mm assistant port was routinely closed with a Carter-Thompson.

Using a mailed survey, we assessed information regarding the hernia type, location on a body diagram, and any postoperative hernia repair. Only men that answered the survey question about whether or not they had developed a hernia were included in the analysis. Hernias that occurred pre-RARP were excluded from the analysis. We also reviewed the patients' medical records for demographic, clinical, operative, and outcome characteristics. The time elapsed between date of surgery and July 15, 2013 (date that all surveys were mailed), was used to calculate the time since RARP.

Recorded data at the time of RARP included age, American Society of Anesthesiologists (ASA) score, smoking status, body mass index (BMI), operative time, intraoperative/postoperative complications, pathological stage, drain type (Jackson Pratt, penrose or none), blood loss, prostate weight, prior abdominal surgery, prior herniorrhaphy, prior laparoscopic cholecystectomy, prior appendectomy, prior colon surgery, and any other prior abdominal surgeries.

The Wilcoxon Rank Sum test, Chi-square test, and pooled t-tests were used to compare those who reported a postoperative incisional hernia with those who reported no hernia. Exact P values were obtained for the Chi-square test in the case of small expected frequencies. Multivariate logistic regression models were fit where variables were

considered for inclusion if the univariate P values from Table 3 were ≤0.20. 95% Wald confidence intervals for odds ratios were obtained. Models with interaction terms were also considered. The fit of logistic regression models was assessed with Hosmer-Lemeshow tests and plots of model diagnostics. The SAS System for Windows version 9.3 was used for statistical analysis. Statistical significance was defined by a two-sided P value <0.05.

3. Results

We identified 1,587 patients who underwent RARP and data provided by 577 patients (36%) that returned our mailed survey were analyzed. Analysis of these 577 patients with a mean follow-up of 5.05 years revealed 48 (8.3%) patients with an incisional hernia. The hernias were diagnosed at (median) 1.2 years (IQR 0.5–2.9; range .01–9.1) after RARP.

On the body diagram, 48 patients indicated that at least one hernia was located at an incisional site, with one patient reporting two; one at an umbilical site and the other at a port site. In twelve patients that reported an incisional hernia, the actual location of the hernia was too unclear on the body diagram to report; however these were included in the total for calculation of incidence. Of the 49 total incisional hernias, 71% (35/49) were umbilical and 4% (2/49) were other ports. Both other port hernias were at the 12 mm lateral port site. Upon further review of the 35 umbilical site hernias, only one was by a surgeon who routinely used a transverse incision at the supraumbilical port site.

23 men (4%) with incisional hernias had repair of 24 incisional hernias, 22 of these men had an umbilical (extraction site) hernia repaired. The 2 hernias repaired at other sites were both the 12 mm lateral port. One patient had an incisional hernia at both sites and they were repaired simultaneously.

Of all men that returned a survey, 48/577 (8.3%) developed at least one inguinal hernia. Those patients who reported only a groin hernia and those whose reported date of hernia occurred before RARP were excluded; as a result, the number of subjects used for analysis to compare incisional hernia patients with no hernia patients was 532 (Table 1). Men with postoperative groin and inguinal hernias were included in the analysis. Of the 532 patients, the mean age was 61.5 ± 6.7 years (median 62, range 42–78), and the mean BMI was 27.80 (median 27.12, range 16.66 to 55.5). 413/525 (78.7%) had stage T2 prostate cancer. 13/532 (2.4%) had any intraoperative complications and 58/532 (11%) reported postoperative complications.

The incisional hernia (N = 48) patients were compared to those that did not develop a hernia (N = 484) on 18 potential risk factors for developing an incisional hernia after RARP. In the incisional hernia/no hernia groups, years since RARP were 4.32 ± 2.59 and 5.12 ± 2.62, respectively.

No statistically significant differences were found in preoperative diabetes, smoking, pathological stage, age, operative time, blood loss, drain type, and intraoperative and/or postoperative complications between patients with incisional hernias and those without hernias (Table 3). Of note, when we classified patients into 3 groups based on

TABLE 1: Patient characteristics and surgical data for 532 patients with no hernia or incisional hernia.

	N	Mean ± SD (range)
Age (years)	528	61.5 ± 6.7 (42–78)
BMI		
Median (range)	530	27.2 (16.7–55.5)
Years since RARP	531	5.05 ± 2.62 (0.63–10.64)
		N (%)
ASA classification	513	
1		24 (4.7)
2		382 (74.5)
3		102 (20.0)
4		2 (0.4)
Prior herniorrhaphy	528	100 (18.9)
Intraoperative complication	531	13 (2.4)
Hemorrhage		1
Bladder injury		9
Epigastric artery laceration		1
Robot malfunction		2
Postoperative complication (Grade I or II Clavien classification)	532	58 (11)
Pathological stage	525	
T2		413 (79)
T3		112 (21)

TABLE 2: Patients classified by BMI and incisional hernia status.

	Incisional hernia N (%)	No hernia N (%)	Total
Normal/underweight (BMI < 25 kg/m^2)	6 (4.7%)	121 (95.3%)	127 (24.0%)
Overweight (25 kg/m^2 ≤ BMI < 30 kg/m^2)	28 (10.6%)	237 (89.4%)	265 (50%)
Obese (BMI ≥ 30 kg/m^2)	14 (10.1%)	124 (89.9%)	138 (26.0%)
Total	48 (9.1%)	482 (90.9%)	530

BMI (normal/underweight (BMI < 25 kg/m^2), overweight (25 kg/m^2 ≤ BMI < 30 kg/m^2), and obese (BMI ≥ 30 kg/m^2)), there was a lower rate of incisional hernia in the normal/underweight (4.7%) group while the hernia rates in the overweight (10.6%) and obese (10.1%) groups were similar ($P = 0.15$) (Table 2). Although the rate of incisional hernia was lower in normal/underweight men, the sample size was not powered to show statistical significance.

Interestingly, 17% (8/48) in the incisional hernia group and 10.3% (50/484) in the no hernia group had postoperative complications ($P = 0.22$, OR = 1.74, 95% CI for OR: (0.66, 4.04)). However, of those postoperative complications surgical site infection was not common as only 2 patients reported a surgical site infection in the no hernia group (2/464 = 0.4%) and none were reported in the incisional hernia group.

There were indications of increasing hernia rates with worse ASA physical status ($P = 0.096$). Additionally, median prostate weight was higher (45 versus 38 grams; $P = 0.001$) in the incisional hernia group compared to the no hernia group. Even though there were no statistically significant differences

in prior abdominal surgery, herniorrhaphy, appendectomy, colon surgery, or any other prior abdominal surgeries between the two groups, a higher proportion of incisional hernia patients had a history of laparoscopic cholecystectomy when compared to the no hernia group (12.5% (6/48) versus 4.6% (22/480); $P = 0.033$, OR = 2.97, 95% CI for OR: (0.93, 8.10)).

Four variables were considered for inclusion in logistic regression models based on univariate P values and the absence of zero frequencies, which precluded fitting the model. BMI was modeled as categories (underweight/normal, overweight, and obese) rather than continuous, given the lack of fit indicated with the Hosmer-Lemeshow test. For ASA class, patients with unknown status were excluded and ASA was modeled as a continuous predictor. Our chosen model includes effects of prostate weight and whether or not the patient had a prior cholecystectomy. Larger prostate weight and history of prior cholecystectomy were associated with higher proportions of incisional hernia (Table 4). The estimated effects of these variables as measured by odds ratios are similar in the univariate logistic regressions

TABLE 3: Comparison of incisional hernia versus no hernia groups on potential risk factors.

	Incisional hernia N (%)	No hernia N (%)	P value
Diabetes	4/48 (8.3)	55/478 (11.5)	0.64
Past or current smoking	24/48 (50.0)	219/476 (46.0)	0.65
Prior abdominal surgery	18/48 (37.5)	153/479 (31.9)	0.33
Prior herniorrhaphy	9/48 (18.8)	91/480 (19.0)	1.00
Prior cholecystectomy	6/48 (12.5)	22/480 (4.6)	0.033
ASA classification	N = 48	N = 462	
1	0 (0.0)	24 (5.2)	
2	35 (72.9)	347 (75.1)	0.096
3	13 (27.1)	89 (19.3)	
4	0 (0.0)	2 (0.4)	
Intraoperative complication	0/48 (0.0)	13/483 (2.7)	0.14
Drain type	N = 46	N = 470	
None	2 (4.4)	16 (3.4)	
JP	35 (76.1)	338 (71.9)	0.68
Penrose	9 (19.6)	116 (24.7)	
Postoperative complication (Grade I or II Clavien classification)	8/48 (16.7)	50/484 (10.3)	0.22
Pathological stage			
T2	38/48 (79.2)	375/477 (78.6)	1.00
T3	10/48 (20.8)	102/477 (21.4)	
Age (years)			
Mean ± SD	62.46 ± 6.93	61.38 ± 6.69	0.29
Operative time (hours)			
Median (range)	3.23 (1.88–4.72)	3.27 (1.6–9.22)	0.30
Blood loss (mL)			
Median (range)	100 (10–500)	100 (10–1200)	0.60
BMI			
Median (range)	27.15 (20.7–42.9)	27.1 (16.7–55.5)	0.18
Prostate weight (grams)			
Median (range)	45.0 (17–92)	38 (13–139)	0.001

for each variable separately, a multivariate logistic regression with four variables (Model 1: prostate weight, prior cholecystectomy, ASA, and BMI category), and a logistic regression with just prostate weight and prior cholecystectomy status (Model 2); these odds ratios are displayed in Table 4. Adjusting for prostate weight, the odds of incisional hernia for men with prior cholecystectomy are estimated to be 3.1 times the odds for men without prior cholecystectomy. Adjusting for prior cholecystectomy status, for every increase in prostate weight of five grams, the odds of incisional hernia increase by 13 percent.

4. Discussion

As one of the mainstays of treatment for clinically localized prostate cancer, complications of the RARP such as urinary incontinence and erectile dysfunction have been well described. However, an often overlooked complication that can contribute significantly to morbidity when incurred is incisional hernias. The cumulative incidence of incisional

hernia in large open abdominal surgery ranges from 9% to 19% [3, 14, 17, 18].

This analysis of more than 550 RARP patients operated on by various surgeons revealed a relatively high incidence of incisional hernias at 8.3%. These results do not compare favorably with previously reported results in several large series ranging from 0.2% to 4.8% [5–13]. However, as the incidence of incisional hernias increases with time, many of these series may be underreporting their true incidence due to inadequate follow-up. Blatt and colleagues [5] reported a 1.9% incisional/inguinal hernia rate at 4 months of follow-up. Furthermore, they failed to make a distinction between incisional and inguinal hernias. Menon et al. [6] followed 2,652 patients for a median of 36 months, but complications were not broken down to calculate the rate of incisional hernia. Martinez-Pineiro and colleagues [7] reported a 3% incisional hernia rate in 600 patients but failed to define the time of follow-up. Similarly, Chiong et al. [8] reported a 0.9% incisional hernia rate in 441 patients without identifying the follow-up time. Our large series of 577 RARP patients with

TABLE 4: Differences in incisional hernia rates as measured by odds ratios from logistic regression models.

Variable	Model 1 OR (95% CI)	Model 2 OR (95% CI)
Prostate weight (5 gm increases)	1.13 (1.04, 1.22)	1.13 (1.05, 1.22)
Prior cholecystectomy	2.75 (1.03, 7.35)	3.10 (1.17, 8.20)
ASA	1.492 (0.81, 2.74)	
BMI category:		
Overweight versus normal/underweight	2.16 (0.86, 5.44)	
Obese versus overweight	0.88 (0.44, 1.78)	
Obese versus normal/underweight	1.90 (0.69, 5.21)	

Model 1 contains main effects for prostate weight, prior cholecystectomy, ASA class, and BMI category. Model 2 contains main effects for prostate weight and prior cholecystectomy.
Odds ratios for prostate weight are for a five gram increase. OR = odds ratio; 95% CI = Wald 95% CI from logistic regression.

long term follow-up (mean of 5.05 years; range of 0.63–10.64 years) raises concerns about the underreporting of incisional hernia after RARP, as the higher incidence of incisional hernia is significant enough to warrant preoperative counseling.

Supporting the possibility of previously unrecognized incidence is a recent report using the SEER database that identified a 5.3% reoperative rate for incisional hernia repair after RARP at median follow-up of 3.1 years [15]. Notably, even though this rate of actual repair was higher than previously reported, the incidence of incisional hernia is likely even higher since not all incisional hernias lead to repair. The rate of reoperative repair from our study (4%) compares similarly with this large series. With a significant portion of patients requiring surgical revision of incisional hernias, urologists need to make their patients more aware of this potential complication when counseling patients for RARP.

With regard to predicted risk factors of incisional hernia such as diabetes, smoking, and BMI, statistical analysis failed to detect any significant difference between the two groups. However, when we classified patients into groups based on BMI, there was a lower rate of incisional hernia in the normal/underweight group (4.7%), whereas the hernia rates in the overweight (10.6%) and obese (10.1%) groups were higher. This can be interpreted as normal weight and is a protective factor compared to being overweight and obese. This study had an inadequate sample size precluding definitive demonstration of being overweight or obese as a significant risk factor for incisional hernia. Nonetheless, obesity remains a recognized risk factor for incisional hernia, as previous studies have identified it as an independent risk factor for incisional hernia formation [13, 19, 20]. Obese patients increased incisional hernia risk is attributed to the difficulty in fascial closure and elevated intra-abdominal pressure [21]. Moreover, these patients are at a higher risk of wound dehiscence predisposing to incisional hernia formation [22]. Additionally, there was a trend towards increasing hernia rates with worsening ASA physical status, albeit not statistically significant.

When comparing prostate weights in those with an incisional hernia and those without, we did find that men with

incisional hernias had statistically significant larger prostates (medians 45 versus 38 grams; $P = 0.001$). As the umbilical incision is often extended to facilitate extraction of the specimen, prostate weight is likely a marker for incision size and particular care should be exercised in closing the fascia in patients with larger specimens. When necessary, the skin incision should likewise be extended to allow appropriate fascial closure.

Additionally, a higher proportion of incisional hernia patients had a history of laparoscopic cholecystectomy when compared to the no hernia group. It is interesting and worth noting that these two procedures share a common specimen extraction site, namely, the umbilical port site. In patients who have undergone previous laparoscopic cholecystectomy, repeat specimen extraction at the same site may contribute to weakening of the periumbilical fascia. This is indirectly supported elsewhere as incisional hernias have been reported to occur more commonly with increasing port size and in cases that use the port site for tissue extraction as in RARP [10]. It is reasonable to consider the potentially deleterious effect that repeat extractions at the same site may have on fascial integrity, and this appears to be an area in need of further investigation.

Regarding surgical technique, all patients in our series had closure of the supraumbilical incision in an interrupted fashion. Yet there is debate in minimally invasive surgery, as some recommend closing the supraumbilical incision in an interrupted suturing technique [11], while others favor the continuous approach [23]. A superior approach between these two has not been clearly elucidated with regards to limiting subsequent hernia formation.

At our institution trocar placement for a RARP traditionally includes a 5 mm port, three 8 mm ports, and another 12 mm lateral port. Both port site hernias in our series involved the 12 mm lateral port sites. The current results are consistent with a large systematic review of 19 studies, which showed that the incidence of trocar site hernias ranged from 0 to 5.2%, with an overall estimated incidence of 0.5% [24]. Review of the literature on laparoscopic surgery shows some authors recommending that all 12 mm port sites be closed [8, 25, 26]. However, controversy exists as others suggest that bladeless trocars, including the 12 mm ports, do not necessitate routine fascial closure. Rubenstein and colleagues reported no incisional hernias when they did not close the fascia of 12 mm ports in 112 port sites [27]. Additionally, Kang et al. reported no lateral 12 mm port site hernia in 498 patients where only the fascia of 12 mm midline port site was closed [10]. Despite these findings, closure of all 12 mm ports in our institution is routine.

Although our study is one of the largest reviews of postoperative incisional hernias in RARP patients with a mean follow-up of 5 years, it has limitations. Self-report of hernias is subject to error especially given the time frame between the surgery and survey completion. Survey questions may have been misinterpreted by the patient and limitations such as missing data are inherent with medical record review. Additionally, we had a relatively low questionnaire response rate of 36%, the effect of which is difficult to determine. With our high incisional hernia rate, it is possible that symptomatic patients were more apt to participate in our survey, or inversely that asymptomatic patients remain further undiagnosed. Regrettably we were unable to compare patient characteristics between responders and nonresponders and the possibility of selection bias cannot be excluded. Notwithstanding, those responding do represent a fairly sizeable number of patients and the data generated does point to both specimen size and prior cholecystectomy as significant risk factors for umbilical hernia formation, for which significance remained on multivariate analysis.

With regard to predisposing factors, we were unable to evaluate all technical factors, such as entry techniques, trocar design, and suture. All but one surgeon in our institution used a vertical incision at the supraumbilical camera port site. In an effort to reduce the rate of incisional hernias at the umbilicus, Beck and colleagues recently noted a significant reduction in midline camera port incisional hernias with the use of a transverse incision (0.6%) over a vertical incision (5.3%) [13]. The type of suture used to close the supraumbilical incision varied by surgeon and included nonabsorbable as well as absorbable suture. A large meta-analysis of randomized controlled trials of abdominal fascial closures showed level 1 evidence that there is a lower rate of incisional hernia when using a nonabsorbable suture [23]. Incisions were all closed with interrupted suture however. Our inability to evaluate proposed risk factors such as prior laparoscopic cholecystectomy and larger median prostate independent of other potential risk factors such as supraumbilical incision orientation and type of suture is a limitation of the study.

5. Conclusion

This study raises concerns about underreporting of incisional hernia after RARP. It is a complication often requiring surgical revision, and as such merits inclusion in preoperative counseling. Umbilical extraction site is not only where incisional hernias most likely occur but also where the vast majority of hernias significant enough to warrant repair are located. Factors such as larger prostate weight and previous laparoscopic procedures such as cholecystectomy directly affect the umbilical extraction site and may predispose to incisional hernia at this location.

Disclosure

Jason Hafron is a speaker for Myriad and Genomic. He is a trial investigator for Dendreon, Oncocell, and Cellay. He is also on the advisory board for Astellas. Kenneth M. Peters is a consultant for Medtronic, Taris, and Stimguard.

Conflict of Interests

The authors declare that there is no conflict of interests regarding the publication of this paper.

Acknowledgment

The authors acknowledge the Ministrelli Program for Urology Research and Educatio (MPURE).

References

[1] V. R. Patel and A. Sivaraman, "Current status of robot-assisted radical prostatectomy: progress is inevitable," *Oncology*, vol. 26, pp. 616–619, 2012.

[2] D. G. Murphy, M. Kerger, H. Crowe, J. S. Peters, and A. J. Costello, "Operative details and oncological and functional outcome of robotic-assisted laparoscopic radical prostatectomy: 400 cases with a minimum 12 months follow up," *European Urology*, vol. 55, no. 6, pp. 1358–1367, 2009.

[3] S. T. Brown and P. B. Goodfellow, "Transverse verses midline incisions for abdominal surgery," *Cochrane Database of Systematic Reviews*, no. 4, Article ID CD005199, 2005.

[4] D. Dindo, N. Demartines, and P.-A. Clavien, "Classification of surgical complications: a new proposal with evaluation in a cohort of 6336 patients and results of a survey," *Annals of Surgery*, vol. 240, no. 2, pp. 205–213, 2004.

[5] A. M. Blatt, A. Fadahunsi, C. Ahn et al., "Surgical complications related to robotic prostatectomy: prospective analysis," *The Journal of Urology*, vol. 181, no. 4, article 353, 2009.

[6] M. Menon, A. Shrivastava, S. Kaul et al., "Vattikuti institute prostatectomy: contemporary technique and analysis of results," *European Urology*, vol. 51, no. 3, pp. 648–658, 2007.

[7] L. Martinez-Pineiro, F. Cáceres, C. Sánchez et al., "Learning curve of laparoscopic radical prostatectomy in a university teaching hospital: experience after the first 600 cases," *European Urology Supplements*, vol. 5, no. 1, pp. 914–924, 2006.

[8] E. Chiong, P. K. Hegarty, J. W. Davis, A. M. Kamat, L. L. Pisters, and S. F. Matin, "Port-site hernias occurring after the use of bladeless radially expanding trocars," *Urology*, vol. 75, no. 3, pp. 574–580, 2010.

[9] V. R. Patel, K. J. Palmer, G. Coughlin, and S. Samavedi, "Robot-assisted laparoscopic radical prostatectomy: perioperative outcomes of 1500 cases," *Journal of Endourology*, vol. 22, no. 10, pp. 2299–2305, 2008.

[10] D. I. Kang, S. H. Woo, D. H. Lee, and I. Y. Kim, "Incidence of port-site hernias after robot-assisted radical prostatectomy with the fascial closure of only the midline 12-mm port site," *Journal of Endourology*, vol. 26, no. 7, pp. 848–851, 2012.

[11] A. Fuller, A. Fernandez, and S. E. Pautler, "Incisional hernia after robot-assisted radical prostatectomy—predisposing factors in a prospective cohort of 250 cases," *Journal of Endourology*, vol. 25, no. 6, pp. 1021–1024, 2011.

[12] B. M. Lin, M. E. Hyndman, K. E. Steele et al., "Incidence and risk factors for inguinal and incisional hernia after laparoscopic radical prostatectomy," *Urology*, vol. 77, no. 4, pp. 957–962, 2011.

[13] S. Beck, D. Skarecky, K. Osann, R. Juarez, and T. E. Ahlering, "Transverse versus vertical camera port incision in robotic radical prostatectomy: effect on incisional hernias and cosmesis," *Urology*, vol. 78, no. 3, pp. 586–590, 2011.

[14] M. Mudge and L. E. Hughes, "Incisional hernia: a 10 year prospective study of incidence and attitudes," *British Journal of Surgery*, vol. 72, no. 1, pp. 70–71, 1985.

[15] S. V. Carlsson, B. Ehdaie, C. L. Atoria, E. B. Elkin, and J. A. Eastham, "Risk of incisional hernia after minimally invasive and open radical prostatectomy," *The Journal of Urology*, vol. 190, no. 5, pp. 1757–1762, 2013.

[16] H. Tonouchi, Y. Ohmori, M. Kobayashi, and M. Kusunoki, "Trocar site hernia," *Archives of Surgery*, vol. 139, no. 11, pp. 1248–1256, 2004.

[17] L. A. Israelsson and T. Jonsson, "Incisional hernia after midline laparotomy: a prospective study," *European Journal of Surgery*, vol. 162, no. 2, pp. 125–129, 1996.

[18] P. J. Osther, P. Gjode, B. B. Mortensen, P. B. Mortensen, J. Bartholin, and F. Gottrup, "Randomized comparison of polyglycolic acid and polyglyconate sutures for abdominal fascial closure after laparotomy in patients with suspected impaired wound healing," *British Journal of Surgery*, vol. 82, no. 8, pp. 1080–1082, 1995.

[19] R. Veljkovic, M. Protic, A. Gluhovic, Z. Potic, Z. Milosevic, and A. Stojadinovic, "Prospective clinical trial of factors predicting the early development of incisional hernia after midline laparotom," *Journal of the American College of Surgeons*, vol. 210, no. 2, pp. 210–219, 2010.

[20] T. E. Bucknall, P. J. Cox, and H. Ellis, "Burst abdomen and incisional hernia: a prospective study of 1129 major laparotomies," *British Medical Journal*, vol. 284, no. 6320, pp. 931–933, 1982.

[21] G. M. Eid and J. Collins, "Application of a trocar wound closure system designed for laparoscopic procedures in morbidly obese patients," *Obesity Surgery*, vol. 15, no. 6, pp. 871–873, 2005.

[22] R. P. Merkow, K. Y. Bilimoria, M. D. McCarter, and D. J. Bentrem, "Effect of body mass index on short-term outcomes after colectomy for cancer," *Journal of the American College of Surgeons*, vol. 208, no. 1, pp. 53–61, 2009.

[23] N. C. F. Hodgson, R. A. Malthaner, and T. Østbye, "The search for an ideal method of abdominal fascial closure: a meta-analysis," *Annals of Surgery*, vol. 231, no. 3, pp. 436–442, 2000.

[24] F. Helgstrand, J. Rosenberg, and T. Bisgaard, "Trocar site hernia after laparoscopic surgery: a qualitative systematic review," *Hernia*, vol. 15, no. 2, pp. 113–121, 2011.

[25] Z. Shaher, "Port closure techniques," *Surgical Endoscopy*, vol. 21, no. 8, pp. 1264–1274, 2007.

[26] E. J. Kouba, J. S. Hubbard, E. Wallen, and R. S. Pruthi, "Incisional hernia in a 12-mm non-bladed trocar site following laparoscopic nephrectomy," *Urologia Internationalis*, vol. 79, no. 3, pp. 276–278, 2007.

[27] J. N. Rubenstein, L. W. Blunt Jr., W. W. Lin, H. M. User, R. B. Nadler, and C. M. Gonzalez, "Safety and efficacy of 12-mm radial dilating ports for laparoscopic access," *BJU International*, vol. 92, no. 3, pp. 327–329, 2003.

28

Pathological Characteristics of Primary Bladder Carcinoma Treated at a Tertiary Care Hospital and Changing Demographics of Bladder Cancer in Sri Lanka

S. Sasikumar,[1] K. S. N. Wijayarathna,[1] K. A. M. S. Karunaratne,[2] U. Gobi,[1] A. Pathmeswaran,[3] and Anuruddha M. Abeygunasekera[1]

[1]*Urology Unit, Colombo South Teaching Hospital, 10350 Dehiwala, Sri Lanka*
[2]*Department of Pathology, Colombo South Teaching Hospital, 10350 Dehiwala, Sri Lanka*
[3]*Department of Public Health, Faculty of Medicine, University of Kelaniya, 11010 Ragama, Sri Lanka*

Correspondence should be addressed to S. Sasikumar; msssasii@gmail.com

Academic Editor: Fabio Campodonico

Objectives. The aim was to compare demographics and pathological features of bladder carcinoma treated in a urology unit with findings of previous studies done in Sri Lanka. *Materials and Methods.* Data of newly diagnosed patients with bladder cancer in a tertiary referral centre from 2011 to 2014 were analysed. Data on bladder cancers diagnosed from 1993 to 2014 were obtained from previous publications and Sri Lanka Cancer Registry. *Results.* There were 148 patients and mean age was 65 years. Male to female ratio was 4.1 : 1. Urothelial carcinoma (UC) was found in 89.2% of patients. Muscle invasion was noted in 35% of patients compared to 48.4% two decades ago. In patients with UC, 16.5% were found to have pT_1 high grade tumour. It was 5.3% from 1993 to 2000. Pure squamous cell carcinoma was found in 8.1% of patients while primary or de novo carcinoma in situ (not associated with high grade pT_1 tumours) was seen in one patient only. *Conclusions.* The percentage of squamous carcinoma is higher among Sri Lankan patients while primary carcinoma in situ is a rarity. The percentage of muscle invasive disease has decreased while the percentage of pT_1 high grade tumours has increased during the last two decades in Sri Lanka.

1. Introduction

Sri Lanka is an island nation in South Asia, the others being India, Pakistan, Bangladesh, Nepal, Bhutan, and Maldives. Twenty-three urological surgeons serve the country's population of 20 million. Sri Lanka has been categorized as a middle income country recently and has a National Health Service which is free at the point of delivery. Though National Health Service provides healthcare to the vast majority of people, there are private sector hospitals which provide services to the more affluent. Average life expectancy at birth is 75 years in Sri Lanka and the country spends 3.3% of its gross domestic product for health [1]. Prostate and bladder cancers contribute to most of the urological cancers in Sri Lanka [2].

Bladder cancer is the seventh most common malignancy worldwide and the fourth common cancer in men [3]. In South Asia, reported rate of bladder cancer is about 2.1 per 100 000 [3]. In Sri Lanka it is 0.8 per 100 000 according to the Cancer Registry data compiled by the National Cancer Control Programme of Sri Lanka (NCCPSL) which is based on patients registered at oncology units of the country [2]. Hence incidence of bladder cancer appears to be low in Sri Lanka compared to rates in other South Asian countries such as India (3.2 per 100 000) and Karachi, Pakistan (8.9 per 100 000) [4, 5]. In Delhi, India, the age adjusted bladder cancer incidence reaches 5.8/100 000 [6].

Bladder cancer shows a male predominance with a sex ratio of 3 : 1 [3]. The spectrum of bladder cancer is diverse, but the majority (nearly 90%) are urothelial tumours. The other tumours are squamous cell carcinoma, adenocarcinoma, and rare varieties like small cell carcinoma. Clinical stage and grade are the two most important determinants of the prognosis of bladder cancer [7]. Previous studies show varying results in relation to sex ratio, proportion of muscle invasive disease, and histological types of bladder cancer in Sri Lanka and in neighbouring South Asian countries [2, 8–18]. Therefore the aims of our study were to identify the clinical and pathological characteristics of bladder cancer treated at a single urology unit in a tertiary hospital of Sri Lanka and to identify changes in demographics and pathological features of bladder carcinoma during the last two decades in Sri Lanka by perusing already published data. Since Sri Lankan Cancer Registry data is based only on patients registered at oncology units of the country, we aimed to compare its data with the data obtained from urology units of Sri Lanka to determine the accuracy and reliability of the available data regarding bladder cancer in Sri Lanka.

2. Materials and Methods

This descriptive study was performed on newly diagnosed primary bladder cancer patients at a urology unit of a tertiary care hospital (Colombo South Teaching Hospital, Sri Lanka) between 1 January 2011 and 31 December 2014. The data were collected from the bladder cancer register maintained in the unit. All consecutive patients who underwent their first transurethral resection of bladder tumour in the unit were included in the study. Pathological grading was assessed according to the World Health Organisation (WHO) and International Society of Urological Pathology (ISUP) classification 2004 [19]. Every attempt was taken to perform a complete resection of the tumour during the first surgery. Once the histology was available, those who did not have muscle tissue in the specimen were scheduled to have re-resection in six weeks' time. Thereafter patients were referred to the oncologist for appropriate further treatment. A contrast enhanced CT scan of kidneys, ureter, and bladder (KUB) was done in patients with muscle invasive disease.

All publications on bladder cancer in Sri Lanka after 1993 were identified by searching PubMed database as well as by perusing Sri Lankan journals manually which are not indexed in PubMed. Data on clinical and histopathological features of bladder cancers diagnosed from 1993 to 2014 were obtained from those publications and Sri Lanka Cancer Registry [2, 8–13, 20]. There were only three urology units in 1993 and by the end of 2014 there were 16 urology units treating bladder cancers in Sri Lanka. Statistical analysis was done using the Chi-square test. A $p < 0.05$ was considered statistically significant. Approval for the study was obtained from the Ethics Committee of the Institute.

3. Results

There were 148 patients with newly diagnosed primary bladder malignancies during the study period of four years. One urachal carcinoma and one inflammatory myofibroblastic tumour of the bladder treated during the study period were not included in the study. Two more patients had metastatic deposits in the bladder from a breast carcinoma and a melanoma. They were also excluded from the study. Average age of the study cohort was 65 years (range 28–88) and 91% were more than 50 years old (Figure 1). The mean age was

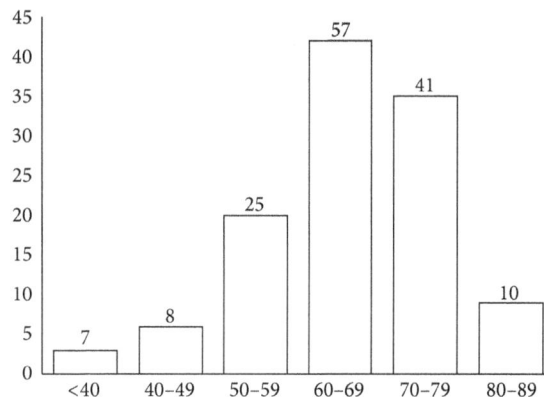

FIGURE 1: Age distribution of patients with bladder cancer.

similar to that of other studies done in Sri Lanka from 1993 to 2011 (Table 1).

There were 119 men with a male to female ratio of 4.1 : 1. The male to female ratio was 5.5 : 1 and 9 : 1 in two studies done at National Hospital of Sri Lanka (NHSL) [11, 12]. Haematuria was the most common clinical presentation encountered in 81% (120/148) of patients. Others presented with lower abdominal pain (7%), lower urinary tract symptoms (7%) and found incidentally (5%). The initial investigation which indicated the diagnosis was urinary tract ultrasonography in 115 (77.7%) patients.

There were 132 (89.2%) urothelial tumours (Table 2). The proportion of urothelial tumours in the previous studies done in urology units of Sri Lanka ranges from 90.9% to 97% (Table 2). However according to the Cancer Registry maintained by NCCPSL, only 72% and 69% were urothelial tumours during the period from 2001 to 2005 and in 2006, respectively [10, 13]. This difference was statistically significant ($p < 0.05$).

Staging could not be completed in 5 patients with urothelial carcinoma as they could not come for re-resection at six weeks when there was inadequate muscle in the initial specimen. Therefore 127 patients with urothelial carcinoma were included in the analysis for staging. Majority (54.3%) of the urothelial tumours were in the T_1 stage (Table 3). About 35% of the staged patients had muscle invasive disease. According to the study done by Goonewardena et al. at NHSL from 1993 to 2000, 48.4% were muscle invasive tumours at initial presentation (Table 1) [11]. According to the data from the Cancer Registry of the NCCPSL, 94% had muscle invasive disease (Table 3) [10].

There were 21 high grade malignancies among the 69 T_1 stage urothelial tumours (Table 3). Therefore in our study, the percentage of pT_1 high grade tumour among urothelial cancers was 16.5% and is closer to the findings of a study done at NHSL in 2010 which was 18% [9]. A study done in the same urology unit of the NHSL from 1993 to 2000 showed the pT_1 high grade tumour to be only 5.3% and this difference was statistically significant ($p < 0.005$) [11]. Among muscle invasive urothelial cancers, 86.4% (38/44) were high grade tumours.

TABLE 1: Summary of results from published studies on bladder cancer in Sri Lanka.

Study (Time period of study and authors)	1993–2000 Goonewardena et al. [11]	2000-2001 Perera et al. [12]	2001–2005 Ranasinghe et al. [10] and NCCPSL [20]	2006 NCCPSL [13]	2007 NCCPSL [2]	2009 Sathesan et al. [8]	2010 Prabath et al. [9]	2011–2014 Present study
Male : female ratio	5.5 : 1	9 : 1	4 : 1	3 : 1	3.2 : 1	3.1 : 1	3.7 : 1	4.1 : 1
Average age	64	Not available	Median age group 62–64	65	Median age group 65–69	Median age 65	Median age 67.5	65
Urothelial carcinoma	93.4%	96%	72%	69.5%	79%	97%	90.9%	89.2%
Squamous carcinoma	3%	Not available	9%	9%	8%	0%	6.1%	8.1%
Adeno carcinoma	1.3%	Not available	3%	5%	4%	0%	0%	1.4%
Muscle invasive tumour	48.4%	30.9%	94%	Not available	Not available	37.3%	21.2%	35%
Primary carcinoma-in-situ	None	Not available	1.9%	None	None	None	None	0.7%
pT_1 high grade tumour	5.3%	Not available	Not available	Not available	Not available	3%	18%	16.5%
Total number of patients	301	139	637	131	151	35	33	148

NCCPSL = Cancer Registry of National Cancer Control Programme of Sri Lanka.

TABLE 2: Histological classification of tumours included in the study cohort.

Tumour type	Number
Urothelial tumours ($n = 132$)	
Infiltrating urothelial carcinoma	105
With squamous differentiation	11
With glandular differentiation	1
Micropapillary	1
Noninvasive urothelial neoplasms (14)	
Urothelial carcinoma in situ	1
Noninvasive papillary urothelial carcinoma, low grade	12
Noninvasive papillary urothelial neoplasm of low malignant potential	1
Squamous neoplasms ($n = 12$)	
Squamous cell carcinoma	12
Glandular neoplasms ($n = 2$)	
Adenocarcinoma (enteric type)	2
Mesenchymal tumours ($n = 1$)	
Leiomyosarcoma	1
Haematopoietic and lymphoid tumours ($n = 1$)	
Lymphoma (large B cell)	1
Total	**148**

Urothelial carcinoma with squamous differentiation was found in 11 (7.4%) of patients and all those patients were found to have muscle invasive and high grade tumour in our study. There were one urothelial tumour with glandular differentiation and one micropapillary variety. Among noninvasive urothelial carcinomas there was one primary (de novo) urothelial carcinoma in situ and one noninvasive papillary urothelial neoplasm of low malignant potential in our study (Table 3). Cancer Registry data from 2001 to 2005

shows only 10 cases (1.9%) of carcinoma in situ of the bladder [20]. None of the other published studies done in Sri Lanka show any cases of primary or de novo urothelial carcinoma in situ of the bladder (Table 1). Therefore primary carcinoma in situ not associated with pT_1 high grade tumours is extremely rare in Sri Lanka.

Squamous cell carcinoma was present in 8.1% (12/148) of patients. None of the patients with squamous cell carcinoma had bladder stones at the time of diagnosis while only one had

Pathological Characteristics of Primary Bladder Carcinoma Treated at a Tertiary...

221

TABLE 3: Different pT stages of urothelial tumours.

Stage	Number
pT_a ($n = 14$)	
Low grade	12
High grade	2
pT_1 ($n = 69$)	
Low grade	48
High grade	21
$\geq pT_2$ ($n = 44$)	
Low grade	6
High grade	38
Uncertain	5
Total	**132**

surgery for bladder stones done 20 years ago. Furthermore they had not travelled outside Sri Lanka. Although the percentage of urothelial tumours in the present study was similar to published data from other urology units, the percentage of squamous cell carcinoma in the present study (8.1%) was significantly higher ($p = 0.009$) than the percentage (3%) reported from NHSL (Table 1) [11, 12]. According to the Cancer Registry, percentage of squamous cell carcinoma in Sri Lanka was 9% which was closer to the percentage of the present study [2, 13].

In the present study there were two patients (1.4%) with adenocarcinoma of bladder, which was in par with the 1.3% of the study done at NHSL [11]. Both were of enteric type. There was one lymphoma and immunohistochemistry showed it to be a large B cell lymphoma. A 34-year-old female patient had a leiomyosarcoma of the bladder.

4. Discussion

The average age at diagnosis of bladder cancer patients in Sri Lanka is similar to that of India which is around 65 [15]. In Pakistan the mean age of bladder cancer is around 55–58 years [17, 18]. In the present study male to female ratio was 4.1 : 1, compared to the ratio of 3 : 1 quoted worldwide [3, 21]. In India the male to female ratio is 8.6 : 1 [16]. All Sri Lankan studies show a higher male preponderance similar to other South Asian countries than described in the western countries [16–18]. Low prevalence of smoking among women in Sri Lanka could be the reason for this difference [1].

The proportion of urothelial tumours among bladder cancers in our study cohort (89.2%) is less than those of India and Pakistan which are over 95% [15–18]. The reason for this is the higher percentage of squamous cell carcinoma seen in Sri Lanka. In the western world the percentage of squamous cell carcinoma among bladder cancers is around 1–3%, depending on the ethnicity of the population [16, 22]. The present study involving 148 patients and data from National Cancer Registry show a significantly higher percentage (around 8%) of squamous cell carcinoma. Even in neighbouring India percentage of squamous cell carcinoma among bladder cancers is low [16]. While the percentage of urothelial carcinoma and adenocarcinoma remain the same among studies, the reason

for the significantly high percentage of squamous cell carcinoma of the bladder among patients treated outside NHSL is unclear. Since schistosomiasis is not found in Sri Lanka, the reason for high percentage of squamous cell carcinoma of bladder is only speculative. One plausible explanation could be the agrochemicals that are being used commonly in Sri Lanka by its semiurban and rural populations. Sri Lanka has one of the highest rates of pesticide use in the world and is believed to be a reason for the high incidence of chronic kidney disease of uncertain origin in Sri Lanka [23, 24].

Stage pT_1 high grade urothelial tumour also known as high grade lamina-invasive bladder cancer is unique in its aggressive behaviour [25]. It shows a high recurrence rate and commonly progresses to invasive disease [26]. The percentage of pT_1 high grade tumours has increased over the last two decades in Sri Lanka (Table 1). One possible reason for this difference could be the change in the pathological grading system over the years from 1973 WHO classification to 2004 WHO classification. The 1973 WHO classification which was used in the earlier study had three different grades of anaplasia (G1, G2, and G3 or high grade) while the 2004 WHO classification which was used in the present study has only two grades of anaplasia (low and high grades).

According to a study done at NHSL from 1993 to 2000, the percentage of muscle invasive tumours at initial presentation was 48.4% but the corresponding value was 35% in the present study (Table 1) [11]. The percentage of muscle invasive disease in our study (35%) is similar to that of Manipur in India (36.36%) and Pakistan (37.6%) [14, 18]. This gradual decline in the percentage of muscle invasive tumours could be due to the early diagnosis of the disease due to improving healthcare facilities and urological services in Sri Lanka. It is known that the depth of tumour invasion in the bladder wall could be time dependent [27].

Urothelial tumours with squamous or adenodifferentiation are more aggressive and are at a higher stage at initial presentation [28]. In the present study there were eleven patients with squamous differentiation and one patient with glandular differentiation and all patients had muscle invasive, high grade tumours at presentation. Percentage of adenocarcinoma among patients with bladder cancer in Sri Lanka is in par with the percentage seen in the western world which is around 2% [29]. However the occurrence of primary carcinoma in situ not associated with pT_1 high grade tumours in the bladder appears to be extremely rare in Sri Lanka similar to India [14]. The reason for the very low incidence of primary carcinoma in situ in South Asian countries is unknown. A protective factor in the South Asian diet rich in spices or a genetic variation is a possible reason.

Many patients with noninvasive bladder cancer do not seek services of oncology units of Sri Lanka. They prefer to stay away from oncology units due to sociocultural reasons and stigma attached to cancer patients in South Asian countries like Sri Lanka. Hence their data are not included in the Cancer Registry of the NCCPSL. This could be the reason for the unusually high rate of muscle invasive disease and the lower percentage of urothelial tumours in the Cancer Registry of the NCCPSL when compared to data from urology units of the country.

Maintaining a comprehensive bladder Cancer Registry is essential to analyse the changing patterns of prevalence, incidence, survival, and mortality of malignancies. The different findings among the institutional studies need to be compared with nationwide trends. As the National Cancer Registry is based on data collected from oncology units and reporting of cancers by clinicians is not mandatory in the country, the data seems to be incomplete as evidenced by our analysis which shows significant differences in the patterns of the Cancer Registry and those of urology units. In Sri Lanka initial surgical management (transurethral resection of bladder tumour) of bladder tumours is always done in urology units and data from urology units are more likely to be representative in relation to clinicopathological characteristics. Therefore conclusions should not be made purely based on Cancer Registry data of Sri Lanka. Until a comprehensive electronic database is established, it is important for individual urology units in Sri Lanka to maintain their own cancer audits. It is time for all cancer patients in Sri Lanka to be referred to oncologists during treatment irrespective of the stage. When Sri Lankan healthcare planners use data, they must rely on a combination of data from Cancer Registry as well as individual units. Otherwise interpretations made could be erroneous and biased. Therefore with comparatively high smoking rates [1] and possible underreporting to oncology units, the incidence of bladder cancer is likely to be higher than the reported rate (0.8 per 100 000) in the National Cancer Registry of Sri Lanka.

In conclusion, the percentage of muscle invasive disease has decreased while the percentage of pT_1 high grade tumours has increased during the last two decades in Sri Lanka. The incidence of squamous cell carcinoma is higher among Sri Lankan patients with bladder carcinoma while primary carcinoma in situ is a rarity. The reasons for some of these differences are uncertain and warrant further research in the identified areas.

Conflict of Interests

The authors declare that there is no conflict of interests.

References

[1] World Health Organization, *World Health Statistics 2014*, World Health Organization, Geneva, Switzerland, 2014.

[2] *Cancer Incidence Data: Sri Lanka Year 2007*, National Cancer Control Programme, 2013.

[3] J. Ferlay, H. R. Shin, F. Bray, D. Forman, C. Mathers, and D. M. Parkin, "GLOBOCAN 2008: cancer incidence and mortality worldwide," IARC CancerBase no. 10, International Agency for Research on Cancer, Lyon, France, 2010, http://globocan.iarc.fr.

[4] T. Rastogi, S. Devesa, P. Mangtani et al., "Cancer incidence rates among South Asians in four geographic regions: India, Singapore, UK and US," *International Journal of Epidemiology*, vol. 37, no. 1, pp. 147–160, 2008.

[5] Y. Bhurgri, A. Bhurgri, S. H. Hassan et al., "Cancer incidence in Karachi, Pakistan: first results from Karachi Cancer Registry," *International Journal of Cancer*, vol. 85, no. 3, pp. 325–329, 2000.

[6] V. Raina, B. B. Tyagi, and N. Manoharan, *New Delhi: 2002-2003. Cancer Incidence and Mortality in Delhi UT-Urban Delhi Cancer Registry*, Dr. BR Ambedkar Institute Rotary Cancer Hospital, All India Institute of Medical Sciences, New Delhi, India, 2003.

[7] M. V. Khochikar, "Rationale for an early detection program for bladder cancer," *Indian Journal of Urology*, vol. 27, no. 2, pp. 218–225, 2011.

[8] B. Sathesan, A. P. I. Prabath, and S. A. S. Goonewardena, "Urological malignancies: one-year audit from a tertiary referral centre," *Sri Lanka Journal of Urology*, vol. 10, pp. 24–27, 2009.

[9] A. P. I. Prabath and S. A. S. Goonewardena, "Pattern of urological malignancies in 2010—an audit from a tertiary referral centre," *Sri Lanka Journal of Urology*, vol. 11, no. 1, pp. 30–35, 2010.

[10] W. K. B. Ranasinghe, D. de Silva, M. V. C. de Silva et al., "Incidence of bladder cancer in Sri Lanka: analysis of the cancer registry data and review of the incidence of bladder cancer in the South Asian population," *Korean Journal of Urology*, vol. 53, no. 5, pp. 304–309, 2012.

[11] S. A. S. Goonewardena, W. A. S. De Silva, and M. V. C. De Silva, "Bladder cancer in Sri Lanka: experience from a tertiary referral center," *International Journal of Urology*, vol. 11, no. 11, pp. 969–972, 2004.

[12] N. D. Perera, "Characterisation of a bladder cancer cohort in a urological unit." *The Ceylon medical journal*, vol. 47, no. 3, p. 102, 2002.

[13] National Cancer Control Programme, *Cancer Incidence Data: Sri Lanka Year 2006*, 2012.

[14] R. S. Laishram, P. Kipgen, S. Laishram, S. Khuraijam, and D. C. Sharma, "Urothelial tumors of the urinary bladder in manipur: a histopathological perspective," *Asian Pacific Journal of Cancer Prevention*, vol. 13, no. 6, pp. 2477–2479, 2012.

[15] B. R. Roy, M. Sristidhar, G. Debasish, B. Keya, and K. Dilip, "An epidemiological study of cases of urothelial carcinoma of urinary bladder in a tertiary care centre," *Journal of Krishna Institute of Medical Sciences University*, vol. 2, no. 1, pp. 82–88, 2013.

[16] P. Gupta, M. Jain, R. Kapoor, K. Muruganandham, A. Srivastava, and A. Mandhani, "Impact of age and gender on the clinicopathological characteristics of bladder cancer," *Indian Journal of Urology*, vol. 25, no. 2, pp. 207–210, 2009.

[17] M. Rafique and A. A. Javed, "Clinico-pathological features of bladder carcinoma: experience from a tertiary care hospital of Pakistan," *International Urology and Nephrology*, vol. 38, no. 2, pp. 247–250, 2006.

[18] Z. Ahmed, S. Muzaffer, M. Khan et al., "Transitional cell carcinomas of the urinary bladder. A histopathological study," *The Journal of the Pakistan Medical Association*, vol. 52, no. 9, pp. 396–398, 2002.

[19] J. N. Eble, G. Sauter, J. I. Epstein, and I. A. Sesterhenn, Eds., *World Health Organization Classification of Tumors. Pathology and Genetics of Tumors of the Urinary System and Male Genital Organs*, IARC Press, Lyon, France, 2004.

[20] National Cancer Control Programme, *Cancer Incidence Data: Sri Lanka Year 2001–2005*, 2009.

[21] S. L. Johansson and S. M. Cohen, "Epidemiology and etiology of bladder cancer," *Seminars in Surgical Oncology*, vol. 13, no. 5, pp. 291–298, 1997.

[22] D. J. Grignon, M. N. El-Bolkainy, B. J. Schmitz-Dräger, R. Simon, and J. E. Tyczynski, "Squamous cell carcinoma," in *World Health Organisation Classification of Tumours. Pathology*

and Genetics of Tumours of the Urinary System and Male Genital Organs, J. N. Eble, G. Sauter, J. I. Epstein, and I. A. Sesterhenn, Eds., pp. 124–126, IARC Press, Lyon, France, 2004.

[23] N. Jayatilake, S. Mendis, P. Maheepala, and F. R. Mehta, "Chronic kidney disease of uncertain aetiology: prevalence and causative factors in a developing country," BMC Nephrology, vol. 14, no. 1, article 180, 2013.

[24] S. Jayasinghe, "Chronic kidney disease of unknown etiology should be renamed chronic agrochemical nephropathy," MEDICC Review, vol. 16, no. 2, pp. 72–74, 2014.

[25] A. Mandhani, "Proactive approach to treat high-grade lamina-invasive bladder cancer," Indian Journal of Urology, vol. 27, no. 2, pp. 233–237, 2011.

[26] T. Lebret, D. Bohin, Z. Kassardjian et al., "Recurrence, progression and success in stage Ta grade 3 bladder tumors treated with low dose bacillus Calmette-Guerin instillations," The Journal of Urology, vol. 163, no. 1, pp. 63–67, 2000.

[27] D. M. A. Wallace, R. T. Bryan, J. A. Dunn, G. Begum, and S. Bathers, "Delay and survival in bladder cancer," British Journal of Urology International, vol. 89, no. 9, pp. 868–878, 2002.

[28] A. Billis, A. A. Schenka, C. C. O. Ramos, L. T. Carneiro, and V. Araújo, "Squamous and/or glandular differentiation in urothelial carcinoma: prevalence and significance in transurethral resections of the bladder," International Urology and Nephrology, vol. 33, no. 4, pp. 631–633, 2001.

[29] E. Jacobo, S. Loening, J. D. Schmidt, and D. A. Culp, "Primary adenocarcinoma of the bladder: a retrospective study of 20 patients," The Journal of Urology, vol. 117, no. 1, pp. 54–56, 1977.

29

Reduced Cardiovascular Capacity and Resting Metabolic Rate in Men with Prostate Cancer Undergoing Androgen Deprivation: A Comprehensive Cross-Sectional Investigation

Bradley A. Wall,[1,2] Daniel A. Galvão,[2] Naeem Fatehee,[2] Dennis R. Taaffe,[2,3] Nigel Spry,[2,4,5] David Joseph,[2,4,5] and Robert U. Newton[2,6]

[1]*School of Psychology and Exercise Science, Murdoch University, Murdoch, WA 6150, Australia*
[2]*Exercise Medicine Research Institute, Edith Cowan University, Joondalup, WA 6027, Australia*
[3]*School of Medicine, University of Wollongong, Wollongong, NSW 2522, Australia*
[4]*Department of Radiation Oncology, Sir Charles Gairdner Hospital, Nedlands, WA 6009, Australia*
[5]*Faculty of Medicine, University of Western Australia, Nedlands, WA 6009, Australia*
[6]*Centre for Clinical Research, The University of Queensland, Herston, QLD 4006, Australia*

Correspondence should be addressed to Bradley A. Wall; b.wall@murdoch.edu.au

Academic Editor: In Ho Chang

Objectives. To investigate if androgen deprivation therapy exposure is associated with additional risk factors for cardiovascular disease and metabolic treatment-related toxicities. *Methods*. One hundred and seven men (42–89 years) with prostate cancer undergoing androgen deprivation therapy completed a maximal graded objective exercise test to determine maximal oxygen uptake, assessments for resting metabolic rate, body composition, blood pressure and arterial stiffness, and blood biomarker analysis. A cross-sectional analysis was undertaken to investigate the potential impact of therapy exposure with participants stratified into two groups according to duration of androgen deprivation therapy (<3 months and ≥3 months). *Results*. Maximal oxygen uptake (26.1 ± 6.0 mL/kg/min versus 23.2 ± 5.8 mL/kg/min, $p = 0.020$) and resting metabolic rate (1795 ± 256 kcal/d versus 1647 ± 236 kcal/d, $p = 0.005$) were significantly higher in those with shorter exposure to androgen deprivation. There were no differences between groups for peripheral and central blood pressure, arterial stiffness, or metabolic profile. *Conclusion*. Three months or longer exposure to androgen deprivation therapy was associated with reduced cardiorespiratory capacity and resting metabolic rate, but not in a range of blood biomarkers. These findings suggest that prolonged exposure to androgen deprivation therapy is associated with negative alterations in cardiovascular outcomes. Trial registry is: ACTRN12609000200280.

1. Introduction

Androgen deprivation therapy (ADT) is a commonly used treatment for prostate cancer [1]. Although ADT improves prostate cancer survival, a number of studies have reported associations between ADT and treatment-related toxicities, such as increased risk of cardiovascular disease (CVD) and metabolic complications which can compromise survival and quality of life [2–4]. Moreover, several toxicities have been reported to be present soon after initiation of treatment. For example, increased arterial stiffness and adverse body compositional changes were associated with increasing

insulin concentrations after 6 months of ADT treatment suggestive of impaired insulin sensitivity [5], and others have reported increases in serum insulin levels after only 3 months of ADT exposure [6]. ADT-related decline in physical function, grip strength, and self-reported physical function has been previously reported by Alibhai et al. [7] when compared with non-ADT controls; ADT users also had worse role physical function, bodily pain, and vitality. Importantly, these reductions in objective and self-reported measures of physical function were apparent within the first 3 months of initiating ADT treatment and persisted for at least 12 months.

Metabolic implications of long-term ADT have been previously explored by Basaria et al. [3], who found men receiving >12 months ADT developed insulin resistance and hyperglycaemia, independent of age and body mass index (BMI). In addition, long-term ADT has been associated with diabetes and metabolic syndrome [8]. Keating et al. [9] were the first to report higher risks of cardiovascular and metabolic complications as well as sudden cardiac death in prostate cancer patients receiving ADT, whilst short-term ADT treatment was significantly associated with greater risks of disease and the elevated risks persisted in men on longer duration therapy [9]. Given the association between cardiorespiratory fitness and CVD mortality [10], the measurement of aerobic capacity can significantly improve the risk classification for CVD mortality [11]. While previous research has predominantly used surrogate measures of cardiorespiratory fitness such as the six-minute walk test (6 MWT) or 400 m walk [7, 12], directly assessing aerobic capacity in ADT-treated men will further our understanding of the cardiovascular risks associated with this form of treatment. In this study, we report for the first time potential differences in relation to patients ADT exposure using objective measures of aerobic capacity, resting metabolic rate, blood pressure, arterial stiffness, and blood biomarkers. We hypothesized that longer-term ADT would lead to compromised aerobic capacity and metabolic parameters hence posing a greater risk for the development and progression of cardiovascular and metabolic diseases.

2. Methods

2.1. Participants. 272 patients with prostate cancer were screened for participation in a 12-month exercise trial [13] from February 2009 to August 2011 in Perth, Western Australia, and Brisbane, Queensland. 109 patients declined participation or were excluded for the following main reasons: declined to participate, too far to travel, unable to fit in with work, unable to obtain general practitioner/physician consent, and bone metastatic disease. In this report, we present the results from baseline assessment of a subgroup of 107 patients who undertook testing including cardiorespiratory capacity by October 2010. This study was approved by the University Human Research Ethics Committee and all participants provided signed informed consent.

All participants underwent assessment for cardiorespiratory capacity, resting metabolic rate, peripheral and central blood pressure and arterial stiffness, and markers of metabolic health.

2.2. Cardiorespiratory Capacity. Participants performed a standardised progressive maximal walking test (Bruce Protocol) on a motorized treadmill supervised by a physician. Expired respiratory gases were collected (Parvo Metabolic Measuring System, Sandy, UT, USA) to determine maximal oxygen uptake (the maximal amount of oxygen that can be consumed and utilised, VO_{2max}). A plateau in oxygen consumption was used as the criterion for achieving VO_{2max}; if no plateau occurred, then a respiratory exchange ratio (RER) of ≥ 1.1 was used. If the subject achieved no plateau in oxygen consumption or a RER value < 1.1 their data were

excluded. This direct assessment of peak oxygen consumption is considered the gold standard outcome of cardiorespiratory fitness or aerobic capacity [14]. The coefficient of variation for repeated maximal exercise tests is approximately 4% [15]. Blood pressure was measured during the last minute of each 3-minute stage via manual auscultatory technique.

2.3. Resting Metabolic Rate. Resting metabolic rate (RMR) was measured via respiratory gas analysis over 20 minutes. A 5-minute period that showed an oxygen consumption with a coefficient of variation of <10% was selected for analysis [16]. The coefficient of variation for RMR is <3%.

2.4. Resting Blood Pressure and Arterial Stiffness. Brachial blood pressure was recorded at the dominant arm in triplicate via a validated oscillometric device (HEM-705CP, Omron Corporation, Japan) [17]. Applanation tonometry (SPC-301, Millar Instruments, Houston, Texas, USA) was used to measure radial artery pressure waveforms at the right arm. A generalised transfer function was applied to obtain the central pressure waveform at the ascending aorta. Pulse wave analysis was used to determine central blood pressure and indices of arterial stiffness, performed using SphygmoCor version 6.1 software (AtCor Medical, Sydney, Australia). Assessing central blood pressure using this method has been validated against invasive techniques [18]. The augmentation index (AIx) refers to the ratio of augmentation to central pulse pressure, expressed as a percentage, and measures systemic arterial stiffness. Variability has been previously reported as 0.3 mmHg for central systolic pressure and 1.5% for the AIx. Carotid-to-radial pulse wave velocity was measured by collecting arterial pressure waves at both the carotid and radial locations. The reported coefficient of variation for forearm (radial) pulse wave velocity is 2.9% whilst the brachial pulse wave velocity coefficient of variation is 7.7% [19].

2.5. Metabolic Syndrome. Patients were classified as having metabolic syndrome if they met three of the following five criteria according to the Adult Panel III Criteria [20]: (1) plasma glucose level more than 110 mg/dL, (2) serum triglyceride levels ≥ 150 mg/dL, (3) serum high density lipoprotein less than 40 mg/dL, (4) waist circumference greater than 102 cm, and (5) blood pressure $\geq 135/80$ mmHg. Patients on antihypertensive and antilipid medications were also considered positive for the respective criterion.

2.6. Other Measures. Venous blood samples (2×8.5 mL) were obtained from the antecubital vein with whole blood analysed for haemoglobin A1C (HbA1C, %) whilst the remaining blood was separated and analysed for testosterone, insulin, prostate specific antigen, triglycerides, LDL cholesterol, HDL cholesterol, total cholesterol, glucose, and C-reactive protein. All blood variables were analysed commercially by accredited Australian National Association of Testing Authorities laboratories (Pathwest Laboratory Medicine, WA).

Whole body bone mineral-free lean mass and fat mass, trunk fat, and body fat percentage were assessed by dual

TABLE 1: Subject characteristics for the short- and longer-term androgen deprivation groups.

Variable	<3 months Mean ± SD n = 57	≥3 months Mean ± SD N = 50	Mean difference (95% CI)	p value
Age (years)	67.6 ± 8.9	69.9 ± 9.7	−2.3 (−5.9, 1.3)	0.395
Prostate specific antigen (ng·mL^{-1})	1.2 ± 1.7	1.4 ± 2.6	−0.2 (−1.1, 0.7)	0.659
Gleason Score	7.6 ± 0.8	7.7 ± 1.4	−0.1 (−0.6, 0.6)	0.985
Testosterone (pg·mL^{-1})	1.3 ± 1.5	1.5 ± 3.4	−0.2 (−1.2, 0.8)	0.651
Height (cm)	172.2 ± 6.4	172.7 ± 6.3	−0.5 (−3.2, 2.1)	0.648
Body mass (kg)	85.7 ± 13.6	83.4 ± 14.0	2.3 (−3.1, 7.8)	0.105
Body mass index (kg·m^2)	28.9 ± 4.3	28.0 ± 3.9	0.9 (−0.7, 2.4)	0.215
Waist circumference (cm)	99.2 ± 12.1	100.3 ± 12.9	−0.9 (−5.5, 3.9)	0.737

energy X-ray absorptiometry (DEXA, Hologic Discovery A, Waltham, MA, USA). In addition, appendicular lean mass was calculated as the sum of upper and lower limb lean mass. The coefficient of variation for body composition measures is <1%.

2.7. Statistical Analysis. Sample size calculations for the initial RCT [13] resulted in a requirement for 65 subjects per group at the commencement of the study. For the principal analyses in this report, we had 80% power to detect a significant difference in METS and similarly for VO_{2max} in absolute (L/min) and relative terms (mL/kg/min), and 87% for RMR in kcal/24 hr.

Analyses were performed using the Statistical Package for Social Sciences version 18.0 software (PASW, Chicago, IL, USA). Normality of the data was assessed using the Kolmogorov-Smirnov test. The analyses included standard descriptive statistics, Student's independent t-tests, and Pearson's chi-square test for categorical variables. Potential differences between patients on <3 months or ≥3 months on ADT were undertaken based on the previous prospective work by Alibhai and colleagues [7] which showed that even short-term treatment leads to substantial deterioration in physical function. All tests were two-tailed and an alpha level of 0.05 was applied as the criterion for statistical significance. Results are reported as the mean ± standard deviation.

3. Results

3.1. Subject Characteristics. Characteristics for all participants were age 68.6 ± 8.8 kg; height 172.4 ± 6.3 cm; and body mass 84.0 ± 13.7 kg. Mean ADT duration was 2.0 ± 0.0 and 7.1 ± 6.2 months for the shorter and longer groups, respectively. There were no significant differences in any subject characteristics (Table 1) or lean and fat mass (Table 2) based on ADT exposure.

3.2. Cardiorespiratory Capacity. 91 (85%) of the participants were able to achieve the desired criteria for VO_{2max} with no difference between groups in their ability to achieve VO_{2max}. Maximal oxygen consumption was significantly higher in the shorter ADT duration group when presented

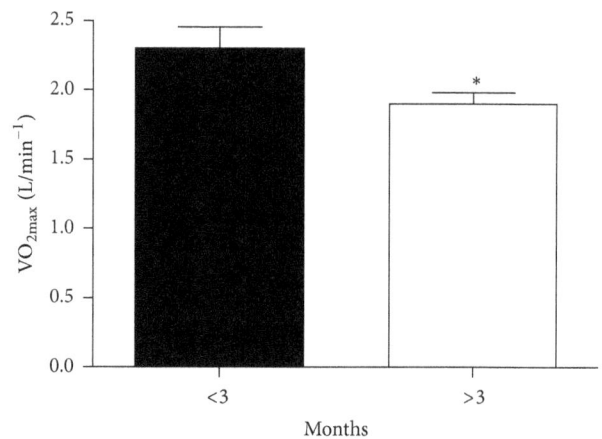

FIGURE 1: Absolute VO_{2max} values (mean ± SE) for the short- and longer-term androgen deprivation groups. ∗ denotes significant difference versus <3 months.

in absolute (L/min^{-1}) ($p = 0.035$) (Figure 1) or relative terms (mL/kg/min^{-1}) ($p = 0.020$) (Table 3). Corresponding metabolic equivalents were also significantly higher in the shorter duration ADT group ($p = 0.02$). Whilst test duration was not statistically significant, shorter duration group exhibited an additional 54 seconds ($p = 0.080$) of walking endurance.

3.3. Resting Metabolic Rate. There was a significant difference observed in RMR with the shorter duration group recording a significantly higher ($p = 0.005$) RMR in absolute terms and relative to body mass RMR ($p = 0.017$) compared to the longer duration group (Table 3). Whilst not statistically significant ($p = 0.079$), RMR relative to lean body mass was 1.3 kcal/lean kg/24 hr higher in those with shorter ADT exposure.

3.4. Central Blood Pressure. There were no differences between short and longer ADT exposure in any of the central or peripheral blood pressure variables or central augmentation index (Table 3). Further, there was no difference in pulse wave velocity between groups (Table 3).

TABLE 2: Body composition and blood markers for the short- and longer-term androgen deprivation groups.

Variable	<3 months Mean ± SD $n = 57$	≥3 months Mean ± SD $N = 50$	Mean difference (95% CI)	p value
Lean tissue mass (kg)				
Whole body	60.1 ± 7.5	58.0 ± 8.6	2.1 (−1.0, 5.2)	0.184
Appendicular	25.6 ± 3.3	24.5 ± 3.9	1.1 (−0.3, 2.5)	0.112
Fat mass (kg)				
Whole body	23.1 ± 7.3	24.6 ± 8.3	−1.5 (−4.5, 1.4)	0.307
Trunk	12.4 ± 4.5	12.9 ± 5.8	−0.5 (−2.5, 1.5)	0.627
Body fat %	26.4 ± 5.1	28.3 ± 5.2	−1.9 (−4.0, 0.1)	0.053
Blood markers				
HbA1C (%)	6.4 ± 3.7	6.1 ± 1.0	0.3 (−0.8, 1.3)	0.638
Testosterone (pg·mL^{-1})	1.3 ± 1.5	1.5 ± 3.4	−0.2 (−1.2, 0.8)	0.651
Prostate specific antigen (ng·mL^{-1})	1.2 ± 1.7	1.4 ± 2.6	−0.2 (−1.1, 0.7)	0.659
Insulin (mU/L)	11.2 ± 6.7	9.2 ± 4.3	2.0 (−0.3, 4.2)	0.085
Triglycerides (mmol/L)	1.3 ± 0.6	1.4 ± 0.7	−0.1 (−0.3, 0.1)	0.393
LDL cholesterol (mmol/L)	2.8 ± 0.9	2.9 ± 1.0	−0.1 (−0.5, 0.3)	0.575
HDL cholesterol (mmol/L)	1.3 ± 0.4	1.4 ± 0.4	−0.1 (−0.3, 0.1)	0.269
Total cholesterol (mmol/L)	4.7 ± 1.1	4.9 ± 1.0	−0.2 (−0.6, 0.2)	0.287
Glucose (mmol/L)	5.5 ± 1.1	5.9 ± 1.9	−0.4 (−1.0, 0.2)	0.216
C-reactive protein (mg/L)	2.9 ± 3.3	2.5 ± 2.0	0.4 (−0.7, 1.5)	0.469

HbA1C: glycated haemoglobin; LDL: low density lipoprotein; HDL: high density lipoprotein.

3.5. Metabolic Profile. No significant differences were observed between short and longer ADT exposure in any of the blood markers analysed (Table 2). Whilst not statistically significant, insulin was 19.6% higher in the shorter duration group (p – 0.085).

3.6. Metabolic Syndrome Variables. According to National Cholesterol Education Program Adult Treatment Panel III, 20.3% of the acute group and 13.5% of the chronic group were classified as having metabolic syndrome ($p = 0.337$). However, there were no significant differences observed between groups for fasting plasma glucose ($p = 0.998$), serum triglycerides ($p = 0.874$), serum HDL ($p = 0.815$), waist circumference ($p = 0.994$), or hypertension ($p = 0.093$).

4. Discussion

We examined the difference between patients on either short- or longer-term ADT across a variety of cardiovascular and metabolic parameters to determine if additional therapy time exposure is associated with accumulating CVD risk factors or metabolic treatment-related toxicities. Those exposed to ADT for a longer period of time had a lower cardiorespiratory capacity and RMR suggesting that longer ADT duration is associated with decline in cardiovascular capacity and aspects of metabolic function.

The maximal aerobic exercise testing protocol used in this study has been shown to be safe and feasible in this population [21]. To our knowledge, this is the first research

study to directly measure VO$_{2max}$ in men on ADT to investigate the effect duration of treatment has on cardiorespiratory capacity. Our findings demonstrate that there are differences in cardiorespiratory capacity between men on shorter- and longer-term ADT. The VO$_{2max}$ of the shorter duration ADT group was 21% higher than the longer exposed group, which has important implications when considering that the low levels of cardiorespiratory fitness have been associated with a markedly increased risk of premature death from all causes and in particular CVD in all populations including healthy older men and those with established cardiovascular disease [10]. Conversely, an increase in cardiorespiratory fitness is associated with a reduced risk of CVD [22]. No differences were observed in any of the blood pressure parameters in relation to ADT exposure.

ADT exposure time appears to influence resting energy expenditure with those men on longer duration ADT having a lower RMR. Fat-free mass plays a major role in the variance of RMR amongst individuals [23], with more recent research suggesting that both fat-free mass and fat mass significantly influence RMR [24]. Whilst no significant differences in any body composition values were reported, it is likely that the combined effects of the nonsignificant differences in lean body mass (2 kg) and fat mass (1.5 kg) contributed to this significant reduction in resting energy expenditure in the longer ADT exposure group. A reduced RMR with continuing ADT exposure would contribute to the accumulation of adipose tissue if dietary intake remained unchanged.

When exploring additional CVD risk factors, metabolic syndrome has been widely used as a surrogate marker for

TABLE 3: Resting and maximal cardiorespiratory values and hemodynamic and pulse wave analysis parameters for the short- and longer-term androgen deprivation groups.

Variable	<3 months Mean ± SD n = 57	≥3 months Mean ± SD N = 50	Mean difference (95% CI)	p value
VO_{2max} (L/min^{-1})*	2.3 ± 1.0	1.9 ± 0.6	0.4 (0.1, 0.7)	0.035
VO_{2max} (mL/kg/min^{-1})*	26.1 ± 6.0	23.2 ± 5.8	2.9 (0.5, 5.3)	0.020
VO_{2max} (METS)*	7.5 ± 1.7	6.6 ± 1.6	0.9 (0.1, 1.5)	0.020
Test duration (mins)	8.5 ± 2.8	7.6 ± 2.6	0.9 (−0.1, 2.1)	0.080
Resting metabolic rate (kcal/24 hr)*	1795 ± 256	1647 ± 236	147 (46, 249)	0.005
Relative total body mass Resting metabolic rate (kcal/kg/24 hr)*	21.5 ± 3.0	20.0 ± 2.6	1.5 (0.3, 2.7)	0.017
Relative lean body mass Resting metabolic rate (kcal/lean kg/24 hr)	30.5 ± 3.2	29.2 ± 4.1	1.3 (−0.2, 2.9)	0.079
Peripheral SBP (mmHg)	150.9 ± 19.9	149.0 ± 19.4	1.9 (−5.8, 9.6)	0.624
Peripheral DBP (mmHg)	85.6 ± 12.1	84.5 ± 10.4	1.1 (−3.4, 5.6)	0.626
Peripheral MAP (mmHg)	108.4 ± 15.0	107.2 ± 12.8	1.2 (−4.3, 6.7)	0.669
Central SBP (mmHg)	139.1 ± 21.1	138.7 ± 20.2	0.4 (−7.7, 8.5)	0.922
Central DBP (mmHg)	86.8 ± 12.3	85.5 ± 10.6	1.3 (−3.2, 5.8)	0.571
Central MAP (mmHg)	108.9 ± 16.1	107.2 ± 12.8	1.7 (−4.1, 7.5)	0.557
Peripheral augmentation index (AIx, %)	83.5 ± 13.0	86.5 ± 13.9	−3.0 (−8.3, 2.3)	0.261
Central augmentation pressure (mmHg)	15.4 ± 8.2	16.7 ± 9.6	−1.3 (4.8, 2.1)	0.445
Augmentation load (mmHg)	14.3 ± 5.0	14.6 ± 4.9	−0.3 (−2.3, 1.6)	0.732
Central augmentation index (AIx, %)	140.4 ± 17.8	144.4 ± 19.6	−4.0 (−11.3, 3.3)	0.281
Pulse wave velocity (m/s)	10.0 ± 1.4	10.0 ± 1.8	0.0 (−0.6, 0.7)	0.983

VO_{2max}: maximal oxygen uptake; METS: metabolic equivalents; SBP: systolic blood pressure; DBP: diastolic blood pressure; MAP: mean arterial pressure; AIx: augmentation index.
* refers to a significant difference between <3 months and ≥3 months.

CVD. In our study, 20.3% and 13.5% of the shorter and longer ADT exposure groups, respectively, met the criteria for metabolic syndrome. These values are lower than the 55% of ADT-treated prostate cancer patients previously reported by Braga-Basaria et al. [25] but similar to non-ADT-treated prostate cancer patients (22%) and control subjects (20%) reported in the same study [25]. Waist circumference and hypertension appear to be the two most common cardiovascular risk factors present in both groups, demonstrating that these risk factors are present irrespective of the treatment duration.

Whilst not measured in the present study, physical activity levels are known to exert large influences on aerobic capacity and functional performance. Previous research in breast cancer patients has demonstrated that physical activity levels are significantly reduced following cancer diagnosis and during treatment [26, 27] and these reductions in physical activity negatively alter energy balance. We have recently reported that only ~12% of Australian prostate cancer survivors are meeting sufficient exercise levels (150 min of

moderate intensity or 75 min of strenuous exercise per week and twice weekly resistance exercise) [28]. It is possible that in the current study physical activity levels were reduced following diagnosis and either they continued to decline as treatment time progressed or the side effects associated with declining physical activity levels did not present until later in treatment which may have contributed to the differences observed in aerobic fitness and RMR.

It was somewhat surprising that we observed no differences in the measured blood biomarkers or central blood pressure in relation to ADT exposure. With regard to the blood biomarkers, it may be that testosterone suppression has such a rapid effect, shown by the increased serum insulin levels previously reported by Dockery et al. [6] after only 3 months of ADT, which leads us to believe that these biomarkers may have stabilised within the first three months.

The strength of this study is that we directly measured VO_2 during a maximum exercise stress test (gold standard assessment for aerobic capacity) rather than use of surrogate measures such as the 400 meters or 6 MWT as well as assessments of RMR and central blood pressure. A limitation of this study is that patients were only assessed at a single time point during their treatment; hence, we were unable to continually monitor each participant as treatment time progressed. Further, the cross-sectional nature of the study does not permit us to infer causality; however, it provides initial evidence of decline in aerobic capacity measured objectively and it could be clinically meaningful to patients but needs further validation in prospective studies. However, it should be recognised that men in this study were volunteers for an exercise trial and therefore are not representative of all men with prostate cancer undergoing ADT. Lastly, given the exploratory nature of the study, we did not adjust for multiple comparisons [29] and, as a result, cannot discount the possibility that 1-2 of the significant differences may have been a chance finding.

5. Conclusion

In conclusion, we found that patients exposed to longer duration ADT had reduced cardiorespiratory capacity and RMR and these could have clinical meaningful implications. The exact mechanisms remain unclear as to why these cardiovascular parameters are further declining as the treatment time progresses and should be determined in future mechanistic studies. Intervention strategies to preserve cardiovascular capacity and RMR such as exercise medicine interventions have significant potential to counteract these forms of decline.

Conflict of Interests

The authors declare that they have no conflict of interests.

Acknowledgments

The data presented in this paper are from a randomized clinical trial funded by the National Health and Medical Research Council, Project Grant AppID 534409. Daniel A. Galvão received fund from the Cancer Council Western Australia Research Fellowship and Movember New Directions Development Award obtained through Prostate Cancer Foundation of Australia's Research Program.

References

[1] G. W. Chodak, "Comparing treatments for localized prostate cancer—persisting uncertainty," *The Journal of the American Medical Association*, vol. 280, no. 11, pp. 1008–1010, 1998.

[2] M. R. Smith, J. S. Finkelstein, F. J. McGovern et al., "Changes in body composition during androgen deprivation therapy for prostate cancer," *Journal of Clinical Endocrinology and Metabolism*, vol. 87, no. 2, pp. 599–603, 2002.

[3] S. Basaria, D. C. Muller, M. A. Carducci, J. Egan, and A. S. Dobs, "Hyperglycemia and insulin resistance in men with prostate carcinoma who receive androgen-deprivation therapy," *Cancer*, vol. 106, no. 3, pp. 581–588, 2006.

[4] D. A. Galvão, N. A. Spry, D. R. Taaffe et al., "Changes in muscle, fat and bone mass after 36 weeks of maximal androgen blockade for prostate cancer," *BJU International*, vol. 102, no. 1, pp. 44–47, 2008.

[5] J. C. Smith, S. Bennett, L. M. Evans et al., "The effects of induced hypogonadism on arterial stiffness, body composition, and metabolic parameters in males with prostate cancer," *Journal of Clinical Endocrinology and Metabolism*, vol. 86, no. 9, pp. 4261–4267, 2001.

[6] F. Dockery, C. J. Bulpitt, S. Agarwal, M. Donaldson, and C. Rajkumar, "Testosterone suppression in men with prostate cancer leads to an increase in arterial stiffness and hyperinsulinaemia," *Clinical Science*, vol. 104, no. 2, pp. 195–201, 2003.

[7] S. M. H. Alibhai, H. Breunis, N. Timilshina et al., "Impact of androgen-deprivation therapy on physical function and quality of life in men with nonmetastatic prostate cancer," *Journal of Clinical Oncology*, vol. 28, no. 34, pp. 5038–5045, 2010.

[8] S. Basaria, "Androgen deprivation therapy, insulin resistance, and cardiovascular mortality: an inconvenient truth," *Journal of Andrology*, vol. 29, no. 5, pp. 534–539, 2008.

[9] N. L. Keating, A. J. O'Malley, and M. R. Smith, "Diabetes and cardiovascular disease during androgen deprivation therapy for prostate cancer," *Journal of Clinical Oncology*, vol. 24, no. 27, pp. 4448–4456, 2006.

[10] J. Myers, M. Prakash, V. Froelicher, D. Do, S. Partington, and J. Edwin Atwood, "Exercise capacity and mortality among men referred for exercise testing," *The New England Journal of Medicine*, vol. 346, no. 11, pp. 793–801, 2002.

[11] S. Gupta, A. Rohatgi, C. R. Ayers et al., "Cardiorespiratory fitness and classification of risk of cardiovascular disease mortality," *Circulation*, vol. 123, no. 13, pp. 1377–1383, 2011.

[12] D. A. Galvão, D. R. Taaffe, N. Spry, D. Joseph, and R. U. Newton, "Combined resistance and aerobic exercise program reverses muscle loss in men undergoing androgen suppression therapy for prostate cancer without bone metastases: a randomized controlled trial," *Journal of Clinical Oncology*, vol. 28, no. 2, pp. 340–347, 2010.

[13] R. U. Newton, D. R. Taaffe, N. Spry et al., "A phase III clinical trial of exercise modalities on treatment side-effects in men receiving therapy for prostate cancer," *BMC Cancer*, vol. 9, no. 1, article 210, 2009.

[14] W. R. Thompson, N. F. Gordon, and L. S. Pescatello, Eds., *ACSM's Guidelines for Exercise Testing and Prescription*, Lippincott Williams & Wilkins, 8th edition, 2010.

[15] E. T. Howley, D. R. Bassett Jr., and H. G. Welch, "Criteria for maximal oxygen uptake: review and commentary," *Medicine and Science in Sports and Exercise*, vol. 27, no. 9, pp. 1292–1301, 1995.

[16] C. Compher, D. Frankenfield, N. Keim, and L. Roth-Yousey, "Best practice methods to apply to measurement of resting metabolic rate in adults: a systematic review," *Journal of the American Dietetic Association*, vol. 106, no. 6, pp. 881–903, 2006.

[17] E. O'Brien, F. Mee, N. Atkins, and M. Thomas, "Evaluation of three devices for self-measurement of blood pressure according to the revised British Hypertension Society Protocol: the Omron HEM-705CP, Philips HP5332, and Nissei DS-175," *Blood Pressure Monitoring*, vol. 1, no. 1, pp. 55–61, 1996.

[18] A. L. Pauca, M. F. O'Rourke, and N. D. Kon, "Prospective evaluation of a method for estimating ascending aortic pressure from the radial artery pressure waveform," *Hypertension*, vol. 38, no. 4, pp. 932–937, 2001.

[19] S. Nottin, G. Walther, A. Vinet et al., "Reproducibility of automated pulse wave velocity measurement during exercise.

Running head: Pulse wave velocity during exercise," *Archives des Maladies du Coeur et des Vaisseaux*, vol. 99, no. 6, pp. 564–568, 2006.

[20] Expert Panel on Detectio, Evaluation, and Treatment of High Blood Cholesterol in Adults, "Executive summary of the third report of the National Cholesterol Education Program (NCEP) Expert panel on detection, evaluation, and treatment of high blood cholesterol in adults (Adult Treatment Panel III)," *Journal of the American Medical Association*, vol. 285, no. 19, pp. 2486–2497, 2001.

[21] B. A. Wall, D. A. Galvão, N. Fatehee et al., "Maximal exercise testing of men with prostate cancer being treated with ADT," *Medicine and Science in Sports and Exercise*, vol. 46, no. 12, pp. 2210–2215, 2014.

[22] C. E. Barlow, L. F. DeFina, N. B. Radford et al., "Cardiorespiratory fitness and long-term survival in 'low-risk' adults," *Journal of the American Heart Association*, vol. 1, no. 4, Article ID e001354, 2012.

[23] R. L. Weinsier, Y. Schutz, and D. Bracco, "Reexamination of the relationship of resting metabolic rate to fat-free mass and to the metabolically active components of fat-free mass in humans," *The American Journal of Clinical Nutrition*, vol. 55, no. 4, pp. 790–794, 1992.

[24] A. M. Johnstone, S. D. Murison, J. S. Duncan, K. A. Rance, and J. R. Speakman, "Factors influencing variation in basal metabolic rate include fat-free mass, fat mass, age, and circulating thyroxine but not sex, circulating leptin, or triiodothyronine," *American Journal of Clinical Nutrition*, vol. 82, no. 5, pp. 941–948, 2005.

[25] M. Braga-Basaria, A. S. Dobs, D. C. Muller et al., "Metabolic syndrome in men with prostate cancer undergoing long-term androgen-deprivation therapy," *Journal of Clinical Oncology*, vol. 24, no. 24, pp. 3979–3983, 2006.

[26] M. L. Irwin, D. Crumley, A. McTiernan et al., "Physical activity levels before and after a diagnosis of breast carcinoma," *Cancer*, vol. 97, no. 7, pp. 1746–1757, 2003.

[27] W. Demark-Wahnefried, V. Hars, M. R. Conaway et al., "Reduced rates of metabolism and decreased physical activity in breast cancer patients receiving adjuvant chemotherapy," *American Journal of Clinical Nutrition*, vol. 65, no. 5, pp. 1495–1501, 1997.

[28] D. A. Galvão, R. U. Newton, R. A. Gardiner et al., "Compliance to exercise-oncology guidelines in prostate cancer survivors and associations with psychological distress, unmet supportive care needs, and quality of life," *Psycho-Oncology*, vol. 24, no. 10, pp. 1241–1249, 2015.

[29] K. J. Rothman, "No adjustments are needed for multiple comparisons," *Epidemiology*, vol. 1, no. 1, pp. 43–46, 1990.

30

Can CT Virtual Cystoscopy Replace Conventional Cystoscopy in Early Detection of Bladder Cancer?

Sachin Abrol, Ankush Jairath, Sanika Ganpule, Arvind Ganpule, Shashikant Mishra, Ravindra Sabnis, and Mahesh Desai

Muljibhai Patel Urological Hospital, Dr. Varendra Desai Road, Nadiad, Gujarat 387001, India

Correspondence should be addressed to Ankush Jairath; ankushjairath@rediffmail.com

Academic Editor: Maxwell V. Meng

Aim. To correlate findings of conventional cystoscopy with CT virtual cystoscopy (CTVC) in detecting bladder tumors and to evaluate accuracy of virtual cystoscopy in early detection of bladder cancer. *Material and Method.* From June 2013 to June 2014, 50 patients (46 males, four females) with history and investigations suggestive of urothelial cancer, with mean age 62.76 ± 10.45 years, underwent CTVC by a radiologist as per protocol and subsequently underwent conventional cystoscopy (CPE) the same day or the next day. One urologist and one radiologist, blinded to the findings of conventional cystoscopy, independently interpreted the images, and any discrepant readings were resolved with consensus. *Result.* CTVC detected 23 out of 25 patients with bladder tumor(s) correctly. Two patients were falsely detected as negative while two were falsely labeled as positive in CTVC. Virtual and conventional cystoscopy were comparable in detection of tumor growth in urinary bladder. The sensitivity, specificity, positive predictive value, and negative predictive value of virtual cystoscopy were 92% each. *Conclusion.* CTVC correlates closely with the findings of conventional cystoscopy. Bladder should be adequately distended and devoid of urine at the time of procedure. However, more studies are required to define the role of virtual cystoscopy in routine clinical practice.

1. Introduction

The most common cancer of the lower urinary tract is bladder tumor, with recurrence as one of its main troublesome features associated depending upon different stages and grades [1, 2]. Therefore, close monitoring of the patients is required at regular intervals. The mainstay of diagnosis and follow-up of bladder neoplasia as of now is conventional cystoscopy [1] but it is an invasive procedure. Replacing invasive diagnostic procedures with noninvasive sensitive and specific imaging techniques is a growing trend in medicine today.

With computer assisted rapid image acquisition and three-dimensional image reconstruction by commercially available software, virtual reality imaging has been developed. This can be applied to many organs including the colon, stomach, bronchus, and bladder [3–8]. Because of its simple luminal morphology, relatively small volume, and absence of involuntary peristalsis, urinary bladder may possibly be an ideal intra-abdominal organ for virtual endoscopy [9].

The accuracy of detecting bladder lesions (<1 cm) by computed tomography virtual cystoscopy (CTVC) has been variously reported ranging within 60–100% [7, 10–12]. Even bladder lesions <5 mm have also been reportedly detected by some authors utilizing CTVC [13–15], while others have found the visualization of such lesions to be difficult [10]. This technology is considered safe for bladder cancer follow-up with detection rates comparable to conventional cystoscopy.

Conventional cystoscopy (CPE) on the other hand is invasive and time consuming and, especially in males, the evaluation of bladder neck and narrow neck diverticular tumors is limited. In addition, there is risk of urinary sepsis and urethral injury, which can lead to late urethral strictures [5] so virtual cystoscopy can play increasing role as a first-line screening test to evaluate patients at risk of bladder cancer or who present with symptoms like hematuria in near future.

In this study we report our experience with CTVC in detecting bladder tumors in terms of sensitivity, specificity, positive predictive value, and negative predictive value.

2. Patients and Methods

2.1. Patients. After getting informed consent and obtaining ethics committee approval, all patients with history and investigations suggestive of urothelial cancer who serially presented in outpatient department from June 2013 to June 2014 were included in the study. The age ranged from 30 to 83 years (mean age 62.76 ± 10.45 years), 46 were males, and four were females. A focused history examination, urine analysis/culture/cytology for malignant cells, renal function tests, and ultrasonography of kidney, ureters, and bladder (KUB) region, was performed in all the patients. Out of the 50 patients, 21 patients had presented to our outpatient department first time with gross painless hematuria and symptoms suggestive of bladder tumor and the remaining 29 patients were already proven cases of bladder tumor that had undergone TURBT and were admitted for follow-up check cystoscopy.

2.2. Technique. Virtual cystoscopy began drainage of residual urine by placing a 12 fr Foleys catheter into the bladder. It was then insufflated with 300–400 mL of room air using 60 cc syringe and clamp, according to the bladder capacity and tolerance. In few cases, the catheter was withdrawn to the distal penile urethra so that the urethra may also be visualized at the time of virtual cystoscopy. Initially, a scout view was obtained to locate the bladder and confirm its adequate distention with the patient in the supine position. Subsequently, single breath hold CT was performed with Multidetector CT (Bright speed, GE Health care) with 1 mm collimation, 120 KV, 250 mA, and 7–10 mm/sec table speed. Images were reconstructed at 1.25 mm intervals by using the minimal field of view measured from the inner aspect of the middle of the pelvis. The procedure was repeated with the patient in prone position using the same CT parameters. The data was then analyzed using software for interactive intraluminal navigation with a volume rendering algorithm. One urologist and one radiologist, blinded to the findings of conventional cystoscopy, independently interpreted the images, and any discrepant readings were resolved with consensus. Using the multiplanar reformation from the source images, the central observation point was defined in the middle of the bladder. The camera of the virtual cystoscopy was placed in the center of the bladder and thereafter advanced to each quadrant and the findings were then evaluated from various angles.

The number, size, location, and morphological features of the lesions were evaluated and virtual images were obtained with the patients in both the prone and the supine positions. Each lesion was then classified as polypoidal lesion, a sessile mass, or wall thickening. A discrete lesion was considered polypoidal if it was taller than it was wide, while a sessile mass was defined as a lesion that was wider at the base. A lesion was characterized as wall thickening when there was elevation of the bladder wall without a discrete mass.

Subsequently, each of the patients underwent conventional cystoscopy (CPE) the same day or the next day. The urologists, who were not preminded with virtual cystoscopic findings, performed cystoscopic examinations using rigid wide angle telescopes. They were instructed to determine the number, location, and morphology of the bladder lesions by drawing or video-recording.

CPE findings were used as reference standard to evaluate the sensitivity, specificity, positive predictive value, and negative predictive value of CTVC for detection of bladder tumors.

3. Result

Out of 50 patients included in the study, twenty-one (21) patients were evaluated for gross painless hematuria and the remaining twenty-nine (29) patients were already proven cases of bladder tumor who had undergone TURBT in our institution previously and were on follow-up check cystoscopy. Out of 21 patients evaluated for hematuria, transitional cell carcinoma, benign prostate hyperplasia, and cystitis were diagnosed in 17, 2, and 2 patients, respectively, on CPE. New growths were detected in 8 out of 29 patients undergoing check CPE.

Both CTVC and CPE were well tolerated by all the patients without any complications. Images in 45 out of 50 virtual cystoscopies were of excellent or good quality, with adequate bladder distention and minimum residual urine. Images in 5 patients were suboptimal due to inadequate bladder distention and moderate residual urine.

CTVC detected 23 out of 25 patients with bladder tumor(s) correctly (Table 1(a)). Out of two patients who were falsely detected as negative on virtual cystoscopy, one patient had a sessile tumor measuring around 1.0 cm on right lateral wall on CPE and CTVC diagnosed it as normal while another patient with 1 cm tumor near bladder neck was not picked on CTVC probably due to residual urine. Two patients were falsely labeled as positive in CTVC. In one patient, two lesions of 0.3 mm were suspected on the right lateral wall, near the previous site of TURBT, but no lesion was found on CPE. This was due to inadequate bladder distention and bladder trabeculations present in this patient which led to the misinterpretation of findings. In another patient who was labeled as bladder tumor at bladder neck by CTVC, only prostatomegaly was detected on CPE.

A total of 80 tumor lesions were detected in 25 positive patients in CPE. Single tumor was found in thirteen patients, two lesions were detected in two patients, and more than two were found in ten patients. Other than one CIS and four other tumors which were missed on CTVC, all other tumor lesions were identified with accuracy with regard to position and distribution as on CPE.

Morphologically, identified tumors were categorized into three types, papillary in 60 lesions, sessile in nineteen, and CIS in one. In the present study, virtual and conventional cystoscopy were comparable in detection of tumor growth in urinary bladder. The tumor size ranged from 0.2 cm to 5.0 cm in maximum dimension.

Among the visualized 80 tumors, 31 were located at the right lateral wall (Figures 1(a)-1(b)), sixteen on left lateral wall, twelve at the posterior wall, ten at the base, six at the dome, and four lesions in the diverticulum (Figure 1(c)) and one was a case of CIS.

TABLE 1: (a) Tumor detection in patients with bladder tumors: taking CPE as reference standard, CTVC falsely detects two patients with tumor lesion out of twenty-five with no lesion on CPE. Similarly, CTVC fails to detect two patients out of twenty-five with lesion positive on CPE. (b) Depicting the sensitivity and specificity of CTVC for bladder tumor detection.

(a)

Parameter	Positive result (tumor detected) (N)	Negative result (tumor not detected) (N)	True positive (N)	True negative (N)	False positive (N)	False negative (N)
CPE*	25	25	25	25	0	0
CTVC**	25	25	23	23	2	2

*CPE: cystopanendoscopic examination was taken as reference standard, N: number of patients, and **CTVC: computed tomography virtual cystoscopy.

(b)

Parameter	Sensitivity	Specificity	Ppv	Npv
CTVC	92%	92%	92%	92%

Ppv: positive predictive value and Npv: negative predictive value.

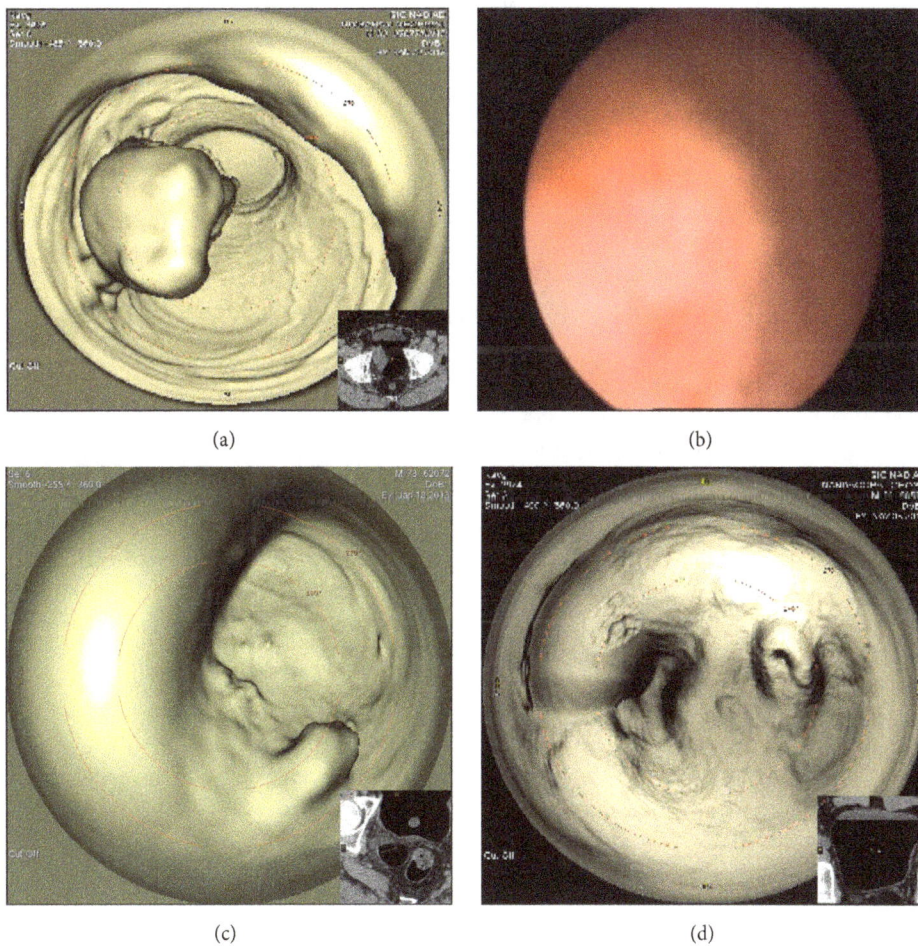

(a)

(b)

(c)

(d)

FIGURE 1: (a-b) Large right lateral wall growth in a patient presenting with gross painless hematuria on CTVC and CPE, respectively. (c) CTVC image of inside the bladder diverticulum showing papillary lesions. (d) Follow-up case of TCC bladder with normal findings on CTVC.

Other results were shown in Tables 1(b), 2(a)-2(b), and 3.

4. Discussion

Bladder cancer is one of the most common urological malignancies, with the need for long-term follow-up. Because bladder tumors have a tendency towards multifocality and recurrence, it seems very important to find out diagnostic techniques that are less invasive and at the same time highly sensitive.

Although several imaging techniques like intravenous urography, ultrasound, CT, and magnetic resonance imaging

TABLE 2: (a) Number of tumors detected in patients: taking CPE as reference standard, out of 80 tumors detected on CPE, CTVC was able to detect 75 tumors accurately while five tumors were missed. Four tumors were falsely detected as positive on CTVC which were actually not present on CPE. (b) Depicting the sensitivity and specificity of CTVC in patients with respect to number of tumors detected.

(a)

Parameter	CTVC positive	CTVC negative
CPE* positive	75	5
CPE negative	4	25

*CPE: cystopanendoscopic examination was taken as reference standard and CTVC: computed tomography virtual cystoscopy.

(b)

Parameter	Sensitivity	Specificity	Ppv	Npv
CTVC	94.90%	83.30%	93.75	86.21

Ppv: positive predictive value and Npv: negative predictive value.

TABLE 3: Number of bladder growths detected by virtual and conventional cystoscopies according to size.

Size of tumor	≥1 cm	0.3–1.0 cm	<0.3 cm
CPE ($n = 80$)	19	58	2 + CIS
CTVC ($n = 75$)	19	56	0

CIS: carcinoma in situ.

have been used for detecting bladder tumor, none of them may be completely sensitive in all aspects. While overall CT may be a useful radiological tool, its sensitivity appears to be low particularly for detection of small bladder lesions. More negative findings on CT may warrant further evaluation with conventional CPE [3, 4, 16].

Conventional CPE has traditionally served as the reference standard for detecting intravesical lesions [3, 5]. However, CPE has some limitations. The evaluation of bladder neck, anterior wall, and diverticulum (narrow neck) is difficult. Primary intradiverticular carcinomas are rare but diagnosis is often difficult with conventional method [6, 17–19]. Marked hematuria is another factor that limits the technical success of cystoscopy, thereby decreasing its reliability. Cystoscopy is performed under general or local anesthesia and it is an invasive and uncomfortable procedure for the patient and complications like infection, bladder perforation, scarring, and stricture of urethra have been observed [3, 6].

Recently introduced virtual endoscopy seems to be an advantageous tool to detect and evaluate bladder lesions. Virtual endoscopy has been most widely applied to the imaging of colon and many investigators report its feasibility in the detection of colorectal polyps [20, 21]. After the first report of virtual cystoscopy in study by Vining et al., there have been a lot of studies on the utility of virtual cystoscopy of bladder. Urinary bladder is a good organ for virtual cystoscopy because of its simple luminal morphology, relatively small volume, and absence of involuntary peristalsis. Therefore, virtual cystoscopic rendering of bladder takes less

time to navigate and does not require great skill on the part of operator [4, 5, 22]. According to a study by Kim et al., virtual cystoscopy was found superior to multiplanar reconstruction and source CT images for lesion detection in contrast material filled bladder [21].

A recent meta-analysis of 26 studies done by Qu et al. has reported pooled sensitivity and specificity of virtual cystoscopy to be 93.9% and 98.1%, respectively [23]. CTVC is a relatively noninvasive emerging tool in the diagnostic armamentarium of bladder pathology.

CTVC in our study was obtained by combined use of supine and prone images, as reported by others [9, 16, 24, 25]. We calculated the data patientwise as well as lesionwise. Both sensitivity and specificity in our study turned out to be 92%. As the multiplicity of the bladder tumors may change the treatment plan, we analyzed sensitivity and specificity of CTVC in detecting number of tumors (Table 2(a)). While sensitivity (94.9%) increases, specificity decreases to 83.3% (Table 2(b)).

Three-dimensional images generated from volumetric data obtained from helical CT imaging were used in our study. Since the work published by Vining et al. [4], there have been several studies that discussed the utility of VC in bladder lesions [5, 6, 22, 26, 27]. To date, two techniques that use either air or contrast material to fill bladder have been used for VC [4, 5, 26, 27]. The results obtained from intravenous contrast media were adequately similar to those obtained with air contrast. However, presence of faint artifacts within obtained images when using IV contrast makes the images obtained from air contrast clearer and sharper.

In our study, we found that virtual cystoscopy is a feasible technique for use in detection of bladder lesions greater than 3 mm. Narumi et al. [27] identified 77% of lesions smaller than 10 mm. Fenlon et al. [25] identified all the lesions smaller than 10 mm in their study of 13 patients. However, these studies retrospectively evaluated bladder lesions that had been confirmed on CPE.

Though all patients tolerated the CTVC procedure well, still our study lacked any objective data with respect to tolerance of the procedure in form of pain scores or validated questionnaire. This could be included as an objective in future multicenter trial. Also, we did not record the exact timing to complete the CTVC procedure (including patient preparation, instillation of air, CT imaging, processing of the acquired data, and analysis) which forms one of the limitations of our study. Further randomized studies will be needed to validate and define the role of CTVC in routine practice.

5. Conclusion

(1) CT virtual cystoscopy correlates closely with the findings of conventional cystoscopy in our study.

(2) The sensitivity, specificity, positive predictive value, and negative predictive value of virtual cystoscopy were 92% each, in our study.

The salient procedure points noted in our study are as follows:

(a) The bladder should be adequately distended at the time of procedure; otherwise, crumpling of wall may give artefacts in the study.

(b) The bladder should be devoid of urine at the time of examination. Virtual cystoscopy should be done both in supine and in prone positions.

(c) In grossly trabeculated bladder, small papillary growth may be overlooked, so close inspection is required.

(d) The dictum followed should be a systematic inspection of bladder starting by keeping centre of bladder as the region of interest and moving systematically from normal to abnormal area/surface.

Conflict of Interests

The authors declare that there is no conflict of interests regarding the publication of this paper.

Acknowledgment

The authors thank Upendra Prajapati (Chief Radiology Technician, Muljibhai Patel Urological Hospital, NADIAD).

References

[1] A. Jemal, R. C. Tiwari, T. Murray et al., "Cancer statistics, 2004," *CA: A Cancer Journal for Clinicians*, vol. 54, no. 1, pp. 8–29, 2004.

[2] Z. Kirkali, T. Chan, M. Manoharan et al., "Bladder cancer: epidemiology, staging and grading, and diagnosis," *Urology*, vol. 66, no. 6, pp. 4–34, 2005.

[3] J. K. Kim, J. H. Ahn, T. Park, H. J. Ahn, C. S. Kim, and K.-S. Cho, "Virtual cystoscopy of the contrast material-filled bladder in patients with gross hematuria," *American Journal of Roentgenology*, vol. 179, no. 3, pp. 763–768, 2002.

[4] D. J. Vining, R. J. Zagoria, K. Liu, and D. Stelts, "CT cystoscopy: an innovation in bladder imaging," *American Journal of Roentgenology*, vol. 166, no. 2, pp. 409–410, 1996.

[5] J. H. Song, I. R. Francis, J. F. Platt et al., "Bladder tumor detection at virtual cystoscopy," *Radiology*, vol. 218, no. 1, pp. 95–100, 2001.

[6] M. Lämmle, A. Beer, M. Settles, C. Hannig, H. Schwaibold, and C. Drews, "Reliability of MR imaging-based virtual cystoscopy in the diagnosis of cancer of the urinary bladder," *American Journal of Roentgenology*, vol. 178, no. 6, pp. 1483–1488, 2002.

[7] J. Y. Yun, H. J. Ro, J. B. Park et al., "Diagnostic performance of CT colonography for the detection of colorectal polyps," *Korean Journal of Radiology*, vol. 8, no. 6, pp. 484–491, 2007.

[8] S. C. Chen, D. S. K. Lu, J. R. Hecht, and B. M. Kadell, "CT colonography: value of scanning in both the supine and prone positions," *American Journal of Roentgenology*, vol. 172, no. 3, pp. 595–599, 1999.

[9] R. Yadav and R. Kumar, "Virtual versus real cystoscopy," *Indian Journal of Urology*, vol. 23, no. 1, pp. 85–86, 2007.

[10] K. Inamoto, K. Kouzai, T. Ueeda, and T. Marukawa, "CT virtual endoscopy of the stomach: comparison study with gastric fiberscopy," *Abdominal Imaging*, vol. 30, no. 4, pp. 473–479, 2005.

[11] Y. Lacasse, S. Martel, A. Hébert, G. Carrier, and B. Raby, "Accuracy of virtual bronchoscopy to detect endobronchial lesions," *Annals of Thoracic Surgery*, vol. 77, no. 5, pp. 1774–1780, 2004.

[12] H. Arslan, K. Ceylan, M. Harman, Y. Yilmaz, O. Temizoz, and S. Can, "Virtual computed tomography cystoscopy in bladder pathologies," *International Braz J Urol*, vol. 32, no. 2, pp. 147–154, 2006.

[13] V. Panebianco, M. Osimani, D. Lisi et al., "64-Detector row CT cystography with virtual cystoscopy in the detection of bladder carcinoma: preliminary experience in selected patients," *Radiologia Medica*, vol. 114, no. 1, pp. 52–69, 2009.

[14] D. Y. Josephson, E. Pasin, and J. P. Stein, "Superficial bladder cancer: part 1. Update on etiology, classification and natural history," *Expert Review of Anticancer Therapy*, vol. 6, no. 12, pp. 1723–1734, 2006.

[15] J. Schmidbauer and G. Lindenau, "Follow-up of nonmuscle invasive transitional cell carcinoma of the bladder: how and how often?" *Current Opinion in Urology*, vol. 18, no. 5, pp. 504–507, 2008.

[16] T. M. Bernhardt and U. Rapp-Bernhardt, "Virtual cystoscopy of the bladder based on CT and MRI data," *Abdominal Imaging*, vol. 26, no. 3, pp. 325–332, 2001.

[17] S. M. Durfee, L. H. Schwartz, D. M. Panicek, and P. Russo, "MR imaging of carcinoma within urinary bladder diverticulum," *Clinical Imaging*, vol. 21, no. 4, pp. 290–292, 1997.

[18] W. T. Stephenson, F. F. Holmes, M. J. Nobel, and K. B. Gerald, "Analysis of bladder carcinoma by subsite. Cystoscopic location may have prognostic value," *Cancer*, vol. 66, no. 7, pp. 1630–1635, 1990.

[19] J. Baniel and T. Vishna, "Primary transitional cell carcinoma in vesical diverticula," *Urology*, vol. 50, no. 5, pp. 697–699, 1997.

[20] A. K. Hara, C. D. Johnson, J. E. Reed et al., "Detection of colorectal polyps with CT colography: initial assessment of sensitivity and specificity," *Radiology*, vol. 205, no. 1, pp. 59–65, 1997.

[21] J. K. Kim, S.-Y. Park, H. S. Kim, S. H. Kim, and K.-S. Cho, "Comparison of virtual cystoscopy, multiplanar reformation, and source CT images with contrast material-filled bladder for detecting lesions," *American Journal of Roentgenology*, vol. 185, no. 3, pp. 689–696, 2005.

[22] C. Yazgan, S. Fitoz, C. Atasoy, K. Turkolmez, C. Yagci, and S. Akyar, "Virtual cystoscopy in the evaluation of bladder tumors," *Clinical Imaging*, vol. 28, no. 2, pp. 138–142, 2004.

[23] X. Qu, X. Huang, L. Wu, G. Huang, X. Ping, and W. Yan, "Comparison of virtual cystoscopy and ultrasonography for bladder cancer detection: a meta-analysis," *European Journal of Radiology*, vol. 80, no. 2, pp. 188–197, 2011.

[24] J. R. Fielding, L. X. Hoyte, S. A. Okon et al., "Tumor detection by virtual cystoscopy with color mapping of bladder wall thickness," *Journal of Urology*, vol. 167, no. 2, pp. 559–562, 2002.

[25] H. M. Fenlon, T. V. Bell, H. K. Ahari, and S. Hussain, "Virtual cystoscopy: early clinical experience," *Radiology*, vol. 205, no. 1, pp. 272–275, 1997.

[26] E. M. Merkle, A. Wunderlich, A. J. Aschoff et al., "Virtual cystoscopy based on helical CT scan datasets: perspectives and limitations," *British Journal of Radiology*, vol. 71, pp. 262–267, 1998.

[27] Y. Narumi, T. Kumatani, Y. Sawai et al., "The bladder and bladder tumors: imaging with three-dimensional display of helical CT data," *American Journal of Roentgenology*, vol. 167, no. 5, pp. 1134–1135, 1996.

31

The Use of Flaps and Grafts in the Treatment of Urethral Stricture Disease

Eric S. Wisenbaugh and Joel Gelman

University of California, Irvine, 333 City Boulevard West, Suite No. 1240, Orange, CA 92868, USA

Correspondence should be addressed to Eric S. Wisenbaugh; eric.wisenbaugh@gmail.com

Academic Editor: Miroslav L. Djordjevic

The use of various grafts and flaps plays a critical role in the successful surgical management of urethral stricture disease. A thorough comprehension of relevant anatomy and principles of tissue transfer techniques are essential to understanding the appropriate use of grafts or flaps to optimize outcomes. We briefly review these principles and discuss which technique may be best suited for a given anterior urethral stricture, depending on the location and length of the stricture, the presence or absence of an intact corpus spongiosum, and the availability of adequate and healthy penile skin.

1. Introduction

1.1. Principles of Tissue Transfer. The two broad categories of tissue transfer are flaps and grafts. A flap refers to tissue that is transferred with its native blood supply intact, while a graft refers to tissue removed from its donor site without its native blood supply and relies on establishing new circulation through a process termed "take." This process consists of two separate 48-hour phases: imbibition is the initial phase in which the graft is directly absorbing nutrients from the graft recipient bed; this is followed by inosculation, during which new blood supply is established.

1.2. Blood Supply to the Urethra and Penile Skin. Detailed knowledge of the blood supply to the penile skin and corpus spongiosum is mandatory for successful tissue transfer. The healthy urethra within the corpus spongiosum has dual blood supply: it receives antegrade flow directly from the paired bulbar arteries and retrograde flow from the terminal branches of the dorsal arteries, which communicates with the corpus spongiosum in the glans penis (Figure 1). Although there are also small perforating vessels between the corpora cavernosa and corpus spongiosum, this is a minor contribution. This robust dual blood supply all within the corpus spongiosum allows aggressive mobilization of the spongiosum off of the corporal bodies without compromising the blood supply to the urethra. However, the distal blood supply to the corpus spongiosum is compromised in cases of hypospadias, especially more severe forms, or after prior repair and after urethroplasty. In these cases, wide mobilization may compromise the blood supply to the urethra and create ischemic stenosis.

The penile skin receives its blood supply from branches of the superficial external pudendal artery. These branches travel just underneath the dartos fascia in an axial pattern, which provides reliable blood flow to skin flaps that are elevated on this fascial layer; hence these are referred to as fasciocutaneous flaps. There is also random blood supply achieved through the subdermal plexus, although this is much less dependable and not ideal for the survival of the flap (Figure 2).

1.3. Graft Material. The use of grafts in urethral reconstruction has been described since the late 19th century but was not popularized until Devine et al. began using full thickness penile skin grafts in 1961 [1]. This "patch graft" technique was historically the substitution procedure of choice, although it has now largely been supplanted by buccal mucosal grafts (BMG), split thickness skin grafts, and, in some cases, lingual grafts.

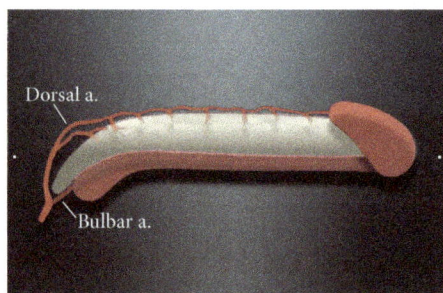

FIGURE 1: The dual blood supply to the urethra.

Buccal mucosal grafts have many advantages over penile skin and other materials which have led to their widespread use in recent years. These grafts are readily available and easily harvested and have more favorable vascular characteristics, including a rich submucosal plexus that facilitates good take. Additionally, buccal mucosa is nonhirsute and has an epithelial surface that is already well suited to a "wet" environment. As would be expected, long-term success rates with the use of BMG appear to be superior to penile skin grafts [2]. The use of lingual mucosa, while not as commonly used, is very similar in histology to buccal mucosa and has been described with very similar success rates [3].

1.4. Flap Techniques. Penile skin flaps, when used correctly, are a reliable and time-tested tool for urethral reconstruction. In the absence of prior flap surgery, penile skin (foreskin and distal penile skin in particular) is nonhirsute, has reliable axial vascular supply, and can be well mobilized and used to cover long urethral defects. Various flaps have been described, which can be elevated from ventral or dorsal skin and taken in either the longitudinal or transverse direction.

Orandi first described his ventral, longitudinal flap for penile urethral strictures using a lateral pedicle in 1968 with good results [4]. One disadvantage of this type of flap, however, is that if the stricture involves the proximal part of the pendulous or any part of the bulbar urethra, hair-bearing skin is involved in the reconstruction which can lead to recurrent infections and stone formation. For strictures isolated to the fossa, Jordan reported the use of a smaller, ventral penile skin flap that can be rotated onto the incised urethral opening [5].

For longer strictures, Quartey and McAninch have both described methods of obtaining transverse penile/preputial island flaps [6, 7]. These transverse flaps are versatile and hairless and can supply enough tissue to cover near panurethral defects. Furthermore, they involve a circumcision type incision with minimal disfigurement of the penis.

1.5. Grafting Techniques. Several techniques have been described, the two most common of which are the dorsal and ventral onlay grafts. The dorsal onlay approach was first described by Monseur in 1980 in which he incised the dorsal surface of the strictured urethra and sutured the edges directly to the corpora cavernosa to heal by secondary intention; this was later modified by Barbagli who used a

penile skin or buccal graft to fill the defect [8, 9]. The ventral onlay graft was first described by Devine with the use of a full-thickness "patch graft" of penile skin and then later was modified to use with buccal mucosa [1, 10]. Several other grafting techniques have been described and will be detailed throughout this paper.

2. Selecting the Right Technique

Selecting the appropriate technique for each patient is highly individualized and dependent on multiple factors. The optimal repair will depend on the length and location of the stricture, the presence or absence of healthy, abundant penile skin, and whether or not the corpus spongiosum is intact. Incorporating all of these considerations can make the decision-making process quite complex; however, the proper selection of tissue transfer technique is paramount to success. Our aim is to provide a logical, easily comprehensible approach to the appropriate selection of grafts and flaps in urethral reconstruction.

3. Tissue Transfer to the Glans and Fossa Navicularis

Our approach to strictures of the glans and fossa navicularis is summarized in Figure 3. If a stricture is truly limited to the glans penis alone (meatal stenosis), a simple meatotomy is the procedure of choice. However, distal strictures often either extend into the fossa navicularis or are limited to the fossa. These strictures are often best treated with a one-stage flap repair as long as there is abundant and healthy penile skin. When this is not the case, as in cases of prior penile flap surgery or in cases of lichen sclerosus (LS) also known as balanitis xerotica obliterans (BXO), then a two-stage repair with buccal mucosa grafting is more appropriate given the prohibitively high recurrence rates when using skin in these situations [11, 12]. Alternatively, the patient may simply elect for an extended meatotomy if he believes that the resulting ventral displacement of the meatus is cosmetically acceptable and prefers a simple procedure.

Although multiple flap techniques have been described, we prefer the ventral transverse island flap as initially described by Jordan for this location [5]. This technique involves incising the urethra ventrally through the stricture, elevating a transverse skin island on a broad pedicle of dartos fascia, and inverting the flap onto the defect prior to closure (Figure 4). This technique has been demonstrated to be highly successful, with Jordan reporting success in all 23 patients who did not have LS with an average follow-up of 10 years. Of note, the success was only 50% (6/12 patients) in those who had LS, reaffirming the recommendation against using penile skin in these cases [12].

Grafts are used by some authors for one-stage repairs of strictures involving the glans and fossa navicularis with dorsal graft placement [13]. Others place buccal mucosa grafts as ventral onlays using the glans wings as the graft bed [14, 15]. However, we do not believe that these techniques in our hands obtain the same caliber of patency (24–30 French)

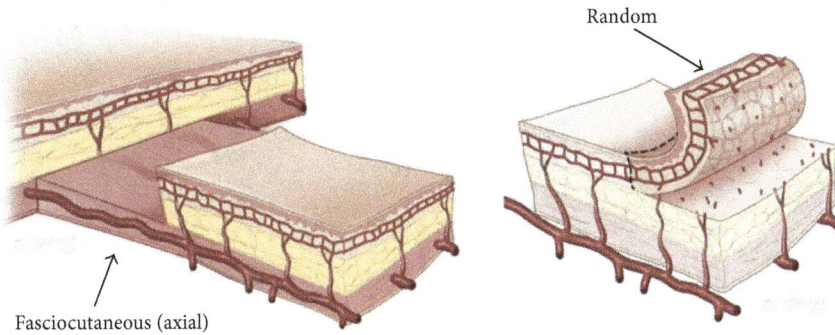

FIGURE 2: Axial and random flaps.

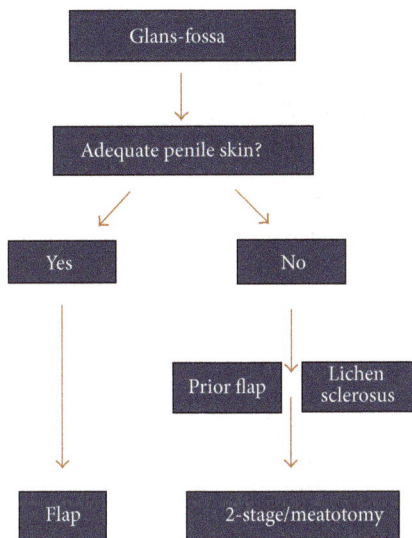

FIGURE 3: Treatment algorithm for strictures of the fossa navicularis.

that can be achieved with ventral flaps or staged repairs. Most importantly, however, it should be emphasized that the priority of the repair is relief of obstruction; thus the caliber of the repair, regardless of technique, should not be compromised by aggressively attempting to bring the meatus all the way to the tip of the glans.

4. Tissue Transfer to the Penile Urethra and Bulbar Urethra

The repair of penile and bulbar urethral strictures that are not amenable to EPA can be performed with grafts, flaps, or staged procedures, depending on whether the corpus spongiosum is intact and whether there is sufficient penile skin, as summarized in the algorithm in Figure 5. There is some debate about at what length an EPA should be avoided in favor of a tissue transfer technique, as lengthy excisions can lead to a tethered penis and tension on the anastomosis. In general, strictures in the penile urethra and distal bulbar urethra are only highly amenable to EPA when they are

short (i.e., less than 2 cm), whereas primary repairs without undue tension can be achieved for longer proximal bulbar strictures. In this location, maneuvers including separation of the corporal bodies and detachment of the bulb from the perineal body are options, and EPAs have been described for strictures up to 5 cm long in this location [16].

4.1. When the Corpus Spongiosum Is Intact. There is general consensus that strictures of the penile urethra not amenable to excisional repair are best repaired with a dorsal onlay graft, as the spongiosum even when intact is tenuous in this area and does not supply a reliable vascular bed to a ventrally placed graft [17]. Prior to the popularization of BMG, skin flaps were preferred as the most reliable approach when available. Dorsally placed buccal grafts, however, have also been demonstrated in multiple studies to provide very reliable results and are more durable and better suited to the "wet" environment than penile skin [17, 18]. Moreover, with the use of dorsal buccal grafting, the dorsal aspect of the urethra is supported by the corporal bodies, and the ventral and lateral native urethra is supported by intact corpus spongiosum, which will likely prevent both fistula formation and diverticular change.

Strictures of the bulbar urethra have generated considerably more debate as to the optimal location and technique of graft placement. There is an anatomical difference between the penile urethra and bulbar urethra with regard to the ventral spongiosum. As the urethra moves proximally, it becomes more dorsally located so that the spongiosum becomes thicker and more robust ventrally, thus providing a potentially suitable vascular bed for graft take.

Some authors prefer the ventral approach as it limits urethral mobilization with preservation of cavernosal-spongiosal perforating arteries [19]. In addition, the ventral approach is often considered to be less technically challenging with shorter operative times. Even Barbagli, who developed the dorsal onlay graft, has noted preference for the ventral approach in certain situations: if the dorsal aspect of the urethra is scarred down to the corpora from prior surgery or if the stricture extends proximally beyond the triangular ligament [20].

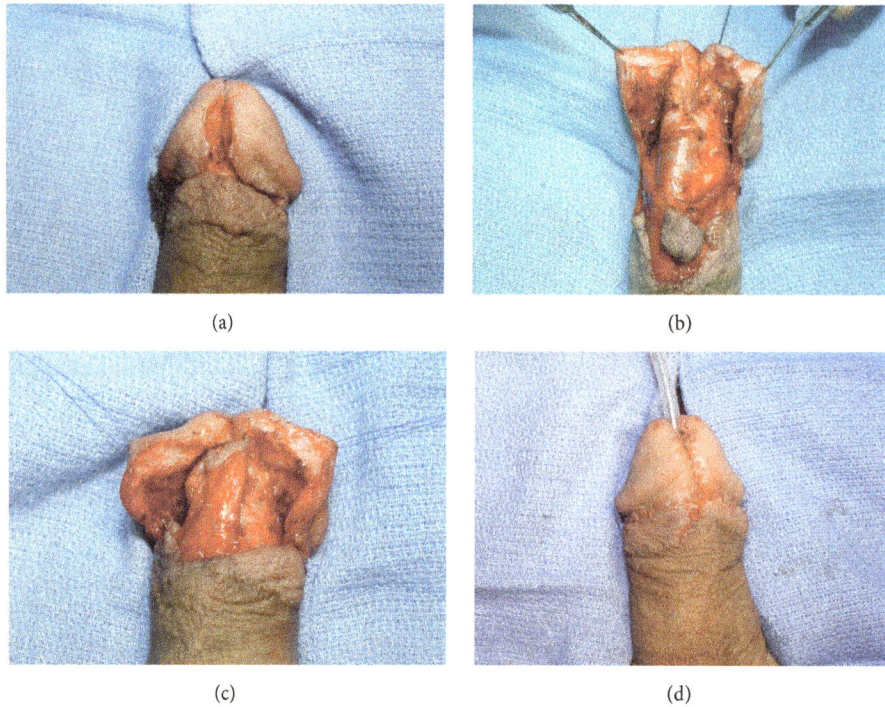

FIGURE 4: (a) An extended meatotomy is made through the stricture. (b) Glans wings are mobilized and a ventral flap is isolated. (c) The ventral flap has been rotated onto the defect. (d) Immediate appearance after closure.

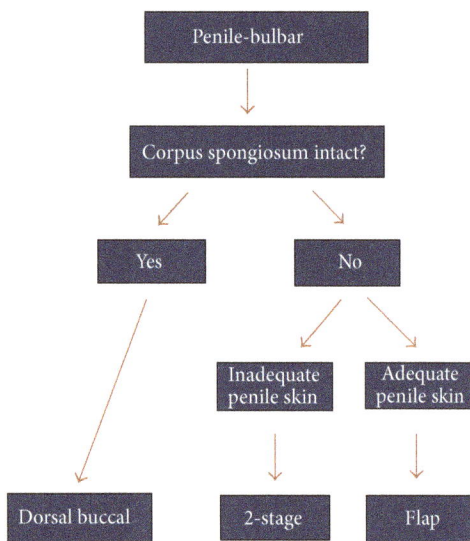

FIGURE 5: Treatment algorithm for strictures of the penile urethra and bulbar urethra.

However, several advantages exist to the dorsal approach, including the fact that the graft can be spread fixated to the corpora cavernosa, which supplies a consistently reliable graft bed that is not affected by spongiofibrosis. This spread-fixation, which cannot be accomplished with the ventral approach, also maximizes the surface area of the graft that is in direct contact with its vascular bed. This optimizes the conditions for graft take and allows for a widely patent lumen, ideally up to 30 French. Additionally, the use of a dorsal approach may reduce the incidence of postvoid dribbling, which has been shown in at least one retrospective study to be more prominent with the ventral approach [21].

Fueling the controversy is the fact that there have not been any randomized controlled trials to compare these two techniques, and the evidence that does exist is limited by its retrospective nature and conflicting results. One early comparison of 71 patients concluded that the dorsal onlay method was superior (5% versus 14% failure rates), but no statistical analysis was performed [22]. In contrast, Barbagli et al. retrospectively compared 17 ventral, 27 dorsal, and 6 lateral bulbar urethroplasties and found a success rate (defined by lack of subsequent treatment at mean follow-up of 42 moths) of 83%, 85%, and 83%, respectively [21]. More recently, a group of authors published a multicenter series with extended follow-up (median of 118 months) and found very similar success rates between the two techniques (80.2% of 81 patients with dorsal onlay compared to 81.5% of 130 patients with ventral onlay (n = 130)) [2]. However, we advise caution before concluding that these results are equivalent because each patient was carefully selected for the procedure they received and therefore the inherent selection bias prohibits this study from providing a decisive comparison. Another large retrospective study compared 62 ventral onlay cases with 41 dorsal onlay cases and reported equivalent outcomes with failure rates of 19% and 17%, respectively, at a mean follow-up of 36 months. However, the authors admit a selection bias as dorsal onlay procedures are reserved for more complicated strictures at their institution [19]. A recent systematic review of published series showed very little difference between the two techniques. The published ventral onlay series success rates ranged from 83% to 100% with an average of 88.84%, while the reviewed dorsal onlay series successes ranged from 73% to 100% with an average of 88.37% [17].

An additional technique was described in 2001 by Asopa et al., in which they were able to access the dorsal aspect of the urethra via a ventral urethrotomy and then excise an elliptical portion of the dorsal urethra and apply a dorsal "inlay" graft in its place before retubularizing the urethra [23]. The benefit of this approach is to combine the advantages of having a dorsally placed graft laying on the corporal graft bed while avoiding division of the perforating arteries that occurs during urethral mobilization to maintain maximal blood supply. This technique has been evaluated by several authors with results that compare to the historical results for the ventral and dorsal onlay approaches [17].

While the debate between these techniques is likely to continue until higher level evidence emerges, we prefer the dorsal approach at our institution for the variety of reasons mentioned above.

4.2. When the Corpus Spongiosum Is Not Intact. In cases where the spongiosum is not intact, such as in hypospadias, a one-stage graft is not recommended as the blood supply to the urethra will be severely compromised once it is fully mobilized. In these cases, whether it involves the penile or bulbar urethra, a skin flap is more appropriate as long as there is adequate and healthy penile skin. Transverse fasciocutaneous penile/preputial skin flaps can provide excellent coverage and have achieved good to excellent results in the published literature. In his initial description, McAninch obtained flaps up to 15 cm with no stricture recurrence in 10 patients with strictures which are 8–21 cm long and a mean follow-up of 14 months [24]. A subsequent publication of his long-term data revealed a success rate of 87% in 54 patients [25]. A review by Wessells and McAninch evaluated nine studies, all with at least one year of follow-up, and found that success rates ranged from 77% to 95%, with an average of 85.5% [18].

When there is not enough healthy skin, such as in cases of LS or prior flap surgery, a two-staged approach is more appropriate (Figure 6).

5. Special Situations

In certain complex cases with a segment of obliterated or near-obliterated urethra, there is not an adequate urethral plate to perform a ventral or dorsal onlay graft. If these are short strictures, they are best treated by excision with primary anastomosis (EPA). However, in such cases when the stricture is too long for an EPA, an augmented anastomosis can be considered. This technique, initially described by Turner-Warwick, involves excising the stricture, placing a graft dorsally, and then reanastomosing the native urethral edges ventrally [26]. Yet even this technique can be limited by length, with the longest stricture treated with this technique in one prominent series being of only 2 cm [27].

In patients with longer obliterative segments, an EPA or augmented anastomotic repair may not be feasible. Additionally, in patients who have already failed urethroplasty or have a history of hypospadias, strictures that would otherwise be technically amenable to one of these repairs may be at risk of urethral ischemia with urethral transection. For this small subset of patients, a more involved and creative approach may be necessary. Tabularized grafts and flaps have been attempted but have significantly high failure rates, reportedly up to 58%; therefore other techniques are needed to repair these challenging cases [14, 28].

5.1. Graft/Flap Combination. A more successful method to treat these strictures is with the combination of a dorsal buccal graft to augment or replace the inadequate urethral plate, followed by a penile skin flap onlay reconstruction (Figure 7). This was initially described by Morey in 2001 for single stage circumferential tissue transfer in 2 patients with penile urethral strictures [29]. A larger series of 12 patients was subsequently published with a success rate of 92% defined as wide patency documented by cystoscopy 4 months after surgery with subsequent follow-up that averaged 39 months [30].

The graft and flap combination can also be used for panurethral strictures that are too long for repair with BMG even when bilateral grafts are harvested. This technique typically involves using as much BMG as possible in the proximal aspects of the stricture and then using a penile skin flap to repair the remainder of the stricture distally [31, 32].

5.2. Combined Dorsal/Ventral Buccal Grafting. If penile skin is not available for a flap, then a combination of a dorsal and ventral BMG may be used. Such a combination approach was initially described by Palminteri et al. who used the Asopa technique to place a dorsal inlay graft and then place a ventral onlay graft in the ventral urethrotomy to obtain additional area within the new lumen [33]. However, this description was not targeted to obliterative strictures as the technique relies on a native urethra wide enough to be sutured to both grafts. Gelman and Siegel recently reported results from our institution on a series of 18 patients who had segments of total or near-total obliteration of their urethras and underwent combined ventral and dorsal buccal grafting for a 1-stage repair. The technique involves a dorsal incision without transection of the mobilized urethra, thereby preserving the continuity of the blood supply within the spongy tissue. Buccal mucosa is quilted dorsally to the corporal bodies in the standard dorsal onlay fashion. Additional buccal mucosa can then be quilted to the dorsally incised, nontransected corpus spongiosum in continuity with the distally and proximally spatulated urethra. The repair is then completed by approximating dorsal and ventral buccal mucosal graft segments (Figure 8). We feel the strengths of this technique include being able to leave the robust ventral spongy tissue intact and being able to place quilting sutures to secure the graft firmly to its bed. In this series with a mean follow-up of 50 months, the success rate was 94% (100% after the single failure underwent an internal urethrotomy) [34]. Although this needs to be

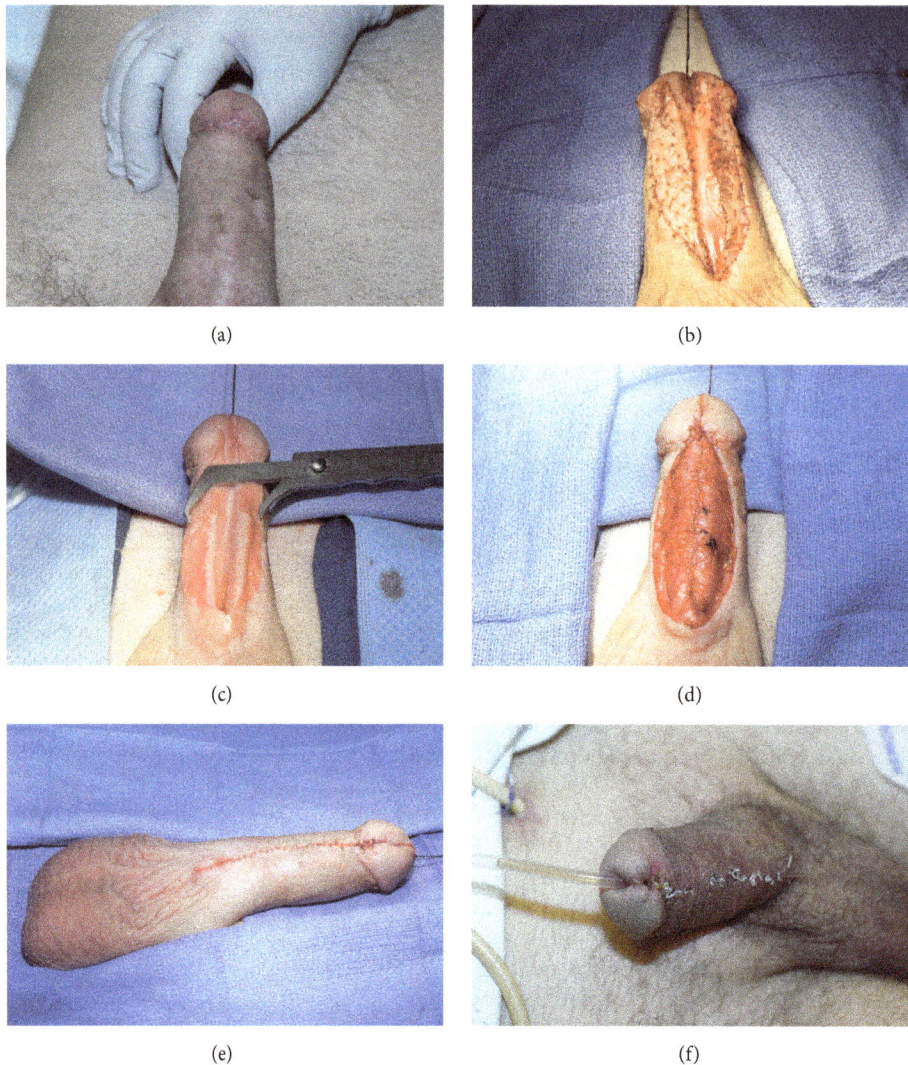

FIGURE 6: A 2-stage repair performed for a patient with a fossa and penile urethral stricture. (a) Demonstration of inadequate penile skin. (b) BMG quilted on either side of the opened urethral plate. (c) The urethral plate is now very adequate after healing of 1st stage. (d) Tubularization of new urethral plate. (e and f) Postoperative appearance immediately after closure and 3 weeks postoperatively.

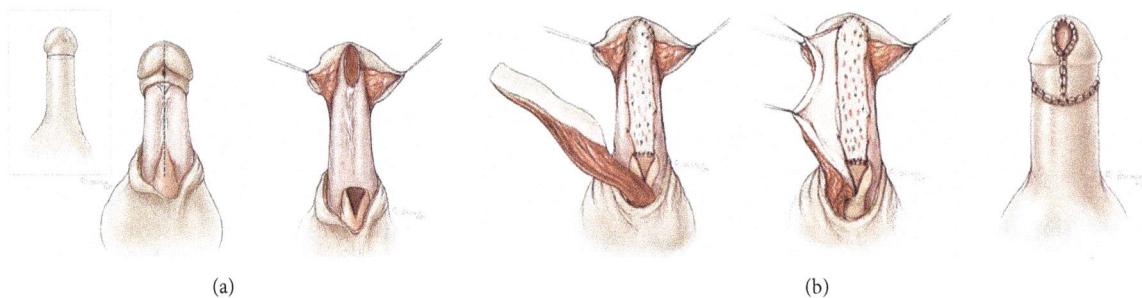

FIGURE 7: Graft/flap combination. (a) The obliterated urethra is incised proximally until a healthy, widely patent lumen is encountered. (b) The buccal graft is spread fixated to the corpora cavernosa, after which a penile skin flap is rotated ventrally onto the graft to create a new lumen. In cases where there is a deficiency of urethra within the fossa and a lack of a groove within the glans penis, a defect is created and the BMG is extended into the glans.

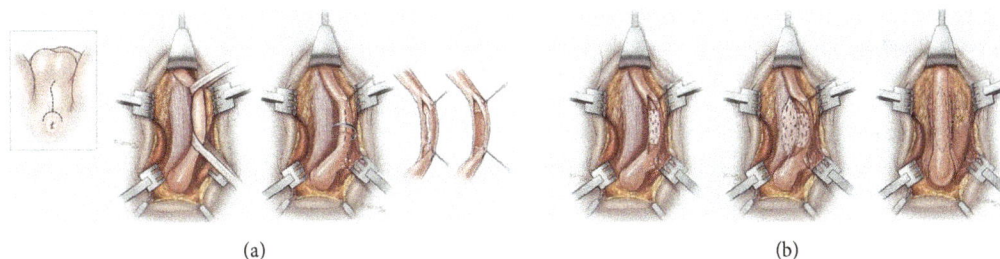

(a)   (b)

FIGURE 8: Dorsal and ventral buccal graft combination. (a) The urethra is mobilized and incised dorsally and healthy ventral spongiosum is exposed. (b) A buccal graft is spread fixated to the spongiosum where the obliterated segment was located, and an additional buccal graft is applied to the corpora cavernosa before the edges are anastomosed for retubularization.

validated by other studies, it remains a promising technique for some of the most challenging cases.

6. Summary

The use of grafts and flaps in the treatment of urethral stricture disease remains an indispensable tool in the armamentarium of the reconstructive urologist. While success rates are very difficult to compare between various techniques at this time, all of the current techniques mentioned appear to be highly successful for appropriately selected patients. The decision on which technique to use is dependent on a variety of factors. For strictures involving the fossa navicularis, the use of a penile skin flap provides excellent coverage while leaving a widely patent lumen. A meatotomy or two-stage repair should be considered if the penile skin is unhealthy or deficient. For strictures of the penile or bulbar urethra, we prefer the dorsal buccal approach as long as the corpus spongiosum is intact and reserve the use of a flap for when the spongiosum is not intact or a two-stage repair if the penile skin will not allow a flap to be used. Randomized controlled trials will likely be necessary to definitively recommend one technique over another, but until that time, it is imperative for the surgeon to be comfortable with all of the described techniques to individualize the treatment approach for each patient.

Conflict of Interests

The authors declare that there is no conflict of interests regarding the publication of this paper.

References

[1] P. C. Devine, J. R. Wendelken, and C. J. Devine Jr., "Free full thickness skin graft urethroplasty: current technique," *Journal of Urology*, vol. 121, no. 3, pp. 282–285, 1979.

[2] G. Barbagli, S. B. Kulkarni, N. Fossati et al., "Long-term followup and deterioration rate of anterior substitution urethroplasty," *The Journal of Urology*, vol. 192, no. 3, pp. 808–813, 2014.

[3] S. K. Das, A. Kumar, G. K. Sharma et al., "Lingual mucosal graft urethroplasty for anterior urethral strictures," *Urology*, vol. 73, no. 1, pp. 105–108, 2009.

[4] A. Orandi, "One-stage urethroplasty: 4-year followup," *The Journal of Urology*, vol. 107, no. 6, pp. 717–719, 1972.

[5] G. H. Jordan, "Reconstruction of the fossa navicularis," *The Journal of Urology*, vol. 138, no. 1, pp. 102–104, 1987.

[6] J. K. M. Quartey, "One-stage penile/preputial island flap urethroplasty for urethral stricture," *Journal of Urology*, vol. 134, no. 3, pp. 474–475, 1985.

[7] J. W. McAninch, "Reconstruction of extensive urethral strictures: circular fasciocutaneous penile flap," *Journal of Urology*, vol. 149, no. 3, pp. 488–491, 1993.

[8] J. Monseur, "L'elargissement de l'uretre au moyen du plan sus uretral. Bilan après 13 ans sur 219 cas," *Journal d'Urologie*, vol. 6, p. 439, 1980.

[9] G. Barbagli, C. Selli, A. Tosto, and E. Palminteri, "Dorsal free graft urethroplasty," *The Journal of Urology*, vol. 155, no. 1, pp. 123–126, 1996.

[10] A. F. Morey and J. W. McAninch, "When and how to use buccal mucosal grafts in adult bulbar urethroplasty," *Urology*, vol. 48, no. 2, pp. 194–198, 1996.

[11] I. Depasquale, A. J. Park, and A. Bracka, "The treatment of balanitis xerotica obliterans," *British Journal of Urology International*, vol. 86, no. 4, pp. 459–465, 2000.

[12] R. Virasoro, E. A. Eltahawy, and G. H. Jordan, "Long-term follow-up for reconstruction of strictures of the fossa navicularis with a single technique," *BJU International*, vol. 100, no. 5, pp. 1143–1145, 2007.

[13] S. B. Kulkarni, P. M. Joshi, and K. Venkatesan, "Management of panurethral stricture disease in India," *The Journal of Urology*, vol. 188, no. 3, pp. 824–830, 2012.

[14] J. S. Wiener, R. W. Sutherland, D. R. Roth, and E. T. Gonzales Jr., "Comparison of onlay and tubularized island flaps of inner preputial skin for the repair of proximal hypospadias," *The Journal of Urology*, vol. 158, no. 3, pp. 1172–1174, 1997.

[15] P. Chowdhury, P. Nayak, S. Mallick, S. Gurumurthy, D. David, and A. Mossadeq, "Single stage ventral onlay buccal mucosal graft urethroplasty for navicular fossa strictures," *Indian Journal of Urology*, vol. 30, no. 1, pp. 17–22, 2014.

[16] R. P. Terlecki, M. C. Steele, C. Valadez, and A. F. Morey, "Grafts are unnecessary for proximal bulbar reconstruction," *The Journal of Urology*, vol. 184, no. 6, pp. 2395–2399, 2010.

[17] A. Mangera, J. M. Patterson, and C. R. Chapple, "A systematic review of graft augmentation urethroplasty techniques for the treatment of anterior urethral strictures," *European Urology*, vol. 59, no. 5, pp. 797–814, 2011.

[18] H. Wessells and J. W. McAninch, "Current controversies in anterior urethral stricture repair: free-graft versus pedicled skin-flap reconstruction," *World Journal of Urology*, vol. 16, no. 3, pp. 175–180, 1998.

[19] B. D. Figler, B. S. Malaeb, G. W. Dy, B. B. Voelzke, and H. Wessells, "Impact of graft position on failure of single-stage bulbar urethroplasties with buccal mucosa graft," *Urology*, vol. 82, no. 5, pp. 1166–1170, 2013.

[20] G. Barbagli, "Buccal mucosal graft urethroplasty," in *Urethral Reconstructive Surgery*, S. B. Brandes, Ed., Current Clinical Urology, pp. 119–136, Humana Press, New York, NY, USA, 1st edition, 2008.

[21] G. Barbagli, E. Palminteri, G. Guazzoni, F. Montorsi, D. Turini, and M. Lazzeri, "Bulbar urethroplasty using buccal mucosa grafts placed on the ventral, dorsal or lateral surface of the urethra: are results affected by the surgical technique?" *The Journal of Urology*, vol. 174, no. 3, pp. 955–958, 2005.

[22] D. E. Andrich, C. J. Leach, and A. R. Mundy, "The Barbagli procedure gives the best results for patch urethroplasty of the bulbar urethra," *BJU International*, vol. 88, no. 4, pp. 385–389, 2001.

[23] H. S. Asopa, M. Garg, G. G. Singhal, L. Singh, J. Asopa, and A. Nischal, "Dorsal free graft urethroplasty for urethral stricture by ventral sagittal urethrotomy approach," *Urology*, vol. 58, no. 5, pp. 657–659, 2001.

[24] J. W. McAninch, "Reconstruction of extensive urethral strictures: circular fasciocutaneous penile flap," *The Journal of Urology*, vol. 149, no. 3, pp. 488–491, 1993.

[25] K. J. Carney and J. W. McAninch, "Penile circular fasciocutaneous flaps to reconstruct complex anterior urethral strictures," *Urologic Clinics of North America*, vol. 29, no. 2, pp. 397–409, 2002.

[26] R. Turner-Warwick, "Principles of urethral reconstruction," in *Reconstructive Urology*, G. Webster, Ed., vol. 2, p. 609, Blackwell Scientific, Boston, Mass, USA, 1993.

[27] M. L. Guralnick and G. D. Webster, "The augmented anastomotic urethroplasty: indications and outcome in 29 patients," *The Journal of Urology*, vol. 165, no. 5 I, pp. 1496–1501, 2001.

[28] J. W. McAninch and A. F. Morey, "Penile circular fasciocutaneous skin flap in 1-stage reconstruction of complex anterior urethral strictures," *The Journal of Urology*, vol. 159, no. 4, pp. 1209–1213, 1998.

[29] A. F. Morey, "Urethral plate salvage with dorsal graft promotes successful penile flap onlay reconstruction of severe pendulous strictures," *The Journal of Urology*, vol. 166, no. 4, pp. 1376–1378, 2001.

[30] J. Gelman and W. Sohn, "1-stage repair of obliterative distal urethral strictures with buccal graft urethral plate reconstruction and simultaneous onlay penile skin flap," *The Journal of Urology*, vol. 186, no. 3, pp. 935–938, 2011.

[31] J. N. Warner, I. Malkawi, M. Dhradkeh et al., "A multiinstitutional evaluation of the management and outcomes of long-segment urethral strictures," *Urology*, vol. 85, no. 6, pp. 1483–1488, 2015.

[32] R. K. Berglund and K. W. Angermeier, "Combined buccal mucosa graft and genital skin flap for reconstruction of extensive anterior urethral strictures," *Urology*, vol. 68, no. 4, pp. 707–710, 2006.

[33] E. Palminteri, G. Manzoni, E. Berdondini et al., "Combined dorsal plus ventral double buccal mucosa graft in bulbar urethral reconstruction," *European Urology*, vol. 53, no. 1, pp. 81–90, 2008.

[34] J. Gelman and J. A. Siegel, "Ventral and dorsal buccal grafting for 1-stage repair of complex anterior urethral strictures," *Urology*, vol. 83, no. 6, pp. 1418–1422, 2014.

Permissions

All chapters in this book were first published in ART by Hindawi Publishing Corporation; hereby published with permission under the Creative Commons Attribution License or equivalent. Every chapter published in this book has been scrutinized by our experts. Their significance has been extensively debated. The topics covered herein carry significant findings which will fuel the growth of the discipline. They may even be implemented as practical applications or may be referred to as a beginning point for another development.

The contributors of this book come from diverse backgrounds, making this book a truly international effort. This book will bring forth new frontiers with its revolutionizing research information and detailed analysis of the nascent developments around the world.

We would like to thank all the contributing authors for lending their expertise to make the book truly unique. They have played a crucial role in the development of this book. Without their invaluable contributions this book wouldn't have been possible. They have made vital efforts to compile up to date information on the varied aspects of this subject to make this book a valuable addition to the collection of many professionals and students.

This book was conceptualized with the vision of imparting up-to-date information and advanced data in this field. To ensure the same, a matchless editorial board was set up. Every individual on the board went through rigorous rounds of assessment to prove their worth. After which they invested a large part of their time researching and compiling the most relevant data for our readers.

The editorial board has been involved in producing this book since its inception. They have spent rigorous hours researching and exploring the diverse topics which have resulted in the successful publishing of this book. They have passed on their knowledge of decades through this book. To expedite this challenging task, the publisher supported the team at every step. A small team of assistant editors was also appointed to further simplify the editing procedure and attain best results for the readers.

Apart from the editorial board, the designing team has also invested a significant amount of their time in understanding the subject and creating the most relevant covers. They scrutinized every image to scout for the most suitable representation of the subject and create an appropriate cover for the book.

The publishing team has been an ardent support to the editorial, designing and production team. Their endless efforts to recruit the best for this project, has resulted in the accomplishment of this book. They are a veteran in the field of academics and their pool of knowledge is as vast as their experience in printing. Their expertise and guidance has proved useful at every step. Their uncompromising quality standards have made this book an exceptional effort. Their encouragement from time to time has been an inspiration for everyone.

The publisher and the editorial board hope that this book will prove to be a valuable piece of knowledge for researchers, students, practitioners and scholars across the globe.

List of Contributors

Anthony Kodzo-Grey Venyo
Department of Urology, North Manchester General Hospital, Delaunays Road, Crumpsall, Manchester, UK

Wei Shen Tan and John D. Kelly
Division of Surgery and Interventional Science, UCL Medical School, University College London, 74 Huntley Street, LondonWC1E 6AU, UK
Department of Urology, University College London Hospital, 16-18Westmoreland Street, LondonW1B 8PH, UK

Benjamin W. Lamb
Department of Urology, University College London Hospital, 16-18Westmoreland Street, LondonW1B 8PH, UK

Wajahat Aziz and M. Hammad Ather
Section of Urology, Department of Surgery, Aga Khan University, P.O. Box 3500, Stadium Road, Karachi 74800, Pakistan

Rishi Modh, Peter Y. Cai, Alyssa Sheffield and Lawrence L. Yeung
Department of Urology, University of Florida College of Medicine, Gainesville, FL 32608, USA

Waleed Al Taweel
Department of Urology, King Faisal Hospital and Research Center, Riyadh 11211, Saudi Arabia

Raouf Seyam
Department of Urology, King Faisal Hospital and Research Center, Riyadh 11211, Saudi Arabia
Faculty of Medicine, Suez Canal University, Ismailia, Egypt

Satinder Pal Aggarwal, Shivam Priyadarshi, Vinay Tomar, S. S. Yadav, Goto Gangkak, Nachiket Vyas, Neeraj Agarwal and Ujwal Kumar
SMS Medical College and Hospital, Jaipur 302004, India

Ünal Bakal and Mehmet Sarac
Department of Pediatric Surgery, Faculty of Medicine, Firat University, 23119 Elazig, Turkey

Musa AbeG
Department of Pediatric Surgery, Faculty of Medicine, Adiyaman University, 23119 Elazig, Turkey

Erdal Alkan, Mehmet Murad Basar, Oguz Acar and Mevlana Derya Balbay
Department of Urology, Memorial Şişli Hospital, Şişli, Istanbul, Turkey

Ali Saribacak
Department of Urology, Konak Hospital, Izmit, Turkey

Ahmet Oguz Ozkanli
Department of Anesthesiology, Memorial Şişli Hospital, Şişli, Istanbul, Turkey

Andres F. Correa, Katherine Theisen, Matthew Ferroni, Jodi K. Maranchie, Ronald Hrebinko, Benjamin J. Davies and Jeffrey R. Gingrich
Department of Urology, University of Pittsburgh Medical Center, 3471 5th Avenue, Suite 700 Kaufmann Building, Pittsburgh, PA 15213, USA

Joel Gelman and Eric S. Wisenbaugh
University of California, Irvine, 333 City Boulevard West, Suite 1240,Orange, CA 92868, USA

Krishnan Venkatesan
Department of Urology, MedStar Washington Hospital Center, 110 Irving Street NW, Suite 3B 19, Washington, DC 20010, USA

Dmitriy Nikolavsky
Department of Urology, State University of New York Upstate Medical University, 750 East Adams Street, Syracuse, NY 13210, USA

Stephen Blakely
Division of Urology, University of Colorado, 12605 E. 16th Avenue, Aurora, CO 80045, USA

Matthias Beysens, Willem Oosterlinck, Anne-Françoise Spinoit, Piet Hoebeke, Karel Decaestecker and Nicolaas Lumen
Department of Urology, Ghent University Hospital, 9000 Ghent, Belgium

Enzo Palminteri
Center for Urethral and Genital Surgery, 52100 Arezzo, Italy

Philippe François
Department of Urology, CH Mouscron, 7700 Mouscron, Belgium

Francisco E. Martins
Department of Urology, Hospital Santa Maria, University of Lisbon, School of Medicine, 1600-161 Lisbon, Portugal
ULSNA-Hospital de Portalegre, 7300-074 Portalegre, Portugal

Natalia Martins
ULSNA-Hospital de Portalegre, 7300-074 Portalegre, Portugal

Sanjay B. Kulkarni and Pankaj Joshi
Kulkarni Reconstructive Urology Center, Pune 411038, India

Jonathan Warner
City of Hope Medical Center, Duarte, CA 91010, USA

Essam-Elden M. Mohammed
Dermatology and Andrology Department, Faculty of Medicine, Al-Azhar University, Assiut, Egypt

Eman Mosad and Asmaa M. Zahran
Clinical Pathology Department, South Egypt Cancer Institute, Assiut University, Assiut, Egypt

Diaa A. Hameed
Urology Department, Faculty of Medicine, Assiut University, Assiut, Egypt

Emad A. Taha
Dermatology and Andrology Department, Faculty of Medicine, Assiut University, Assiut, Egypt

Mohamed A. Mohamed
Gynaecology and Obstetric Department, Faculty of Medicine, Al-Azhar University, Assiut, Egypt

Timothy D. Lyon, Thomas W. Fuller, Benjamin J. Davies, Jeffrey R. Gingrich, Ronald L. Hrebinko, Jodi K. Maranchie and Tatum V. Tarin
Department of Urology, University of Pittsburgh, Pittsburgh, PA, USA

Nicholas J. Farber
Division of Urology, Rutgers Robert Wood Johnson Medical School, New Brunswick, NJ, USA

Leo C. Chen
University of Pittsburgh School of Medicine, Pittsburgh, PA, USA

Jennifer M. Taylor
Department of Urology, Baylor College of Medicine, Houston, TX, USA

Nikolaos Mertziotis, Christos Kyratsas and Andreas Konandreas
Iaso General Hospital, 264 Messogeion Avenue, 15562 Athens, Greece

Diomidis Kozyrakis
General Hospital of Volos, 134 Polimeri Street, 38222 Volos, Greece

Anthony Kodzo-Grey Venyo
North Manchester General Hospital, Department of Urology, Delaunays Road Crumpsall, Manchester, UK

Fouad Aoun, Ksenija Limani, Alexandre Peltier, Marc Zanaty and Roland van Velthoven
Department of Urology, Jules Bordet Institute, Université Libre de Bruxelles, 1000 Brussels, Belgium

Alexandre Chamoun, Marc Vanden Bossche, QuentinMarcelis and Thierry Roumeguère
Department of Urology, Erasme Hospital, Université Libre de Bruxelles, 1070 Brussels, Belgium

Iyad Khourdaji, Jacob Parke and Avinash Chennamsetty
Beaumont Health System, Department of Urology, 3601W.Thirteen Mile Road, Royal Oak, MI 48073, USA

Frank Burks
Beaumont Health System, Department of Urology, 3601W.Thirteen Mile Road, Royal Oak, MI 48073, USA
Oakland University William Beaumont School of Medicine, 216O'DowdHall, 2200 N. Squirrel Road, Rochester, MI 48309, USA

C. Browne, N. F. Davis, E. Mac Craith, G. M. Lennon, D. W. Mulvin, D. M. Quinlan and D. J. Galvin
Department of Urology, St. Vincent's University Hospital, Dublin 4, Ireland

Gerard P. Mc Vey
Department of Radiation Oncology, St. Vincent's University Hospital, Dublin 4, Ireland

Timothy D. Lyon, Omar M. Ayyash, Matthew C. Ferroni, Kevin J. Rycyna and Mang L. Chen
Department of Urology, University of Pittsburgh School of Medicine, Pittsburgh, PA 15213, USA

Vinita Rathi, Sachin Agrawal, Shuchi Bhatt and Naveen Sharma
University College of Medical Sciences and Guru Teg Bahadur Hospital, Dilshad Garden, Delhi 110095, India

Hiroyuki Yamanaka, Kazuhide Makiyama, Kimito Osaka and Yoshinobu Kubota
Department of Urology, Yokohama City University, Yokohama 236-0004, Japan

Manabu Nagasaka and Masato Ogata,
Mitsubishi Precision Co., Ltd., Kamakura 247-8505, Japan

Takahiro Yamada
Graduate School of Environment and Information Sciences, Yokohama National University, Yokohama 240-8501, Japan

Anthony Kodzo-Grey Venyo
Department of Urology, North Manchester General Hospital, Delaunays Road, Manchester, UK

Henry Okafor and Dmitriy Nikolavsky
Department of Urology, Upstate Medical University, 750 East Adams Street, Syracuse, NY 13210, USA

Zaher Bahouth, Sarel Halachmi, Gil Meyer, Ofir Avitan, Boaz Moskovitz and Ofer Nativ
Department of Urology, Bnai Zion Medical Center, 3339414 Haifa, Israel
Faculty of Medicine, Technion-Israel Institute of Technology, 3200003 Haifa, Israel

Avinash Chennamsetty, Luke Edwards and Kim A. Killinger
Beaumont Health System, Department of Urology, Royal Oak, MI 48073, USA

Jay Hollander, Kenneth M. Peters and Jason Hafron
Beaumont Health System, Department of Urology, Royal Oak, MI 48073, USA
Oakland University William Beaumont School of Medicine, Rochester, MI 48309, USA

Scott Pew and Behdod Poushanchi
Oakland University William Beaumont School of Medicine, Rochester, MI 48309, USA

Mary P. Coffey
Beaumont Health System, Department of Biostatistics, Research Institute, Royal Oak, MI 48073, USA

S. Sasikumar, K. S. N. Wijayarathna, U. Gobi and AnuruddhaM. Abeygunasekera
Urology Unit, Colombo South Teaching Hospital, 10350 Dehiwala, Sri Lanka

K. A. M. S. Karunaratne
Department of Pathology, Colombo South Teaching Hospital, 10350 Dehiwala, Sri Lanka

A. Pathmeswaran
Department of Public Health, Faculty of Medicine, University of Kelaniya, 11010 Ragama, Sri Lanka

Bradley A. Wall
School of Psychology and Exercise Science, Murdoch University, Murdoch,WA 6150, Australia
Exercise Medicine Research Institute, Edith Cowan University, Joondalup,WA 6027, Australia

Daniel A. Galvão and Naeem Fatehee
Exercise Medicine Research Institute, Edith Cowan University, Joondalup, WA 6027, Australia

Dennis R. Taaffe
Exercise Medicine Research Institute, Edith Cowan University, Joondalup, WA 6027, Australia
School of Medicine, University of Wollongong, Wollongong, NSW2522, Australia

Nigel Spry and David Joseph
Exercise Medicine Research Institute, Edith Cowan University, Joondalup, WA 6027, Australia
Department of Radiation Oncology, Sir Charles Gairdner Hospital, Nedlands, WA 6009, Australia
Faculty of Medicine, University of Western Australia, Nedlands, WA 6009, Australia

Robert U. Newton
Exercise Medicine Research Institute, Edith Cowan University, Joondalup, WA 6027, Australia
Centre for Clinical Research,The University of Queensland, Herston, QLD 4006, Australia

Sachin Abrol, Ankush Jairath, Sanika Ganpule, Arvind Ganpule, Shashikant Mishra, Ravindra Sabnis and Mahesh Desai
Muljibhai Patel Urological Hospital, Dr. Varendra Desai Road, Nadiad, Gujarat 387001, India

Eric S. Wisenbaugh and Joel Gelman
University of California, Irvine, 333 City Boulevard West, Suite No. 1240, Orange, CA 92868,USA

www.ingramcontent.com/pod-product-compliance
Lightning Source LLC
Chambersburg PA
CBHW080505200326
41458CB00012B/4097